Integrative Women's Health

Integrative Medicine Library

Published and Forthcoming Volumes

SERIES EDITOR

Andrew Weil, MD

Integrative Women's Health

EDITED BY

Victoria Maizes, MD

Executive Director
Arizona Center for Integrative Medicine
Associate Professor of Medicine, Family Medicine and Public Health
University of Arizona Health Sciences

Tieraona Low Dog, MD

Director of the Fellowship
Arizona Center for Integrative Medicine
Clinical Associate Professor of Medicine
University of Arizona Health Sciences

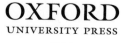

OXFORD
UNIVERSITY PRESS
2010

OXFORD
UNIVERSITY PRESS

Oxford University Press, Inc., publishes works that further
Oxford University's objective of excellence
in research, scholarship, and education.

Oxford New York
Auckland Cape Town Dar es Salaam Hong Kong Karachi
Kuala Lumpur Madrid Melbourne Mexico City Nairobi
New Delhi Shanghai Taipei Toronto

With offices in
Argentina Austria Brazil Chile Czech Republic France Greece
Guatemala Hungary Italy Japan Poland Portugal Singapore
South Korea Switzerland Thailand Turkey Ukraine Vietnam

Published by Oxford University Press, Inc.
198 Madison Avenue, New York, New York 10016
www.oup.com

Oxford is a registered trademark of Oxford University Press

Library of Congress Cataloging-in-Publication Data
Women's integrative health / [edited by] Victoria Maizes, Tieraona Low Dog.
p. ; cm. — (Weil integrative medicine library)
Includes bibliographical references and index.
ISBN 978-0-19-537881-8
1. Women—Health and hygiene.   2. Integrative Medicine.   I. Maizes, Victoria.
II. Low Dog, Tieraona.   III. Series.
[DNLM: 1. Women's Health.   2. Integrative Medicine. WA 309.1 W8728 2010]
RA778.W773 2010
613'.04244—dc22
2009020487

3 5 7 9 8 6 4 2
Printed in the United States of America
on acid-free paper

In honor of my mother Hannah Maizes (of blessed memory) and father Isaac Maizes whose love and support are the foundation for this work and everything else I do.
—Victoria

I dedicate this work to the women who have shaped my life, my grandmothers Jessie and Josephine, my mother Vivian, and Kiara my daughter. From you I have learned the magic, mystery and wonder of being female. I feel your strength and love flow through me, inspiring all that I do. Yours is the sweetest of debts and one that I will never be able to repay.
—Tieraona

FOREWORD

ANDREW WEIL, MD

Series Editor

As the only male contributor to this excellent volume on *Integrative Women's Health*, I feel both honored and intimidated.

Throughout history, medicine was a fraternal guild that excluded women. As recently as 1964, when I entered my first year at Harvard Medical School, my class of 125 included only 12 women. Even into the 20th century, women were considered unfit for the profession, and very few were allowed to become doctors. Of course, times have greatly changed, with female students now often outnumbering males in colleges of medicine. But the influence of centuries of tradition lingers in medical thinking and practice.

Ancient Greek physicians, the godfathers of Western medicine, thought female patients were peculiarly prone to disorders that simulated genuine dysfunction of internal organs. They called this class of ailments "hysteria," from their word for uterus (*hystera*), believing that the womb could detach from its moorings and travel elsewhere in the body, pressing on the diaphragm, throat, or other structures to cause symptoms. In their view, the probable cause of uterine wandering was that the organ became light and dry as a result of lack of sexual intercourse.

It is now 2,000 years later, and here is the definition of *hysteria* in a contemporary edition of Webster's Revised Unabridged Dictionary:

Hys*te"ri*a\, n. [NL.: cf. F. hyst['e]rie. See Hysteric.] (Med.) A nervous affection, occurring almost exclusively in women, in which the emotional and reflex excitability is exaggerated, and the will power correspondingly diminished, so that the patient loses control over the emotions, becomes the victim of imaginary sensations, and often falls into paroxism or fits.

Note: The chief symptoms are convulsive, tossing movements of the limbs and head, uncontrollable crying and laughing, and a choking sensation as if a ball were lodged in the throat. The affection presents the most varied symptoms, often simulating those of the gravest diseases, but generally curable by mental treatment alone.

In fact, even into our times, male physicians have tended to dismiss the somatic complaints of female patients as hysterical, especially when symptoms are generalized, vague, and difficult to diagnose.

When the first anti-anxiety drugs came on the market in the middle of the past century, they seemed just right for managing the disordered emotionality of women that was believed to be the cause of their headaches, listlessness, and various aches and pains. I have one pharmaceutical advertisement from the period in my files that shows a clearly hysterical woman—just the sort of patient you would not want to have to deal with—under the banner, "Emotional Crisis? Calm her immediately with injectable Valium (diazepam)!" In the 1960s, the manufacturer of Ritalin (methylphenidate) targeted women in a noteworthy series of ads in leading journals. On the left-hand page of each two-page spread was a black-and-white photograph of a depressed housewife contemplating a sink full of dirty dishes, a messy living room, or some other household disaster. "What can you do for this patient?" the physician–reader was asked. "Write 'Ritalin' on your prescription pad!" was the answer on the adjoining page— this over a full-color photograph of the same woman, now cheerful and energetic, standing proudly by spotlessly clean dishes or an ordered living room. The unwritten subtext was clear: Here is an easy way to get rid of complaining female patients, who take up your time, probably have nothing really wrong with them, and are so emotionally unbalanced that they are likely not even doing their housework.

The first oral contraceptive pills were becoming popular when I did my clinical rotations as a medical student. I remember a preceptor I had—a cocky, young internist—who urged us to prescribe them not just for contraception. "You know these women who just never feel right?" he told us. "You just put them on the pill, and they feel like a million bucks." In my OB/GYN rotation, I assisted in a lot of hysterectomies, many of them not necessary by today's standards. Hysterectomy was the "final solution" to female complaints.

How much have things changed? Today we experience a booming antidepressant industry; when we look back will we see it as any different from the Valium or Ritalin chapters? At the same time, there is growing acknowledgment that men and women are different and that the differences extend beyond reproduction to physiology and virtually every organ system. While female reproductive physiology is undeniably complex, it does not sufficiently explain why women are at greater risk for autoimmune disorders, process information differently in the brain, or react differently to pharmaceutical drugs than men. As the caregivers in our society, women experience particular forms of stress. Yet women throughout the world live longer than men; why they do is unknown. Gender-based medicine is a nascent field and it is growing.

Women have been vocal about their desire to be seen as more than just physical bodies. They have pushed for a broader view of health and wellness. Women are the major consumers of health care consumers and are also much more health conscious than men in our society. They take better care of themselves and are more likely to seek professional help for symptoms that demand attention. Women are the chief buyers of books about health and self-care, and women's magazines have been major outlets for information on these subjects. Over the past few decades, women have led the consumer movement for holistic and alternative medicine, because they are more open than men to natural therapies, mind/body interventions, and the healing traditions of other cultures. That consumer movement, which is still gaining strength, laid the foundation for acceptance of integrative medicine.

Integrative medicine, as this series of volumes from Oxford University Press demonstrates, has much broader goals than simply bringing alternative and complementary therapies into the mainstream. It aims to restore the focus of medicine on health and healing, especially on the human organism's innate capacity for maintaining and repairing itself; to foster whole-person medicine that includes the mental/emotional and spiritual dimensions of human life; to train physicians to attend to all aspects of lifestyle in working with patients; and to protect the practitioner/patient relationship as a key contributor to the healing process. Because integrative medicine stresses the individuality of patients and encourages real partnerships between doctors and patients, it is able to recognize and discard the limiting, paternalistic attitudes, and concepts that have dominated medicine for centuries and give women's health issues the attention and care they demand.

As women have moved toward equality with men in the medical profession, both in terms of numbers and status, the field of women's health has come into its own. I believe that integrative medicine and women's health are a perfect fit. Therefore, it gives me great pleasure to introduce this outstanding compilation of practical information on *Integrative Women's Health*. The editors are long-time friends and colleagues. Drs. Victoria Maizes and Tieraona Low Dog are leading voices in the emerging field of women's integrative health. Victoria Maizes, a pioneer graduate of the integrative medicine fellowship that I founded at the University of Arizona, has been the executive director of the Arizona Center for Integrative Medicine for the past decade. Dr. Tieraona Low Dog, one of the world's leading authorities on botanical medicine and dietary supplements, is director of the Arizona Center's Fellowship program. I congratulate them for the excellence of their editorial work and thank them for asking me to add my words to theirs.

PREFACE

VICTORIA MAIZES AND TIERAONA LOW DOG

We are delighted to present *Integrative Women's Health*—the first such text created for health professionals. It is our hope that you will find it of great value as you care for your patients. As the largest group of health care consumers, women have made it abundantly clear that they desire a broader, more integrative approach to their care. In response to this need, we have elected to cover both women's reproductive health and those conditions that manifest differently in women. Thus, in the chapters that follow you will find perspectives on aging, spirituality and sexuality, integrative approaches to premenstrual syndrome, pregnancy, menopause, fibroids, and endometriosis as well as specific recommendations for the treatment of cardiovascular disease, rheumatoid arthritis, HIV, depression, and cancer in women.

We honor the clinical experience and heartfelt connection with clinicians and their patients. We have intentionally designed this book to present the latest scientific evidence within a clinically relevant framework. Woven together are conventional treatments, mind–body interventions, nutritional strategies, acupuncture, manual medicine, herbal therapies, and dietary supplements. Careful attention is given to the art of medicine; clinical pearls include language that helps motivate patients, questions that enhance a health history, and the spiritual dimensions of care. Thus, unlike many primers on women's health that emphasize either an alternative or conventional approach—this text is truly integrative.

While gender-specific medicine is growing as a field, it tends to focus on the biological differences between men and women and, at times, turns normal life events such as pregnancy and menopause into medical problems that need to be managed. We have encouraged our authors to convey, in their chapters, care that addresses not only the medical issue at hand but also the woman's body, mind, and spirit; acknowledging the therapeutic relationship that exists between patient and provider, and making use of the best of conventional and complementary medicine. To this end, we have intentionally chosen only female authors as a tribute to the growing influence of women providers and their unique perspective.

It has been a great joy working together to conceptualize, write, edit, and birth this text. We pass it on to you hoping that you will find a life-affirming perspective that honors the many paths to healing.

ACKNOWLEDGMENTS

We are very grateful to all the women who authored the chapters for this book; your passion for the fields of integrative medicine and women's health is felt in every written word. We would like to thank all of the fellows, faculty, directors, and staff at the Arizona Center for Integrative Medicine who have served as partners in helping to transform our medical system. We are profoundly appreciative of our many wonderful teachers and mentors who have shared their stories, time, teachings, ideas, and wisdom with us throughout the course of our lives. To our families, we owe the deepest gratitude for all their love and support. And finally, we would like to honor Andrew Weil, MD, whose voice and vision initiated this field and inspired us all.

CONTENTS

III   Reproductive Health

IV   Common Illnesses in Women

CONTRIBUTORS

Priscilla Abercrombie, RN, NP, PhD, AHN-BC
Assistant Clinical Professor
UCSF School of Nursing
Department of Community Health Systems
Women's Health Center
San Francisco General Hospital
and
Founder
Women's Health & Healing
San Francisco, CA

Lise Alschuler, ND, FABNO
President
American Association of Naturopathic Physicians
Naturopathic Specialists, LLC
Scottsdale, AZ

Patricia K. Ammon, MD
Private Practice
Integrative Family Medicine
Ridgway, CO

Iris R. Bell, MD, PhD
Professor of Family and Community Medicine, Psychiatry, Psychology, Medicine, and Public Health
Department of Family and Community Medicine
The University of Arizona College of Medicine
Tucson, AZ

Rita Benn, PhD
Director Education
Integrative Medicine
Department of Family Medicine
and
Assistant Research Scientist
Institute for Research on Women and Gender
University of Michigan
Ann Arbor, MI

Sarah L. Berga, MD
James Robert McCord Professor and Chairman
Department of Gynecology and Obstetrics
Emory University
Atlanta, GA

Bridget S. Bongaard, MD, FACP
Fellow in Integrative Medicine
Director of the Integrative Medicine
  Service Line
CMC-Northeast Medical Center
Concord, NC

Ann Marie Chiasson, MD, MPH, CCFP
Assistant Clinical Professor of
  Medicine
Arizona Center for Integrative
  Medicine
University of Arizona
and
Medical Director
Valor Hospice and Palliative Care
and
Medical Director
The Haven, Rehabilitation Center for
  Women
Tucson, AZ

MargEva Morris Cole, MD
Clinical Associate Professor
Division, Durham Obstetrics and
  Gynecology
Department of Obstetrics and
  Gynecology
Duke University Medical Center
Durham, NC

Beate Ditzen, PhD
Assistant Professor
University of Zurich
Department of Psychology
Zurich, Switzerland

Marlene P. Freeman, MD
Perinatal and Reproductive Psychiatry
  Program
Department of Psychiatry
Massachusetts General Hospital
Harvard Medical School
Boston, MA

Louise Gagné, MD
Clinical Assistant Professor
Department of Community Health and
  Epidemiology
University of Saskatchewan
Saskatoon, Canada

Mary Hardy, MD
Medical Director
Simms/Mann-UCLA Center for
  Integrative Oncology
Jonsson Comprehensive Cancer Center
University of California
Los Angeles, CA

Cheryl Hawk, DC, PhD
Vice President of Research and
  Scholarship
Cleveland Chiropractic College
Kansas City, MO and Los Angeles, CA

Bettina Herbert, MD, FAAPMR
Clinical Instructor
Department of Rehabilitation
  Medicine
Department of Emergency Medicine
Jefferson-Myrna Brind Center of
  Integrative Medicine
Jefferson Medical College
Jefferson University Hospital
Philadelphia, PA

Lana L. Holstein, MD
Founder
Intimacy Growth Associates
Tucson, AZ

Tori Hudson, ND
Clinical Professor
National College of Natural Medicine
Bastyr University
and
Medical Director, A Woman's Time
Portland, OR

Raheleh Khorsan
Research Associate
Military Medical Research and
   Integrative Medicine
Samueli Institute
Irvine, CA

Wendy Kohatsu, MD
Assistant Clinical Professor
Department of Family and Community
   Medicine
University of California
San Francisco, CA
and
Director
Integrative Medicine Fellowship
Santa Rosa Family Medicine Residency
Santa Rosa, CA

Vivian A. Kominos, MD, FACC
Heart Specialists of Central Jersey, LLP
Assistant Clinical Professor of
   Medicine
Robert Wood Johnson Medical School
New Brunswick, NJ

Karen E. Konkel, MD
Private Practice
Towson, MD

Naomi Lam, MD
Integrative Psychiatrist
Osher Center for Integrative Medicine
and
Assistant Clinical Professor
Department of Psychiatry
University of California, San Francisco
San Francisco, CA

Beverly Lanzetta, PhD
Research Scholar
Religious Studies/Feminist Research
   Institute
University of New Mexico
Albuquerque, NM

Patricia Lebensohn, MD
Associate Professor of Clinical
   Family and Community Medicine
Department of Family and
   Community Medicine
University of Arizona
Tucson, AZ

Roberta Lee, MD
Vice Chair
Department of Integrative Medicine
Beth Israel Medical Center
and
Director
Integrative Medicine Fellowship
New York, NY

Tammy L. Loucks, MPH
Director for Research Projects
Department of Gynecology and
   Obstetrics
Emory University
Atlanta, GA

Susan Love, MD, MBA
President
Dr. Susan Love Research Foundation
Santa Monica, CA

Tieraona Low Dog, MD
Director of the Fellowship
Arizona Center for Integrative
    Medicine
and
Clinical Assistant Professor
Department of Medicine
University of Arizona Health Sciences
    Center
Tucson, AZ

Elizabeth R. Mackenzie, PhD
Lecturer
School of Arts and Sciences
and
Fellow
Center for Spirituality and the Mind
and
Associate Fellow
Institute on Aging
University of Pennsylvania
Philadelphia, PA

Victoria Maizes, MD
Executive Director
Arizona Center for Integrative
    Medicine
and
Associate Professor
Medicine, Family Medicine, and Public
    Health
University of Arizona
Tucson, AZ

Nisha J. Manek, MD, MRCP (UK)
Assistant Professor of Medicine
Division of Rheumatology
Department of Internal Medicine
Mayo Clinic College of Medicine
Rochester, MN

Kelly McCann, MD, MPH & TM
Program Development Director
Integrative Medicine and Wellness
    Program
Hoag Memorial Hospital Presbyterian
Newport Beach, CA

Leslie McGee RN, LAc
Diplomate in Acupuncture
Diplomate in Chinese Herbology
    (NCCAOM)
East-West Acupuncture & Chinese
    Herbs
Tucson, AZ

Daphne Miller, MD
Associate Clinical Professor Adjunct
Department of Family and Community
    Medicine
University of California, San Francisco
and
Private Family Practice
San Francisco, CA

Dixie J. Mills, MD
Medical Director
Dr. Susan Love Research Foundation
Santa Monica, CA

Pamela A. Pappas, MD, MD(H)
Private Practice
Scottsdale, AZ
and
Clinical Faculty
American Medical College of
    Homeopathy
Phoenix, AZ

Premal Patel, MD
Integrative Health Consultant
Fort Worth, TX

Jacquelyn M. Paykel, MD, FACOG
Department of Obstetrics and
    Gynecology
Riverside Medical Group
Williamsburg, VA

Joanne L. Perron, MD, FACOG, RYT
Postdoctoral Fellow
Program on Reproductive Health and
    the Environment
Department of Obstetrics, Gynecology,
    and Reproductive Sciences
University of California
San Francisco, CA

Sudha Prathikanti, MD
Integrative Psychiatrist
Osher Center for Integrative Medicine
and
Associate Clinical Professor
Department of Psychiatry
University of California
San Francisco, CA

Birgit Rakel, MD
Assistant Professor
Department of Family and Community
    Medicine
Department of Emergency Medicine
Thomas Jefferson University Hospital
Myrna Brind Center of Integrative
    Medicine
Philadelphia, PA

Melinda Ring, MD, FACP
Assistant Professor of Clinical
    Medicine
Northwestern University Feinberg
    School of Medicine
and
Medical Director
Center for Integrative Medicine and
    Wellness
Northwestern Memorial Physicians
    Group
Chicago, IL

Cynthia A. Robertson, MD, FACP
Voluntary Clinical Instructor
Department of Family and
    Preventative Medicine
University of California
San Diego School of Medicine
San Diego, CA

Carolyn Coker Ross, MD, MPH
Clinical Assistant Professor of
    Medicine
Arizona Center for Integrative
    Medicine
University of Arizona, Tucson, AZ
Eating Disorder
Addiction Medicine and Integrative
    Medicine Consultant
Denver, CO

PART I

Lifestyle

1

Philosophy of Integrative Women's Health

VICTORIA MAIZES AND TIERAONA LOW DOG

Women are healers, the holders of rituals, and the determiners of family life. Mothers, sisters, daughters, wives, and friends, our many relationships often define us as powerfully as our occupations. We have experienced triumphs and losses, joys and sorrows, and we bear the hidden scars and treasured trophies as our stories.

We believe that health care professionals who explore the fullness of women's lives are best able to provide them with the finest possible health care. Understanding a woman's beliefs, intuitions, and preferences for care allows us to form a healing partnership with the woman. By acknowledging the value of the partnership, we bring our presence fully to the interaction, desiring to understand the woman who sits across from us. Together we craft a unique treatment plan that fits this woman, her story, at this moment in time.

Each woman who comes to us has a story to tell. Our professional life is enriched when we listen to these stirring narratives. We provide our patient with the opportunity to hear her own story, sometimes for the very first time, and serve as witness to her triumphs and challenges. As the story unfolds, connections can be made, insights gained, and the foundation for healing is laid. An intimacy develops, which is one of the supreme privileges of being a healer, as we receive the story.

The root of health is hale or whole. We adopt the World Health Organization's broader definition of health: "Health is not only the absence of infirmity and disease but also a state of physical, mental and social well-being." The purpose of medicine, then, is to restore wholeness. To do so may require an investigation into all factors that may be interfering with healing. Our recognition that impediments may arise from body, mind, spirit, and emotions leads us to value a broader history.

A myriad of questions that deepen connection and understanding are drawn upon to augment a conventional medical history. "What is most important to you at this point in your life" is revealing. "Tell me about a typical day" outlines the pattern of a woman's life. "Imagine that a decade has gone by, what would you like to have accomplished" exposes a longer trajectory. "What gives you a sense of joy?" may reveal a hobby that lights the teller's eyes and spirit. "What are your strengths" is another question that deepens our understanding of our patient's character. When a woman finds it challenging to answer, a follow-up question, "what would your friends say they adore about you" may elicit more information. In some settings, it can be revealing to ask "What is your belief about what happens after we die?" When a woman says, "There is nothing more," or "I'd like to believe in an afterlife but I don't," a follow-up question might be gently posed such as "Have you ever had an experience of awe or mystery, something you just can't explain?" And at times remarkable experiences are then shared.

This broader set of questions will later create a framework for a broader set of treatment options. Perhaps journaling is called for if a woman is unclear as to what she wishes to unfold. When there is barely a moment of quiet in the depiction of a typical day, rest or meditation can be included. A crisis of spirit can be identified and may require a referral to priest, minister, or spiritual director.

It is our passionate belief that there are multiple routes to healing. An integrative practitioner possesses a larger tool box and is cognizant of many treatment options beyond pharmaceutical approaches. Numerous tools can be found in the chapters that follow. But integrative medicine is not simply about learning to use new treatment options. It is about a different way of being with a patient.

The integrative provider seeks to understand her patients' beliefs, honors them, and weighs them as she suggests treatment recommendations. As women use health care, their decisions are often influenced by the needs of others and their observation of others. Therefore, it is essential to ask women "What is your belief about…" For example, one woman choosing to use hormonal replacement therapy (HRT) for her menopausal symptoms tells us "I want to continue to take hormones because they keep me looking young." Another patient says nearly the opposite "Every time I swallow one of those pills I feel as if I am feeding a breast tumor." These two women and every other woman who come to us for healing have a unique set of experiences and beliefs that informs their decisions. Integrative medicine honors and validates such beliefs.

A 72-year-old woman calmly shares her life story filled with tremendous challenges. She has overcome the loss of her mother at 14, the death of her 37-year-old son, years of alcoholism in her husband, and a personal history of breast cancer. Her story provides a natural segue to inquire into her spiritual history. When asked what has given her the strength to carry on, she describes her deep connection to the Catholic Church. "It is her faith," she says, "that has allowed her to survive." Rather than being broken by these many losses, it has drawn her closer to God, her husband, and her friends.

Women have the capacity to see the sacred in everyday life. In sunrises, in the changing colors of the mountain in the deserts, and in the laughter of a child, women may be reminded of the ineffable. Women frequently are holders of the family rituals. Faith, religion, and spirituality are often their core sources of strength. In seeking to understand our patients, it is vital to capture this part of women's history.

Eliciting history is a reductive exercise. Over the course of a complete history, we ask about the parts of the story, the organ systems, and the details of a particular condition's history. In an integrative medicine encounter, what follows is a holistic function. It is often useful to briefly summarize what we have heard and understood. For example, we might say "You are a 42-year-old woman with a wonderful marriage, two children that you adore, a strong commitment to your spiritual practice, and a ten year history of rheumatoid arthritis. While the arthritis is controlled with ibuprofen and enbrel, you are eager to see whether nutritional changes would allow you to reduce your dose as you are concerned about long term use of your medications." When hearing her own story, our patient's motivation may get stronger; she can correct any error, or add to the list of concerns. It also provides an opportunity to emphasize her strengths, thereby reinforcing her ability to make necessary changes. Assembling this summary is a synthetic process. Not only do we reveal interconnections between symptoms, we remind ourselves and our patients of our fundamental wholeness.

The vastness of our toolbox in integrative medicine helps us in many ways, not least of which is the mindset that we always have something to offer. Should one intervention be unsuccessful, there is always another that can be attempted, leaving a hopeful perspective. Where Western medicine has been unsuccessful, a traditional Chinese medicine or Ayurvedic approach might offer a unique therapeutic strategy.

Our philosophical orientation is to look for roots of the illness. When recognizable patterns emerge, they provide guidance for treatment recommendations in novel conditions. For example, many diseases have inflammation as an underlying root cause. A treatment plan, which combines an antiinflammatory diet and herbs and mind–body approaches that help mitigate stress thereby reducing inflammation, can serve as a cornerstone of treatment in a disease for which there is not yet a solid body of evidence.

We are struck by how frequently the synergism of multiple, simple, low-tech interventions can be a powerful medicine. A 53-year-old woman with gastroesophageal reflux who has been treated for some time with proton pump inhibitors (PPI) comes to the clinic for advice. The PPI work well, but she is concerned about the long-term risks of the medication including iron deficiency anemia, B12 deficiency, hip fractures, and community-acquired pneumonia. She had tried to stop taking PPI more than once but had experienced a rebound set of symptoms that forced her back to the medication. In our clinic, we advise eliminating triggers of acid reflux in the diet, a trial off dairy, and the use of botanical remedies such as deglycyrrhized licorice (DGL) and dietary supplements including D-limonene. We question her about sources of stress and her coping skills. A simple breathing exercise that elicits the relaxation response is taught. Gradually, she is able to taper off PPI, then her supplements, and manages her symptoms with only occasional DGL.

As health care providers, there is always something we can do to be of service. Our very calling to medicine sets us apart from others who may be repelled by human suffering. Instead we lean in, seeking to be of help. From our simple presence, to serving as a witness to a woman's life experiences, to offering information about options, to teaching a quieting practice, to laying on our hands with a healing intent, to prescribing medications, or performing surgery, to caring for the dying, we can serve in a multitude of ways.

Suggested Reading

Maizes V, Koffler K, Fleishman, S. Revisiting the health history: an integrative approach. *Adv Mind Body Med.* Winter 2002;18(2):32–34.

Miller WR, Rollnick S. *Motivational Interviewing: Preparing People for Change.* 2nd ed. New York: Guilford Press; 2002.

Muller W. *How Then Shall We Live: Four Simple Questions That Reveal the Beauty and Meaning of Our Lives.* New York: Bantam Books; 1996.

Remen, RN. *Kitchen Table Wisdom.* New York: Riverhead Books; 1996.

Walsh, R. *Essential Spirituality: The 7 Central Practices to Awaken Heart and Mind.* New York: John Wiley and Sons, Inc; 1999.

2

Nutrition

WENDY KOHATSU

CASE STUDY

Helen is a 29-year-old busy professional woman who approached me for care to address her concerns of weight gain. She had gained weight steadily over the past 2 years and felt it was affecting her energy levels and causing more fatigue. Helen was a frequent soda drinker, and due to her hectic work schedule tended to eat big meals, when she could, at her desk. Typically, she complained of being "ravenous" by the time she got home for dinner and then indulged in overeating. Helen felt trapped in a vicious cycle.

Together, we worked on a plan to restructure her diet and exercise plan. I advised her to phase out soft drinks, and space out her calories with regular healthy snacks between meals to avoid binge eating. Helen added a healthy snack between 3 and 4 pm-usually a ¼ cup of nuts, a couple of whole grain crackers with hummus or hard-boiled egg, or low-fat plain yogurt with fresh fruit. Also, we discussed the Okinawan philosophy of *hara hachi bu* ["eat until you are eight parts [out of ten] full"]—stopping when nearly 8/10 full and paying attention to hunger and satiety signals. Helen also committed to one yoga class per week, and walking her dogs for 20 minutes a couple of days after work.

Eight months after adopting this gradual lifestyle change, her weight dropped from 173 to 161 pounds, and in another 8 months down to 153 pounds, dropping her BMI from 27.1 to a healthy 23.6. Helen is happy with her weight and lifestyle and notes that she has more energy with moderating her carb intake and increasing protein. She is also willing to explore incorporating new healthy foods and exercise into her daily life.

Introduction

Nutrition is a cornerstone of health, and food is necessary for energy, growth, repair, and renewal. Hippocrates' dictum "Let food be thy medicine and medicine be thy food" applies equally to men and women. The subject of nutrition is vast; emphasis in this chapter is placed on whole diets and providing practical tips for incorporating nutrition into a medical practice.

Basics

A brief review of the basics of nutrition—carbohydrates, proteins, fats, and water—follows; micronutrients including vitamins and minerals will not be covered in this chapter.

KEY INFORMATION

Carbohydrates ("carbs") provide the bulk of the body's energy needs and are available in the form of starches, sugars, and fibers. When evaluating the health benefits of carbohydrates, the following questions are important to address:

1. How processed is the carbohydrate?
2. What is the fiber content?
3. What is the glycemic index/load?
   - *Processed or unprocessed carbohydrates.* Wheat can be served as a cracked whole grain entree or as bleached white flour in a cookie. Unfortunately, refining strips away the nutrient-dense bran and germ, and 70%–80% of the iron, folate, fiber, B vitamins, magnesium, and zinc, which do not always get added back via "enrichment" (Sizer and Whitney 2006). In women, whole grain intake, but not refined carbohydrates, decreases the risk of type 2 diabetes (de Munter et al. 2007).
   - *Fiber.* Fibers are commonly described as being soluble (dissolves in water) or insoluble (roughage). Soluble fibers—such as pectins and gums—found in oatbran, fruits, legumes, seaweed, and psyllium

lower serum cholesterol by reducing the absorption of dietary cholesterol. Insoluble fibers—such as cellulose and lignin—found in wheat bran and fruit skins increase the sense of fullness, slow the rate of absorption of food across the small intestine, slow the rise in blood glucose levels, and act as bulking agents. Both soluble and insoluble fibers are valuable and are often found together in the same food. Whole oats, prunes, and black beans contain roughly equal amounts of soluble as insoluble fiber. Women should aim for 20 to 35 g of total fiber per day from whole grains, fruits, and vegetables.

- The glycemic index (GI) is a measure of how quickly a carbohydrate food raises blood sugar levels. The scale ranges from 1 to 100, with 100 representing pure glucose. Fiber, protein, and fats in food slow the rate of absorption of carbohydrates and the subsequent rise in blood glucose. Fructose, the most abundant sugar found in fruits, goes through a different metabolic pathway and takes a longer time to raise blood sugar.

- Foods with an index value ≥ 70 are considered high glycemic, 56–69 medium glycemic, and ≤ 54 low glycemic. Foods naturally high in fiber have a lower GI, as do foods that are less processed. Studies have shown a decreased risk of diabetes and cardiovascular disease with low GI diets, and preliminary data suggest a decreased risk of colon and breast cancers as well (Jenkins et al. 2002).

Numerous scientists have criticized the glycemic index as it alone does not represent true values of carbohydrates. A related, but more practical measure is the glycemic load (GL), which takes into account the *amount* of carbohydrates in a typical serving size plus its GI. GL values ≥ 20 are considered high glycemic load, 11–19 medium load, and ≤ 10 a low load. For example, pasta has a medium-level GI, but is so dense in carbohydrate calories that the GL is high at 27. The carbs in watermelon have a high GI of 72; however, watermelon contains only a small amount of carbohydrate, making its GL low at 4. It is recommended that women incorporate more low GL foods into their diets (Table 2.1).

Clinical Pearl

Think of GI/GL as a tool for comparing carbohydrates. When counseling patients, I use the analogy of "food as fuel." Eating low GL foods (with more fiber, naturally occurring fat, etc.) provides more consistent and sustained energy (Figure 2.1 blue dotted line in the graph) than ingesting the same amount of

Table 2.1. International Table of Glycemic Index and Glycemic Load Values: 2002

Food Items	Glycemic Index [Glucose = 100] High GI ≥ 70 Med GI 56–69 Low GI ≤ 55	Glycemic Load High GL ≥ 20 Med GL 11–19 Low GL ≤ 10
White baguette	95	15
Cornflakes	92	24
Watermelon	72	4
Rye crackers, wholegrain	63	11
Spaghetti, white	61	27
Cracked whole wheat bread	58	12
Apple, raw	40	6
Garbanzo beans	28	8
Black beans	20	5
Agave nectar	11	1

Source: From Foster-Powell K, Holt SH, Brand-Miller JC. *Am J Clin Nutr.* 2002;76:5–56.

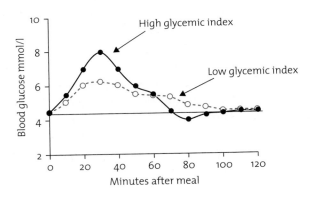

FIGURE 2.1. Glycemic index curve.

high-GL carbs and having the fuel supply spike and then crash 90 minutes later (Figure 2.1, black line where sugar drops).

To simplify the discussion, choose carbs that are whole grain (require chewing), include at least 5 servings of vegetables and fruit, and aim for total of 25 g of fiber per day.

Proteins

MINIMAL PROTEIN NEEDS

A common dietary concern for many women is getting enough protein. The average American diet however provides an ample or even excessive amount of protein. The recommended daily allowance (RDA) of protein in women aged 13 and older (excluding pregnancy) is 46 g/day. For girls aged 4–18 years, the RDA is closer to 1.0 g/kg/d due to increased protein needs. For reference, a 3-ounce (size of a deck of cards) serving of chicken breast provides about 23 g of protein, ½ cup of firm tofu provides 20 g, and one slice of whole grain bread about 4 g. Eating a well-balanced diet should provide plenty of protein for women and girls.

OPTIMAL PROTEIN AMOUNT

The optimal amount of protein varies with health status (i.e., less for women with kidney disease), activity (more protein may be advantageous during resistance training), and age. U.S. Guidelines recommend 0.8 g protein/kg of *ideal* body weight per day, thus for a fit 70 kg/154 lb woman, this would equal 56 g of protein. The World Health Organization (WHO) recommends 10%–15% of total caloric intake as protein.

Another important consideration is the source of protein: animal or plant. Animal proteins, particularly red meat, may raise homocysteine levels and can be high in saturated fat. Plant sources of protein tend to be high in fiber, potassium, folate, and magnesium. Plant-based diets are associated with lower risk of chronic disease, including cardiovascular disease (Hu 2003) and cancer (Byers et al. 2001), whereas a diet high in red meat (one serving per day) increases the risk of diabetes (Fung et al. 2004).

BOTTOM LINE ON PROTEINS

Two to three servings of high-quality, protein-rich foods per day are adequate to meet most women's needs. If consuming animal protein, emphasize fish, chicken, and turkey, while limiting red meat to 1 to 2 times per week. Plant sources of protein (legumes and nuts) are excellent choices and should be considered.

Soy—A Quick Word About Soy

Soy contains a full complement of essential amino acids, making it a complete protein. It also contains isoflavones (genistein, daidzein, glycitein), compounds that can act as weak estrogens or antiestrogens. Large epidemiologic studies in Asian countries have shown that lifelong, traditional consumption of soy may offer some protection against menopausal symptoms, breast cancer, and osteoporosis (Zhang et al. 2005). However, studies on soy and soy isoflavones in Western populations and animals have yielded inconsistent results (Nelson et al. 2006; Trock et al. 2006). Eating whole soyfoods likely poses less of a risk than highly concentrated soy supplements (Messina and Loprinzi 2008).

For women with breast cancer, research studies fail to convincingly indicate if soy intake is beneficial. Some human studies showing positive effects of soy indicate that early soy consumption (during adolescence or lifelong) can help prevent breast cancer (Shu et al. 2001). Much less is known about soy consumption in women at high risk for, or those who currently have, breast cancer. At traditional daily dietary levels (<40 mg isoflavones or 1 to 1.5 soyfood servings), soy does not seem to exacerbate breast cancer (Messina and Loprinzi 2001, Messina and Wood 2008), but most oncologists err on the side of caution and recommend avoiding it. Furthermore, since soy binds to the estrogen receptor, it is especially recommended that women avoid eating all soy products when taking tamoxifen or anastrozole (Arimidex).

The Skinny on Fats

There are three major categories of dietary fats—saturated, monounsaturated, and polyunsaturated—based on the number of double bonds within the lipid molecule. All fats found in nature are composite fats. For example, olive oil is 77% monounsaturated, but also contains 14% saturated fat and 9% polyunsaturated fats (Figure 2.2).

High-quality fats are essential in the diet. Research has highlighted the importance of eliminating *trans*-fats, limiting saturated fats, and increasing monounsaturated fats, especially olive oil. Extra-virgin olive oil contains antioxidants, LDL-lowering sterols, and favorably affects antiinflammatory mediators (Perona et al. 2006). Due to its high monounsaturated content, olive oil is less susceptible to conversion to *trans*-fatty acids.

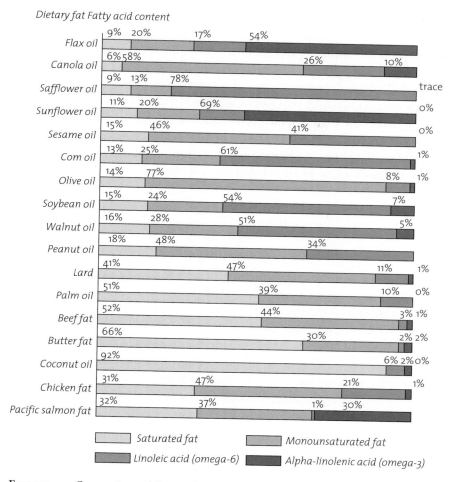

Dietary fat Fatty acid content

FIGURE 2.2. Comparison of dietary fats.
Source: Becoming Vegetarian, V. Melina, B. Davis, V. Harrison. Book Publishing Company, Summertown TN 1995.

Trans-fats increase serum levels of lipoprotein (a) and triglycerides (Mauger et al. 2003), as well as inflammatory mediators in women. Foods containing *trans*-fats should be eliminated from the diet (Mozaffarian et al. 2004). Substituting olive oil for butter and other saturated fats in cooking is a healthy choice. For high-temperature cooking (> 400° F), oils with a higher smoke point, such as grapeseed oil or organic canola oil, can be used.

Omega-3 fatty acids have been shown to decrease cardiac death, stroke, and all-cause mortality (Breslow 2006; Wang et al. 2006) and reduce the risk of certain cancers (Larsson et al. 2004). Research shows that these essential fatty acids play a role in depression (Lin and Su 2007) and may be beneficial for premenstrual syndrome (PMS) and menopausal hot flushes (Bourre 2007).

Omega-3 fats include plant sources such as flaxseed, hempseed, walnuts, and canola, and animal sources such as fatty fish and specialty eggs. Fish oils, in particular, have high concentrations of eicosapentaenoic acid (EPA) and docosahexaenoic acid (DHA), which are the most biologically active omega-3 fats. Plant sources have high amounts of alpha linolenic acid, of which only about 10% is converted to EPA and DHA.

Women should eat 2 to 3 servings of fatty fish per week in order to obtain adequate omega-3 fats, and if not, consider supplementation with purified fish oils containing EPA and DHA.

Water

The Institute of Medicine recommends that women consume nine cups of total beverages per day. But as requirements vary according to activity level, health status, geographical location, and so on, women should drink enough water to quench their thirst so that they produce colorless or slightly yellow-colored urine (Institute of Medicine 2004). Tea, herbal tisanes, and coffee can be added to daily fluid intake, although there is an initial small diuretic effect with caffeine. Sugar-sweetened beverages are associated with obesity and their intake should be minimized (Malik et al. 2006). Hydration is important for weight loss as women can mistake hunger for thirst signals.

Girls (>4 years) need approximately 50 to 60 mL water/kg body weight (Whitmire 2004). This is roughly the number of ounces equivalent to two-thirds of their body weight in pounds. So, a child weighing 36 pounds needs 24 ounces of water. When girls reach the age of 10 to 12 years, their water needs approach that of adults.

Diets Women Should Know About

- Mediterranean-based diet
- Anti-inflammatory diet
- Low-carbohydrate diet
- Elimination diet

WHAT IS A MEDITERRANEAN DIET?

The Mediterranean diet is based on traditional eating patterns of the Mediterranean region (Trichopoulou 2001) that emphasizes olive oil as the primary fat, high intake of fruit, vegetables, whole grains, moderate fish intake, moderate wine consumption, and limited consumption of red meat and saturated fat. It has a favorable balance of polyunsaturated omega-6:omega-3 fatty acids of 2 to 4:1, whereas in the typical U.S. diet, this ratio is closer to 10 to 20:1. Excessive amounts of omega-6 fats are proinflammatory, adversely affecting eicosanoid and cytokine pathways and altering gene expression. Fish, locally consumed wild greens, herbs, and walnuts (all sources of omega-3 fats) help contribute to a more favorable, antiinflammatory balance (Manios et al. 2006).

When combined with a healthy lifestyle, the Mediterranean-based diet has been shown to decrease all-cause mortality in women. Data from the large American Association of Retired Persons (AARP) prospective study (Mitrou et al. 2007) show that all-cause mortality for women dropped by 20%. Similarly, the Healthy Ageing: A Longitudinal Study in Europe (HALE) study, confirmed that adherence to a Mediterranean diet and healthy lifestyle is associated with a >50% lower rate of all-cause and cause-specific mortality in healthy men and women more than 70 years of age (Knoops et al. 2004).

Cardiovascular Disease

The Lyon Heart Study reported that the Mediterranean-type diet reduced the risk of a second heart attack in people who had a previous heart attack (De Lorgeril et al. 1999). The Lyon diet was high in fruits, vegetables, whole grains, with increased intake of legumes and fish. Forty percent of calories were from fat (olive oil and special high monounsaturated spread), as compared to controls who consumed a 30% fat "heart-healthy" diet. There was a 70% reduction in cardiac morbidity in the experimental group and the trial was stopped early. Similarly, in the GIZZI-Prevenzione study (Barzi et al. 2003), there was a 50% reduction of death in participants with high Mediterranean dietary scores compared to those in the lowest quartile. Of note, it appears that women with coronary artery disease (CAD) may be more responsive to the Mediterranean diet than men (Chrysohoou et al. 2003).

Cancer

The overall cancer incidence in Mediterranean countries is lower than in northern European countries, the United Kingdom, and the United States. Several studies show that much of this may be attributable to dietary factors. The Lyon Diet Heart study was also analyzed for its impact on cancer; a 61% decrease in cancer incidence was noted in a short time frame (De Lorgeril et al. 1998). Another study (Trichopoulou et al. 2000) calculated that up to 25% of colorectal cancer, 15% of breast cancer, and 10% of pancreas and endometrial cancers could be prevented if

Western populations shifted to the traditional healthy Mediterranean diet. High intake of monounsaturated fatty acids (chiefly derived from olive oil and seed oils) may be protective against breast cancer and conversely, high intakes of starch and saturated fat may increase risk (Franceschi and Favero 1999).

Obesity

The Mediterranean diet has been associated with reduced obesity and risk of metabolic syndrome (Bes-Rastrollo et al. 2006; Panagiotakos et al. 2006). In a randomized, controlled trial on weight loss, despite a higher fat content (35% compared to 20%), participants eating a Mediterranean-based diet lost 4.1 kg, compared to the control group who gained nearly 3 kg over 18 months (McManus et al. 2001). The palatability of higher fat diet may be the reason for greater long-term adherence—it tastes good, hunger signals are quieted, and people are satisfied. Women with diabetes following a Mediterranean diet had 23% higher levels of adiponectin, a hormone secreted by fat cells that is inversely correlated with body fat percentage (Mantzoros et al. 2006).

In a summary of the research concerning the Mediterranean diet, Dr. Walter Willett from the Harvard School of Public Health concludes that in nonsmoking individuals with regular physical activity, "over 80% of coronary heart disease, 70% of stroke, and 90% of type 2 diabetes can be avoided by healthy food choices that are consistent with the traditional Mediterranean diet" (Willett 2006).

WHAT IS AN ANTI-INFLAMMATORY DIET?

It is now believed that chronic inflammation is the common pathophysiologic pathway underlying CAD, asthma, arthritis, Alzheimer's disease, autoimmune disorders, and some cancers. Obesity, saturated fat, *trans*-fat, and an inadequate amount of omega-3 fats have been shown to increase inflammatory biomarkers such as C-reactive protein (CRP), interleukin 6 (IL-6), and tumor necrosis factor (TNF) (Basu et al. 2006; Simopoulos 2002). An *anti-inflammatory* diet increases dietary intake of foods that decrease inflammation, while reducing foods that increase inflammation. The Mediterranean diet is also an anti-inflammatory diet, showcasing fruits and vegetables, whole grains, healthy fats, and fish.

Dr. Andrew Weil has published a patient-friendly and illustrative anti-inflammatory food pyramid (see http://www.drweil.com/drw/u/ART02995/Dr-Weil-Anti-Inflammatory-Food-Pyramid.html). This plan also features berries, Asian mushrooms, soy, tea, and dark chocolate.

WHAT ABOUT LOW-CARBOHYDRATE DIETS?

Popular diets vary in their carbohydrate recommendations: less than 10% of total calories (Atkins), 40% (Zone), 55%–60% (LEARN), and 65%–75% (Ornish). The Atkins-type low-carb diets have been very popular since the late 1990s and are particularly promoted for weight loss. A 2003 systematic review of low-carb diets reported that weight loss was associated with lower total caloric intake, and increased duration on a diet but not reduced carbohydrate content (Bravata et al. 2003). The low-carb diets did not show significant adverse effects on cholesterol, fasting glucose, insulin levels, or blood pressure as originally feared.

After this review, two 12-month studies were published. The first compared weight loss in obese participants randomized to four different diets: Atkins, Zone, Weight Watchers, and Ornish. Each popular diet modestly reduced body weight in the range of 2.1 to 3.3 kg (4.6 to 7.3 pounds) at the end of 1 year. No significant difference was found *between* diet plans, and weight loss was associated with greater adherence to *any* plan (Dansinger et al. 2005).

The second 12-month randomized trial compared four isocaloric diets with varying amounts of carbohydrate—low (Atkins), moderate (Zone and LEARN), high (Ornish)—in overweight and obese women in free-living conditions (Gardner et al. 2007). Those on the Atkins low-carbohydrate plan lost significantly more weight (–4.7 kg) than any of the other diets (range –1.6 to –2.2 kg) with no adverse effects seen in lipids, fasting glucose, or insulin levels. There was considerable regression with the Ornish high-carb group moving from 63% to 52% of calories as carbs and the low-carb Atkins group eating 18% to 35% as carbs, but still a significant difference was noted at 12 months. During this interval, the women also lowered their reported intake by 250 to 500 calories/day.

If women can adhere to a reduced-calorie, low-carbohydrate diet (35% of calories as carbs, roughly 138 g/day carbs), significantly greater weight loss can occur. Longer-term sustainability and maintenance of weight loss still need to be proven, especially as there was a strong trend toward regaining weight as women started to increase their carbohydrate intake during the second 6 months of the trial.

For a more comprehensive review of carbs, protein, fat, water, vitamins, and minerals, refer to *Nutrition—Concepts and Controversies*, 11th edition, and Krause's *Food, Nutrition and Diet Therapy* textbooks.

THE ELIMINATION DIET

The elimination diet is a clinical tool rather than a diet, per se. It is defined as "an investigational short-term or possible lifelong eating plan that omits one or more foods suspected or known to cause an adverse food reaction or allergic response" (Mahan and Escott-Stump 2004). Food allergy or intolerance may play a significant role in many chronic conditions including migraines, asthma, otitis media, skin conditions, attention-deficit-hyperactive disorder (ADHD), arthritis, autoimmune diseases, and more. Clinical trials using food elimination diets have reported improvement rates as high as 58% for atopic dermatitis, 71% for irritable bowel syndrome (IBS), and 90% for migraines (Rindfleisch 2007). Commonplace symptoms such as dyspepsia, flatulence, chronic fatigue, skin rashes, joint aches, and pains have all been linked to food sensitivities. Many integrative practitioners consider addressing dietary sensitivities as a critical first step to symptom amelioration.

Major food triggers include

- Dairy products
- Wheat and other gluten-like grains
- Eggs
- Corn
- Soy and soy products
- Peanuts
- Citrus fruits
- Yeast
- Refined sugars
- Artificial additives, preservatives and colorings

While immediate IgE hypersensitivity allergies or anaphylaxis to foods are obvious, delayed hypersensitivity reactions (typically, IgG or IgA) can be so subtle that they tend to be dismissed. Conventional laboratory tests such as RAST, ELISA, and provocation tests are not very sensitive for food-induced allergies. An empiric elimination diet is not only straightforward and cost-effective but it is specific to the individual being tested.

Phases of the Elimination Diet

Elimination phase. All suspected foods are omitted from the diet (i.e., refined sugar, dairy products, wheat, etc.) for 10 to 14 days. Clinical symptoms are monitored for resolution. For example, a woman may notice that she is less fatigued or bloated while eliminating dairy products from her diet.

Reintroduction or challenge phase. Suspect food triggers are reintroduced one at time into the diet to see if symptoms recur. For example, fatigue or bloating returns when the aforementioned woman resumes eating dairy.

The theory behind the elimination diet is simple, but as most of our diet consists of composite foods (e.g., pizza = bread + tomato sauce + cheese/dairy + various meat and vegetable toppings), it is often hard to practice. Women must be taught to read labels carefully to identify hidden sources of allergens. For example, casein, lactose, and whey are all dairy products. Women testing for wheat/gluten sensitivity must avoid the usual suspect foods such as breads, cookies, pasta, and cereals as well as the myriad of foods made with wheat, including "modified food starch," beer, caramel coloring, soy sauce, and more. [for detailed list, visit www.celiac.com and search using the keywords "unsafe ingredients"]. Though the elimination diet requires diligence and patience, when properly done, the results can be extremely beneficial.

A modified elimination diet is when *one* suspect food at a time is avoided for 10 to 14 days and then rotated back into the diet (Rockwell 1999). It takes longer to test all the individual foods however is more practical in children and for those who are reluctant to undergo the drastic dietary changes called for in the full elimination diet.

The Organic Controversy

More questions than answers arise when evaluating the scientific evidence for organic food. Consumers pay 10%–40% more for certified organic food (Winter and Davis 2006) because they perceive it as safer, more nutritious, and environmentally friendly. Studies show that organically grown crops have significantly higher levels of vitamin C, iron, magnesium, phosphorus, and lower nitrates than conventionally grown crops (Worthington 2001). While nitrates have been linked to the formation of carcinogenic N-nitroso compounds, the trace amount present on produce has not been directly linked to increased cancer incidence. The long-term cumulative effects of dietary nitrates have not been adequately assessed in humans. One study assessed urinary levels of organophosphate (OP) in children. It found that those consuming organic fruits, vegetables, and juices had six times less OP metabolite concentrations. The authors concluded that adhering to an organic diet would drop children's exposure level from "uncertain" to "negligible" risk based on U.S. Environmental Protection Agency's levels (Curl et al. 2003).

ANIMAL PRODUCTS

By USDA definition, organic meat, poultry, eggs, and dairy products must come from animals that are not given growth hormones or routine antibiotics. It is estimated that 70% of the total amount of antibiotics used in the United States are given to poultry, swine, and beef cattle (Mellon et al. 2000). These antibiotic "food additives" are given as growth promoters and to compensate for crowded animal conditions that place livestock at risk of infections. A major public health concern arising from these practices is the increase in antibiotic resistance.

In one study (White et al. 2001), 20% of 200 meat samples from supermarkets contained Salmonella, 84% were resistant to at least one antibiotic, and 53% were resistant to at least three antibiotics. Sixteen percent of the isolates were resistant to ceftriaxone, the drug of choice for treating salmonellosis in children. The World Health Organization, the American Public Health Association, and the Union of Concerned Scientists have confirmed that overuse of antibiotics in livestock contribute the antibiotic resistance affecting humans and have called for their cessation (APUA 2002; Wegener et al. 2003).

Cattle producers often inject their livestock with bovine somatotropin (bST), a growth hormone that artificially increases milk production and lean tissue growth. The FDA does not require testing of food products for traces of it. Canada and the European Union ban the use of bST in milking cows because it stimulates insulin-like growth factor I (IGF-I) in the cows, raising questions about its potential effects in humans.

Mercury in Fish

Although a source of high-quality protein, fish often swim in waters contaminated with heavy metals such as cadmium, lead, mercury, and other pollutants such as polychlorinated biphenyls (PCBs), dioxins, and DDT. Large predatory fish that eat other fish accumulate higher levels of contaminants in their flesh. Fish highest in mercury include king mackerel, swordfish, shark, tilefish, orange roughy, grouper, and tuna. Some of the safest fish are tilapia, anchovies, and wild salmon. A helpful Web site for further information is http://www.cfsan.fda.gov/~frf/sea-mehg.html from Food and Drug Administration (FDA) and the U.S. Environmental Protection Agency.

Top 12 foods to get organically grown (CHEC, 2008)

- Peaches
- Apples
- Pears
- Winter squash
- Green beans
- Grapes

- Strawberries
- Raspberries
- Spinach
- Potatoes
- Tomatoes
- Cantaloupe

Organophosphate residues, DDT by-products, and other products listed as endocrine disruptors or carcinogens were found in significant amounts in these foods. Since OP residues tend to concentrate in fat, it may be prudent to get most if not all of your food oils (olive oil, butter, etc.) as organic.

Nutrition for Girls

- Iron deficiency
- Bone health
- Childhood obesity

IRON DEFICIENCY IN GIRLS

Despite an abundant food supply in the United States, iron deficiency is relatively common, affecting 7% of U.S. toddlers. Marrow stores from birth are diminished by 6 to 9 months of age, and as babies grow older, many are switched from iron-rich breast milk or formula to cow's milk. Studies have linked iron deficiency with lower school performance scores (Halterman et al. 2001). Iron deficiency precedes anemia, and even without anemia, iron deficiency impairs central nervous system (CNS) function including mental performance. Iron deficiency has been defined as abnormal levels of 2 of 3 measures: serum ferritin, free erythrocyte protoporphyrin, and transferrin saturation. Hemoglobin should also be checked.

As girls attain puberty, iron intake needs to increase due to skeletal muscle growth and menstruation. Girls 4 to 8 years of age need 10 mg/day of iron, increasing to 11–15 mg/day for menstruating girls. Iron is better absorbed from animal than plant sources. Certain legumes and vegetables are high in iron, however 50%–80% higher intake is needed to offset the decreased absorption; vitamin C enhances plant iron absorption. Since many adolescent girls do not eat iron-rich foods, and as many as 16% have been found to be deficient (MMWR 2002), iron supplementation may be required (Table 2.2).

Table 2.2. Iron from Food

Food	Iron (mg)
Clams, ¼ cup	11.2
Beef liver, 3 oz	5.3
Baked beans, 1 cup	5.0
Molasses, blackstrap 1 tbsp	5.0
Bean burrito, 1	2.5
Rice, enriched 1 cup	2.3
Spaghetti with tomato sauce	2.3
Oatmeal, unfortified	1.6
Spinach fresh, 1 cup	1.5
Fortified cereal, ready-to-eat	1.0 – 10+

BONE HEALTH

Adolescence is a critical time for bone development; 45% of the skeletal mass is added during this time (Lytle 2002). Eighty-five percent of adolescent girls have inadequate calcium intake. This, combined with low physical activity and increased soft drink intake, spells trouble for their bones in the future.

Food sources high in calcium include dairy products, broccoli, tofu, almonds, and legumes. While dairy products are an excellent source of calcium, it is intriguing that countries with the highest dairy intake also have the highest rates of osteoporosis. Cruciferous vegetables contain easily absorbed calcium, however, leafy greens such as spinach and chard contain oxalic acid, which inhibits calcium absorption. Vitamin D and weight-bearing exercise are also critical for proper bone development and maintenance. Girls 4 to 8 years old need 800 mg calcium/day; ages 9 to 18 need 1300 mg/day. When supplementing, calcium carbonate is best absorbed in an acidic environment (with meals is ideal), while calcium citrate does not need to be taken with food (Table 2.3).

A QUICK WORD ON CHILDHOOD OBESITY

Rates of childhood obesity have grown alarmingly fast. In 2004, 17% of American children and adolescents were obese (Ogden et al. 2006), putting them at risk for developing diabetes, hypertension, and cardiovascular disease.

Table 2.3. Calcium from Food

Food Source	Calcium (mg)
Yogurt, plain low fat 8 oz.	415
Tofu, firm 1 cup	408
Sardines with bones, 3 oz.	324
Orange juice, calcium-fortified, 8 fl oz.	300
Milk, 8 fl oz.	300
Tahini, 2 tbsp	128
Broccoli, cooked 1 cup	94
Almonds, ¼ cup	89

The average American child sees 30,000 TV commercials per year, many of them promoting high-calorie, high fat, and sugar-laden foods (Wiecha et al. 2006). Watching TV over 4 h/day increases the risk for obesity (Coon and Tucker 2002), so it is recommended to limit TV watching to no more than 2 h/day and for parents to be proactive in monitoring what their children watch. On the positive side, studies show that familiarity with vegetables increases their consumption in children (Cooke 2007) and so early exposure to healthy foods is important. Not surprisingly, the dietary habits of parents rub off on their children, so whole families can benefit from healthy eating patterns (Moag-Stahlberg et al. 2003).

Top Tips from Clinical Experience

- Weight loss guidelines recommend that obese women with BMI >35 cut out 500+ calories/day. Women with a BMI of 26–35 should reduce caloric intake by 300–500 calories/day.
- Successful "losers" engage in frequent exercise, eat an estimated 1800 kcal/day, eat breakfast, and self-monitor their weight (Wing and Phelan 2005).
- Double vegetable intake, half your refined carb intake—eat an open-faced sandwich with one piece of bread and have a small green salad, or a side of fresh vegetables. Stir in a cup of chopped leafy greens to a bowl of soup.
- Mindful eating + *hara hachi bu*—another clinical pearl I teach patients is to simply check in with their level of hunger. Okinawan longevity is

well-known, and one of their sayings, *hara hachi bu*, simply translates as "eat until you are eight parts [out of ten] full" (Willcox et al. 2001). This simple wisdom advises us to avoid stuffing our stomachs until they are bursting at the seams. It also teaches us be mindful of how much we eat and how are bodies are feeling. Often, we can be satisfied with less.

- Healthy snacks under 200 calories—chopped vegetables (carrots, snow peas, cauliflower, radishes, cucumbers), one-quarter measuring cup of nuts, 2 whole grain rye crackers with hummus, mini-portions of leftover dinner, medium apple with 2 teaspoons of almond butter, half banana with 2 teaspoons of peanut butter, one 8-ounce cup of low-fat plain yogurt with half-cup fresh or frozen blackberries, 2-ounce string cheese, 2-inch square of smoked tofu with veggies. Have patients create their own snacks.
- Chocolate—dark chocolate is rich in antioxidants as well as mood-enhancing phenylethylamine and anandamides. Despite its high saturated fat content, dark chocolate does not raise low-density lipoprotein (LDL), and indeed may lower it. A study showed that dark chocolate can lower blood pressure (Taubert et al. 2007). A small portion (about 1-inch flat square) of dark (70% cocoa or more) can be a healthy and happy treat.
- Watch out for sodium intake—One tablespoon of table salt is packed with 2400 mg sodium, already exceeding the recommended total daily sodium intake of 2300 mg for healthy adults (USDA Dietary Guidelines for Americans 2005).

Summary

- Eat whole, unprocessed foods with low glycemic load.
- Quality and quantity of fats, carbs, and proteins matter.
- Following a traditional Mediterranean diet or anti-inflammatory diet is a powerful medicine and has been proven to prevent or mitigate the onset or occurrence of multiple chronic diseases.
- Eat mindfully (*hara hachi bu*) and savor your food.
- Get adequate sleep—sleep deprivation decreases leptin, a satiety hormone produced by fat cells, and increases ghrelin, a hunger-increasing hormone (Knutson and Van Cauter 2008).
- For girls, check for iron deficiency, investigate to ensure adequate nutrient intake, and also determine level of activity/TV watching.

Resources for Integrative Providers

- Brigham and Women's Web site (http://www.brighamandwomens. org/patient/nutritionRich.aspx#)
  Free online handout on food sources of common nutrients, example: B6 from banana, avocado, rice bran, brown rice, oatmeal, soybeans, etc.
- The Live Strong Web site (http://www.livestrong.com)
  This is an easy-to-use online calorie and fitness tracker, is available for free. Great option is that you can add your own food: www.thedailyplate. com
- Portion size Web site (http://hp2010.nhlbihin.net/portion/)
  The National Heart Lung and Blood Institute of the NIH has a great downloadable Web site to teach people about portion size of foods: http://hp2010.nhlbihin.net/portion
- *Eat, Drink, & Weigh Less* by Mollie Katzen and Walter Willett (2006 Hyperion, New York): An excellent, no-nonsense, reader-friendly book with helpful tips and recipes to help people lose weight.
- *Nutrition – Concepts and Controversies,* 11th edition, by F. Sizer and E. Whitney (Thomson Wadsworth 2006, Belmont, CA). Basic textbook aimed at college level, but good review of nutrition basics in simple language.
- For excellent evidence-based information about vegetarian and vegan diets, read *Becoming Vegetarian* and *Becoming Vegan* by Vesanto Melina and Brenda Davis.

REFERENCES

Alliance for Prudent Use of Antibiotics (APUA). The Need to Improve Antimicrobial Use in Agriculture: Ecological and Human Health Effects; also published in Clinical Infectious Diseases 2002 (Vol 34, Supplement 3). http://www.tufts.edu/med/apua/Ecology/faair.html. Accessed December 15, 2008.

Barzi F, Woodward M, Marfisi RM, et al. GISSI-Prevenzione Investigators. Mediterranean diet and all-causes mortality after myocardial infarction: results from the GISSI-Prevenzione trial. *Eur J Clin Nutr.* 2003;57(4):604–611.

Basu A, Devaraj S, Jialal I. Dietary factors that promote or retard inflammation. *Arterioscler Thromb Vasc Biol.* 2006;26:995–1001.

Bes-Rastrollo M, Sanchez-Villegas A, de la Fuente C, et al. Olive oil consumption and weight change: the SUN prospective cohort study. *Lipids.* 2006;41(3):249–256.

Bourre JM. Dietary omega-3 fatty acids for women. *Biomed Pharmacother.* 2007;61(2–3):105–112.

Bravata DM, Sanders L, Huang J, et al. Efficacy and safety of low-carbohydrate diets: a systematic review. *JAMA*. 2003;(14):1837–1850.

Breslow JL. n-3 fatty acids and cardiovascular disease. *Am J Clin Nutr*. 2006;83(6 Suppl):1477S–1482S.

Byers T, Nestle M, McTiernan A, et al. American Cancer Society 2001 Nutrition and Physical Activity Guidelines Advisory Committee. American Cancer Society guidelines on nutrition and physical activity for cancer prevention: reducing the risk of cancer with healthy food choices and physical activity. *CA Cancer J Clin*. 2002 Mar-Apr;52(2):92–119.

Children's Health Environmental Coalition Website. http://www.checnet.org/HEALTHEHOUSE/education/quicklist-detail.asp?Main_ID=241. Accessed October 10, 2008.

Chrysohoou C, Panagiotakos DB, Pitsavos C, et al. Gender differences on the risk evaluation of acute coronary syndromes: the CARDIO2000 study. *Prev Cardiol*. 2003;6(2):71–77.

Cooke L. The importance of exposure for healthy eating in childhood: a review. *J Hum Nutr Diet*. 2007;20(4):294–301.

Coon KA, Tucker KL. Television and children's consumption patterns. A review of the literature. *Minerva Pediatr*. 2002;54(5):423–436.

Curl CL, Fenske RA, Elgethun K. Organophosphorus pesticide exposure of urban and suburban preschool children with organic and conventional diets. *Environ Health Perspect*. 2003;111:377–382.

Dansinger ML, Gleason JA, Griffith JL, et al. Comparison of the Atkins, Ornish, Weight Watchers, and Zone diets for weight loss and heart disease risk reduction: a randomized trial. *JAMA*. 2005;293:43–53.

de Munter JS, Hu FB, Spiegelman D, et al. Whole grain, bran, and germ intake and risk of type 2 diabetes: a prospective cohort study and systematic review. *PLoS Med*. 2007 Aug;4(8):e261.

De Lorgeril M, Salen P, Martin JL, Monjaud I, Boucher P, Mamelle N. Mediterranean dietary pattern in a randomized trial. Prolonged survival and possible reduced cancer rate. *Arch Intern Med*. 1998;158:1181–1187.

De Lorgeril M, Salen P, Martin JL, et al. Mediterranean diet, traditional risk factors, and the rate of cardiovascular complications after myocardial infarction: final report of the Lyon Diet Heart Study. *Circulation*. 1999;779–785.

Franceschi S, Favero A. The role of energy and fat in cancers of the breast and colon-rectum in a southern European population. *Ann Oncol*. 1999; 10 Suppl 6:61–63.

Fung TT, Schulze M, Manson JE, Willett WC, Hu FB. Dietary patterns, meat intake, and the risk of type 2 diabetes in women. *Arch Intern Med*. 2004;164(20):2235–2240.

Gardner CD, Kiazand A, Alhassan S, et al. Comparison of the Atkins, Zone, Ornish, and LEARN diets for change in weight and related risk factors among overweight premenopausal women: the A TO Z Weight Loss Study: a randomized trial. *JAMA*. 2007;297(9):969–977.

Halterman JS, Kaczorowski JM, Aligne CA, et al. Iron deficiency and cognitive achievement among school-aged children and adolescents in the United States. *Pediatrics*. 2001;107(6):1381–1386.

Hu FB. Plant-based foods and prevention of cardiovascular disease: an overview. *Am J Clin Nutr.* 2003;78(3):544S–551S.

Institute of Medicine. Standing Committee on the Scientific Evaluation of Dietary Reference Intakes, Food and Nutrition Board, 2004.

Jenkins DJ, Kendall CW, Augustin LS, et al. Glycemic index: overview of implications in health and disease. *Am J Clin Nutr.* 2002;76 (suppl):266S–273S.

Knoops KT, deGroot LC, Kromhout D, et al. Mediterranean diet, lifestyle factors, and 10-year mortality in elderly European men and women. *JAMA.* 2004;292(12):1433–1439.

Knutson KL, Van Cauter E. Associations between sleep loss and increased risk of obesity and diabetes. *Ann N Y Acad Sci.* 2008;1129:287–304.

Larsson SC, Kumlin M, Ingelman-Sundberg M, Wolk A. Dietary long-chain n-3 fatty acids for the prevention of cancer: a review of potential mechanisms. *Am J Clin Nutr.* 2004;79(6):935–945.

Lin PY, Su KP. A meta-analytic review of double-blind, placebo-controlled trials of anti-depressant efficacy of omega-3 fatty acids. *J Clin Psychiatry.* 2007;68(7):1056–1061.

Lytle L. Nutritional issues for adolescents. *JADA.* 2002;102:S8.

Mahan LK, Escott-Stump S, eds. *Krause's Food, Nutrition and Diet Therapy.* 11th ed. Philadelphia: WB Saunders, 2004.

Malik VS, Schulze MB, Hu FB. Intake of sugar-sweetened beverages and weight gain: a systematic review. *Am J Clin Nutr.* 2006 Aug;84(2):274–288.

Manios Y, Detopoulou V, Visioli F, Galli C. Mediterranean diet as a nutrition education and dietary guide: misconceptions and the neglected role of locally consumed foods and wild green plants. *Forum Nutr.* 2006;59:154–170.

Mantzoros CS, Williams CJ, Manson JE, et al. Adherence to the Mediterranean dietary pattern is positively associated with plasma adiponectin concentrations in diabetic women. *Am J Clin Nutr.* 2006;84(2):328–335.

Mauger JF, Lichtenstein AH, Ausman LJ, et al. Effect of different forms of dietary hydrogenated fats on LDL particle size. *Am J Clin Nutr.* 2003;78(3):370–375.

McManus K, Antinoro L, Sacks F. A randomized controlled trial of a moderate-fat, low-energy diet compared with a low fat, low-energy diet for weight loss in overweight adults. *Intl J of Obesity.* 2001;25:1503–1511.

Mellon M. *Hogging It: Estimates of Antimicrobial Abuse in Livestock.* Cambridge, MA: Union of Concerned Scientists, 2000.

Messina MJ, Loprinzi CL. Soy for breast cancer survivors: A critical review of the literature. *J Nutr.* 2001;131:3095S–3108S.

Messina MJ, Wood CE. Soy isoflavones, estrogen therapy, and breast cancer risk: analysis and commentary. *Rev Nutr J.* 2008;7:17.

Mitrou PN, Kipnis V, Thiebaut AC, et al. Mediterranean dietary pattern and prediction of all-cause mortality in a US population: results from the NIH-AARP Diet and Health Study. *Arch Intern Med.* 2007;167(22):2461–2468.

MMWR, Iron Deficiency—United States 1999–2000; *MMWR.* 2002;51(40):897–901.

Moag-Stahlberg A, Miles A, Marcello M. What kids say they do and what parents think kids are doing: The ADAF/Knowledge Networks 2003 Family Nutrition and Physical Activity Study. *J Am Diet Assoc.* 2003;103(11):1541–1546.

Mozaffarian D, Pischon T, Hankinson SE, et al. Dietary intake of trans fatty acids and systemic inflammation in women. *Am J Clin Nutr*. 2004;79(4):606–612.

Nelson HD, Vesco KK, Haney E, et al. Nonhormonal therapies for menopausal hot flashes: systematic review and meta-analysis. *JAMA*. 2006;295:2057.

Ogden CL, Carroll MD, Curtin LR, et al. Prevalence of overweight and obesity in the United States, 1999–2004. *JAMA*. 2006;295(13):1549–1555.

Panagiotakos DB, Chrysohoou C, Pitsavos C, et al. Association between the prevalence of obesity and adherence to the Mediterranean diet: the ATTICA study. *Nutrition*. 2006;22(5):449–456.

Perona JS Cabello-Moruno R, Ruiz-Gutierrez V. The role of virgin olive oil components in the modulation of endothelial function. *J Nutr Biochem*. 2006;17(7):429–445.

Rindfleisch JA. Adverse food reactions and the elimination diet. In: Rakel D, ed. *Integrative Medicine*. 2nd ed. Philadelphia, PA: Saunders Elsevier, 2007.

Rockwell SJ. Rotation diet: a diagnostic and therapeutic tool. In: Pizzorno JE, Murray MT, eds. *Textbook of Natural Medicine*. Edinburgh: Churchill Livingstone, 1999.

Shu XO, Jin F, Dai Q, et al. Soyfood intake during adolescence and subsequent risk of breast cancer among Chinese women. *Cancer Epidemiol Biomark Prev*. 2001;10:483–488.

Simopoulos AP. Omega-3 fatty acids in inflammation and autoimmune diseases. *J Am Col Nutr*. 2002;21(6):495–505.

Sizer F, Whitney E. Consumer corner: refined, enriched and whole-grain foods. Chap 4. The carbohydrates. In: Sizer F, Whitney E, ed. *Nutrition—Concepts and Controversies*. 11th ed. Belmont, CA: Thomson Wadsworth, 2006: 116–118.

Taubert D, Roesen R, Lehmann C, et al. Effects of low habitual cocoa intake on blood pressure and bioactive nitric oxide: a randomized controlled trial. *JAMA*. 2007;298(1):49–60.

Trichopoulou A, Lagiou P, Kuper H, et al. Cancer and Mediterranean dietary traditions. *Cancer Epidemiol Biomarkers Prev*. 2000;9(9):869–873.

Trichopoulou A. Mediterranean diet: the past and the present. *Nutr Metab Cardiovasc Dis*. 11(4 Suppl):1–4, 2001.

Trock BJ, Hilakivi-Clarke L, Clarke R. Meta-analysis of soy intake and breast cancer risk. *J Natl Cancer Inst*. 2006; 98:459.

Wang C, Harris WS, Chung M, et al. n-3 Fatty acids from fish or fish-oil supplements, but not alpha-linolenic acid, benefit cardiovascular disease outcomes in primary- and secondary-prevention studies: a systematic review. *Am J Clin Nutr*. 2006;84(1):5–17.

Wegener HC. Antibiotics in animal feed and their role in resistance development. *Curr Opin Microbiol*. 2003;(6):439–445.

Weil A. http://www.drweil.com/drw/u/ART02995/Dr-Weil-Anti-Inflammatory-Food-Pyramid.html Accessed January 14, 2009.

White DG, Zhao S, Sudler R, et al. The isolation of antibiotic-resistant Salmonella from retail ground meats. *NEJM*. 2001;345(16):1147–1154.

Whitmire SJ. Water, electrolytes and acid-base balance. Chap 6. In: Mahan LK, Escott-Stump S, eds. *Krause's Food, Nutrition and Diet Therapy*. 11th ed. Philadelphia: WB Saunders, 2004.

Wiecha JL, Peterson KE, Ludwig DS, et al. When children eat what they watch: impact of television viewing on dietary intake in youth. *Arch Pediatr Adolesc Med.* 2006;160(4):436–442.

Willcox BJ, Willcox DC, Suzuki M. *The Okinawa Program.* New York: Clarkson Potter/ Publishers, 2001.

Willett WC. The Mediterranean diet: science and practice. *Public Health Nutr.* 2006; 9(1A):105–110.

Wing RR, Phelan S. Long-term weight loss maintenance. *Am J Clin Nutr.* 2005;82(suppl):222S–225S.

Winter CK, Davis SF. Organic foods. *J Food Sci.* 2006;71(9):R117–R124.

Worthington V. Nutritional quality of organic versus conventional fruits, vegetables, and grains. *J Altern Comp Med.* 2001;7(2):161–173.

Zhang X, Shu XO, Li H, et al. Prospective cohort study of soy food consumption and risk of bone fracture among postmenopausal women. *Arch Intern Med.* 2005;165:1890.

3

Dietary Supplements

MARY HARDY

Case Study: A Tale of Two Patients

PATIENT ONE

Sally had heard about the benefits of calcium and vitamin D in newspapers and from her friends, but her intake was low because she restricted dairy products in her diet due to lactose intolerance. She rightly decided that she would need to take a supplement to get enough of these two nutrients. On her first trip to the store, she was so overwhelmed by the number and variety of available products that she gave up and did nothing. During our next office visit, she raises these questions: How do I decide what supplements are right for me? How can I tell if a product is of good quality? How do I know which one to pick?

PATIENT TWO

Lisa was a young woman with a hormone-sensitive breast cancer who had developed elevated liver enzymes since she was started on tamoxifen. After questioning her more closely, her oncologist discovered that Lisa was taking dietary supplements (DS) during active treatment—a startling revelation for the doctor! At the request of the oncologist, I saw Lisa in order to determine if her increased liver enzymes were due to her supplements, her tamoxifen, or a combination of both. At my request, the patient

30

brought all her medication (prescription and over-the-counter) and supplements to her first visit with me.

Lisa brought in four shopping bags of supplements, over 30 products that she faithfully took every day, firm in the belief that these would keep her cancer from returning. This was much more than what her oncologist had thought. Lisa had decided what to take after reading a wide variety of information from books and the internet as well as questioning friends, family, and clerks at her local health food store for their suggestions and ideas. She was so afraid of a recurrence that she grasped anything with any potentially positive information. Needless to say, she was spending hundreds of dollars a month on her supplements, as well as contributing to her elevated liver function tests.

These two, apparently very different patients, demonstrate common challenges that women using DS face. They were using supplements as part of a self-care program, initially without involvement from their health care provider. An open-minded provider, well informed about issues and opportunities inherent in DS use, would be able to help women design an appropriate strategy for DS use and integrate it into their overall medical plan.

Introduction

Dietary supplements (DS) are used by most Americans, with more than 70% according to some surveys (Timbo et al. 2009). In women, use is generally higher (84% in a cohort of elderly female HMO members) (Gordon and Schaffer 2005), and has been increasing over time. The National Health and Nutrition Examination Survey (NHANES) shows that use of combined DS has grown in the general population from 23% in 1999 to 40% in 2005 (Rock 2007). Increases in the 5 years following the passage of Dietary Supplement Health and Education Act (DSHEA), 1994–1999, were especially steep; for example, they rose in elderly women from 14% to more than 45% (Wold et al. 2005).

Women comprise the majority of DS users and they generally direct use for the rest of their family. To adequately counsel women using DS, providers must understand how and why women decide to use DS as well as how DS are regulated in the United States and the implications for quality, safety, and efficacy. (For information regarding the use of DS for specific conditions, please refer to the appropriate chapter in this text.)

Utilization of Dietary Supplements by Women

Women use a variety of DS including products specifically related to women's health, such as black cohosh, or evening primrose oil, as well as others for less gender-specific uses such as glucosamine and St. John's wort (Wold et al. 2005). Multiple vitamin formulations (MV) and/or multiple vitamin/mineral (MVM) are by far the most commonly used DS (Rock 2007) followed by vitamins E and C, calcium alone, zinc with folic acid, vitamin B12, and vitamins D and A (Kaufman et al. 2002). These patterns of use are relatively stable year to year. Herbal medicine use is less frequent (17%–30% in most surveys) (Gardiner, Graham et al. 2007), and more variable over time. Finally, some popular DS such as fish oil and glucosamine do not fit into any of these categories.

> When evaluating a multivitamin, it is helpful to first look at the vitamin A to assure there is no preformed vitamin A—the label would say retinol or retinyl palmitate. Mixed carotenoids of 10,000 to 15,000 IU daily is best and beta carotene alone is the second best. For postmenopausal women, barring special indications, there should be no iron. Next look at the Vitamin E, there should be about 400 IU of natural mixed tocopherols. Other general recommendations include: vitamin C, 200 mg a day, no more than selenium 200 µg, folic acid 400 µg, and at least vitamin D3 1,000 IU.

Consumers of DS frequently take multiple products and use them for extended periods of time. For example, an elderly cohort reported taking an average of three nonvitamin, nonmineral (NVNM) DS for more than 2 years (Wold et al. 2005). While vitamin and mineral preparations were the most commonly used supplement (84%) by the elderly, almost 60% also used a DS that was not MV or calcium. In addition, 25% reported using herbal medications (Gordon and Schaffer 2005). Use increased over time when measured longitudinally in an elderly cohort from 5% at beginning of the study to 30% after more than 15 years (Knudtson et al. 2007).

While the typical DS user is a well-educated, middle-aged white woman with a high socioeconomic status, DS use is also high in multiple ethnic groups and within lower socioeconomic groups, as supported by data from the Multiethnic Cohort Study that evaluated the use among African-Americans, Latinos, Native Americans, Native Hawaiians, and Caucasians. On average, half of the cohort used MV/ MVM supplements, with highest use reported by Caucasians (57%) and lowest by Native Hawaiians (37%) (Park et al. 2008). In a recent survey, 50%

of Hispanics and Asians, 41% of whites, and only 22% of African-Americans reported using herbs (Kuo et al. 2004). Despite financial constraints, indigent patients are high utilizers of DS. In a survey at a large urban clinic serving, the indigent 37% of the 311 responders reported using a wide variety of DS for a broad range of medical conditions (Clay et al. 2006).

Reasons for Using Dietary Supplements

Illness prevention and symptom reduction were the most common reasons that the Canadian women gave for their use of DS (Pakzad et al. 2007). Elders also reported using DS for arthritis and memory improvement as well as for general health and well-being (Wold et al. 2005). Some consumers take supplements to counteract the effects of negative health behaviors, such as eating junk food or smoking, or to mitigate the adverse events of sustained stress. Women might also substitute a "safe" DS for a prescription drug with a higher perceived risk (Nichter and Thompson 2006). DS may be used to substitute for expensive or unavailable medical care, particularly in patients with lower socioeconomic status (Gardiner, Graham et al. 2007).

In addition, users often have overarching philosophical positions that are consonant with DS use (Nichter and Thompson 2006). Health enhancement is one of the most commonly held beliefs by DS consumers. More than half of respondents to a national survey agreed that DS are good for health and well-being (Blendon et al. 2001).

Supplement users often cite the declining quality of the food supply and inability to get sufficient nutrition from diet as a reason to use DS. Interestingly, trend data for common garden crops has shown significant declines in the last half of the twentieth century for vitamins A, C, thiamine, riboflavin, and niacin as well as protein, calcium, phosphorus, and iron (Davis et al. 2004). Equally troubling is the fact that most people don't meet the goals of *Healthy People 2010*, of a minimum of two fruits and three vegetables servings daily. According to Center for Disease Control data from the 2005 Behavioral Risk Factor Surveillance System, only 32.6% ate fruit more than two times per day while less than 27% ate vegetables more than three times per day (MMWR 2005). Sadly, this level of intake has been fundamentally unchanged since 1994 despite public health messages encouraging increased intake (Blanck et al. 2008).

Dietary supplement use accounts for a significant portion of dietary intake of many important nutrients in the United States (Rock 2007; Archer et al. 2005). Diet plus supplements significantly increases dietary intake of iron and folic acid as well as vitamins A, C, E, and niacin (Archer et al. 2005). In NHANES III, 90% of women had inadequate intake of folate and vitamin E from food sources and over half of the smokers consumed inadequate amounts of vitamin C (Arab et al. 2003). When compared to Hispanic and Caucasian women, African-American women have the lowest dietary intake of calcium, vitamin D, folic acid, and vitamin B6 (Arab et al. 2003). Inadequate intake may be especially problematic for at-risk groups including the elderly (Sebastian et al. 2007), adolescents (Stang et al. 2000), pregnant women (Haugen et al. 2008), and women who are dieting.

Ironically, DS users tend to consume more nutrients from food than nonusers (Rock 2007; Sebastian et al. 2007; Stang et al. 2000). For example, the diets of adolescent DS users were higher in most key nutrients than nonusers (Dwyer et al. 2001). In the elderly, belief in the importance of following a healthy diet was a consistent predictor of supplement use (Sebastian et al. 2007). Elderly users in a longitudinal study also had healthier habits and fewer comorbid conditions (Knudtson et al. 2007).

Dietary Supplement Use in Conditions of Special Interest to Women

PREGNANCY

Nutrient demands of pregnancy are high and it has been estimated that without supplementation up to 75% of pregnant women would be deficient in at least one vitamin (Kontic-Vucinic et al. 2006). In some surveys, the use of prenatal vitamins is as high as 89.2% (Refuerzo et al. 2005). However, there has been a decline in the percentage of women of childbearing age taking DS containing at least 400 mcg of folic acid from 40% in 2004 to 33% in 2005 (MMWR 2005). Young women of childbearing age (18–24) have a low awareness of the importance of folic acid consumption (61%) as well as the lowest reported use (30%) (MMWR 2008). Even women actively planning pregnancy were not taking adequate amounts of folic acid either in diet or through DS (Hilton 2007).

In pregnant women, use of DS, besides prenatal vitamins, is low at about 13%, and 75% informed their primary care provider of their use. Relief from nausea and vomiting was cited as the most common reason for use, and ginger was one of the most commonly used DS (Tsui et al. 2001; Buckner et al. 2005). There is a growing body of evidence suggesting the importance of calcium, vitamin D, and omega-3 fatty acids, particularly docosahexaenoic acid, during pregnancy, yet the intake for all three may be low in many pregnant women. For more detailed information regarding specific supplement usage in pregnancy, refer to Chapter 14.

MENOPAUSE

Reports regarding the risk benefit ratio of hormone replacement therapy (HRT) have raised concerns among women and health care providers. It has also generated interest in the effectiveness and safety of DS for managing menopausal symptoms. A survey of more than 400 postmenopausal women reported that 65% were current users of DS and 19% were former users (Albertazzi et al. 2002). Evening primrose oil and multiple vitamins were cited as most commonly used supplements in a survey of 147 DS women attending a menopause clinic; most use of DS occurred without consulting providers (Gokhale et al. 2003). Herbal medicine users reported more menopausal symptoms than nonusers, and almost 70% of them felt that their herbal medicines were helpful (Dailey et al. 2003). Herbs most commonly used for relief of menopausal symptoms include black cohosh (*Actaea racemosa*), soy (*Glycine max*), red clover (*Trifolium pratense*), dong quai (*Angelica sinensis*), and chaste tree (*Vitex agnus-castus*).

OSTEOPOROSIS

Women are at higher risk and account for 75% of the 10 million cases of osteoporosis in the United States. Dietary intake of calcium and vitamin D is insufficient for most Americans. Fifty nine percent of women report eating less than two servings of dairy per day (Dawson-Hughes et al. 2002), and only 40% of the participants in the NHANES survey met the minimum adequate intake levels for calcium. In addition, only 48% of the respondents reported using a calcium supplement (Ma et al. 2007). Even when the diagnosis of osteoporosis is made, use of calcium and vitamin D remains low. In a survey of elderly nursing home patients with osteoporosis, only 66% were prescribed calcium and 58% vitamin D (Kamel 2004). In the United States, the adequate intake levels for women are 1300 mg/day from age 9 to18, 1000 mg/day from age 19 to 50, and 1200 mg/day from age 50 onward. Vitamin D supplements are an inexpensive and reliable way to ensure an optimum concentration. For most adult women, at least 1000 IU of vitamin D3 per day is recommended, though the adequate intake levels are only 200 IU/day for women aged 19–50, 400 IU/day for women aged 51–70, and 600 IU/day for those over 70 years of age.

CANCER

Dietary supplements are very often used by women with breast and gynecological cancers. Indole-3-carbinol, a compound found in cruciferous vegetables and its biologically active congener diindolylmethane (DIM) as well as vitamin D3 are commonly used DS by women hoping to reduce the risk of recurrence of estrogen-driven cancers (Gissel et al. 2008; Mulvey et al. 2007; Hardy 2008). Use of complementary therapies may be as high as 90% during cancer treatment, with DS representing a major proportion of all use (Yates et al. 2005; Molassiotis et al. 2006). Many oncologists are concerned about DS usage, especially antioxidants, while undergoing chemotherapy or radiation. A recent review concluded that their use should be discouraged because of the possibility of tumor protection and reduced survival (Lawanda 2008). The majority (53%) of women being tested for genetic risk of developing breast cancer reported using DS to decrease their risk (DiGianni et al. 2003). Physicians are usually unaware of their patients' use of DS and there are currently no evidence-based guidelines to assist them when counseling high risk women or breast cancer survivors (Velicer and Ulrich 2008).

Information Resources, Disclosure, and Decision Making Regarding Dietary Supplement Use

Women often do not disclose their use of DS to their health care providers. Reasons cited for nondisclosure include expectation of a negative response (Tasaki et al. 2002) and the perception that providers do not have the requisite knowledge about DS (Blendon et al. 2001). Assessment of a cohort of health care practitioners taking an online herbal course supported these assertions rating providers knowledge of herbal DS as only moderate and noting that their communication skills in this area were poor (Kemper et al. 2006).

Clerks in health food store frequently dispense advice regarding the use of DSs, even in customers with significant medical conditions. Eighty-nine percent of health food store clerks gave advice to researchers posing as an 8-week pregnant women with nausea (Buckner et al. 2005). Although ginger, a safe and effective remedy for this indication, was recommended most frequently, less than 4% of the time did clerk recommendations agree with the medical literature either in dose or product type. Fifteen percent of the time, products were recommended which are contraindicated in pregnancy. Likewise, recommendations were made for the treatment of depression (Glisson et al. 2003) and breast cancer in every instance tested (Mills et al. 2003).

Women frequently turn to their friends and family to advise them regarding DS use (Nichter and Thompson 2006). Many elders cite mail order information as the most common source of DS information (Wold et al. 2007). The internet represents a major source of information for consumers about health in general and DS in particular (Nichter and Thompson 2006). Patients and physicians have difficulty distinguishing unbiased from biased web sites (Bauer et al. 2003). The majority of web sites analyzed in a recent survey (76%) were retail sites selling product and 81% of these made one or more health claim in violation of current regulations.

While scientific evidence is very important to health care providers, it carries less weight with consumers. A number of large clinical trials of multiple vitamin/antioxidant combinations have been negative with respect to mortality reduction in healthy populations (Bjelakovic et al. 2008) and the US Preventative Services Task Force reports no benefit in reduction of cardiovascular risk or mortality from any single vitamin or combination (Morris and Carson 2003). Thus, physicians often use DS as placebos for their patients (Tilburt et al. 2008). Consumers, in contrast, are generally skeptical of scientific evidence, especially with regard to lack of efficacy (Nichter and Thompson 2006). Belief in efficacy of DS is so strong that almost three quarters of current users reported that they would continue to use their herbs even if scientific studies were negative (Kuo et al. 2004).

Dietary Supplement Regulation

The regulation of DS in the United States is unique within the global regulatory community and many of the issues associated with DS sales in the United States are the result of the provision of this regulatory structure. DS manufacture and sales are regulated by the Dietary Supplement Health and Education Act (DSHEA) of 1994 which was drafted by Congress in order to secure consumer access to high quality DS. A recent survey revealed that physician knowledge of DS regulation was limited and most did not know where to report adverse events (Ashar et al. 2007). Consumers also demonstrated poor knowledge when questioned about information on the DS label (Miller 2004).

Three provisions of DSHEA engender the most concern and confusion. First, only structure function claims, for example those claims that support the normal structure or function of the body, are allowed (Wollschlaeger 2003). DS are expressly forbidden to use "drug" claims, for example those that intend to diagnose, treat, cure, or prevent any disease. This may lead to vague terms such as "supports a healthy immune system" as opposed to "treats the common cold." This regulatory requirement creates a troublesome paradox between what can be claimed versus how products are researched by scientists and perceived by the public. Research generally does not assess structure function claims and patients are adept at "decoding" structure function claims into their disease-based counterparts (Knudtson et al. 2007). Second, all DS ingredients sold on the market before the passage of DSHEA (October 1994) are presumed to be safe and no premarket approval is required. The FDA has the right to remove any unsafe DS from the market, but the burden of proof is on the agency (Wollschlaeger 2003). Third, while regulations regarding good manufacturing processes have been required since the passage of DSHEA, they are only being implemented now. These rules are designed to assure the identity, purity, quality, strength and composition of DS (Crowley and FitzGerald 2006). It is expected that they will address some of the product quality problems identified in the DS industry in the past.

Quick tips for reading supplement labels

- On vitamins and minerals, look carefully at the percent daily value (%DV) and the serving size. To get 100% of the daily value you might need to take one or three tablets per day. As most people prefer to take fewer pills, this can affect adherence.
- Also, note that a single nutrient may be present in a number of different supplements. Include all amounts in all supplements when assessing for adequate or excessive amounts.
- Remember the %DV is a simplification of the recommended daily allowance and does not take into account age or gender. You must help your patient understand how much she needs to take.
- Some products contain nutrients for which a daily value has not been established (i.e., boron, herbs, etc.). Confirm that the amounts included make sense and are not excessive.
- For most vitamins and minerals, encourage women not to exceed 70%–100% of the daily value in their dietary supplements to avoid excessive intake.
- Encourage women to discard vitamins/minerals after the expiration date has passed.
- DS products should all contain the manufacturer/distributor name and contact information.
- Products that contain quality seals on their labels from the United States Pharmacopeia (USP), National Sanitation Foundation (NSF), or Consumer Labs (CL), indicate that the manufacturer has had their product independently tested for quality and purity by a third party.

Safety Concerns with Dietary Supplements

Consumers generally perceive DS as safe (Nichter and Thompson 2006). Over half of women in a recent survey agreed in the theory that DS might have adverse effects, but 66% of them would not associate observed adverse effects with a DS (Albertazzi et al. 2002). Incidence of reported adverse events was higher when DS and prescription medication were used concurrently.

Clinician's concerns revolve largely around issues of adverse events arising from allergy, contamination/adulteration of the DS, or interaction with conventional medications. Allergy (immediate hypersensitivity) has been reported with herbal medicines but is not commonly seen. Adulteration has been reported particularly in ethnic or imported products (Saper et al. 2008). Chinese patent medicines have been found to contain pharmaceutical drugs or heavy metals (Ko 2006). Ayurvedic products have also been shown to be high in a variety of heavy metals (Saper et al. 2008). Misidentification or substitution of a less toxic, for a more toxic herb, has occurred. On rare occasions this has led to serious adverse outcomes as in the case of using *Aristolochia* species in place of the safer *Stephania* herb (Debelle et al. 2008), which led to numerous cases of acute renal failure and late onset of genitourinary cancers.

Interaction of DS with conventional medicine is an oft cited concern for providers. Rates of concurrent use of prescription medication with herbal/DS range from 16% to 21% (Kaufman et al. 2002; Gardiner et al. 2006). In a large national survey, 72% of herb users were also using prescription drugs and 84% were using over the counter preparations (Gardiner, Graham et al. 2007). Concurrent DS and medication use is of particular concern in the elderly where, according to one survey, 52% of this population was taking DS and prescriptions concurrently (Qato et al. 2008). In fact, some patients may preferentially combine herbal and prescribed medication. Respondents in a survey of multi-ethnic herbal medicine users reported that 40% believed that combining herbs with drugs had a synergistic effect Kuo et al. 2004.

Authoritative information on dietary supplement-drug interaction is scarce, but concern exists for drugs that are critical or have a narrow therapeutic index (Yetley 2007). Anticoagulant medications, especially warfarin, were the drugs are most often identified as having highest risk for DS/drug interactions (Qato et al. 2008). Despite the identification of theoretical interactions, relatively few events are documented. During a 5 year retrospective chart review of elderly DS/drug users in which 142 potential interactions were noted, no specific events were identified (Wold et al. 2005). In a prospective survey of patients attending an urban outpatient clinic in California, 15% out of 804 patients were found to be concurrently using herbs (Bush et al. 2007). Although 85 potential interactions were noted, only 12 possible interactions were identified. These were all rated as mild and largely involved the use of a traditional medicine/food, nopal (prickly pear cactus) contributing to hypoglycemia in diabetic patients.

Product Quality and Variety

One of the most overwhelming aspects of the DS industry for patients and providers is the variety and number of available DS. In a survey of over 26,000 multiethnic subjects in Los Angeles and Hawaii, more than 1200 different products were used (Murphy et al. 2007). These products represented wide variations in composition and concentration of ingredients. Variability may be highest for herbal products both because of the greater variability inherent in botanical materials as well as significant differences in formulation.

In a study conducted on single ingredient herb supplements obtained from both retail and internet outlets, variation between different batches at a single company was relatively low (Krochmal et al. 2004). However, much larger differences were seen between various products of the same herb from different companies. Instruction for use (dosage) also varied significantly between companies for the same herb as well.

Conclusions and Recommendations

Dietary supplement use is highly prevalent in women throughout their life spans and across a broad array of conditions and diseases. Women often don't disclose their use of DS to the health care team and therefore, it is recommended that inquiries about DS use must be made at all patient encounters. Adequate intake of folic acid should be investigated for women of child bearing age and for adequate calcium and vitamin D intake for women at risk of osteoporosis.

Questioning should be nonjudgmental in order to encourage full disclosure. Assessing the reasons for supplement usage and asking about information sources used by the patient, allows for much clearer insight into use. Respect for a woman's worldview and support for her efforts towards health enhancement is recommended.

Due to the high degree of variability in products, it is critical to look at the actual labels in order to most accurately determine intake. One must document all products used in the medical chart and be alert for potential adverse effects and herb-drug interactions, as well as therapeutic benefit.

Avoid blanket, negative declarations about DS. This does not discourage use, but rather damages provider credibility. However, when specific concerns

The following questions can help clinicians assess a woman's beliefs, cultural practices, and use of DS:

- Many women use vitamins or herbal remedies to improve their health or treat medical problems. What is your experience? If the response confirms use then what are your goals and how do you think they are working?
- How did you learn about using vitamins or herbal remedies?
- Would you be willing to bring your vitamins or herbal remedies with you to your next appointment so that we could look at them together?

about DS use arise, especially if safety is the issue, sharing this information with your patient can change behavior. Engaging women in this manner will optimize her health and well-being.

Helpful Resources for DS evidence, safety, and dose

- The National Center for Complementary and Alternative Medicine, NCCAM (www.nccam.nih.gov)

Look for the Alerts and Advisories, treatment information, resources, and links to other organizations (FDA, AHRQ, ODS etc.). (Free)

- Office of Dietary Supplements, ODS (ods.od.nih.gov/index.aspx)

Very helpful site; under Health Information you will find excellent DS fact sheets. (Free)

- Health Canada (http://www.hc-sc.gc.ca)

The Canadian government regulates natural health products in Canada licensing products with proof of safety and efficacy. This is a very helpful site—it lists products licensed in Canada and has helpful monographs.

Other Web Sites

- American Botanical Council (www.herbalgram.org)

The American Botanical Council is a nonprofit, international member-based organization providing education using science-based and traditional information on herbal medicine. The web site offers an excellent online bookstore and an Herb Clip service summarizing current research articles and an educational resource section offering continuing education credits for health care professionals.

- Natural Medicines Comprehensive Database (www.naturaldatabase. com)

Herbal Monographs include extensive information about common uses, evidence of efficacy and safety mechanisms, interactions, and dosage. Also continuing medical education (CME), listserv, and interactions information available. (Subscription available)

- Natural Standard (www.naturalstandard.com)

This is an independent collaboration of international clinicians and researchers who created a database which can be searched by complementary and alternative medicine subject or by medical condition. CME available. Quality of evidence is graded for each supplement. (Subscription available)

- Consumer Labs (www.consumerlabs.com)

Evaluates commercially available DS for composition, purity, bioavailability, and consistency of products. Part of the web site is free. More in-depth reports of product quality are available by subscription.

REFERENCES

Albertazzi P, Steel SA, Clifford E, Bottazzi M. Attitudes towards and use of dietary supplementation in a sample of postmenopausal women. *Climacteric.* 2002;5(4):374–382.

Arab L, Carriquiry A, Steck-Scott S, Gaudet MM. Ethnic differences in the nutrient intake adequacy of premenopausal US women: results from the Third National Health Examination Survey. *J Am Diet Assoc.* 2003;103(8):1008–1014.

Archer SL, Stamler J, Moag-Stahlberg A, et al. Association of dietary supplement use with specific micronutrient intakes among middle-aged American men and women: the INTERMAP Study. *J Am Diet Assoc.* 2005;105(7):1106–1114.

Ashar BH, Rice TN, Sisson SD. Physicians' understanding of the regulation of dietary supplements. *Arch Intern Med.* 2007;167(9):966–969.

Bardia A, Nisly NL, Zimmerman MB, Gryzlak BM, Wallace RB. Use of herbs among adults based on evidence-based indications: findings from the National Health Interview Survey. *Mayo Clin Proc.* 2007;82(5):561–566.

Bauer B, Lee M, Wahner-Roedler D, Brown S, Pankratz S, Elkin P. A controlled trial of physicians' and patients' abilities to distinguish authoritative from misleading complementary and alternative medicine Web sites. *J Cancer Integr Med.* 2003;1(1):48–54.

Bjelakovic G, Nikolova D, Gluud LL, Simonetti RG, Gluud C. Antioxidant supplements for prevention of mortality in healthy participants and patients with various diseases. *Cochrane Database Syst Rev.* 2008(2):CD007176.

Blanck H, Gillespie C, Kimmons J, Seymour J, Serdula M. Trends in fruit and vegetable consumption among U.S. men and women, 1994–2005. *Prev Chronic Dis.* 2008;5:1–9.

Blendon RJ, DesRoches CM, Benson JM, Brodie M, Altman DE. Americans' views on the use and regulation of dietary supplements. *Arch Intern Med.* 26, 2001;161(6):805–810.

Buckner KD, Chavez ML, Raney EC, Stoehr JD. Health food stores' recommendations for nausea and migraines during pregnancy. *Ann Pharmacother.* 2005;39(2):274–279.

Bush TM, Rayburn KS, Holloway SW, et al. Adverse interactions between herbal and dietary substances and prescription medications: a clinical survey. *Altern Ther Health Med.* 2007;13(2):30–35.

Clay PG, Glaros AG, Clauson KA. Perceived efficacy, indications, and information sources for medically indigent patients and their healthcare providers regarding dietary supplements. *Ann Pharmacother.* 2006;40(3):427–432.

Crowley R, FitzGerald LH. The impact of cGMP compliance on consumer confidence in dietary supplement products. *Toxicology.* 2006;221(1):9–16.

Dailey R, Neale A, Northrup J, West P, Schwartz K. Herbal product use and menopause symptom relief in primary care patients: a MetroNet study. *J Womens Health (Larchmt).* 2003;12(7):633–641.

Davis DR, Epp MD, Riordan HD. Changes in USDA food composition data for 43 garden crops, 1950 to 1999. *J Am Coll Nutr.* 2004 Dec;23(6):669–682.

Dawson-Hughes B, Harris SS, Dallal GE, Lancaster DR, Zhou Q. Calcium supplement and bone medication use in a US Medicare health maintenance organization. *Osteoporosis Int.* 2002;13(8):657–662.

Debelle F, Vanherweghem JL, Nortier JL. Aristolochic acid nephropathy: a worldwide problem. *Kidney Int.* 2008;74(2):158–169.

DiGianni LM, Kim HT, Emmons K, Gelman R, Kalkbrenner KJ, Garber JE. Complementary medicine use among women enrolled in a genetic testing program. *Cancer Epidemiol Biomarkers Prev.* 2003;12(4):321–326.

Dwyer JT, Garcea AO, Evans M, et al. Do adolescent vitamin-mineral supplement users have better nutrient intakes than nonusers? Observations from the CATCH tracking study. *J Am Diet Assoc.* 2001;101(11):1340–1346.

Gardiner P, Graham R, Legedza AT, Ahn AC, Eisenberg DM, Phillips RS. Factors associated with herbal therapy use by adults in the United States. *Altern Ther Health Med.* 2007;13(2):22–29.

Gardiner P, Graham RE, Legedza AT, Eisenberg DM, Phillips RS. Factors associated with dietary supplement use among prescription medication users. *Arch Intern Med.* Oct 9, 2006;166(18):1968–1974.

Gardiner P, Kemper KJ, Legedza A, Phillips RS. Factors associated with herb and dietary supplement use by young adults in the United States. *BMC Complement Altern Med.* 2007;7:39.

Gissel T, Rejnmark L, Mosekilde L, Vestergaard P. Intake of vitamin D and risk of breast cancer—a meta-analysis. *J Steroid Biochem Mol Biol.* 2008;111:195–199.

Glisson JK, Rogers HE, Abourashed EA, Ogletree R, Hufford CD, Khan I. Clinic at the health food store? Employee recommendations and product analysis. *Pharmacotherapy.* 2003;23(1):64–72.

Gokhale L, Sturdee D, Parsons A. The use of food supplements among women attending menopause clinics in the West Midlands. *J Br Menopause Soc.* 2003;9(1):32–35.

Gordon NP, Schaffer DM. Use of dietary supplements by female seniors in a large Northern California health plan. *BMC Geriatr.* 2005;5:4.

Hardy ML. Dietary supplement use in cancer care: help or harm. *Hematol Oncol Clin North Am.* 2008;22(4):581–617, vii.

Haugen M, Brantsaeter AL, Alexander J, Meltzer HM. Dietary supplements contribute substantially to the total nutrient intake in pregnant Norwegian women. *Ann Nutr Metab.* 2008;52(4):272–280.

Hilton JJ. A comparison of folic acid awareness and intake among young women aged 18–24 years. *J Am Acad Nurse Pract.* 2007;19(10):516–522.

Kamel H. Underutilization of calcium and vitamin D supplements in an academic long-term care facility. *J Am Med Dir Assoc.* 2004;5(2):98–100.

Kaufman DW, Kelly JP, Rosenberg L, Anderson TE, Mitchell AA. Recent patterns of medication use in the ambulatory adult population of the United States: the Slone survey. *JAMA.* 2002;287(3):337–344.

Kemper KJ, Gardiner P, Gobble J, Woods C. Expertise about herbs and dietary supplements among diverse health professionals. *BMC Complement Altern Med.* 2006;6:15.

Knudtson MD, Klein R, Lee KE, et al. A longitudinal study of nonvitamin, nonmineral supplement use: prevalence, associations, and survival in an aging population. *Ann Epidemiol.* 2007;17(12):933–939.

K. R. Safety of ethnic imported herbal and dietary supplements. *Clin Toxicol (Phila).* 2006;44(5):611–616.

Kontic-Vucinic O, Sulovic N, Radunovic N. Micronutrients in women's reproductive health: I. Vitamins. *Int J Fertil Womens Med.* 2006;51(3):106–115.

Krochmal R, Hardy M, Bowerman S, et al. Phytochemical assays of commercial botanical dietary supplements. *Evid Based Complement Alternat Med.* 2004;1(3):305–313.

Kuo GM, Hawley ST, Weiss LT, Balkrishnan R, Volk RJ. Factors associated with herbal use among urban multiethnic primary care patients: a cross-sectional survey. *BMC Complement Altern Med.* 2004;4:18.

Lawanda BD, Kelly KM, Ladas EJ, Sagar SM, Vickers A, Blumberg JB. Should supplemental antioxidant administration be avoided during chemotherapy and radiation therapy? *J Natl Cancer Inst.* 2008;100:773–783.

Ma J, Johns RA, Stafford RS. Americans are not meeting current calcium recommendations. *Am J Clin Nutr.* 2007;85(5):1361–1366.

Miller MF, Bellizzi KM, Sufian M, Ambs AH, Goldstein MS, Ballard-Barbash R. Dietary supplement use in individuals living with cancer and other chronic conditions: a population-based study. *J Am Diet Assoc.* 2008;108(3):483–494.

Mills E, Ernst E, Singh R, Ross C, Wilson K. Health food store recommendations: implications for breast cancer patients. *Breast Cancer Res.* 2003;5(6):R170–R174.

Miller CK, Russell T. Knowledge of dietary supplement label information among female supplement users. *Patient Educ Couns.* 2004 Mar;52(3):291–296.

MMWR. Use of dietary supplements containing folic acid among women of childbearing age—United States. *Morb Mortal Wkly Rep.* 2005 Sep30;54(38):955–958.

MMWR. Fruit and vegetable consumption among adults—United States, 2005. *Morb Mortal Wkly Rep.* 2007 Mar 16;56(10):213–217.

MMWR. Use of supplements containing folic acid among of childbearing age. *Morb Mortal Wkly Rep.* 2008 Jan 11;57(1):5–8.

Molassiotis A, Ozden G, Platin N. Complementary and alternative medicine use in patients with head and neck cancers in Europe. *Eur J Cancer Care (Engl).* 2006;15(1):19–24.

Monmaney T. Remedy's U.S. sales zoom, but quality control lags. *Los Angeles Time.* August 31, 1998.

Morris CA, Avorn J. Internet marketing of herbal products. *JAMA.* 2003;290(11):1505–1509.

Morris CD, Carson S. Routine vitamin supplementation to prevent cardiovascular disease: a summary of the evidence for the U.S. Preventive Services Task Force. *Ann Intern Med.* 2003;139(1):56–70.

Mulvey L, Chandrasekaran A, Liu K, et al. Interplay of genes regulated by estrogen and diindolylmethane in breast cancer cell lines. *Mol Med.* 2007 ;13(1–2):69–78.

Murphy SP, White KK, Park SY, Sharma S. Multivitamin-multimineral supplements' effect on total nutrient intake. *Am J Clin Nutr.* 2007;85(1):280S–284S.

Nichter M, Thompson JJ. For my wellness, not just my illness: North Americans' use of dietary supplements. *Cult Med Psychiatry.* 2006;30(2):175–222.

Pakzad K, Boucher BA, Kreiger N, Cotterchio M. The use of herbal and other non-vitamin, non-mineral supplements among pre- and post-menopausal women in Ontario. *Can J Public Health.* 2007;98(5):383–388.

Park SY, Murphy SP, Martin CL, Kolonel LN. Nutrient intake from multivitamin/mineral supplements is similar among users from five ethnic groups: the Multiethnic Cohort Study. *J Am Diet Assoc.* 2008;108(3):529–533.

Qato DM, Alexander GC, Conti RM, Johnson M, Schumm P, Lindau ST. Use of prescription and over-the-counter medications and dietary supplements among older adults in the United States. *JAMA.* 2008;300(24):2867–2878.

Refuerzo JS, Blackwell SC, Sokol RJ, et al. Use of over-the-counter medications and herbal remedies in pregnancy. *Am J Perinatol.* 2005;22(6):321–324.

Rock CL. Multivitamin-multimineral supplements: who uses them? *Am J Clin Nutr.* Jan 2007;85(1):277S–279S.

Saper R, Phillips R, Sehgal A, et al. Lead, mercury, and arsenic in US- and Indian-manufactured Ayurvedic medicines sold via the Internet. *JAMA.* 2008;300(8):915–923.

Satia-Abouta J, Kristal AR, Patterson RE, Littman AJ, Stratton KL, White E. Dietary supplement use and medical conditions: the VITAL study. *Am J Prev Med.* 2003;24(1):43–51.

Sebastian RS, Cleveland LE, Goldman JD, Moshfegh AJ. Older adults who use vitamin/mineral supplements differ from nonusers in nutrient intake adequacy and dietary attitudes. *J Am Diet Assoc.* 2007;107(8):1322–1332.

Stang J, Story MT, Harnack L, Neumark-Sztainer D. Relationships between vitamin and mineral supplement use, dietary intake, and dietary adequacy among adolescents. *J Am Diet Assoc.* 2000;100(8):905–910.

Tasaki K, Maskarinec G, Shumay D, Tatsumura Y, Kakai H. Communication between physicians and cancer patients about complementary and alternative medicine: exploring patients' perspective. *Psychooncology.* 2002;11(3):212–220.

Tilburt JC, Emanuel EJ, Kaptchuk TJ, Curlin FA, Miller FG. Prescribing "placebo treatments": results of national survey of US internists and rheumatologists. *BMJ.* 2008;337:a1938.

Timbo BB, Ross MP, McCarthy PV, Lin CT. Dietary supplements in a national survey: prevalence of use and reports of adverse events. *J Am Diet Assoc.* 2006;106(12):1966–1974.

Tsui B, Dennehy CE, Tsourounis C. A survey of dietary supplement use during pregnancy at an academic medical center. *Am J Obstet Gynecol.* 2001;185(2):433–437.

Use of dietary supplements containing folic acid among women of childbearing age—United States, 2005. *MMWR.* 2005;54(38):955–958.

Use of supplements containing folic acid among women of childbearing age—United States, 2007. *MMWR.* 2008;57(1):5–8.

Velicer CM, Ulrich CM. Vitamin and mineral supplement use among US adults after cancer diagnosis: a systematic review. *J Clin Oncol.* 2008;26:665–673.

Wold RS, Lopez ST, Yau CL, et al. Increasing trends in elderly persons' use of nonvitamin, nonmineral dietary supplements and concurrent use of medications. *J Am Diet Assoc.* 2005;105(1):54–63.

Wold RS, Wayne SJ, Waters DL, Baumgartner RN. Behaviors underlying the use of non-vitamin nonmineral dietary supplements in a healthy elderly cohort. *J Nutr Health Aging.* 2007 Jan–Feb;11(1):3–7.

Wollschlaeger B. The dietary supplement and health education act and supplements: dietary and nutritional supplements need no more regulations. *Int J Toxicol.* 2003;22(5):387–390.

Yates J, Mustian K, Morrow G. Prevalence of complementary and alternative medicine use in cancer patients during treatment. *Support Care Cancer.* 2005;13(10):806–811.

Yetley EA. Multivitamin and multimineral dietary supplements: definitions, characterization, bioavailability, and drug interactions. *Am J Clin Nutr.* 2007;85(1):269S–276S.

4

Physical Activity

PATRICIA LEBENSOHN

Physical Activity and Women's Health

"Life is like riding a bicycle. To keep your balance you must keep moving."

—*Albert Einstein*

As the primary caregivers in most societies, women of all ages struggle to keep balance in their lives. When it comes to taking care of themselves, women have trouble prioritizing what is good for their health and what is needed from them to care for others in their families, communities, and workplaces. In my family medicine practice, for almost 20 years I have heard the same reasons from women about why it is hard for them to be physically active: no time, too tired, hard to get motivated, physical limitations, unsafe neighborhoods, and so on.

In my late twenties, I was at the same place as most of my patients—going through medical school and residency, and starting a family had prevented me from being physically active for years. Then, at age 27, I was diagnosed with thyroid cancer. This wake-up call motivated me toward a path of making physical activity a priority in my life. The primary motivation then was to be able to have a long and healthy life to be available to my family. Physical activity has given me not only the physical and mental sense of well-being I have today, but it has also allowed me to become a member of a community of physically active women and empowered me to have a positive outlook when facing the challenges of the complex world we live in.

This chapter reviews the general recommendations for physical activity and exercise for healthy women, providing specific guidelines for those with common medical conditions. It also addresses important issues to discuss with our patients as we encourage them to get motivated to start and maintain regular physical activity as part of their lifestyle.

The Burden of Physical Inactivity in Women

Throughout their lifecycle, women are less physically active than their male counterparts. In the United States, less than 50% of all women meet the physical activity goal based on the Healthy People 2010 recommendation of 30 minutes of moderate physical activity at least 5 days a week (CDC 2007).

Thirty-eight million women in the United States have cardiovascular disease, the leading cause of death for women. And even though cardiovascular death has decreased over the past 20 years, obesity and type 2 diabetes are on the rise in the U.S. female population (Centers for Disease Control and Prevention Web site: http://www.cdc.gov/nchs/hus.htm). Multiple studies support regular physical activity for both primary and secondary prevention of cardiovascular disease (Ellekjaer et al. 2000; Gregg et al. 2003; He et al. 2001; Hu et al. 2000; Kushi et al. 1997; Lee et al. 2001; Manson et al. 2002; Paganini-Hill and Barreto 2001; Rockhill et al. 2001; Weller and Corey 1998).

In addition to cardiovascular benefit, physical activity may prevent or ameliorate type 2 diabetes mellitus (Folsom et al. 2000; Hsia et al. 2005; Hu et al. 1999; Hu et al. 2003; Kriska et al. 2003; Weinstein et al. 2004), breast cancer (Breslow et al. 2001; McTiernan 2003; Rockhill et al. 1999; Sesso et al. 1998; Tehard et al. 2006; Thune et al. 1997), colon cancer (Martinez et al. 1997), and possibly lung, endometrial, ovarian, and other cancers (Brown et al. 2007) as well as osteoporosis (Borer 2005; Ondrak and Morgan 2007; Schwab and Klein 2008). Physically active women are expected to have fewer symptoms of depression and anxiety. Moderate physical activity also improves chronic pain syndromes such as osteoarthritis and fibromyalgia (Jones et al. 2005).

The following definitions will help health care professionals speak a common language as they develop patient-centered recommendations.

- *Physical activity*: Bodily movement produced by the contraction of skeletal muscle that substantially increases energy expenditure above the resting level (U.S. Department of Health and Human Services 1996).
- *Exercise*: A category of physical activity that is planned, structured, repetitive, and designed to improve one or more aspects of physical fitness (U.S. Department of Health and Human Services, 1996).

- *Physical fitness*: The ability to carry out daily tasks with vigor and alertness, without undue fatigue and with ample energy to enjoy leisure-time pursuits and to meet unforeseen emergencies. Performance-related components of fitness include agility, balance, coordination, power, and speed. Health-related components of physical fitness include body composition, cardiorespiratory function, flexibility, and muscular strength/endurance.

One framework used to counsel patients about exercise is to develop an exercise prescription advising the frequency, intensity, time, and type (acronym FITT) of physical activity. Age, level of fitness, medical conditions and physical limitations, ethnicity, culture, and social context also need to be addressed for the recommendation to be initiated and maintained over time (Speck and Harrell 2003).

Recommendations

The following recommendations are consistent with guidelines for prevention of cardiovascular disease in women (Centers for Disease Control and Prevention: http://www.cdc.gov/physicalactivity/everyone/guidelines/adults.html). These recommendations are the same for adult males and females:

- 150 minutes (2:30 hours) each week of moderate-intensity aerobic activity
  or
- 75 minutes (1:15 hours) each week of vigorous-intensity activity
  or
- 7–15 Metabolic equivalents (METs)/week

In addition to aerobic exercise, women should include muscle-strengthening activities of all major muscle groups—legs, hips, back, abdomen, chest, shoulders, and arms—two or more days a week (see Table 4.1). For women who need to maintain or lose weight, the recommendation is 60–90 minutes of moderate exercise for most days of the week. Recommendations for girls and adolescents are at least 60 minutes of physical activity for most days.

For pregnant women without contraindications, the recommendation is to continue similar levels of physical activity as prior to pregnancy. For inactive pregnant women, it is recommended to start slow and build up to 150 minutes a week of moderate aerobic physical activity. Walking and swimming are excellent choices during pregnancy. Yoga enhances strength and flexibility training

Table 4.1. Glossary of Exercise Terminology

Exercise intensity:
Generally expressed as a percentage of either HR (heart rate) or VO_2 (volume of oxygen uptake). Since VO_2 is not practical to measure in the practitioner's office, heart rate is generally used.

Heart rate reserve (HRR):
Maximal heart rate (HR_{max}) observed during a symptom-limited exercise stress test minus the resting heart rate (HR rest). A percentage of the HRR range is added to the HR at rest to determine a target heart rate (THR) range to be used during exercise.

Target heart rate (THR):
For most individuals 50%–85% HRR added to the HR at rest is generally recommended. For deconditioned individuals, 50% HRR may be more appropriate for beginning exercise. Physically active individuals may require higher intensities to achieve improvements in their conditioning.

Max heart rate (HR_{max}):
Can be calculated using the following formula:
   Sedentary women 226 – age
   Fit women 211– (age/2)

Metabolic equivalents (METs):
Useful units when recommending exercise. By definition, 1 MET is the amount of oxygen consumed at rest or about 3.5 mL/kg/min. Most people walking 2 mph require 2 METs, and those walking 3 mph require 3–4 METs. Published MET tables describe many activities in terms of the estimated MET requirements (CDC, Physical activity for everyone, 2008: http://www.cdc.gov/physicalactivity/downloads/PA_Intensity_table_2_1.pdf)

Moderate-intensity aerobic activity:
Raises the heartbeat and leaves the person feeling warm and slightly out of breath. It increases the body's metabolism to 3–6 times the resting level (3–6 METs). Brisk walking has an equivalent of 4.5 METs.

Vigorous-intensity aerobic activities:
Enables people to work up a sweat and become out of breath. These activities usually involve sports or exercise such as running or fast cycling. They raise the metabolism to at least 6 times resting level. Activities include rhythmic, repetitive physical exercise that uses large muscle groups at 70% or more of maximum heart rate for age.

Muscle strength or resistance training:
Any exercise that causes the muscles to contract against an external resistance with the expectation of increases in strength, tone, mass, and/or endurance. The external resistance can be provided by dumbbells, free weights, rubber exercise tubing, one's own body weight, bricks, bottles of water, or any other object that causes the muscles to contract. A typical recommendation is 8–15 repetitions of 10 major muscle groups.

(continued)

It is recommended that a woman start with a weight with which she can do 8 repetitions and continue at that weight until she is able to do 15 repetitions. She can then advance the weight and start again with 8 repetitions, increase to 15, and so forth. Yoga, Pilates, and tai chi all include strength-training activities.

Flexibility training:
Range of motion around a joint. Good flexibility can help prevent injuries throughout life. Warm-up and cool-down stretching as well as yoga and tai chi are examples.

to prevent back pain, and breathing exercises could help prepare for the birthing experience. Exercises to avoid while pregnant include activities that involve lying on the back or that put women at risk of falling or abdominal injury, such as horseback riding, soccer, or basketball. It is important to counsel pregnant women to avoid overheating and dehydration when exercising.

Cardiovascular Disease and Physical Activity

There is an inverse relationship between levels of physical activity and cardio-vascular disease (CVD) events in women. Reductions in CVD events in women with physical activity are in the range of 30%–50% despite the fact that changes in individual risk factors are modest; lipids are reduced 5%, blood pressure 3–5 mmHg, and hemoglobin A1c 1% (Hu et al. 2004; Stevens et al., 2002).

Mora et al. (2007) examined the extent to which traditional and novel risk factors explain the cardioprotective benefits of physical activity. Using prospectively collected data from the Women's Health Study, which followed 27,055 initially healthy women for 11 years, they found that even moderate levels of physical activity (at least 600 kcal/week or the equivalent of just over 2 h/week of brisk walking) were associated with 30%–40% relative risk reduction for CVD. A dose response was seen as physical activity increased in intensity and/or duration. Inflammatory and hemostatic biomarkers (high-sensitivity C-reactive protein, fibrinogen, and soluble intracellular adhesion molecule-1) provided the largest contribution to lowered risk (33%), followed by blood pressure (27%), lipids (19%), body mass index (10%), and glucose abnormalities (9%), with minimal contribution from changes in renal function or homocysteine.

Kelley et al. (2005) conducted a meta-analysis of the effects of aerobic exercise on lipids in women. They concluded that aerobic exercise was correlated with reductions of 2% for total cholesterol, 3% for LDL-cholesterol, and 5% for triglycerides; in addition, they observed an increase of 3% in HDL cholesterol.

Another review confirms the multiple benefits of physical activity for women (Brown et al. 2007). Studies revealed 28%–58% risk reduction of cardiovascular

Table 4.2. Examples of Moderate and Vigorous Exercise for Women

Moderate Exercise	Vigorous Exercise
Walking at 3–4.5 mph	Race walking 5 mph
Hiking	Jogging/running
Bicycling less than 9 mph	Bicycling more than 10 mph
Aerobic dancing	High-impact aerobics
Water aerobics	Martial arts
Yoga	Circuit training
Golfing, carrying clubs	Most competitive sports
Tennis doubles	Tennis singles
Recreational swimming	Swimming laps

disease and 14%–46% risk reduction of diabetes. The protective benefits were seen with as little as 60 minutes of moderate-intensity physical activity per week or 4 MET hours (see Table 4.2).

Fisher et al. (2008) evaluated possible pathways through which social support may reduce cardiovascular disease risk in a diverse population of women. Higher social support was positively associated with minutes of physical activity per week, number of days of physical activity per week, and with increased HDL cholesterol. The authors suggest that specific components of social support, including emotional and instrumental components, may be beneficial in improving risk factors for CVD, such as HDL-C.

Physical Activity and Cancer

Epidemiologic studies have shown that breast cancer risk is reduced 30%–40% in highly physically active women compared with inactive women. In a population-based breast cancer case–control study in Poland conducted in 2000–2003, Peplonska et al. (2008) analyzed data on physical activity patterns in 2176 breast cancer cases and 2326 controls. They concluded that moderate to vigorous physical activity levels (6–15 METs/week) during adulthood may reduce breast cancer risk. This applies to activities, including recreational activities, outdoor chores, and occupational tasks (see Table 4.3). The protective effect of moderate/heavy activities occurred independently of menopausal status, body mass index (BMI), family history of breast cancer, and tumor features. Their study suggested that increases in activity levels when a woman is in her fifties might be particularly relevant.

Table 4.3. Examples of Recreational or Occupational Physical Activity that have Similar Energy Expenditure as Moderate and Vigorous Exercise

Moderate recreational or occupational PA	Vigorous recreational or occupational PA
Gardening: raking, bagging leaves	Gardening: digging ditches, swinging an ax
Housework: scrubbing floors, sweeping, washing windows	Housework: pushing heavy furniture, carrying objects up the stairs
Putting groceries away: items less than 50 lb	Grocery shopping while carrying children or carrying 25 lb bags up the stairs
Actively playing with children	Vigorously playing with children, running
Animal care: feeding, grooming farm animals	Animal care, carrying heavy equipment
Waiting tables	Aerobic instructor
Patient care (bathing, dressing, moving patients)	Loading/unloading a truck, firefighting

Source: Adapted from Centers for Disease Control and Prevention: http://www.cdc.gov/physicalactivity/downloads/PA_Intensity_table_2_1.pdf.

Lee (2003) reviewed data from epidemiological studies and concluded that physically active men and women have about a 30%–40% reduction in the risk of developing colon cancer, compared with inactive persons. Although he reports the data are sparse, a minimum of 30 to 60 min/day of vigorous to moderate physical activity is needed to decrease the risk of colon cancer for men and women. There is a dose–response relation, with risk declining further at higher levels of physical activity.

Physical Activity and Depression

Women report both positive and negative affective responses to exercise, which could depend on their own fitness level or health status and the intensity of the physical activity (Anish 2005) (see Table 4.4).

Several studies demonstrate the negative correlation between physical activity and depressive symptoms. Craft et al. (2008) asked 61 women to complete demographic, depression, and exercise-related questionnaires. Women with depressive symptoms reported minimal exercise involvement, numerous barriers to exercise, and low exercise self-efficacy and social support for exercise. The same authors in 2007 reported on a study of two different exercise programs for women with depressive symptoms (Craft et al. 2007). Women were randomly assigned to either a clinic-based or home-based exercise intervention. Both programs were associated with reductions in depressive symptoms and

Table 4.4. Biological and Psychological Mechanisms of Exercise

Biological Mechanisms of Exercise	Psychological Mechanisms of Exercise
Increases in body temperature result in a short-term tranquilizing effect	Exercise resembles a graded task assignment resulting in a sense of mastery as distinct achievements are noted
(Regular exercise) improves stress adaptation via increases in adrenal gland activity	Changes a woman's perception of her physical self and identity in a positive way
Improvements in fitness result in a diminished cardiovascular response to stress	Serves as a form of meditation that triggers an altered and more relaxed state of consciousness
Reduction in resting muscle activity following exercise leads to tension release	Is a form of biofeedback that teaches how to regulate our own autonomic arousal
Exercise enhances the neurotransmission of norepinephrine, serotonin, and dopamine	Provides distraction, diversion, or time away from unpleasant cognition, emotions, and behavior
Exercise results in an increase in circulating B endorphins	Social reinforcement among exercisers may result in improved psychological states

increased physical activity participation, suggesting that even a home-based program can benefit women with depressive symptoms. Using a database of 22,073 college females, Adams et al. (2007) found that both vigorous/moderate exercise and strength training exercise was positively associated with perceived health and negatively associated with depression.

The LEVITY program (Light, Exercise and Vitamin Intervention TherapY) included an exercise component as well as light and vitamins to treat subthreshold depression in women (Brown and Shirley 2005). Twenty minutes a day of moderately paced exercise (60% of maximum heart rate) was recommended 5 days a week. Based on a woman's current level of fitness, varying speeds of walking were required to maintain the target heart rate. For most, it was a brisk pace at which a conversation could be maintained without shortness of breath. With only 20 minutes of exercise, the LEVITY program was able to create a positive impact on mood.

Physical Activity and Diabetes

Exercise and weight reduction are effective in the primary prevention of diabetes mellitus in most women. Exercise increases insulin sensitivity and decreases triglycerides and total cholesterol. Exercise improves glucose tolerance in lean and obese type 2 diabetics under the age of 55 years and in obese patients older than 55 years (Zierath et al. 1992). A recent study by Stewart et al. (2005) determined that in people aged 55 to 75 years, a moderate program of physical exercise could significantly offset metabolic syndrome. A sedentary individual who initiates an exercise program consisting of walking approximately 5 km/day or swimming, running, or biking 30 to 60 min/day reduces the risk of diabetes by 50% (Byyny and Speroff 1996). Exercise even once a week appears to have an effect as evidenced in an 8-year study of women aged 34 to 59 years who had a 16% decrease in the relative risk of diabetes after initiating a once-a-week exercise program (Manson et al. 1991).

Physical Activity and Bone Health

Recent advances in bone biology have established that exercise in the form of short, repetitive mechanical loading leads to the greatest gains in bone strength. As demonstrated by both observational and randomized exercise intervention trials, these gains are best achieved in childhood but can be maintained in adulthood with continued regular weight-bearing exercise. In the later years, there is evidence to support the implementation of balance training to decrease fall risk, especially in elderly patients with low bone mass (Borer 2005; Ondrak and Morgan 2007; Schwab and Klein 2008).

Regular exercise, including resistance training and high-impact activity, contributes to the development of high peak bone mass and may reduce the risk of falls in older women (Hagey and Warren 2008). A study of mature female athletes found that women who regularly engage in high-impact physical activity in the premenopausal years have higher BMD than nonathletic controls (Dook et al. 1997). See Chapter 36 on Osteoporosis for recommendations.

Physical Activity and Menopause

Although many of the chronic illnesses that increase in postmenopausal women are positively affected by physical activity, there is not definitive evidence that activity improves vasomotor symptoms. Van Poppel and Brown (2008) assessed the relationship between changes in physical activity and self-reported menopausal symptoms using data from the Australian Longitudinal Study on Women's Health (http://www.alswh.org.au). Physical activity was not associated with total menopausal symptoms, vasomotor, or psychological symptoms. Weight gain was associated with increased total, vasomotor, and somatic symptoms while weight loss reduced total and vasomotor symptoms.

A Cochrane review found only one small trial assessing the effectiveness of exercise in the management of vasomotor menopausal symptoms (Daley et al. 2007). Exercise was not as effective as hormone replacement therapy (HRT) in this trial. They found no evidence that exercise is an effective treatment relative to other interventions or no intervention in reducing hot flashes and/or night sweats in symptomatic women. While it is important to recommend physical activity for prevention of chronic illness, women should not be given unrealistic expectations regarding the effects on vasomotor symptoms.

Fibromyalgia and Physical Activity

Physical activity relieves many symptoms in fibromyalgia patients; it helps women maintain general fitness, physical function, emotional well-being, and overall health; it also provides women with enhanced feelings of control over their well-being. Forty-six exercise treatment studies with a total of 3035 subjects were reviewed and the strongest evidence is for aerobic exercise (Jones et al. 2006). The greatest effect and lowest attrition occurred in exercise programs that were of lower intensity. Exercise that is of appropriate intensity, self-modified, and symptom-limited is most likely to be of help.

Bircan et al. (2008) compared the effects of aerobic training with a muscle-strengthening program in patients with fibromyalgia. Thirty women with fibromyalgia were randomized to either an aerobic exercise program or a strengthening exercise program for 8 weeks; both programs were similarly effective at improving symptoms, tender point count, fitness, depression, and quality of life. Similar findings were reported by the Ottawa panel (Brosseau et al. 2008).

Challenges to motivating women with fibromyalgia to exercise include that many are deconditioned due to pain and fatigue; many are overweight or obese; and some have become socially isolated. Interventions unique to patients with fibromyalgia include the following:

- Greater exercise adherence occurs when there is greater agreement between patient and physician regarding the patient's level of well-being and when the patient's pain and stress have been addressed (Rooks 2008).
- Physical activity recommendations should be tailored to the individual patient.
- Initial discussions should concentrate around ways to increase physical activity daily; for example, adding walking tasks with or without a pedometer, parking farther away from the destination, using stairs, and engaging in gardening and house cleaning.

Enhancing Motivation

Although the benefits of regular physical activity are vast, less than 50% of U.S. women meet the "Healthy people 2010" recommended guidelines (CDC 2007). The challenge to motivate women to increase their physical activity is twofold. First is the motivation to initiate physical activity and second is the ability to maintain regular physical activity (defined as maintaining the required levels of exercise for more than 6 months) (Marcus et al. 1992).

Maintaining regular, long-term physical activity is critical to achieving its benefits. However, the dropout rate in clinical programs is 50% or greater within the first 6 months (Dishman 1988). Variables that impact motivation were identified in a review article and include demographic, psychological, social environmental, physiologic, health status, and physical activity (Speck and Harrell 2003).

Demographic variables such as age are important considerations when designing studies and developing interventions. Older women exercise at lower levels and less frequently than younger women (Scharff et al. 1999). One study found differing predictors of four types of activity: sports/exercise, active living, household/caregiving, and occupational activities (Sternfeld et al. 1999). Women with the highest levels of both sports/exercise and active living were likely to be white, better educated, younger, without young children at home, with lower BMI, higher self-efficacy, and lower perceived barriers to exercise. Women with the highest level of household/caregiving responsibilities were more likely to be Hispanic, older, married with young children in the home, and not employed. Women with the highest occupational physical activity were likely to be less educated and were current smokers.

In analyses of a national survey, women in all three ethnic classifications— Caucasian, African-American, Mexican-American—had higher percentages of inactivity than men, ranging from 22% to 47% for women and 14% to 32% for men (Crespo et al. 2000). Among women, African-Americans and Mexican-Americans had higher percentages of inactivity than Caucasians in nearly every category of the social class indicators (education, income, occupation, poverty, employment, and marital status).

HEALTH STATUS VARIABLES

In a national survey of ethnically diverse women 40 to 70+ years old ($n = 2912$), the personal barrier "not in good health" was 1 of 11 variables that were significant predictors of being sedentary (King et al. 2000). Heesch et al. (2000)

further analyzed this data and found "bad health" was identified as a frequent barrier to exercise in Caucasian, Native American, and Hispanic subjects in the precontemplation stage of physical activity, but not in African-Americans. Precontemplators were defined as not currently exercising and with no plan to begin exercising in the next 6 months.

PSYCHOLOGICAL VARIABLES

Self-efficacy is the belief that one is capable of performing a specific behavior (Bandura 1986). Self-efficacy is consistently positively correlated with higher levels of physical activity (Piazza et al. 2001; Speck 2001; Sternfeld et al. 1999). Other studies demonstrated that self-efficacy is a predictor of initiation and early adherence to exercise but maintenance is predicted by the interaction of self-efficacy and the type of program (McAuley et al. 1994, Oman and King 1998). When the physical activity is self-selected instead of prescribed by the study design, self-efficacy might play a bigger role in maintenance. Outcome expectation is the belief that performing a specific behavior will lead to a specific outcome and is linked to self-efficacy. Overly optimistic expectations of inexperienced exercisers may lead to disappointment and attrition (Jones et al. 2005).

PHYSICAL ACTIVITY VARIABLES

Aspects of physical activity may be important since negative experiences with a behavior can lead to suppression of the behavior and positive experiences can increase a woman's self-efficacy around that behavior (Bandura 1986). Variables include type of activity and the number of relapses from regular physical activity.

Many studies have shown that walking is an important activity for women. For example, in an Australian survey, more than 60% of women identified walking as their preferred physical activity, 14% identified swimming, and all other activity choices were chosen by less than 10% of the women. Social environmental variables include support of friends and family and social and environmental barriers. In an Australian survey of inactive women (Booth et al. 1997), 19% identified lack of someone to exercise with as a barrier and 35% preferred to exercise with the support of a group. Another study (Wallace et al. 1995) demonstrated that women had better adherence when they exercised with their spouses than alone. However, lower family support predicted higher maintenance. This paradoxical finding could mean that for working women with families, spending time with family is a higher priority than exercising.

The most frequently identified barrier to activity maintenance in women is lack of time due to work and family obligations (Booth et al. 1997; Jaffe et al. 1999). Qualitative studies of barriers to physical activity in both African-American women and Caucasian women found lack of time, motivation, and social support (Nies et al. 1998, 1999). Barriers identified only by African-Americans were lack of childcare, lack of space for exercise in the home, and unsafe neighborhoods. A barrier unique to Caucasian women was poor body image.

RECOMMENDATIONS FOR CLINICIANS

As health care providers, we can empower women to be physically active. We have plenty of evidence—as reviewed in this chapter—of the benefits of regular physical activity for primary and secondary prevention of chronic illnesses. As integrative providers, we have the tools to provide patient-centered care and to elicit the unique needs, preferences, and barriers women of all ages and ethnic backgrounds have around physical activity. We can communicate that even small increments in physical activity, leisure time with family, occupational, structured exercise, or alternative ways of transportation can improve health and well-being.

After my thyroidectomy, when I learned I had cancer with extensive lymph node involvement, I turned to exercise to improve my well-being. The first week, I could hardly jog for 5 minutes. Even those few minutes gave me a sense of well-being and hope and I increased the frequency, intensity, and time as I felt ready. I also added different exercises: swimming, yoga, and biking. Today, at age 50, I am in the best athletic condition of my entire life. I am grateful to feel this way. It is my hope that you will be inspired by this chapter not only to work with your women patients to help them make activity a part of their daily routine but also to be a model for your patients and advocate in your community.

REFERENCES

Adams TB, Moore MT, Dye J. The relationship between physical activity and mental health in a national sample of college females. *Women & Health.* 2007;45(1):69–85.

Anish EJ. Exercise and its effects on the central nervous system. *Curr Sports Med Rep.* 2005;4(1):18–23.

Bandura A. *Social Learning Theory.* Englewood Cliffs, NJ: Prentice Hall; 1986.

Bircan C, Karasel SA, Akgun B, El O, Alper S. Effects of muscle strengthening versus aerobic exercise program in fibromyalgia. *Rheumatol Intl.* 2008;28(6):527–532.

Booth ML, Bauman A, Owen N, Gore CJ. Physical activity preferences, preferred sources of assistance, and perceived barriers to increased activity among physically inactive Australians. *Prev Med.* 1997;26:131–137.

Borer KT. Physical activity in the prevention and amelioration of osteoporosis in women: interaction of mechanical, hormonal and dietary factors. *Sports Med.* 2005;35(9):779–830.

Breslow RA, Ballard-Barbash R, Munoz K, Graubard BI. Long term recreational physical activity and breast cancer in the National Health and Nutrition Examination Survey I Epidemiologic Follow-up Study. *Cancer Epidemiol Biomarkers Prev.* 2001;10:805–808.

Brosse AL, Sheets ES, Lett HS, et al. Exercise and the treatment of clinical depression in adults: recent findings and future directions. *Sports Med.* 2002;32:741–760.

Brosseau L, Wells GA, Tugwell P, et al. Ottawa Panel evidence-based clinical practice guidelines for strengthening exercises in the management of fibromyalgia: part 2. *Phys Therapy.* 2008;88(7):873–886.

Brown MA, Shirley JL. Enhancing women's mood and energy: a research-based program for subthreshold depression using light, exercise, and vitamins. *Holist Nurs Pract.* 2005;19(6):278–284.

Brown WJ, Burton NW, Rowan PJ. Updating the evidence on physical activity and health in women. *Am J Prev Med.* 2007;33(5):404–411.

Byyny RL, Speroff L, Million L. *A Clinical Guide for the Care of Older Women: Primary and Preventive Care.* 2nd ed. Baltimore: Williams & Wilkins; 1996:161–227.

Centers for Disease Control and Prevention (CDC). Prevalence of regular physical activity among adults—United States, 2001 and 2005. *MMWR.* 2007;56(46):1209–1212.Centers for Disease Control and Prevention website, Health, United States 2007 (An annual report on health statistics): http://www.cdc.gov/nchs/hus.htmCenters for Disease Control and Prevention website, Physical Activity for Everyone How much physical activity do you need, 2008: http://www.cdc.gov/physicalactivity/everyone/guidelines/adults.html

Centers for Disease Control and Prevention website, Physical Activity for everyone, Measuring Physical Activity Intensity: http://www.cdc.gov/physicalactivity/downloads/PA_Intensity_table_2_1.pdf

Craft LL, Freund KM, Culpepper L, Perna FM. Intervention study of exercise for depressive symptoms in women. *J Women's Health.* 2007;16(10):1499–1509.

Craft LL, Perna FA, Freund, KM, Culpepper L. Psychosocial correlates of exercise in women with self-reported depressive symptoms. *J Phys Activity Health.* 2008;5(3):469–480.

Crespo CJ, Smit E, Andersen RE, Carter-Pokras O, Ainsworth BE. Race/ethnicity, social class and their relation to physical inactivity during leisure time: results from the Third National Health and Nutrition Examination Survey, 1988–1994. *Am J Prev Med.* 2000;18:46–53.

Daley A, MacArthur C, Mutrie N, Stokes-Lampard H. Exercise for vasomotor menopausal symptoms. *Cochr Database Syst Rev.* 2007;(4):CD006108.

Dishman RK. *Exercise Adherence: Its Impact on Public Health*. Champaign, IL: Human Kinetics; 1988.

Dook JE, James C, Henderson NK, et al. Exercise and bone mineral density in mature female athletes. *Med Sci Sports Exerc*. 1997;29:291–296.

Ellekjaer H, Holman J, Ellekjar E, Vatten L. Physical activity and stroke mortality in women: 10-year follow-up of the Nord-Trondelag Health Survey 1984–1986. *Stroke*. 2000;31:14–18.

Fischer Aggarwal BA, Liao M, Mosca L. Physical activity as a potential mechanism through which social support may reduce cardiovascular disease risk. *J Cardiovascular Nurs*. 2008;23(2):90–96.

Folsom AR, Kushi LH, Hong CP. Physical activity and incident diabetes mellitus in post menopausal women. *Am J Public Health*. 2000;90:134–138.

Gregg EW, Cauley JA, Stone K, et al. Relationship of changes in physical activity and mortality among older women. *JAMA*. 2003;289:2379–2386.

Hagey AR, Warren MP. Role of exercise and nutrition in menopause. *Clin Obstet Gynecol*. 2008;51(3):627–641.

He J, Ogden L, Bazzana L, Vupputuri S, Loria C, Whelton P. Risk factors for congestive heart failure in U.S. men and women: NHANES I epidemiologic follow-up study. *Arch Intern Med*. 2001;161:996–1002.

Heesch KC, Brown DR, Blanton CJ. Perceived barriers to exercise and stage of exercise adoption in older women of different racial/ethnic groups. *Women Health*. 2000;30(4):61–76.

Hsia J, Wu L, Allen C, et al. Physical activity and diabetes risk in post menopausal women. *Am J Prev Med*. 2005;28:19–25.

Hu FB, Li TY, Colditz GA, Willett WC, Manson JE. Television watching and other sedentary behaviors in relation to risk of obesity and type 2 diabetes mellitus in women. *JAMA*. 2003;289:1785–1791.

Hu FB, Sigal RJ, Rich-Edwards JW, et al. Walking compared with vigorous physical activity and risk of type 2 diabetes in women. *JAMA*. 1999;282:1433–1439.

Hu FB, Stampfer MJ, Colditz GA, et al. Physical activity and risk stroke in women. *JAMA*. 2000;283:2961–2967.

Hu FB, Willett WC, Li T, et al. Adiposity as compared with physical activity in predicting mortality among women. *N Engl J Med*. 2004;351:2694–2703.

Jaffe L, Lutter JM, Rex M, Hawkes C, Bucaccio P. Incentives and barriers to physical activity for working women. *Am J Health Promot*. 1999;13:215.

Jones F, Harris P, Waller H, Coggins A. Adherence to an exercise prescription scheme: the role of expectations, self-efficacy, stage of change and psychological well-being. *Br J Health Psychol*. 2005;10(3):359–378.

Jones KD, Adams D, Winters-Stone K, Burckhardt CS. A comprehensive review of 46 exercise treatment studies in fibromyalgia (1988–2005). *Health Qual Life Outcomes*. 2006;4:67.

Kelley GA, Kelley KS, Tran ZV. Aerobic exercise and lipids and lipoproteins in women: a meta-analysis of randomized controlled trials. *J Womens Health (Larchmt)*. 2005;13(10):1148–1164. [Erratum in *J Womens Health (Larchmt)*. 2005;14(2):198.]

King AC, Castro C, Wilcox S, Eyler AA, Sallis JF, Brownson RC. Personal and environmental factors associated with physical inactivity among different racial-ethnic groups of U.S. middle-aged and older-aged women. *Health Psychol.* 2000;19: 354–364.

Kriska AM, Saremi A, Hanson RL, et al. Physical activity, obesity, and the incidence of type 2 diabetes in a high risk population. *Am J Epidemiol.* 2003;158: 669–675.

Kushi LH, Fee RM, Folsom AR, Mink PJ, Anderson KE, Sellers TA. Physical activity and mortality in postmenopausal women. *JAMA.* 1997;277:1287–1292.

Lee IM. Physical activity and cancer prevention—data from epidemiologic studies. *Med Sci Sports Exerc.* 2003;35(11):1823–1827.

Lee IM, Rexrode KM, Cook NR, Manson JE, Buring JE. Physical activity and coronary heart disease in women: is "no pain, no gain" passé? *JAMA.* 2001;285: 1447–1454.

Manson JE, Greenland P, LaCroix AZ, et al. Walking compared with vigorous exercise for the prevention of cardiovascular events in women. *N Engl J Med.* 2002;347: 716–725.

Manson JE, Rimm EB, Stampfer MJ, et al. Physical activity and incidence of non-insulin-dependent diabetes mellitus. *Lancet.* 1991;338:774–778.

Marcus BH, Selby VC, Niaura RS, Rossi JS. Self-efficacy and the stages of exercise behavior change. *Res Q Exerc Sport.* 1992;63:60–66.

Martinez ME, Giovannucci E, Spiegelman D, Hunter DJ, Willett WC, Colditz GA. Leisure time physical activity, body size, and colon cancer in women. *J Nat Cancer Inst.* 1997;89:948–955.

McAuley E, Courneya KS, Rudolph DL, Lox CL. Enhancing exercise, adherence in middle-aged males and females. *Prev Med.* 1994;23:498–506.

McTiernan A, Kooperberg C, White E, et al. Recreational physical activity and the risk of breast cancer in postmenopausal women: the Women's Health Initiative Cohort Study. *JAMA.* 2003;290:1331–1336.

Mora S, Cook N, Buring JE, Ridker PM, Lee IM. Activity and reduced risk of cardiovascular events: potential mediating mechanisms. *Circulation.* 2007;116(19): 2110–2118.

Nies MA, Vollman M, Cook T. Facilitators, barriers, and strategies for exercise in European American women in the community. *Public Health Nurs.* 1998;15: 263–272.

Nies MA, Vollman M, Cook T. African American women's experiences with physical activity in their daily lives. *Public Health Nurs.* 1999;16:23–31.

Oman RF, King AC. Predicting the adoption and maintenance of exercise participation using self-efficacy and previous exercise participation rates. *Am J Health Promot.* 1998;12:154–161.

Ondrak KS, Morgan DW. Physical activity, calcium intake and bone health in children and adolescents. *Sports Medicine.* 2007;37(7):587–600.

Paganini-Hill A, Barreto MP. Stroke risk in older men and women: aspirin, estrogen, exercise, vitamins and other factors. *J Gend Specif Med.* 2001;4(2):18–28.

Peplonska B, Lissowska J, Hartman TJ, et al. Adult lifetime physical activity and breast cancer. *Epidemiology.* 2008;19(2):226–236.

Piazza J, Conrad K, Wilbur J. Exercise behavior among occupational health nurses. *AAOHN J.* 2001;49(2):79–86.

Rockhill B, Willett WC, Hunter DJ, Manson JE, Hankinson SE, Colditz GA. A prospective study of recreational physical activity and breast cancer risk. *Arch Intern Med.* 1999;159:2290–2296.

Rooks DS. Talking to patients with fibromyalgia about physical activity and exercise. *Curr Opin Rheumatol.* 2008;20(2):208–212.

Scharff DP, Homan S, Kreuter M, Brennan L. Factors associated with physical activity in women across the life span: implications for program development. *Women Health.* 1999;29:115–134.

Schwab P, Klein RF. Nonpharmacological approaches to improve bone health and reduce osteoporosis. *Curr Opin Rheumatol.* 2008;20(2):213–217.

Sesso HD, Paffenbarger RS Jr, Lee IM. Physical activity and breast cancer risk in the College Alumni Health Study (United States). *Cancer Causes Control.* 1998;9:433–439.

Speck BJ. Maintenance of regular physical activity in working women. In: Funk S, Tornquist E, Leeman J, eds. Key Aspects, 2001.

Speck, BJ, Harrell JS. Maintaining regular physical activity in women: evidence to date. *J Cardiovascular Nursing.* 2003;18(4):282–291; quiz 292–293.

Sternfeld BS, Ainsworth BE, Quesenberry CP. Physical activity patterns in a diverse population of women. *Prev Med.* 1999;28:313–323.

Stevens J, Cai J, Evenson KR, Thomas R. Fitness and fatness as predictors of mortality from all causes and from cardiovascular disease in men and women in the lipid research clinics study. *Am J Epidemiol.* 2002;156:832–841.

Stewart KJ, Bacher AC, Turner K, et al. Exercise and risk factors associated with metabolic syndrome in older adults. *Am J Prev Med.* 2005;28:9–18.

Tehard B, Friedenreich CM, Oppert JM, Clavel-Chapelon F. Effect of physical activity on women at increased risk of breast cancer: results. 2006

Thune I, Brenn V, Lund E, Gaard V. Physical activity and the risk of breast cancer. *N Engl J Med.* 1997;336:1269–1275.

U.S. Department of Health and Human Services. Physical activity and health: a report of the Surgeon General. Atlanta: U.S. Department of Health and Human Services, Centers for Disease Control and Prevention, National Center for Chronic Disease Prevention and Health Promotion; 1996.

van Poppel MN, Brown WJ. "It's my hormones, doctor"—does physical activity help with menopausal symptoms? *Menopause.* 2008;15(1):78–85.

Wallace J, Raglin J, Jastremski C. Twelve month adherence of adults who joined a fitness program with a spouse vs without a spouse. *J Sports Med Phys Fitness.* 1995;35:206–213.

Weinstein AR, Sesso HD, Lee IM, et al. Relationship of physical activity vs body mass index with type 2 diabetes in women. *JAMA.* 2004;292:1188–1194.

Weller I, Corey P. The impact of excluding non-leisure energy expenditure on the relation between physical activity and mortality in women. *Epidemiology*. 1998;9: 632–635.

Zierath JR, Wallberg-Henriksson H. Exercise training in obese diabetic patients. Special considerations. *Sports Med*. 1992;14:171–189.

5

Mind–Body Therapies

RITA BENN

CASE STUDY

It is hard to get a word in edgewise with Jane. Intense, driven, and successful in her career, she describes herself as a "case study in perceptual motion." Hitting age 50, Jane relates that she suddenly feels more out of control. In the last several months, she has experienced bouts of chest tightness, throat constriction, intermittent waves of panic and increasing states of moodiness. Not wanting to take any medication, Jane enrolls in a mindfulness meditation class offered at the community hospital. She initiates a daily sitting practice and reports feeling a new level of self-awareness and contentment unfolding. She now looks forward to getting home at night to her cushion—the designated spot for sitting quiet. After a few weeks, the physical manifestations of stress and fluctuating moods have lessened in frequency and intensity. While Jane still rushes throughout her day, she describes feeling more present in her activities and will often take intermittent breaks at the office where she shuts her door, closes her eyes and follows her breath for a few minutes. Jane finds that as a result of meditation, she is kinder to herself and to others and better able to cope with her work demands.

Introduction

Mind–body therapies are widely used by the public. The most recent Centers for Disease Control and Prevention (CDC) population-based survey of 31,000 adults reports that over 50% of the population has used some form of mind–body therapy in the past year to support their health (Barnes et al. 2002). Mind–body therapies have the highest usage of all complementary and alternative medicine (CAM) modalities, particularly if prayer is considered as one of these therapies. With prayer excluded, the data suggests that mind–body practices have the second highest use (17%), slightly behind that found for natural products (19%). Aside from prayer, the three most common mind–body therapies used by consumers to support their health are deep breathing exercises, meditation, and yoga.

> I was first introduced to meditation in college. In practicing meditation for the past 25 years, I have come to appreciate how this simple practice of sitting still has helped anchor me to the fullness of the present moment, allowing me to deeply experience a sense of connection to the wholeness that life offers. Meditation has been, and continues to be, a repeated invitation to meet, explore and replenish the relationship to myself and to others.

The purpose of this chapter is to reveal how mind–body practices may optimize health and reduce distress in women. The chapter begins with a description of mind–body therapies and their underlying mechanisms. A discussion of the relationship between health and stress follows. Key findings from systematic reviews on the effectiveness of mind–body therapies along with examples of recent controlled trials are presented. The chapter concludes with implications for clinical practice, suggesting how providers may use mind–body options not only as an adjunctive treatment strategy but for the promotion of health.

Description of Mind–Body Therapies

Mind–body therapies consist of a variety of techniques that have their origins in Asian healing systems, European medical practices, and Western psychological therapies. Meditation, hypnosis, and movement therapies, such as yoga and tai-chi, are some examples. Mind–body therapies share a common assumption that an inner directed experiential practice can alleviate tensions originating in the mind and/or expressed in the body.

The National Center for Complementary and Alternative Medicine (NCCAM) of the National Institutes of Health (NIH) defines mind–body approaches as those "practices that focus on the interactions of the brain, mind, body and behavior, with the intent to use the mind to affect physical functioning and promote health" (NCCAM, accessed 2008). While support groups, cognitive-behavioral approaches, and psychodynamic therapies all meet this definition, this chapter will focus on practices that are considered complementary and alternative by NCCAM. A list of these practices is presented in Table 5.1.

Table 5.1. Descriptions of Common Mind Body Techniques

Mind–Body Technique	Definition
Autogenics	Use of self-guided verbal instructions directed to a specific body function (e.g., my forehead is cool, etc.) in order to alter that physiological response.
Biofeedback	External feedback of bodily measurements (e.g., brain waves, heart rate) provided from a device connected to the skin, heart, or scalp and used to modulate a physiological response. Some common biofeedback approaches are known as EMG, heartmath, or neurofeedback.
Breathwork	The active direction of attention to inhalation and exhalation of the breath, and/or its pacing or volume, to cultivate various states of awareness. Common breathing techniques include deep abdominal breathing, alternate nostril breathing, chaotic breathing and practices known as holotropic breathwork.
Expressive writing	A structured or unstructured process of journaling used to uncover deep thoughts, feelings, and new meanings. Studied practices involve writing 15 minutes daily or several times per week on the effect and meaning of health event or symptoms.
Guided imagery	Directed verbal instructions that invoke sensory images to facilitate awareness and mastery of feelings, emotions, thoughts and tensions. The imagery may include pleasant scenes, physiologically directed functions, mental performance, receptive or metaphoric foci.
Healing Arts Art therapy	The process of using specific media and materials to stimulate awareness, relaxation and/or resolution of feelings, emotions, and conflicts.

(continued)

Table 5.1. (Continued)

Mind–Body Technique	Definition
Dance therapy	The use of choreographed or improvised movement with music to facilitate expression of feelings, emotions, conflicts, tension release, mood alteration and relaxation.
Music therapy	The process of listening to specific musical pieces, using one's voice, or playing instruments to create musical compositions or sounds geared to alleviate physical and psychological symptoms.
Hypnosis	Guided facilitation of ideas, suggestions and mental imagery to induce a state of inner absorption and focused attention that allows for new perceptions and behavior changes to emerge.
Meditation	The process of intentionally directed attention to create a state of inner stillness or awareness that may be facilitated by the use and/or focus of a mantra, word, phrase, sound, image, or breath. There are hundreds of types of meditation practices. Popular forms include Transcendental meditation (TM), mindfulness meditation (also known as Vipassana or insight, mindfulness-based stress reduction (MBSR)), mindfulness–based cognitive therapy (MBCT), loving kindness, relaxation response, and Zen.
Movement-related meditations	
Yoga	A system of practice of various physical postures (asanas) and breathing techniques to align the body's musculoskeletal structure and emotional equilibrium. All yoga stems from hatha yoga. Different schools emphasize various dimensions according to its pre-eminent teacher. Iyengar, Vinyasa, Anasura, Ashtanga, Bikram, and Bhakti yoga are the most common forms.
Tai-Chi	A system of slow coordinated sequences of graceful movements that flow into one another to achieve steadiness in mind and body. Many styles exist (such as Chen, Sun, Wu, and Yang) which vary in terms of intensity and rhythm.
Qi-gong (internal)	A system of slow, gentle, and deliberate circular movements, breathwork and meditation to improve the flow of "Qi" (life force) and emotional stability.
Prayer	The directed focus of a bequest or intention for healing that occurs in personal contemplation originating in religious traditions.
Progressive muscle relaxation (PMR)	The release of emotional and muscular tension through conscious attention of flexing and release of various muscle joints and groups. The term "applied relaxation" uses this technique and breathing.

Often clients ask what form of meditation should they learn. I recommend that individuals use a technique that most resonates with them. Just as there are many different types of physical exercise that have aerobic benefits, there are also a range of meditation practices. Most emphasize inner stillness, using an internal point of focus, such as silently repeating a mantra, following the flow of the breath or body movements, or centering on a loving phrase. Like exercise, it may not matter which technique one uses. The key is to consistently incorporate its practice into one's daily routine.

THEORETICAL MECHANISMS OF ACTION

All mind–body therapies focus on inducing a state of physiological relaxation and stillness. The mental and physical awareness that arises through relaxation can induce positive affective states as well as facilitate recognition of negative emotions and thought patterns that are held outside of everyday consciousness. Over time, individuals may gain insights that can help restore psychological and physical well-being. Mind–body therapies can be thought of as medicine as they engage physiological and psychological processes that reduce distress, facilitate well-being, and promote health (Ader 2007; Jacobs 2001; McEwen and Lasley 2002; Steptoe et al. 2005).

Stress, Positive Affect, and Health Outcomes

The role that stress plays in exacerbating illness has been documented by epidemiological and outcome-based research. Long-term exposure to stress predisposes individuals to (1) increased cardiovascular risk (McEwen and Lasley 2002), resulting in strokes and heart attacks (Wittstein et al. 2005; Williams and Chesney 1993; Irribarren et al. 2000; Mittleman et al. 1995) and (2) weakened immune functioning (McEwen and Lasley 2002; Segerstrom and Miller 2004), resulting in increased inflammation (Weik et al. 2008), greater susceptibility to colds (Cohen et al. 2006), allergies (Hoglund et al. 2006), and a variety of other illnesses (Chandola et al. 2006; Cohen et al. 2007). There are a number of studies that link stress to increased risk of breast, ovarian, and cervical cancers (Fang et al. 2008; Helgesson et al. 2003; Lillberg et al. 2003; Thacker et al. 2006). Using animal models, researchers have shown how catecholamines, glucocorticoids, and other stress hormones influence the progression of cancer by altering the tumor microenvironment (Antonio et al. 2006).

Stress has even been shown to change genomic structures. For example, in individuals overburdened by caregiving, such as mothers whose children have a disability (Eppel et al. 2004), or caregivers for persons with Alzheimer's (Damjanovic et al. 2007), the genomic structures controlling cell division become permanently altered. Blood samples depict shortened telomere length, suggesting premature biological aging.

While prolonged stress has deleterious consequences on physical health, accumulating research demonstrates that positive affect can be protective for health (Cohen et al. 2003; Steptoe 2005). For example, Danner et al. (2001) analyzed the journals of 180 Catholic nuns over their lifetime, and found a positive relationship between expressed positive affect and longevity. A subsequent meta-analysis of 70 published studies ($N = 3481$) showed that psychological well-being is associated with reduced mortality in both healthy and diseased populations (Chida and Steptoe 2008).

THE GENDERED EXPERIENCE OF STRESS

Women report high levels of stress and unhappiness that consequently place them at increased risk for disease. A 2007 national survey ($n = 1848$) indicates that 82% of women perceive that stress negatively impacts their health and well-being (American Psychological Association 2007). Women describe higher levels of stress than men in both psychological symptoms (irritability or anger, nervousness, and lacking energy) and physical symptoms (fatigue, headaches, upset stomach, muscular tension, and change in appetite). It is noteworthy that these same symptoms contribute to 60%–90% of primary care visits (Fava and Sonino 2005).

Women describe a greater number of stressful life events and are more negatively influenced by these events than men, even when their exposure rate is similar (Davis 1999; Tolin and Foa 2006). More women than men indicate that they handle stress poorly (American Psychological Association 2007). As women age, they report less happiness and more dissatisfaction with their lives than do men (Plagnol and Easterlin 2008). A higher prevalence of affective and anxiety disorders has been observed for women over their lifetime as well as during the previous 12-month time periods that were measured (Kessler et al. 1994).

Recent findings suggest a gender-specific neural activation model underlying the stress response (Wang et al. 2007). Researchers observed functional magnetic resonance imaging (fMRI) results of 32 men and women undergoing stressful tasks; the men had increased blood flow to the left orbital frontal cortex, the area presumed to activate resources for the "flight and fight" response, while in women, stress activated the limbic system, the area associated with processing of emotions. Differences in the psychological and neurobiological response to stress may also have implications for the kinds of interventions that providers recommend. Nonpharmacological interventions that access emotional and biobehavioral pathways may have more beneficial effects for women than those that focus on prefrontal areas that emphasize cognitive-focused solutions.

For women, group-based interventions incorporating mind–body instruction may also have added benefit. A "tend-and-befriend" model has been posited to characterize women's need for relationship and support during times of stress (Taylor 2002). Studies of female laboratory animal responses exposed to stress reveal nurturing and affiliative behavior with other animals in contrast to the aggressive or withdrawal responses evident in males (Taylor et al. 2000). Providing a social support structure when learning mind–body therapies may optimize therapeutic effects.

> I have found that stress management groups where women learn mind–body practices are of enormous benefit. Within the safe context of a group, women feel empowered to look at themselves and respond to their physical or mental health challenges in new ways. By experimenting with mind–body practices, they discover an inner voice that reveals information to them from a very deep place of knowing. In listening to themselves and one another, women begin to gain their own sense of agency and to trust their capacity to move forward with their lives.

Mind–Body Therapies on Health Conditions: Evidence

In 2003, Astin and colleagues examined 28 systematic reviews (N = 46,045) of studies on mind–body therapies. The authors concluded that the strength mind–body research compared favorably with other areas of medical research. Gender effects were not discussed in their meta- analysis nor in more recent systematic reviews examining the influence of specific mind–body practices (biofeedback, hypnosis, yoga, tai-chi, qi-gong, guided imagery, meditation, and music therapies) on mental or physical health symptoms (Anderson et al. 2008; Cepeda et al. 2006; Coelho et al. 2007; Grossman et al. 2004; Kirkwood et al. 2005; Lee et al. 2007a, 2007b, 2008; Maratos et al. 2008; Nestoriuc et al. 2008; Pilkington et al. 2005; Rainforth et al. 2006; Roffe et al. 2005; Wang et al. 2004; Yeh et al. 2008). It is particularly surprising that the recent Agency for Healthcare Research and Quality report (Ospina et al. 2007) that evaluated the effects of 65 studies of sitting and movement meditation in patients with hypertension, cardiovascular risk, and substance use, also did not analyze outcomes separately for women and men.

Two recent systematic reviews of mind–body practices did examine the influence of gender on health effects. Manzoni et al. (2008) analyzed 27 studies published from 1997 to 2007 on relaxation training (e.g. meditation, autogenics, progressive muscle relaxation [PMR]) on anxiety. They describe a medium to large effect size for these practices, with applied relaxation,[1] meditation, and PMR showing the highest efficacy. Women showed larger positive pre–post treatment effects than men regardless of the type of treatment.

In a meta-analysis of 146 studies (N = 10,994) that examined the effects of an expressive writing practice[2] with a variety of ill and healthy populations, a small but significant effect size was found for general health, psychological health, physical functioning, perceptions of health, and many immune parameters (Frattaroli, 2006). No differences were found attributable to gender.

PAIN: DYSMENORRHEA AND SURGICAL

For patients with primary and secondary dysmenorrhea, a Cochrane systematic review (Proctor et al. 2007) of five trials (N = 213) found PMR, with or without imagery helpful for spasmodic pain. An unblinded randomized clinical trial (RCT) of 200 women scheduled to undergo breast biopsy or lumpectomy illustrated the benefits of short-term hypnotic induction for alleviation of procedural pain and distress (Montgomery et al. 2007). In this study, investigators compared a 15-minute hypnotic intervention to nondirected empathetic listening and measured the use of analgesia and sedatives as well as self-reported pain, nausea, fatigue, and distress. Patients in the hypnosis group required significantly less anesthesia and reported less surgical pain and other measured side effects; there was no difference in the number of recovery room medications.

PREGNANCY, FERTILITY, AND MENOPAUSE

Systematic reviews examining the effects of mind–body intervention in pregnancy are replete with methodological limitations (Beddoe and Lee 2008). Studies often do not include randomization or controls, and use different measures and end points, such as maternal mood, fear of pain during labor, blood pressure, and gestational age at birth. Three RCTs (n = 110; 58; 31) evaluated the

[1] Applied relaxation consists of deep breathing and PMR.
[2] The writing practice that has been researched involves one to six sessions of private discourse and disclosure regarding feelings surrounding an upsetting event or health trauma.

effect of a specific mind–body therapy (progressive relaxation, guided imagery, or mindfulness meditation) on anxiety using the same measurement tool (Bastini et al. 2005; Teixeira et al. 2005; Vietin and Astin 2008). Two of the studies used 5- to 8-week group-based classes of mind–body techniques while the other provided a single experiential session. Significant pre–post reductions in anxiety were demonstrated with each of the three mind–body therapies.

A Cochrane review of complementary and alternative therapies for pain management during labor reviewed 14 trials ($n = 1537$), 6 of which focused on mind–body therapies (Smith et al. 2006). Of these six, five involved teaching self-hypnosis ($n = 729$) and the sixth ($n = 34$), relaxation through autogenics or Lamaze preparation. The women who had been taught self-hypnosis had diminished requirements for analgesia and epidurals and were more satisfied with their pain management than the controls.

While there is the common belief that anxiety or stress may contribute to fertility issues, there has been little research investigating the influences of mind–body therapies on conception. Alice Domar and her colleagues (2000a, 2000b) used a RCT to compare the efficacy of a 5-year three-arm group-based intervention (multimodal relaxation, social support, and tau; $n = 184$) with women who experienced two years of infertility. The therapies included autogenics, relaxation response meditation, PMR, imagery, and cognitive restructuring. Over time, the standard care arm suffered from significant attrition and required redistribution of participants into the other treatment arms. At 12 months, both treatment arms showed significantly lower levels of psychological distress and higher conception rates than the control; the mind–body group showed greater reduction in distress than the social support group. The conception rate in both treatment groups was, however, remarkably similar, 55% and 54%, as compared to 20% for the control.

Only a few trials have been carried out to explore the influence of mind–body practices during menopause (Nedrow et al. 2006). Chattha et al. (2008) studied the impact of an 8-week, daily yoga therapy program consisting of postures, breathing, and meditation in 120 perimenopausal Indian women randomized to yoga or an exercise control. Significantly decreased vasomotor symptoms and perceived stress were observed for the yoga group. Slow diaphragmatic breathing and a paced respiration practice have been shown to be effective for decreasing the intensity and/or frequency of hot flashes (Irvin et al. 1996; Freedman and Woodard 1992, 1995). Several mind–body therapies may show positive benefits for climeratic symptoms, as slow breathing is a by-product of the relaxation response invoked through mind–body practices. A new multisite research initiative, "Menopause Strategies: Finding Lasting Answers for Symptoms and Health (MsFLASH)," launched in 2008 by the NIH should be able to clarify whether other mind–body therapies may also help with climacteric symptoms (National Institute of Aging 2008).

BREAST CANCER: IMMUNE PARAMETERS, EMOTIONAL DISTRESS

Despite the very high use of mind–body practices among women with cancer (Eschiti 2007; Gansler et al. 2008), there has been no systematic review of their effectiveness for patients receiving treatment for breast cancer. Many studies have examined the impact of guided imagery, writing, and mindfulness-based stress reduction (MBSR) on breast cancer immune parameters, emotional distress, side effects of chemotherapy, and frequency of medical visits (Carlson and Garland 2005; Carlson et al. 2003, 2004, 2007; Low et al. 2006; Stanton et al. 2002; Roffe et al. 2005; Targ and Levine 2002). The small size of the samples and the variable quality of the study designs preclude suggesting one therapy over another.

A recently published RCT assessed the impact of a weekly group-based intervention using PMR with 227 women with stage II breast cancer receiving adjuvant cancer treatment (Andersen 2007a, 2007b). Reductions in emotional distress at four months predicted greater improvement in health at 12 months; the more frequently women practiced relaxation, the greater the reduction in symptoms (Andersen 2007b).

Implications for Clinical Practice

An extensive body of literature supports use of a variety of therapies for women's health conditions, and can help health providers formulate recommendations for their patients. A summary of these techniques and conditions is presented in Table 5.2. Practice guidelines from several professional organizations now include recommendations for specific mind–body therapies. The American College of Cardiology (Vogel et al. 2005), the American Sleep Association (Morgenthaler et al. 2006), the American College of Physicians (Chou and Huffman 2007), the American Pain Society (Chou and Huffman 2007), the American Headache Society (Silberstein 2000), and the American Academy of Neurology (Silberstein 2000) all provide mind–body practice recommendations.

To help women make informed choices, providers need to be able to explain differences in mind–body techniques and suggest ways to learn them. While many excellent and cost-effective educational CDs and DVDs are available, it is also important to guide women to local resources and teachers. Since several treatments may be equally effective in alleviating emotional distress or pain, providers would do well to take into account treatment cost and preference, as well as the patient lifestyle and personality, in developing recommendations.

Table 5.2. Summary of Clinical Evidence

Health Conditions	Level of Evidence		Positive Findings
	Strong	Emerging	
Overall health Psychological health Physical health	Expressive writing (EW) EW; MBSR EW	 MBSR	Small to moderate effect sizes
Chronic pain Back pain Fibromyalgia Rheumatoid Arthritis Cancer symptoms	Multimodal group, Biofeedback Hypnosis PMR	Yoga MBSR	Reduction in pain intensity and distress outcomes-depression
CVD-related	Multimodal group, TM		Reduction in all-cause and cardiac mortality, nonfatal MI recurrences
Hypertension	Multimodal group, TM, PMR Biofeedback, Tai-Chi, Qi-qong		Reduction in SBP and DBP, frequency of medication use
Headaches	Thermal biofeedback Autogenics, PMR		Reduction in headache activity
Incontinence*	Biofeedback		Reduction in episodes
Insomnia	Relaxation, PMR, Biofeedback, Multimodal		Sleep onset latency, total time awake after sleep onset
Mental Health Anxiety Depression (major) (minor)	 Applied relaxation group, meditation, PMR MBCT	 MBSR Music	Reduction in state anxiety Reduction in major depression relapse
Surgical outcomes	Hypnosis, with/without imagery, autogenics	Music	Lesser pain intensity, medication use, length of hospital stay and recovery time

(continued)

Table 5.2. (Continued)

Health Conditions	Level of Evidence		Positive Findings
	Strong	Emerging	
Women's Health Fertility		Multimodal relaxation group; Social support group	Increased conception, decreased emotional distress
PMS	PMR, guided imagery		Decreased pain
Pregnancy	PMR, self-hypnosis		Reduction in anxiety and pharmacological analgesia, more satisfied with labor pain management
Menopause		Yoga	Reduction in hot flashes, vasomotor symptoms, anxiety
Breast cancer		Group with PMR	Reduction in emotional distress' Better immune parameters

* In addition to Astin, see NIH (2007).

Developing a regular mind–body practice, like any new habit, takes time, motivation, patience, and perseverance. For some women, coaching and regular follow-up will help reinforce their efforts. In addition, some women may need monitoring to reduce their dosages of pain or hypertension medications. For example, a recent RCT demonstrated that 80 of 122 patients (both male and female) with elevated hypertension were able to reduce their medications after 16 weeks of practicing mindfulness meditation and relaxation techniques (Dusek et al. 2008).

Health care providers may also want to develop a personal mind–body practice. Studies demonstrate that physicians are more likely to recommend a mind–body practice if they themselves have had some personal experience (Astin et al. 2005, 2006). A study of psychotherapists in training found that psychiatric patients were more satisfied with the course of their therapy and showed less distress if their practitioners practiced Zen meditation (Grepmair et al. 2007a, 2007b).

I often suggest that practitioners develop a brief ritual inbetween seeing their patients in order to help them re-engage and be present with each new person. Before opening or knocking on the door of the next patient, providers can pause and slowly take several deep breaths. Or they can silently repeat the name of the patient they are about to see and direct a simple four-phrase loving-kindness meditation: "May you live in safety. May you be happy. May you be healthy, May you live with ease." Alternatively, thoughts of gratitude after seeing each patient may be brought to awareness. Practitioners can also actively use the hand-washing process as a deliberate point of focus for clearing their mind; paying attention to the flow of the water and sensations touching each finger. Any of these strategies may help providers replenish themselves, refocus, and re-engage with their own healing presence so they can truly be present to each patient.

Summary

Stress is a condition of American life that can adversely affect the health and well-being of women. Research demonstrates that mind–body therapies can mitigate symptoms of stress and facilitate mental and physical health. The absence of gender-based systematic reviews on most mind–body therapies precludes making firm conclusions for the efficacy of one particular technique over another.

For some mind–body therapies, such as meditation or writing, the evidence demonstrates a strong reduction in emotional distress and improved immune function. For others, such as hypnosis, PMR and autogenics, the findings support pain reduction after invasive surgery. With tai-chi, yoga, and guided imagery, the literature is less conclusive, presenting a more heterogeneous picture of mixed findings across a wide spectrum of disorders. Future research will hopefully clarify which patients and conditions may benefit most from use of any one particular technique. But for the time being, there is sufficient evidence for health care providers to recommend mind–body practices to women for disease prevention and health promotion.

REFERENCES

Ader R. ed. *Psychoneuroimmunology*, Vol I and II, 4th ed. New York: Elsevier Academic Press; 2007.

American Psychological Association. Stress in America. http://apahelpcenter. mediaroom.com/file.php/138/Stress+in+America+REPORT+FINAL.doc. Accessed October 24, 2000.

Andersen BL, Farrar WB, Golden-Kreutz D, Emery CF, Glaser R, Crespin T, Carson WE. Distress reduction from a psychological intervention contributes to improved health for cancer patients. *Brain Behav Immun.* 2007a;21(7):953–961.

Andersen BL, Shelby RA, Golden-Kreutz DM. RCT of a psychological intervention for patients with cancer: I. mechanisms of change. *J Consult Clin Psychol.* 2007b;75(6):927–938.

Anderson JW, Liu C, Kryscio RJ. Blood pressure response to transcendental meditation: a meta-analysis. *Am J Hypertens.* 2008;21(3):310–316.

Antonio MH, Lutgendorf SK, Cole SW, et al. The influence of bio-behavioural factors on tumour biology: pathways and mechanisms. *Nat Rev Cancer.* 2006;6(3):240–248.

Astin JA, Shapiro SL, Eisenberg DM, Forys KL. Mind-body medicine: state of the science, implications for practice. *J Am Brd Fam Prac.* 2003;16(2):131–147.

Astin JA, Goddard TG, Forys KL. Barriers to the integration of mind-body medicine: perceptions of physicians, residents, and medical students. *Explore.* 2005;1(4):278–283.

Astin JA, Soeken K, Sierpina VS, Clarridge BR. Barriers to the integration of psychosocial factors in medicine: Results of a national survey of physicians. *J Am Board Fam Med.* 2006;19:557–565.

Barnes PM, Powell-Griner E, McFann K, Nahin RL. Complementary and alternative medicine use among adults: United States, 2002. *Adv Data.* 2004;(343):1–19.

Bastani F, Hidarnia A, Kazemnejad A, Vafaei M, Kashanian M. A randomized controlled trial of the effects of applied relaxation training on reducing anxiety and perceived stress in pregnant women. *J Midwifery Womens Health.* 2005;50(4):e36–40.

Beddoe AE, Lee KA. Mind-body interventions during pregnancy. *J Obstet Gynecol Neonatal Nurs.* 2008;37(2):165–175.

Carlson LE, Garland SN. Impact of mindfulness-based stress reduction (MBSR) on sleep, mood, stress and fatigue symptoms in cancer outpatients. *Int J Behav Med.* 2005;12(4):278–285.

Carlson LE, Speca M, Patel KD, Goodey E. Mindfulness-based stress reduction in relation to quality of life, mood, symptoms of stress, and immune parameters in breast and prostate cancer outpatients. *Psychosom Med.* 2003;65(4):571–581.

Carlson LE, Speca M, Patel KD, Goodey E. Mindfulness-based stress reduction in relation to quality of life, mood, symptoms of stress and levels of cortisol, dehydroepiandrosterone sulfate (DHEAS) and melatonin in breast and prostate cancer outpatients. *Psychoneuroendocrinol.* 2004;29(4):448–474.

Carlson LE, Speca M, Faris P, Patel KD. One year pre-post intervention follow-up of psychological, immune, endocrine and blood pressure outcomes of mindfulness-based stress reduction (MBSR) in breast and prostate cancer outpatients. *Brain Behav Immun.* 2007;21(8):1038–1049.

Cepeda MS, Carr DB, Lau J, Alvarez H. Music for pain relief. *Cochran Database Sys Rev.* 2006, 2:CD004843.

Chandola T, Brunner E, Marmot, M. Chronic Stress at work and metabolic syndrome. *Brit Med J.* 2006;332(7540):521–525.

Chattha R, Raghuram N, Venkatram P, Hongasandra NR. Treating the climacteric symptoms in Indian women with an integrated approach to yoga therapy: a randomized control study. *Menopause.* 2008;15(5):862–870.

Chida Y, Steptoe A. Positive psychological well-being and mortality: a quantitative review of prospective observational studies. *Psychosomatic Med.* 2008;70:741–756.

Chou R, Huffman LH. Nonpharmacologic therapies for acute and chronic low back pain: a review of the evidence for an American Pain Society/American College of Physicians clinical practice guideline. *Ann Intern Med.* 2007;147(7):492–504.

Coelho, H, Canter, P, Ernst, E. Mindfulness-based cognitive therapy: evaluating current evidence and informing future research. *J Consult Clin Psych.* 2007;75(6):1000–1005.

Cohen S, Janicki-Deverts D, Miller GE. Psychological stress and disease. *JAMA.* 2007;298(14):1685–1687.

Cohen S, Doyle WJ, Turner RB, Alper CM, Skoner DP. Emotional style and susceptibility to the common cold. *Psychosomat Med.* 2003;65(4):652–657.

Cohen S, Alper CM, Doyle WJ, Treanor JJ, Turner RB. Positive emotional style predicts resistance to illness after experimental exposure to rhinovirus or influenza a virus. *Psychosom Med.* 2006;68(6):809–815.

Damjanovic AK, Yang Y, Glaser R, et al. Accelerated telomere erosion is associated with a declining immune function of caregivers of Alzheimer's disease patients. *J Immunol.* 2007;179(6):4249–4254.

Danner DD, Snowden DA, Friesen WV. Positive emotions in early life and longevity: findings from the nun study. *J Pers Soc Psychol.* 2001;80:804–813.

Davis M. Is life more difficult on mars or venus? A meta-analytic review of sex differences in major and minor life events. *Soc Behav Med.* 1999:83–97.

Domar AD, Clapp D, Slawsby E, Kessel B, Orav J, Freizinger M. The impact of group psychological interventions on distress in infertile women. *Health Psychol.* 2000a;19(6):568–575.

Domar AD, Clapp D, Slawsby EA, Dusek J, Kessel B, Freizinger M. Impact of group psychological interventions on pregnancy rates in infertile women. *Fertil Steril.* 2000b;73(4):805–811.

Dusek JA, Hibberd PL, Buczynski B, et al. Stress management versus lifestyle modification on systolic hypertension and medication elimination: a randomized trial. *J Altern Complement Med.* 2008;14(2):129–138.

Eppel ES, Blackburn EH, Lin J, et al. Accelerated telomere shortening in response to life stress. *Proc Natl Acad Sci U S A.* 2004;101(49):17312–1735.

Eschiti VS. Lesson from comparison of CAM use by women with female-specific cancers to others: it's time to focus on interaction risks with CAM therapies. *Integr Cancer Ther.* 2007;6(4):313–344.

Fang CY, Miller SM, Bovbjerg DH, et al. Perceived stress is associated with impaired T-cell response to HPV16 in women with cervical dysplasia. *Ann Behav Med.* 2008;35:87–96.

Fava GA, Sonino N. The clinical domains of psychosomatic medicine. *J Clin Psychiatry.* 2005;66(7):849–858.

Freedman RR, Woodard S. Biochemical and thermoregulatory effects of behavioral treatment for menopausal hot flashes. *Menopause*. 1995;2(4):211–218.

Freedman RR, Woodward S. Behavioral treatment of menopausal hot flushes: evaluation by ambulatory monitoring. *Am J Obstet Gynecol*. 1992;167(2):436–439.

Frattaroli J. Experimental disclosure and its moderators: a meta-analysis. *Psychol Bull*. 2006;132(6):823–865.

Gansler T, Kaw C, Crammer C, Smith T. A population-based study of prevalence of complementary methods use by cancer survivors: a report from the American Cancer Society's studies of cancer survivors. *Cancer*. 2008;113(5):1048–1057.

Grepmair L, Mitterlehner F, Loew T, Nickel M. Promotion of mindfulness in psychotherapists in training: preliminary study. *Eur Psychiatry*. 2007a;22(8):485–489.

Grepmair L, Mitterlehner F, Loew T, Bachler E, Rother W, Nickel M. Promoting mindfulness in psychotherapists in training influences the treatment results of their patients: a randomized, double-blind, controlled study. *Psychother Psychosom*. 2007b;76(6):332–338.

Grossman P, Niemann L, Schmidt S, Walach H. Mindfulness-based stress reduction and health benefits. a meta-analysis. *J Psychosom Res*. 2004;57(1):35–43.

Helgesson O, Cabrera C, Lapidus L, Bengtsson C, Lissner L. Self-reported stress levels predict subsequent breast cancer in a cohort of Swedish women. *Eur J Cancer Prev*. 2003;12(5):377–381.

Hoglund CO, Axen J, Kemi C, et al. Changes in immune regulation in response to examination stress in atopic and healthy individuals. *Clin Exp Allergy*. 2006;36(8):982–992.

Irvin JH, Domar AD, Clark C, Zuttermeister PC, Friedman R. The effects of relaxation response training on menopausal symptoms. *J Psychosom Obstet Gynaecol*. 1996;17(4):202–207.

Irribarren C, Sidney S, Bild DE, et al. Association of hostility with coronary artery calcification in young adults: the CARDIA study. Coronary artery risk development in young adults. *JAMA*. 2000;283(19):2546–2551.

Jacobs GD. The physiology of mind-body interactions: the stress response and the relaxation response. *J. Altern Complement Med*. 2001;7 Suppl 1: S83–92.

Jensen M, Patterson DR. Hypnotic treatment of chronic pain. *J Behav Med*. 2006;29(1):95–124.

Kessler RC, McGonagle KA, Zhao S, Nelson CB, Hughes M, Eshleman S, Wittchen HU, Kendler KS. Lifetime and 12-month prevalence of DSM-III-R psychiatric disorders in the United States. Results from the National Comorbidity Survey. *Arch Gen Psychiatry*. 1994;51(1):8–19.

Kirkwood G, Rampes H, Tuffrey V, Richardson J, Pilkington K. Yoga for anxiety: a systematic review of the research evidence. *Br J Sports Med*. 2005;39(12):884–891.

Lee MS, Pittler MH, Ernst E. Tai chi for rheumatoid arthritis: systematic review. *Rheumatol (Oxford)*. 2007;46(11):1648–1651.

Lee MS, Pittler MH, Ernst E. Tai chi for osteoarthritis: a systematic review. *Clin Rheumatol*. 2008;27(2):211–218.

Lee MS, Pittler MH, Guo R, Ernst E. Qigong for hypertension: a systematic review of randomized clinical trials. *J Hypertens*. 2007;25(8):1525–1532.

Lillberg K, Verkasalo PK, Kaprio J, Teppo L, Helenius H, Koskenvuo M. Stressful life events and risk of breast cancer in 10,808 women: a cohort study. *Am J Epidemiol.* 2003;157(5):415–423.

Low CA, Stanton AL, Danoff-Burg S. Expressive disclosure and benefit finding among breast cancer patients: mechanisms for positive health effects. *Health Psychol.* 2006;25(2):181–189.

Manzoni GM, Pagnini F, Castelnuovo G, Molinari E. Relaxation training for anxiety: a ten-years systematic review with meta-analysis. *BMC Psychiatry.* 2008;8:41.

Maratos AS, Gold C, Wang X, Crawford MJ. Music therapy for depression. *Cochrane Database Syst Rev.* 2008;(1):CD004517.

McEwen BS, Lasley EN. *The End of Stress as We Know It.* Washington, DC: Joseph Henry Press; 2002.

Mittleman MA, Maclure M, Sherwood JB, et al. Triggering of acute myocardial infarction onset by episodes of anger. Determinants of Myocardial Infarction Onset Study Investigators. *Circulation.* 1995;92(7):1720–1725.

Montgomery GH, Bovbjerg DH, Schnur JB, et al. A randomized clinical trial of a brief hypnosis intervention to control side effects in breast surgery patients. *J Natl Cancer Inst.* 2007;99(17):1304–1312.

Morgenthaler T, Kramer M, Alessi C, et al. Practice parameters for the psychological and behavioral treatment of insomnia: an update. An American academy of sleep medicine report. *Sleep.* 2006;29(11):1415–1419.

National Center for Complementary and Alternative Medicine. Backgrounder. Mind-Body medicine: an overview. http://nccam.nih.gov/health/backgrounds/mindbody.htm, Accessed September 24, 2008.

National Institute of Aging. New NIH research initiative to test treatments for menopausal symptoms. http://nia.nih.gov/NewsAndEvents/PressReleases/PR20080917menopause. Accessed September 24, 2008

NIH state-of-the science conference statement on prevention of fecal and urinary incontinence in adults. *NIH Consense State Sci.* 2007:12–14:24(1);1–37.

Nedrow A, Miller J, Walker M, Nygren P, Huffman LH, Nelson HD. Complementary and alternative therapies for the management of menopause-related symptoms. *Arch Intern Med.* 2006;166:1453–1465.

Nestoriuc Y, Rief W, Martin A. Meta-analysis of biofeedback for tension-type headache: efficacy, specificity, and treatment moderators. *J Consult Clin Psychol.* 2008;76(3):379–396.

Ospina MB, Bond K, Karkhaneh M. Meditation practices for health: state of the research. *Evid Rep Technol Assess (Full Rep).* 2007;155:1–263.

Pilkington K, Kirkwood G, Rampes H, Richardson J. Yoga for depression: the research evidence. *J Affect Disord.* 2005;89(1–3):13–24.

Plagnol A, Easterlin R. Aspirations, attainments, and satisfaction: life cycle differences between American woman and men. *J Happiness Stud.* 2008. DOI: 10.1007/s10902-008-9106-5.

Proctor ML, Murphy PA, Pattison HM, Suckling J, Farquhar CM. Behavioural interventions for primary and secondary dysmenorrhoea. *Cochrane Database Syst Rev.* 2007(3):CD002248.

Rainforth MV, Schneider RH, Nidich SI, Gaylord-King C, Salerno JW, Anderson JW. Stress reduction programs in patients with elevated blood pressure: a systematic review and meta-analysis. *Curr Hypertens Rep.* 2007; 9(6):520–528.

Roffe L, Schmidt K, Ernst E. A systematic review of guided imagery as an adjuvant cancer therapy. *Psychooncology.* 2005;14(8):607–617.

Segerstrom SC, Miller GE. Psychological stress and the human immune system: a meta-analytic study of 30 years of inquiry. *Psychol Bull.* 2004;130(4):601–630.

Silberstein SD. Practice parameter: evidence-based guidelines for migraine headache (an evidence-based review): report of the Quality Standards Subcommittee of the American Academy of Neurology. *Neurology.* 2000;55(6):754–762. http://www.neurology.org/cgi/content/full/neurology;56/1/142-a.

Smith CA, Collins CT, Cyna AM, Crowther CA. Complementary and alternative therapies for pain management in labour. *Cochrane Database Syst Rev.* 2006(4): CD003521.

Stanton AL, Danoff-Burg S, Sworowski LA. Randomized, controlled trial of written emotional expression and benefit finding in breast cancer patients. *J Clin Oncol.* 2002;20(20):4160–4168.

Steptoe A, Wardle J, Marmot M. Positive affect and health-related neuroendocrine, cardiovascular, and inflammatory processes. *Proc Natl Acad Sci.* 2005;102(18):6508–6512.

Targ EF, Levine EG. The efficacy of a mind-body-spirit group for women with breast cancer: a randomized controlled trial. *Gen Hosp Psych.* 2002; 24(4):238–248.

Taylor SE, Klein LC, Lewis BP, Gruenewald TL, Gurung RA, Updegraff JA. Biobehavioral responses to stress in females: tend-and-befriend, not fight-or-flight. *Psychol Rev.* 2000;107(3):411–429.

Taylor SE. *The Tending Instinct: How Nurturing Is Essential to Who We Are and How We Live.* New York: Holt; 2002.

Teixeira J, Martin D, Prendiville O, Glover V. The effects of acute relaxation on indices of anxiety during pregnancy. *J Psychosom Obstet Gynaecol.* 2005;26(4):271–276.

Thacker PH, Han LY, Kamat AA, et al. Chronic stress promotes tumor growth and angiogenesis in a mouse model of ovarian carcinoma. *Nat Med.* 2006;12(8):939–944.

Tolin DF, Foa EB. Sex differences in trauma and posttraumatic stress disorder: a quantitative review of 25 years of research. *Psychol Bull.* 2006;132(6):959–992.

Vieten C, Astin J. Effects of a mindfulness-based intervention during pregnancy on prenatal stress and mood: results of a pilot study. *Arch Womens Ment Health.* 2008;11(1):67–74.

Vogel JHK, Bolling SF, Costello RB, et al. Integrating complementary medicine into cardiovascular medicine. A report of the American College of Cardiology Foundation Task Force on Clinical Expert Consensus Documents (Writing Committee to Develop an Expert Consensus Document on Complementary and Integrative Medicine). *J Am Col Cardio.* 2005;46(1):184–221.

Wang C, Collet JP, Lau J. The effect of Tai Chi on health outcomes in patients with chronic conditions: a systematic review. *Arch Intern Med.* 2004;164(5):493–501.

Wang J, Korczykowski M, Rao H, et al. Gender difference in neural response to psychological stress. *Soc Cogn Affect Neurosci.* 2007;2(3):227–239.

Weik U, Herforth A, Kolb-Bachofen V, Deinzer R. Acute stress induces proinflammatory signaling at chronic inflammation sites. *Psychosom Med.* 2008; 906–912.

Williams RB, Chesney MA. Psychosocial factors and prognosis in established coronary artery disease. The need for research on interventions. *JAMA.* 1993;270(15):1860–1861.

Wittstein IS, Thiemann DR, Lima JAC, et al. Neurohumoral features of myocardial stunning due to sudden emotional stress. *N Engl J Med.* 2005;352(6):539–548.

Yeh GY, Wang C, Wayne PM, Phillips RS. The effect of tai chi exercise on blood pressure: a systematic review. *Prev Cardiol.* 2008;11(2):82–89.

6

Women, Soul Wounds, and Integrative Medicine

BEVERLY LANZETTA

It should be the obligation of all physicians to respond to, as well as attempt to relieve, all suffering if possible. Therefore, physicians should be able to communicate with their patients about their patients' spirituality as integral to the way their patients cope with suffering. To ask a patient about his or her spiritual beliefs is essential to knowing who the patient is, how the patient copes with illness, and how the patient can heal (Puchalski 1999).

In our various forms of contemporary analysis, we have yet to take a serious look at the effect spiritual suffering and soul wounds exert on women's health. An important fact that impedes the medical profession's recognition of the spiritual implications of women's health has to do with a Western cultural tendency to see suffering as a purely physical response to pain, and to separate the spirit from the body. The effect of this split between the material and spiritual aspects of health continues to have enormous ramifications in physician care and in a woman's capacity for well-being and healing. Despite advances in understanding the cultural, economic, and racial factors that impact health, and the important strides made in recognizing gender in medicine, there continues to be a paucity of research on the more subtle violation to women's spirits and its impact on women's health care. This denial or refusal to discuss soul afflictions blocks women's ability to claim and name themselves as subjects of their own healing and limits the full range of medical options available to health professionals and their patients.

If spirituality is seen as just one more adjunct modality within the various complementary and alternative medical (CAM) options, it truncates the full ability of integrative medicine to actualize its potential as a healing art in two important ways. First, spirituality is selectively incorporated into the integrative model for reasons of understanding, information, or increased empathy between physicians and patients rather than being embraced as a comprehensive perspective on healing, and as an integral system of interpretation, diagnosis, and treatment.

Second, spirituality, when it is incorporated into Western medical models, tends to be researched and applied through a particular evidence-based lens. Research on spirituality in medicine has focused on the effect of external indicators of religious adherence or faith, such as prayer and meditation, or the efficacy of forgiveness, hope, and other virtues on health outcomes. While these studies have helped to expand the range of integrative medicine, they are not designed to take into account the more subtle but powerful care of the soul and wounding of the spirit that in traditional societies, such as the Hopi and Navajo, are always implicated in physical illness.

If integrative medicine recognizes that meaning in one's life is a positive factor in response to illness, then it must take into account how inner wounding effects the totality of women's health and healing. I begin this chapter with a brief overview of current views on spirituality and integrative medicine. I then discuss a specific feminine path to healing—via feminina—and the destructive force of socially sanctioned violence—overt and subtle—against women's souls, and its consequent physical and mental health effects. I end the chapter with positive resources for women's healing, including a description of a distinctive spiritual process of integration, "dark night of the feminine," and some suggestions for health care practitioners.

Spirituality and Integrative Medicine

Integrative medicine, as practiced and defined today, is a vision of health care that focuses on health and healing rather than disease, and values the relationship between patient and physician. It is premised on patients being treated as whole persons—minds and spirits, as well as physical bodies—who participate actively in their own health. Integrative medicine also honors the innate ability of the body to heal and integrates the best of CAM with the best of conventional medicine to facilitate long-term health outcomes (Maizes et al. 2002a, 2002b).

One of the most significant and challenging dimensions of integrative medicine is the inclusion of spirituality in both physicians' and patients' understanding of health and healing. Numerous studies have demonstrated the positive effects prayer and meditation, and religious practice or faith in a higher power, exert on health outcomes, ability to cope with illness, and on patients' reported increase of well-being (Benson and Stark 1997; Bearon and Koenig 1997; Dossey 1993, 1997). Increasingly, the spirituality of medicine—including energy medicine, mind–body medicine, therapeutic touch, homeopathy, and traditional forms of Asian healing modalities—is incorporated into the integrative model.

All of these styles draw on the historical usage of "spirit" as that realm of reality associated with the breath of life. Without the spirit—the animating principle— there is no life. While many religions do not have a word corresponding to the term "spirituality," they nonetheless affirm the holiness of life and the realm of the spirit. Spirituality, then, can be defined as the core or inner life of the person, sometimes called the soul or spirit. In this definition, all beings—human and nonhuman—have an inner life and thus are imbued with spirit (Edmondson 2005; Gabriel 2000; Larson 2003; Massey 1996; Puchalski 2002).

Today, spirituality is used in secular and religious contexts, and is applied across and within disciplines, as well as in medicine and other healing arts. In a sense, spirituality has become a kind of universal code word to indicate the human search for meaning and purpose in life, and as a quest for transcendent truth. In contrast to religion, which is an institutional and culturally determined approach to faith, spirituality is found in all human societies through an individual experience of the divine, a connection to nature, and/or through religious practice.

A spiritual interpretation helps physicians to recognize the spiritual needs and implications of their patients' ills, and thus to refer them to the appropriate professional. It also serves as a point of discussion with patients and a guiding analysis of their physical problems. A spiritual sensibility helps in healing by calling attention to the fact that healing involves physical and spiritual elements. The body may be repaired but the soul may be pained or in need of sustenance. This ability to see the whole person and the type of healing that is required to bring full health is at the heart of the practice of the integrative physician.

The centrality of the spirit in healing and health is being increasingly incorporated into medical school curriculums and by the burgeoning field of integrative medicine. At the same time, integrative medical practice is challenged to understand that spirituality is not another adjunct to medicine proper, another modality to include in the menu of complementary or alternative options. Rather, spirituality is a more fundamental, whole life interpretation, as it is already inscribed in the structure of life itself—the human body, consciousness, and all living organisms. It involves an awareness of the whole person—both physician and patient—as having an inner life or soul, a life that responds to and is sustained by nonmaterial factors. A spiritual perspective in medicine also recognizes that the inner life can sustain wounds and illness, as well as being a source of vitality and change.

Just as other medical and life situations follow stages of transformation, so too does the spirit or soul. In describing the spirit, we must keep in mind that it is not a monolithic, static, or finalized reality. Rather, the spirit is dynamic, continually changing and learning in response to stimuli from the physical, mental, emotional, and psychic realms.

In entering into the privacy and mystery of a person's healing, health professionals observe a depth of experience that is seldom discussed in our culture. There are times in every person's life where changes in spiritual outlook, wounding of the heart, or denial of illness, pain, and death impact on the spiritual journey. Many practitioners are struck by how profoundly people suffer spiritually, and how difficult it is to heal this suffering when there is not a language and a socially sanctioned way of discussing the interior life. Further, physicians express concern that these topics are more suited to clergy, pastors, rabbis, and other religious professionals. Medical researchers also question how spirituality is defined and what role it should play in the overall curriculum of medical students, in medical practice, and in patient care. Foremost among these concerns is whether physicians are crossing an ethical divide by asking patients about their spiritual beliefs, taking spiritual surveys, or including religious practices in health care (Berry 2005; Hall and Curlin 2004; Hall et al. 2004; Post et al. 2000; Sloan 2000, 2006).

Physicians, as well as their patients, move through changes in their spiritual lives, they are illumined, have moments of insight, feel compunction and sorrow, struggle through uncertainty and doubt, suffer loss of prestige or self-identity, and emerge with deeper integration and self-reliance. Because our culture tends to neglect the spiritual suffering or soul wound that underlies the process of healing, it is not part of conventional thought to speak about matters of the heart. Trained to be objective and emotionally neutral, physicians may lack the skills to discuss with patients the embarrassment, shame, or vulnerability that often accompanies illness and healing. The deeper truths of sustaining health may be shrouded in silence and mystery, and in the need for forgiveness and reconciliation. It is in the willingness of physicians and patients to open themselves to these sufferings and fears, and then to share them with others, which is vital to the whole healing process. Thus, it is important for physicians and patients to have permission to address questions of meaning and other significant life issues that traditionally have not been included in medical intake, but are at the core of integrative medicine as a healing art.

Spiritual Suffering and Women's Health

...much of the pain patients experience is not just physical pain, but also spiritual. In fact, from my clinical experience with patients, I have found that spiritual suffering underlies most of the pain that patients and their families experience. Pain is multifactorial: physical, emotional, social, and spiritual. ... the threat to one's physical body can also ... lead to spiritual or existential suffering, which can affect physical pain and manifest as physical symptoms (Puchalski 2006).

Numerous studies of medieval and contemporary women illustrate a female or feminine spiritual consciousness. Whether this consciousness can be ascribed to cultural, historical, or ontological factors is still in question. Nonetheless, without making an essentialist argument, there are tendencies common enough across cultures and historical periods to demarcate the outlines of a feminine spirituality. See Bynum 1984; Bynum 1991; Donnelly 1982; Harvey and Baring 1996; Jantzen 1999, 2000; King 1989, 1993; Newman 1987, 2003; Petroff 1994; Raphael 1996; Wiethaus 1993. Elsewhere, I have coined this spiritual consciousness "*via feminina*" or the way of the feminine, and contend that it speaks to a distinctive female path toward integration and healing (Lanzetta 2005). One historical constant in women's spiritual expression is an emphasis on an embodied, rather than abstract, spirituality. Across cultures and diverse time periods, women consistently name and practice a spirituality of the body, evident through biological life cycles and experiences of birth, menstruation, menopause, and dying. This lived, organic relationship between body, spirit, and nature is present in ancient goddess religions, medieval women mystics, indigenous traditions, as well as in contemporary women today. Attentiveness to the closeness of the spirit in everyday life places further emphasis on the interdependent relationship between body, mind, and spirit in sustaining women's health.

Research on other attributes associated with female spirituality indicate that women describe a more porous sense of self and are more closely attuned to and able to negotiate the permeable boundaries of body and spirit, mind and heart. Current research in neurobiology indicates that the female capacity to be relational, integrative, and holistic also has a biological basis in the brain. Studies indicate that the female brain excels in integrating and assimilating information from the two sides of the brain, recognizing emotional overtones, verbal and social skills and empathy; Alkire et al. 2005; Brizendine 2007; LeVay 1994; Rabinowicz et al. 1999; Sabbatini 2000; Schlaepfer et al. 1995. As a state of consciousness, women's spirituality tends to be relational and "undivided, that is to say, integral and holistic" (King 1989, 1993). It emphasizes qualities of mutuality, intimacy, and receptivity; its expression of the spirit tends to be nurturing, generative, sacrificial, and merciful. Women's spirituality is also bounded by a fierce determination, resiliency, and commitment to children, family, society, and work. Virtues of intimacy, mutuality, communion, and receptivity, often dismissed by material culture as signs of weakness, are distinctive soul strengths that guide women into states of consciousness capable of healing and transforming.

The richness of women's embodied spirituality is evident in their variety and creative expression. Deep founts of healing and soul renewal are found in the impressive panoply of spiritual resources traditionally used by women. From ancient times, women's healing rituals, ceremonies of life, devotional arts, and religious chanting and dance have been sources of strength. Often segregated from male religious privilege, women developed practices of domestic healing, including blessing with oils and water, lighting of candles, tending of sacred fires, intuitive medicine, and herbal cures. Among these many forms, women's communities encouraged reverence for nature and a model of emotional and spiritual nourishment that remain today vital to women's health and ability to overcome illness and other difficult life struggles.

Creating distinctive patterns of female spirituality, women throughout the world find enormous reserves of meaning in religious symbols, archetypes, and rituals. These diverse practices include devotion of Hispanic Catholic women to *Nuestra Señora de Guadalupe*; sacred yarn painting of Huichol Indian women of Mexico; women potters of South India; Eastern Orthodox women iconographers; Jewish women's rituals such as candle lighting and *mikva* (ritual cleansing); traditional rug weaving by Navajo women; Hopi spider women story-telling; vision quest of Lakota women; herbal medicine and spirit healing used by African and Haitian women; and Muslim women's veneration of Bibi Fatima.

In addition to the positive impact women's spirituality can exert on health outcomes, it is vital for health professionals to recognize that women also suffer from certain types of spiritual oppression simply because they are female. By virtue of living in societies that have been historically male-dominated, women in the global community sustain specific types of spiritual sufferings and soul wounds that are not found to the same degree in men. Understanding their causes and alleviation is critical to healing. Studies show that the various forms of personal and social violence—or "intimate violence"—women encounter on a daily basis exert their most profound effects on a woman's inner life or spirit (see Fisher 1988; Fortune 1989; Mananzan et al. 1996; West 1999). Domestic abuse, sexual politics, economic inequalities, and legitimate fear of rape, assault, and other types of intimate violence circumscribe the lives of women and girls on a daily basis. Even women who have never experienced overt physical or sexual violence remain alert to subtle forms of emotional diminishment, social control, or unequal share of child rearing, household and family responsibilities, and care giving.

Recent statistics provide a shocking view of worldwide abuses committed against women in all countries around the globe. "To cite an example, the worldwide economic and social marginalization of women, and their historical status as a permanent underclass are violent acts that rob a woman of self-worth, creating hidden scars in her being. Further, the global dimensions of women's suffering—rape, trafficking in women, wife-beating, bride burning, infanticide of girl babies, as well as the more subtle forms of social, religious, and economic violence" that rob women of dignity—impact on women's capacity to heal and restore themselves to wholeness" (Lanzetta 2005a). Least we think that American women are free of an assault on their integrity, every year in the United States alone, a woman is beaten every 18 minutes, 3 to 4 million are battered each year, and 4,000 beaten to death by their partners (Lanzetta 2005b; Tjaden and Thoennes 2006; UN Department of Public information 1991). Intimate violence is designed to depersonalize women's bodies, rape their souls, and destroy their resistance. This acceptance of the violation of women in the domestic sphere is reflected in shocking acts of violence that dehumanize and objectify women's bodies.

Medical professionals are starting to recognize that abuse and other forms of soul violations are implicated in women's mental, physical, and spiritual health and must become part of their integrative diagnosis and treatment plan (Marcus 2008; Nicolaidis et al. 2004). They are learning that soul injuries and violation of the feminine inevitably impact on women's inner life and physical health. Understanding the causes that generate these soul wounds is essential in designing healing outcomes. Aware of the unequal burden placed on women in societies and religious communities around the world, integrative medicine can advance women's health care by taking into account and analyzing the deeper spiritual causes and consequences of a subtle but equally powerful form of physical and soul illness—the oppression of women's spirit. "I refer to this as *spiritual oppression* and contend its recognition and healing is fundamental to women's health and healing. The core of this stance is that *women's spiritual oppression is the foundation of all her other oppressions*. What harms a woman's soul reverberates in her physical, emotional, and mental spheres, generating suffering in every area of her life." Similarly, violations of a woman's body and diminishment of her social power have a direct impact on the health and integrity of her spirit (Lanzetta 2005c).

What is spiritual oppression? The word "oppression" signifies an unjust exercise of authority or power by one person, group, or institution over another. Because the oppression I am referring to here is spiritual in nature, these varied interactions of personal, societal, and institutional control over women exert their influence beyond external events to invade a woman's psyche, soul, and body. Further, these abuses cannot be fully understood without recognizing how profoundly connected they are to cultural and religious devaluations of women as inferior to men. This fundamental belief in women's spiritual inferiority inevitably permeates the cultural imagination, and contributes to and fosters violent acts against women, as it most often remains unacknowledged and unnamed.

When I say that all forms of women's oppression are fundamentally spiritual oppression, I mean that acts of violence against women—overt or subtle—are directed first and foremost at the core of her nature—her inner life or spirit. Often fueled by unconscious motivations, spiritual oppression is the wrongful violation of the sanctity of a woman's self. Violence against women—personal and structural—can be seen as nothing less than a desire to harm or destroy women's unique and particular embodiment of the spirit.

Corporate forms of oppression are present when the medical community applies a model of Cartesian reductionism to the spiritual implications of women's health; dismisses or denies gender differences in research, diagnosis, and treatment plans; or trivializes women's ailments as symptomatic, psychosomatic, or hysterical. The social structures that allow the unequal distribution of health care and that exploit or dictate women's innate healing abilities effectively possess woman's inner life for they control in what way and in what measure women are valued, and their health concerns taken seriously.

The presence of spiritual suffering in a woman's life is the most significant indicator of her inability to handle illness and quiet the restlessness that divides her soul (see Fisher 1988). Elusive and difficult to grasp, spiritual violence invades the integrity of a woman's psyche and soul at such a primary level that most women cannot recognize or name what has harmed them. Unable to identify the source of their pain, women often blame themselves and develop strategies to protect their oppressors. This quality of soul suffering, which survives at the cost of women's spiritual diminishment, inflicts on women an unequal burden of sin and blame (Fiorenza 1996; Smith 1998; West 1999). Thus, without understanding the subtle ways in which her soul is violated and the fierceness that marks the site of her affliction, an integrative approach is unable to address the full range of women's health care options. Often unspoken, denied, and ridiculed, or dismissed as unimportant and emotional, women's soul wounds must be brought to consciousness to avoid the trivialization of their experience and for healing to occur.

Dark Night of the Feminine and Women's Healing

Within the inner life, a woman finds deep resources of healing. Foremost among these is statistical evidence of women's greater participation in prayer, religion, and other sources of meaning as well as women's capacity for determination, resiliency, and hope. In addition, women often undergo a unique spiritual healing process, what I call the "dark night of the feminine" that moves them from oppression and illness to liberation and healing (Lanzetta 2003a, 2003b, 2005). I have constructed this term from the ancient notion that transformation and healing requires a period of deconstruction or letting-go of old beliefs, wounds, and traumas, followed by an intense period of reintegration and soul healing. My particular usage of the term "dark night" is borrowed from the writings of the sixteenth century Spanish mystic, John of the Cross (John of the Cross 1991).

John depicts the dark night (Spanish, *noche oscura*) as a transformative stage of soul suffering prior to self-integration and divine intimacy. Torn by a wrenching inability to assuage the desolation of this dark passage, a person feels worthless and abandoned in the eyes of society, self, or her religion. Yet the soul is being illuminated by a light so bright it appears dark to the disordered and suffering spirit. The soul cannot see what it is or name what it knows. John says that this dark night is the secret teaching of love in which the soul of a person is released from suffering and is lifted up to a special realization of its original, undivided nature. Using different names and cosmological systems—great death, annihilation, dismemberment—the interior process of spiritual suffering and recognition of soul wounds, followed by the healing light of wisdom and integration, is found in all cultures and religions around the world. While there tends to be a bias in contemporary depictions that the "spirit" or "spirituality" transcends illness, suffering, and disease, this is not, however, the view in traditional religions or civilizations.

The specific attribution of the word "feminine" to dark night experiences indicates that there is another or additional dimension that women face beyond traditional accounts of transformation found in the world's religions. This process of healing specifically locates a woman's struggle to achieve fullness of being within her soul's internalization of the misogyny particular to her world, and of the violation of her womanhood. The night of the feminine is emphasized as a continuum of consciousness that brings women to experience and heal another level of alienation and fragmentation specifically associated with being *female*. This intensification of suffering precludes a break through into a new life of integration in which a woman discovers herself as worthy of healing, and as fundamentally good and whole.

Specific elements of this process include an experience of intense impasse, where a woman is caught between two worlds: she cannot go back to how family, society, or religion defined her, but she cannot go forward to a future as yet unimagined (FitzGerald 1986, 1996). The dark night process also can involve feelings of anguish, grief, and anger; self- and other-betrayal of deep needs and awareness of personal indignities disguised as socially sanctioned forms of women's oppression. Other wounds women have to overcome in the process of healing include the experience of being "nothing"; loss of self-identity or self-worth, often accompanied by self-loathing, guilt, anger, and shame; and internalization of the abuse committed by partners, society, clergy, religions, and family (Fisher 1988a; Friedman 2004; Kobeisy 2004; Mecham 2004).

The addition of the night of the feminine to the vocabulary of healing emphasizes its distinctiveness in a woman's spirituality and refines our understanding of the relationship between the interior life and health. When I say it is a feminine night, I mean women suffer afflictions to their most receptive and intimate nature, both in terms of the negative wounding sustained from violations of women's dignity, and the positive touching of the light of wisdom, which opens her soul to deeper reserves of communion and oneness. It is a dark night of the feminine not only because it occurs in females, but because the experience itself is the healing of the injury women sustain to their integrity of soul. This interior process, whereby a woman consciously or unconsciously experiences the effects of the violation of her body and spirit as female, becomes an essential precursor to her healing and a positive resource in combating illness, pain, suffering, and dying. The term "dark night of the feminine" helps health professionals to realize that even though the causes and conditions of illness may be inscrutable or unknown, the light of wisdom is a powerful healing resource in women's freedom of being and soul healing.

While the "dark night of the feminine" is not explicitly named or perhaps even understood as a spiritual process, physicians recount how women's resistance to healing often is the result of profound feelings of self-loathing, worthlessness, guilt, fear, and grief, fueled by a belief that they have sinned, are being punished by God, or do not deserve to be helped.

To illustrate her conviction that physicians' knowledge of their patients' personal belief systems and spiritual practices can aid in treatment, Christina M. Puchalski, Associate Professor of Medicine at George Washington University School of Medicine, tells this story:

> I once had a patient diagnosed with HIV who felt she had brought the disease on herself, that she had sinned and God was punishing her. As a result, she did not want to go ahead with any treatment plan. I didn't realize why she was so adamant about not taking her medicines until I asked about her spiritual history. Because I asked her I was able to get her help from a trained chaplain. Had I not addressed those issues, I would never have been able to figure out a way to help her (Christina Puchalski cited by Barbara Gabriel 2000).

Suggestions for Integrative Health Care

Awareness of spiritual suffering and soul healing in women is a complex topic that requires new ways of interpreting, diagnosing, and understanding healing of the whole person. Not all medical professionals can or should be prepared for this interior work. Yet, for those who find the more subtle dimensions of health care to be important, it is hoped that the path of *via feminina* and the transformative process of the dark night of the feminine will be of benefit and lead to further research on the profound interrelationship between physical health and spiritual states of consciousness.

Central to the integrative physician is to be of service, and to practice medicine with a loving and compassionate heart. In this way, a rapport is established between the physician and the patient that creates an atmosphere of trust and openness. This is especially important with patients who may be suffering from soul illness or who are confronting a terminal disease. In keeping with the philosophy of doing no harm, the following guidelines may be helpful to physicians and other health providers.

- Be open to a sight and inner wisdom beyond the physical, thus seeing patients as whole people with bodies and souls.
- Consider spirituality as a potentially important component of every patient's physical well-being and mental health.
- Listen to the signs and symptoms of the *inner life.*
- Become aware of your own spirituality, suffering, and ability to deal compassionately with your own and another's pain.
- Raise questions that allow for patient's reflection on their faith or religious beliefs, spiritual suffering, and emotional hopes and fears.
- Respect patient's privacy regarding spirituality and religion; do not impose your beliefs or faith on others.
- Be particularly attentive to subtle forms of spiritual oppression, coercion, and physical and emotional abuse in women.
- Recognize how women's more permeable self and capacity for synthesizing and integration may be implicated in certain types of illness, but also is a source of strength and resiliency.
- Provide female patients with resources for healing and for understanding their journey of *via feminina* and through the "dark night of the feminine."
- Refer patients to other experts, such as chaplains, spiritual directors, social workers, and psychologists when appropriate.
- Allow for and honor mystery.

REFERENCES

Alkire MT, Head K, Yeo A. *Intelligence in Men and Women is a Grey and White Matter*, participated in the study, which was supported in part by the National

Institute of Child Health and Human Development. University of California, Irvine (January 22, 2005). *ScienceDaily*. Retrieved from http://www.sciencedaily.com/releases/2005/01/050121100142.htm.

Bearon LB, Koenig R. Religious cognitions and use of prayer in health and Illness. *Gerontologist*. 30:249–253.

Benson H, Stark M. *Timeless Healing: The Power and Biology of Belief*. New York: Scribner; 1997.

Berry D. Methodological pitfalls in the study of religiosity and spirituality. *West J Nurs Res*. 2005;27(5):628–647.

Brizendine L. *The Female Brain*. New York: Broadway Books; 2007.

Bynum CW. *Fragmentation and Redemption: Essays on Gender and the Human Body in Medieval Religion*. New York: Zone Books; 1991.

Bynum CW. *Jesus as Mother: Studies in the Spirituality of the High Middle Ages*. Berkeley: University of California Press; 1984.

Donnelly DH. The sexual mystic: embodied spirituality. In: Giles ME, ed. *The Feminist Mystic and Other Essays on Women and Spirituality*. New York: Crossroad; 1982:120–141.

Dossey L. *Healing Words: The Power of Prayer and the Practice of Medicine*. San Francisco: Harper San Francisco; 1993.

Dossey L. *Prayer Is Good Medicine: How to Reap the Healing Benefits of Prayer*. San Francisco: Harper San Francisco; 1997.

Edmondson KA, et al. Spirituality predicts health and cardiovascular responses to stress in young adult women. *J Relig Health*. 2005;44:2.

Fiorenza ES. Ties that bind: domestic violence against women. In: Mananzan MJ, Oduyoye MA, Elsa Tamez, et al. eds. *Women Resisting Violence: Spirituality for Life*. Maryknoll, NY: Orbis Books; 1996:39–55.

Fisher K. The problem of anger. In: *Women at the Well: Feminist Perspectives on Spiritual Direction*. New York: Paulist Press; 1988a:154–174.

Fisher K. Violence against women: the spiritual dimension. In: *Women at the Well: Feminist Perspectives on Spiritual Direction*. New York: Paulist Press; 1988:175–192.

FitzGerald C. Impasse and dark night. In: Conn JW ed., *Women's Spirituality: Resources for Christian Development*. New York: Paulist Press; 1986, 1996:410–435.

Fortune MM. The transformation of suffering: a biblical and theological perspective. In: Brown JC, Bohn CR, eds. *Christianity, Patriarchy, and Abuse: A Feminist Critique*. New York: Pilgrim; 1989.

Friedman ME. Shame and illness: a Jewish perspective. *The Yale Journal for Humanities in Medicine*. September 18, 2004.

Gabriel B. Is spirituality good medicine: bridging the divide between science and faith. *AAMC Report*. 2000;9:13.

Hall D, Curlin F. Can physicians' care be neutral regarding religion? *Acad Med*. 2004:79(7):677–679.

Hall D, Koenig H, et al. Conceptualizing "religion": how language shapes and constrains knowledge in the study of religion and health. *Pers Biol Med*. 2004;47(3):386–401.

Harvey A, Baring A. *The Divine Feminine: Exploring the Feminine Face of God Around the World*. Berkeley: Conari Press; 1996.

Jantzen GM. *Becoming Divine: Towards a Feminist Philosophy of Religion*. Bloomington, IN: Indiana University Press; 1999.

Jantzen GM. *Julian of Norwich: Mystic and Theologian*. New York: Paulist Press; 2000.

John of the Cross, "The Dark Night," in *The Collected Works of St. John of the Cross, trans. Kieran Kavanaugh and Otilio Rodriquez*. Washington, DC: Institute of Carmelite Studies; 1991:353–457.

King U. *Women and Spirituality: Voices of Protest and Promise*. University Park, PA: The Pennsylvania State University Press; 1989, 1993.

King U. *Women and Spirituality: Voices of Protest and Promise*. University Park, PA: The Pennsylvania State University Press; 1989, 1993:88.

Kobeisy AN. Shame in the context of illness—an Islamic perspective. *The Yale Journal for Humanities in Medicine*. September 14, 2004

Lanzetta BJ. *Julian and Teresa as Cartographers of the Soul: A Contemplative Feminist Hermeneutic*. Paper delivered American Academy of Religion Annual Meeting, Atlanta, November, 2003a.

Lanzetta BJ. *The Soul of Woman and the Dark Night of the Feminine in St. Teresa of Avila*. Paper delivered American Academy of Religion Western Region (WESCOR), University of California Davis, March, 2003b.

Lanzetta BJ. *Radical Wisdom: A Feminist Mystical Theology*. Minneapolis: Fortress Press; 2005.

Lanzetta BJ. *Radical Wisdom: A Feminist Mystical Theology*. Minneapolis: Fortress Press; 2005a:63.

Lanzetta BJ. *Radical Wisdom: A Feminist Mystical Theology*. Minneapolis: Fortress Press; 2005b;186.

Lanzetta BJ. *Radical Wisdom: A Feminist Mystical Theology*. Minneapolis: Fortress Press; 2005c:68.

Larson DB. Spirituality's potential relevance to physical and emotional health: a brief review of quantitative research. *J Psychol Theol*. 2003;31:1:37–51.

LeVay S. *The Sexual Brain: The Female Brain*. Cambridge, MA: The MIT Press; 1994.

Maizes V, Koffler K, Fleishman S. Revisiting the health history: an integrative medicine approach. *Int J Integr Med*. 2002a;3:7–13.

Maizes V, Schneider C, et al. Integrative medical education: development and implementation of a comprehensive curriculum at the University of Arizona. *Acad Med*. 2002b;77:851–860.

Mananzan MJ, et al. eds. *Women Resisting Violence: Spirituality for Life*. Maryknoll, NY: Orbis Books; 1996.

Marcus EN. Screening for abuse may be key to ending it. *New York Times*, May 20, 2008; http://www.nytimes.com/2008/05/20/health/20abus.html

Nicolaidis C, et al. Violence, mental health and physical symptoms in an academic internal medicine practice. *J Gen Internal Med*. 2004;19.

Massey EA. Affirming spirituality and healing in medicine. *J Past Care*. 1996;50(3):235–237.

Mecham MP. Guilt in the context of illness—a protestant perspective. In Spirituality, Religious Wisdom, and the Care of the Patient (2004), *The Yale Journal of Humanities in Medicine.*

Newman B. *Gods and the Goddesses: Vision, Poetry, and Belief in the Middle Ages.* Philadelphia: University of Pennsylvania Press; 2003.

Newman B. *Sister of Wisdom: St. Hildegard's Theology of the Feminine.* Berkeley, University of California Press; 1987.

Petroff EA. *Body and Soul: Essays on Medieval Women and Mysticism.* New York: Oxford University Press; 1994.Post SG, et al. Physicians and patient spirituality: professional boundaries, competency, and ethics. *Ann Internal Med.* 2000;132(7):578–583.

Puchalski C cited by Barbara Gabriel in, Is spirituality good medicine? Bridging the divide between science and faith. *AAMC Reporter.* 2000:9:13. http://www.aamc.org/newsroom/reporter/oct2000/spirit.htm.

Puchalski CM, Touching the spirit: the essence of healing. *Spiritual Life.* 1999;43(3):154–159. http://www.spiritual-life.org/id30.htm.

Puchalski CM. *A Time for Listening and Caring: Spirituality and the Care of the Chronically Ill and Dying.* New York: Oxford University Press; 2006:21.

Puchalski CM. Forgiveness: spiritual and medical implications. *Yale J Human Med,* 2002. Series "Spirituality, Religious Wisdom, and the Care of the Patient," Yale.

Rabinowicz T, Dean DE, Petetot JM, de Courten-Myers GM. Gender differences in the human cerebral cortex: more neurons in males; more processes in females. *J Child Neurol.* 1999;14(2):98–107.

Raphael M. *Thealogy and Embodiment: The Post-Patriarchal Reconstruction of Female Sacrality.* Sheffield, England: Sheffield Academic Press; 1996.

Russell LM. Spirituality, struggle, and cultural violence. In: Mananzan, et al. eds. *Women Resisting Violence: Spirituality for Life.* Maryknoll, NY: Orbis Books; 1996:62–70.

Sabbatini RME. Are their differences between the Brains of Males and Females? *Mind & Brain: Electronic Magazine on Neuroscience.* Oct–Dec 2000; No. 11.

Schlaepfer TE, Harris GJ, Tien AY, Peng L, Lee S, Pearlson GD. Structural differences in the cerebral cortex of healthy female and male subjects: a magnetic resonance imaging study. *Psychiatry Res.* 1995;61(3):129–135.

Sloan RP. *Blind Faith: The Unholy Alliance of Religion and Medicine.* New York: St. Martin's Press; 2006.

Sloan RP. Field Analysis of the Literature on Religion, Spirituality, and Health, *Metanexus,* http://www.metanexus.net/tarp/pdf/TARP-Sloan.pdf.

Sloan RP. Should physicians prescribe religious activities? *N Engl J Med.* 2000;342(25):1913–1916.

Smith A. Christian conquest and the sexual colonization of native women. In: *Violence Against Women and Children: A Christian Theological Sourcebook.* In: Adams CJ, Fortune MM, ed. New York: Continuum, 1998:377–403.

Tjaden P, Thoennes N. National Institute of Justice and the Centers of Disease Control and Prevention, "Extent, Nature and Consequences of Intimate Partner Violence: Findings from the National Violence Against Women Survey." (2000). U.S.

Department of Justice, Bureau of Justice Statistics, "Intimate Partner Violence in the United States," December 2006.

Traitler-Espiritu R. Violence against women's bodies. In: Mananzan MJ, et al. eds. *Women Resisting Violence: Spirituality for Life.* Maryknoll, NY: Orbis Books; 1996:62–70.

United Nations Department of Public Information. *Women: Challenges to the year 2000.* New York; 1991:67.

West TC. *Wounds of the Spirit: Black Women, Violence, and Resistance Ethics.* New York: New York University Press; 1999.

Wiethaus U, ed. *Maps of Flesh and Light: The Religious Experience of Medieval Women Mystics.* Syracuse, NY: Syracuse University Press, 1993.

PART II

Systems and Modalities

7

Traditional Chinese Medicine

LESLIE McGEE

CASE STUDY

Sally M. was 36 years old and a veteran of 6 years of intrauterine inseminations (IUIs) and seven failed in vitro fertilizations (IVFs), with not a single pregnancy in her quest to have a child. She arrived in my office about 1 month before the 8th IVF was scheduled. She told me that her uterine lining was never more than 6 mm thick for the embryo transfer (a minimum of 8 mm thickness is best for embryo implantation). Sally also told me that she always had a very short and scant 3-day menstrual period and never remembers having any noticeable mid-cycle egg-white quality cervical mucous.

Chinese medicine developed theories describing women's physiology many centuries ago. Long before modern science identified hormones and the hypothalamic-pituitary-adrenal axis, Chinese medicine provided care for women from menarche beyond menopause, and provided insight into the mechanisms of health and disease. Chinese medicine proposes an elaborate theory of women's physiology, which continues to attract modern practitioners and patients with its capacity to restore balance in women's lives.

Acupuncture is the best-known modality of Chinese medicine, but is just one aspect of the full range of treatment options within this system. Women's health issues are usually considered internal medicine conditions, and for these, Chinese herbs, typically in complex and individualized formulations, are utilized. In addition, Chinese medicine practitioners promote lifestyle and diet changes as being fundamental to long-term wellness (Flaws 1997; Maciocia 1998).

Fundamental Theories

Chinese medicine developed over 2000 years ago. Its theories and ideas link human beings and our health with natural phenomenon: heaven and earth, cycles of growth and decline, the seasons, movement and stillness, and every observable process seen in our world, both animate and inanimate. One of the fundamental ideas of Chinese medicine is the theory of yin and yang. Yin and yang are opposite qualities. Yin represents form, substance, stillness, moisture, darkness, the interior, and coolness. Yang represents energy, activity, transformation, heat, the exterior, brightness, and dryness. Yin and yang are clearly opposite qualities, and as such, they are mutually consumptive. For example, yin's moisture can extinguish yang's heat. Or yang's activity can transform yin's stillness and inertia. These qualities translate into the body: our form and substance are yin; the body's metabolic processes are yang. The inside of the uterus is yin. The moment the egg is released from the ovary is yang. Any bodily process or substance can be analyzed in this way.

Paradoxically, it is said that yin and yang are mutually transformative. Extreme yin can transform into yang, and vice versa. For example, the follicular phase in a woman's cycle is considered the yin phase. As yin maximizes there is a sudden transformation to the yang activity of ovulation. In other words, yin and yang can destroy each other, yet they can also become each other. They are opposed, inseparable, yet mutually transformative (Maciocia 2005).

Another fundamental theory of Chinese medicine is the concept of the vital substances. The most significant of these are known as the "three treasures," qi ("chee"), blood, and essence. Qi roughly translates as vital energy and has a yang nature in its functions of moving, warming, and transforming. Blood is dark and fluid, thus more yin, and serves as the substantial nourishment of both body and mind. Essence is a fundamental, highly refined substance, with both yin and yang qualities. It governs growth and reproduction, and declines with age. The body functions and lives through the presence and activities of these substances.

Chinese medicine also theorizes that the body is traversed by a complex web of meridians or channels. Acupuncture points along those meridians are used to adjust the function and balance of the body, using the fine needles of acupuncture or manual stimulation of acupressure.

Over 2000 years ago in the medical classic called *Su Wen—Simple Questions*, Chinese doctors remarked on the stages of life affecting women. Women's lives are governed by the slow maturation and decline of essence in 7 year cycles. They wrote: "The Tian Gui (the heavenly water or menstrual blood) arrives at age 14 (2 × 7) if the Ren vessel is free-flowing and the Chong vessel is exuberant. The menstruation descends periodically, and one can have children…. At 7 × 7, 49 years, the Ren vessel is vacuous and the Chong vessel is debilitated and scanty. The Tian Gui, heavenly water, is exhausted and the pathways are not free-flowing. Thus the body is decrepit and there are no children" (Ting-Liang 1995). Fortunately, decrepitude is not the destiny of every 49 year-old modern woman, but the onset of menopause remains still, on average, at age 49. Imagine if more women saw their menstrual blood as a form of heavenly water!

It is the complex interplay of the three vital substances that governs women's physiology. To be healthy, fertile, and energetic, women need not only an adequate quantity of qi, blood, and essence, but also the proper cyclic movements of these as well. The maturation of essence leads to menarche. The ability of qi to properly move the blood in a monthly fashion, filling and then emptying meridians and the uterus, creates the menstrual cycle. Adequate essence maintains the ovaries and fertility.

The relationship and harmony of yin and yang underscores every aspect of women's health: the balance between energy and restfulness, the proper biphasic curve of the monthly basal body temperature (BBT) chart, and the ground for an easy and predictable monthly cycle. Chinese medicine, without the modern concepts of hormones and biochemistry, describes women's health with clarity and logical consistency.

Pathology in women is analyzed according to the theory of Chinese medicine. Any discomfort unique to women is discussed in the Chinese gynecological literature, both ancient and modern. Treatment is determined not by the disease but by the pattern of disharmony underlying the disease. Thus, for example, there is no single acupuncture or herbal prescription for dysmenorrhea. The pattern underlying the pain must be determined first and then correct treatment chosen.

To take this example further, a careful analysis of the mechanisms of dysmenorrhea and the woman's unique presentation will lead the practitioner to the correct pattern differentiation. From there treatment flows, including acupuncture points, herbal therapies, and lifestyle recommendations. *A Handbook of Menstrual Diseases in Chinese Medicine* (Flaws 1997) lists eight different patterns possible in dysmenorrhea, and each pattern has its unique herbal and acupuncture prescriptions.

Women are often surprised by the inquisitive nature of a good Chinese gynecological assessment. All aspects of the cycle are scrutinized. Regularity, quantity, and quality of blood flow (is it pink, red, purple, brown, thin, thick, clotted?); any cyclic discomforts—both emotional and physical; any pain anywhere in the body that seems linked to the period; and for the menstrual pain itself: does it occur before, during or after the menses, and what is its quality (dull, sharp, fixed, mobile?). Other aspects of a woman's life are also explored such as sleep quality, energy, and digestion. All these questions are asked and their answers ascertained.

Women's health issues treated by Chinese medicine include premenstrual syndrome (PMS), irregular cycles, polycystic ovarian syndrome, dysmenorrhea, endometriosis, vaginal infections, frequent miscarriage, infertility, menopause, and many others. Regular acupuncture and herbal medicine may be needed for many weeks to affect lasting change. Or in some cases, a monthly acupuncture session or herbal formula is adequate. For some women, diet and lifestyle recommendations alone can empower them and restore health.

In Chinese medicine, ideas about connections between different parts of the body are common. For instance, we say the feet are a reflection of the kidney, and the kidney is closely associated with the uterus. Thus, keeping the feet warm is a strategy for keeping the uterus warm and protecting a pregnancy. I often find that infertile women have cold feet, and this informs my diagnosis of their Chinese pattern—cold feet equals deficiency of kidney yang, or the fundamental fire of the body. In modern medicine, cold feet can be associated with hypothyroid function, and optimal thyroid function supports fertility and pregnancy (Poppe 2008). The global phenomenon of these insights was brought home when I asked a Mexican-American client who was hoping to get pregnant to please keep her feet warm, and she told me that her mother had told her to stop walking barefoot on the tile floors once her period started or the cold would enter her uterus and cause menstrual cramps.

Modern Research

In China, a vast resource of literature exists describing the treatment of women with Chinese medicine. Each year, hundreds of Chinese medical journals are published. On the whole, the research methodologies utilized are unsophisticated, leaving the reader with piqued interest and unanswered questions. In spite of this failing, the research suggests avenues that merit further exploration.

One example of research done in China combining Western and Chinese medicine involved 110 infertile women who were divided into two groups. The treatment group received clomiphene and complex Chinese herb formulas adjusted to each of 4 weeks of their cycle. A formula was used for the menstrual period week, another formula for the postmenstrual week, another formula for midcycle, and then another formula for the premenstrual/postinsemination week. The control group received just clomiphene.

Outcome measures included endometrial thickness, cervical mucous, and conception rate. The treatment group had thicker uterine lining, better quality cervical mucous, and a conception rate of 41%. The control group's conception rate was 22% (Jian-Jun 2007).

Western research of Chinese medicine is still in its infancy. One of the strengths of Chinese medicine is the individualized nature of treatment. Researchers are exploring methods that allow treatment to be tailored while also meeting standards of research design and replicability (Schnyer and Allen 2002). Shea explored the arguments within the field contending that randomized controlled trials for research on Chinese medicine are problematic and describes some of the innovations in study design to rectify these issues (Shea 2006). Lao (2008) reviewed randomized clinical trials in acupuncture and explored the challenges in designing adequate controls.

Studies to determine the exact mechanism of acupuncture's effects are also being conducted. Several studies have been completed exploring the idea that acupuncture involves transmission of subtle electrical energies through the meridian system. In reviewing 18 studies, Ahn et al. (2008) found that meridians and acupuncture points had lower electrical impedance and higher capacitance than nearby nonmeridian or nonpoint tissues. Another area of research involves using functional magnetic resonance imaging (fMRI) during acupuncture needling. Lewith et al. (2005) reviewed the fMRI acupuncture research and concluded that specific and largely predictable areas of brain activation occur and often correlate to the traditional Chinese functions attributed to various points.

Most of the research on women's health using Chinese medicine in the West has been done on acupuncture and less often on Chinese herbal interventions. The quality of this research varies considerably. A review of controlled trials of acupuncture for women's reproductive health care concluded that design flaws excluded many studies from their review, but acupuncture for dysmenorrhea and infertility provided the most promising outcomes (White 2003). Acupuncture as a treatment for hot flashes in menopausal women was no better than sham acupuncture according to one study (Vincent 2007). Another study found that acupuncture relieved hot flashes in women getting tamoxifen therapy for breast cancer (Hervik and Mjaland 2008).

Acupuncture for IVF has been the most researched gynecological topic in Western settings. Starting with Paulus in 2002, several randomized clinical trials using acupuncture during IVF cycles have been completed. Data from those trials has been promising in spite of design limitations in several of the studies (Dieterle et al. 2006; Paulus et al. 2002; Smith et al. 2006; Westergaard et al. 2006). Recently the *British Medical Journal* published a systematic review of seven trials with 1366 women undergoing IVF and including acupuncture at the time of embryo transfer. This article concluded that evidence suggests that acupuncture given with embryo transfer improves rates of pregnancy and live births in women undergoing IVF (Manheimer et al. 2008).

Another interesting element of acupuncture practice is that it is far from homogenous in point selection strategies. Several unique acupuncture traditions exist and each has its very different point selection processes and conclusions. The most commonly practiced acupuncture style in the West is traditional Chinese medicine (TCM). Other styles include Japanese meridian therapy (Manaka 1995), classical Chinese style (Van Nghi et al. 2005, 2006), five-element style (Connelly 1992), and various microsystem styles such as Master Tong's method (Tan 1996) and Dr. Ming Qing Zhu's scalp acupuncture system (Dharmananda and Vickers 2000). Thus a salient criticism of the study done by Vincent et al., which concluded that acupuncture was not effective for hot flashes, would be that a Japanese or classical Chinese style acupuncturist would use an entirely different set of points and might have a better clinical outcome. Further research on the strengths of these varied styles is warranted.

There is more agreement and uniformity in the selection of Chinese herbs for women than among point selections. Chinese herbal medicine's framework is well defined by TCM. Pattern differentiation and herb selection have been extensively documented in the Chinese literature and translated into many languages (Sionneau and Gang 1996–2000). Many, if not most, gynecological complaints are treated with complex herb formulas in China and other Asian countries. Thirty-nine trials of Chinese herbs for the treatment of dysmenorrhea were reviewed from Chinese literature (Zhu 2007). Many of these trials had methodological problems, but the reviewers found that Chinese herbs were generally effective against dysmenorrhea, and in some cases rapidly effective. Meiguihua (*Rosa rugosa*) or rosebuds was one single herb found to be effective in a 6-month trial. Most of the formulas used in these trials were typical multiherb, individually tailored prescriptions. Western physicians were advised to seek the expertise of fully trained practitioners of Chinese medicine in order to properly select herbal formulas for individual women.

Clinical trials in progress in the United States, Taiwan, and Hong Kong include studies evaluating the effect of Chinese herbs to reduce the toxicity of chemotherapy in breast cancer patients, a topical Chinese herbal product for vaginal atrophy, comparing hormone therapy with Chinese herbs for endometriosis, and evaluating the single Chinese herb Gu Sui Bu—Drynariae Rhizoma for postmenopausal osteoporosis (clinicaltrials.gov 2008).

Based on my Chinese style assessment, I concluded that Sally's TCM pattern was a combination of yin and blood deficiency, with some blood stasis. Because Sally was receiving extensive pharmaceutical ovarian management and stimulation, she elected to use only acupuncture, and not herbs, to support her chance for pregnancy. Seven acupuncture treatments were given prior to this IVF transfer.

Ultrasound revealed her lining to have improved to an 8 mm thickness with a decent tri-laminar appearance. The day of the embryo transfer, a complex acupuncture protocol was utilized. A single embryo/fetal sac was seen on ultrasound with an uneventful progression until Sally had a miscarriage at 11 weeks. Devastated after this event, Sally decided that she would take a break from the Western approach to her infertility and give Chinese herbs a try. For 2 months, Sally used whole Chinese herbs and consumed them as a cooked decoction. The formula contained herbs to nourish her yin, blood, and essence, and secondarily to rectify the qi and blood.

After about a month on the herbs she returned to her reproductive endocrinologist (RE) and on ultrasound examination he noticed that her uterus looked unusually plump. A month later, when Sally had not resumed ovulating, she decided to do another IVF. The herbs were discontinued while her doctor stimulated her ovaries and recovered a number of eggs. At this time, acupuncture was resumed to support her lining and nourish her yin. The RE followed her uterus on ultrasound and found that its plump condition was maintained and the lining at transfer time was unusually thick for her. Three embryos were transferred and pregnancy occurred. The surprise was that 3 fetal sacs were seen at the first ultrasound. Somehow her uterine lining had become far more hospitable for her embryos! Fortunately, over the next few weeks, first one and then the other embryo faded, and Sally was pregnant with one fetus with a strong heartbeat. Acupuncture was administered every week during the first trimester to support the pregnancy and then tapered to every 3 or 4 weeks for the duration of the pregnancy. Sally had a healthy baby girl at 37 weeks by C-section. When the baby was 8 months old, Sally came in for acupuncture for seasonal allergies and reported that her period resumed at about 4 months and it had changed considerably. She now has a 5 day moderate flow of bright red blood, and fairly abundant, mid-cycle cervical mucous. She is hopeful that she and her husband might be able to conceive without assisted reproductive technology and have a second child.

The language of Chinese medicine gynecology, with its references to yin and yang, essence and heavenly water, may seem quaint and poetic. Chinese medicine proposes that every human being is connected to the universe and our health is affected by climate, season, cycles of day and night, and all natural phenomenon. Dr. Ngyuen Van Nghi, one of the greatest classical Chinese acupuncturists and translator of ancient Chinese texts (Van Nghi et al. 2005, 2006), has stated: "Woman is little nature, a child of heaven and earth, a product of cosmic forces" (Garbacz 2008). This statement captures the essence of Chinese insight into women's health. Chinese medicine recognizes that women, with monthly expression of these natural cycles, are indeed human displays of cosmic forces. The physical, emotional, biochemical, and hormonal reality of a woman's life is connected to heaven and earth, yin and yang, and the ebb and flow of tides and moons. The wisdom of Chinese medicine, using unique concepts and therapies, has a wealth of history behind it and invites further research to explore its reputation as an effective system to enhance women's health.

REFERENCES

Ahn AC, Colbert AP, Anderson BJ, et al. Electrical properties of acupuncture points and meridians: a systemic review. *Bioelectromagnetics.* 2008;29(4):245–256.

Connelly D. *Traditional Acupuncture: The Law of the Five Elements.* 5th ed. Columbia, MD: The Centre for Traditional Acupuncture; 1992.

Dharmananda S, Vickers E. *Synopsis of Scalp Acupuncture.* Portland, OR: Institute for Traditional Medicine; 2000.

Dieterle S, Ying G, Hatzmann W, Neuer A. Effect of acupuncture on the outcome of in vitro fertilization and intracytoplasmic sperm injection: a randomized, prospective, controlled clinical study. *Fertil Steril.* 2006;85(5):1347–1351.

Flaws B. *A Handbook of Menstrual Diseases in Chinese Medicine.* Boulder, CO: Blue Poppy Press; 1997.

Garbacz E. Quoting a lecture by Dr. Ngyuen Van Nghi, reported in "The Acupuncture Energetics of the Normal Female Reproductive System" seminar. Tucson, AZ, May 2008.

Hervik J, Mjaland O. Acupuncture for the treatment of hot flashes in breast cancer patients, a randomized, controlled trial. *Breast Cancer Res Treat.* 2008; [Epub ahead of print].

Lao L. Current status of acupuncture clinical research—challenge and methodology. *Am Acupunct.* 2008;44:26–29.

Lewith GT, White PJ, Pariente J. Investigating acupuncture using brain imaging techniques: the current state of play. *Evid Based Complement Alternat Med.* 2005;2(3):315–319.

Maciocia G. *The Foundations of Chinese Medicine.* 2nd ed. London, UK: Churchill Livingstone; 2005.

Maciocia G. *Obstetrics and Gynecology in Chinese Medicine*. London, UK: Churchill Livingstone; 1998.

Manaka Y. *Chasing the Dragon's Tail*. Brookline, MA: Paradigm Publications; 1995.

Manheimer E, Zhang G, Udoff L, et al. Effects of acupuncture on rates of pregnancy and live birth among women undergoing in vitro fertilization: a systematic review and meta-analysis. *Br Med J*. 2008;336(7643):545–549.

Paulus WE, Zhang M, Strehler E, El-Danasouri I, Sterzik K. Influence of acupuncture on the pregnancy rate in patients who undergo assisted reporoductive therapy. *Fertil Steril*. 2002;77(4):721–724.

Poppe K, Velkeniers B, Glinoer D. Medscape, the role of thyroid auto-immunity in fertility and pregnancy. *Nat Clin Pract Endocrinol Metab*. 2008. [Epub ahead of print].

Schnyer R, Allen J. Bridging the gap in complementary and alternative medicine research: manualization as a means of promoting standardization and flexibility of treatment in clinical trials of acupuncture. *J Altern Complement Med*. 2002;8(5):623–634.

Shea JL. Applying evidence-based medicine: debate and strategy. *J Altern Complement Med*. 2006;12(4):349–350.

Sionneau P, Gang L. *The Treatment of Disease in TCM*. Vols 1–7. Boulder, CO: Blue Poppy Press; 1996–2000.

Smith C, Coyle M, Norman RJ. Influence of acupuncture stimulation on pregnancy rates for women undergoing embryo transfer. *Fertil Steril*. 2006;85(5):1352–1358.

Tan R. *Twelve and Twelve in Acupuncture*. 2nd ed. San Diego, CA: Author; 1996.

Van Nghi N, Viet Dzung T, Recours-Nguyen C. *Huangdi Neijing Lingshu*. Vol 1. Sugar Grove, NC: Jung Tao; 2005.

Van Nghi N, Viet Dzung T, Recours-Nguyen C. *Huangdi Neijing Lingshu*. Vol 2. Sugar Grove, NC: Jung Tao; 2006.

Vincent A, Barton DL, Mandrekar JN, et al. Acupuncture for hot flashes: a randomized sham controlled clinical study. *Menopause*. 2007;14(1):45–52.

Web listings at clinicaltrials.gov, National Institutes of Health, Bethesda, MD, 2008.

Westergaard LG, Mao Q, Krogslund M, Sandrini S, Lenz S, Grinsted J. Acupuncture on the day of embryo transfer significantly improves the reproductive outcome in infertile women: a prospective, randomized trial. *Fertil Steril*. 2006;85(5):1341–1346.

White AR. A review of controlled trials of acupuncture for women's reproductive health care. *J Fam Plann Reprod Health Care*. 2003;(4):233–236.

Zhu X, Proctor M, Bensoussan A, Smith CA, Wu E. Chinese herbal medicine for dysmenorrhea. *Cochrane Database Syst Rev*. 2007;(4):CD005288.

8

Ayurveda

PREMAL PATEL

CASE STUDY

Amy is a 52-year-old financial consultant. She is single, travels four days a week for her job, and often gives up sleep for work. Amy skips breakfast, eats a salad for lunch, and dinner at restaurants. She jogs three times a week. She thrives on competition at work but is facing some insecurity about retirement. She has constipation and flatulence. She is postmenopausal and has been experiencing hot flashes and insomnia. She has been treating her osteoarthritis with ibuprofen as needed.

PHYSICAL EXAMINATION FINDINGS INCLUDE THE FOLLOWING

Prakruti: Pitta predominant, Vata secondary
Vikruti: Vata and Pitta imbalanced
Tongue: Light, white coating (ama) on the back of the tongue

Recommendations

Diet:
- *Eat a warm, sweet breakfast (like oatmeal).*
- *Eat the biggest meal at lunch—warm, cooked, not dry.*
- *Choose soups instead of raw salad.*

Sleep:
- *Set a sleep and wake time, with 7 to 8 hours of sleep.*

- *Take a warm bath before bed.*
- *Massage soles of feet with warm sunflower oil before bed.*

Routine:

- *On weekends at home, perform self-massage with warm oil before shower.*
- *Try swimming and brisk walking instead of jogging.*
- *On weekends, join a yoga class doing restorative poses and pranayama.*

Supplements:

- *Take 2 tablespoons of aloe vera gel three times a day.*
- *Take ½ teaspoon of triphala with warm water every night.*

Introduction

Ayurveda is translated as the "science or knowledge of life." Life, according to Ayurveda, is the inseparable and integral union of mind, body, and spirit. The key in this union is balance. A healthy life is not just one without disease. Health involves a balanced state of the three doshas, the seven bodily tissues, the wastes created by the body, and the digestive fire; it also involves a joyful and content state of the senses, mind, and spirit; and finally, true health exists when one is centered in his or her true self (Lad 1984). This chapter is a brief overview of this healing system, with special attention given to the health of women.

The Five Elements and Three Doshas

Space, air, fire, water, and earth are the classical five elements discussed in Ayurveda. They are different from the elements found in the Periodic Table. Rather, each is a combination of qualities that represent archetypal patterns of behavior. These patterns manifest in human beings with the further aid of three fundamental principles: *vata, pitta, and kapha*—the three *doshas*. It is critical to have some understanding of the relationships between doshas and elements in order to understand health and pathology from an Ayurvedic perspective.

Vata is associated with the space and air elements and governs movement of all kinds. It is required for functions such as physical motion, nerve impulses, thinking, respiration, circulation, ingestion, peristalsis, elimination of wastes, menstruation, and childbirth.

Pitta is associated with fire and water and governs transformation. It is key for any processing to occur in the body, including metabolism, digestion, maintenance of body temperature, comprehension, appetite, and thirst.

Kapha is associated with water and earth, and represents structure and stability. It is essential for growth and nourishment in the body, including physical (bone and muscle) structure, lipid structure, repair and regeneration, lubrication, stamina, sleep, water and electrolyte balance, and memory.

Qualities of Doshas

Vata: Space and Air	Pitta: Fire and Water	Kapha: Earth and Water
Dry	Sharp	Heavy
Light	Penetrating	Cold
Cold	Hot	Dull
Rough	Light	Oily
Subtle	Liquid	Liquid
Mobile	Mobile	Smooth
Clear	Oily	Dense
		Soft
		Static
		Cloudy
		Hard
		Gross

(Lad 2002)

All three doshas exist in all people; what varies is the extent to which they are present and whether or not they are balanced.

Examples of Dosha Balance and Imbalance (Tables 8.1–8.3) (Lad 2002, 2006)

Table 8.1. Vata: Space and Air

General Traits	Imbalanced
Thin	Osteoporosis
Delicate	Osteoarthritis
Narrow eyes–narrow lips	Scoliosis
Variable appetite	Insomnia
Light sleep	Constipation
Creative	Difficulty with attention and concentration
Flexible	

Table 8.2. Pitta: Fire and Water

General Traits	Imbalanced
Medium frame	Hyperacidity
Bright eyes	Skin rashes
Sharp hunger	Inflammation
Passionate	Ulcers
Sharp, probing intellect	Uncontrolled anger/judgment/criticism
	Heat intolerance

Table 8.3. Kapha: Earth and Water

General Traits	Imbalanced
Large frame	Obesity
Strong	High cholesterol
Large eyes	Excess mucus
Thick, smooth skin	Tumors
Steady appetite	Stubborn
Good memory	Possessive
Strong faith	
Compassionate	
Patient	

Balance and Imbalance of the Three Doshas

The balanced state, called prakruti, is the individual's constitution, which is a unique combination of doshas determined for each person at conception and which remains unchanged throughout life. A person's prakruti may be dominant in one dosha, two doshas, or all three doshas (though, again, everyone has all three). As long as one maintains this unique balance, he or she remains healthy and vibrant; this person "ages gracefully." Prakruti also determines a person's experience of the world. For example, when faced with a challenge such as losing a job and finding a new one, a vata-predominant person may respond with creativity or fear and anxiety; a pitta-predominant person may respond with confidence or anger and judgment. And a kapha-predominant person may respond with steadiness or despondency.

While there are advantages and challenges associated with each dosha, no dosha is inherently better or worse. Individuals may make choices that preserve balance as dictated by their prakruti. These choices include diet, daily practices, forms of exercise, emotional digestion, and so on. If these choices exacerbate any of the doshas, pathology begins. When the doshas become increased or decreased, an imbalanced state, called vikruti, comes into existence. It is this imbalance that brings ill health. The goal of healing is to bring one back to his or her unique prakruti. For example, a person with a kapha-predominant prakruti will already have a larger frame, but when that large frame accumulates excess weight, then kapha is increased. However, to return the person to balance, the goal is to return him or her to the healthy large frame, not a thin frame that is more natural for a vata individual.

Agni: The Digestive Fire

Digestion is the root of all health in Ayurveda and agni is the fire responsible for digestion (Caldecott 2006). Food is one part of nourishment, but the sounds, sights, smells, tastes, and textures we experience also create an impact. It is then crucial how we digest these experiences. Witnessing a tragic accident can create a similar sense of unease, indigestion, and difficulty sleeping as ingesting a bad piece of meat can. It is agni's job to transform all food and experiences. If agni is healthy and what is ingested is of good quality, agni can transform it into nourishment for the body, mind, and spirit. If what is ingested is of poor quality, healthy agni can transform it into a form the body can safely expel. When agni is unhealthy, food and experience are not properly transformed. This results in toxic buildup, or *ama*. Ama creates blockages, and tissues can no longer function optimally. Ama is at the root of many imbalances and disease. Physically, ama can manifest in a multitude of ways: sluggish metabolism, lethargy and fatigue, indigestion, odorous breath or wastes (stool, urine, sweat), bodily aches, and lack of mental clarity. A heavy coating on the tongue is one clear physical sign that indicates the presence of systemic ama (Lad 1998).

The key to balancing agni is to protect it and not make it work harder than is required.

SOME BASIC PRACTICAL TIPS INCLUDE THE FOLLOWING

1. Drink warm or at least room temperature liquids—avoid cold and ice.

2. Follow nature—agni is highest when the sun (nature's agni) is highest; eat the heaviest foods/largest meal in the afternoon.
3. Assist the internal fire. If food is cooked and thoroughly chewed, that is less work required of the internal agni.
4. Use warming spices (black pepper, ginger, cinnamon, cardamom, etc.) with foods that are heavier and difficult to digest. To boost agni and decrease ama, try one to two thin one inch slices of ginger with lime juice and a hint of salt.
5. Do not douse the agni with large amounts of liquids around meal-times. For lubrication, drink only occasional sips of warm water with meals.
6. Eat only when hunger is present, and do not overeat.
7. Consume all six tastes in the diet (sweet, sour, salty, pungent, bitter, astringent), favoring those appropriate to any imbalanced dosha.
8. Eat with awareness—do not multitask while eating. Even if the time for a meal is short, give full attention for these few minutes. If the television is on during a mealtime, then agni must multitask in digesting the food as well as processing the images and sounds from the television, and it cannot give full attention to creating optimal nourishment from food.

One is bound to have some exposure to behavior or experiences (through diet, lifestyle, environmental toxins, etc.) that lead to ama formation. Ayurveda calls for cleansing processes to clear this. Daily, the predominant outlet to release ama (and excess doshas) is the gastrointestinal (GI) tract, and regular, healthy bowel movements are considered of utmost importance. This can be achieved naturally or with the help of herbal remedies such as triphala, starting with 1/2 tsp daily at bedtime (or two tablets), and then titrating up or down as needed.

Seasonally, one may consider a complete cleanse. Panchakarma is the predominant method.

Panchakarma

Though this process should be done with a trained professional (as there are indications and contraindications), it is introduced here. It refers to five procedures, each of which predominantly works on specific dosha(s). Traditionally, the five procedures are emesis for kapha imbalances, purgation and bloodletting for pitta imbalances, therapeutic enemas for vata imbalances, and the nasal administration of substances for all three doshas. Other procedures may be added as needed, and specific to women's health, vaginal administration of herbal preparations, called uttara basti, can also be used. Preparation is done for panchakarma using oils (external massage and internal ingestion) and steam. Following the cleanse, rejuvenation is normally required. While this phase is very case dependant, in general, it includes rebuilding agni, a slow resumption of a full diet appropriate to the person's constitution, daily routine practices appropriate for the person's constitution (yoga, pranayama, meditation, etc.), herbs appropriate to any continuing imbalance as well as to tonify/rejuvenate the weaker tissues, slow resumption of appropriate activities (such as work, daily responsibilities, etc.) and exercise, proper sleep health, and stress management (Lad 1984).

The Golden Rule in Creating Balance

The key principle in balancing doshas is to first remove the root cause, and then remedy lingering imbalances with the opposite (Lad 1998). Consider the qualities that are imbalanced, and return them to balance using the opposite qualities. If there is an excess of kapha and/or ama, and the heavy, cold, gross, dense, wet, and static qualities are present, one may present with disorders such as obesity and fibroid tumors. Choose foods and spices that have the opposite qualities: light, warm, subtle, dry, and kindling of agni. Choose activities that help move the stagnation, such as stimulating massage. Choose yoga poses or pranayama (breathing techniques) that stimulate agni and improve metabolism. And choose herbs that also kindle agni and provide what Ayurveda calls "a scraping action," which removes ama.

The Toolbox

Ayurveda has a number of modalities to reestablish balance. Examples include diet, lifestyle, herbs, sense therapies (such as aromatherapy, visualization, music, etc.), meditation, marma (energy points), and detoxification treatments such as panchakarma. Ayurveda also draws on the healing capacities of its sister sciences, such as Yoga (beyond just physical postures, and including pranayama), and Jyotisha (the study of astronomy and astrology).

While balancing each dosha requires a case specific regimen, there are some general guidelines that one can follow using the principle of treating with the opposite qualities (Lad 1984; Miller 1999).

TO BALANCE VATA

1. Routine and rest are crucial. As irregularity and movement are inherent to vata, it must be grounded. Have set sleep and wake times, mealtimes, and so on.
2. Avoid cold, windy, dry weather.
3. Prefer warm, cooked, soft, and easy to digest foods. Include oils in diet, though not as deep fried foods. Also include warming spices.
4. Prefer gentler exercises, including flowing yoga poses that are grounding and strengthen one's core, and swimming in warm water.
5. Prefer naturally sweet, sour, and salty tastes in moderation.
6. Prefer sweet, warm scents like orange, cinnamon, and holy basil; warm colors like deep red, orange, yellow, and green; and gentle, grounding music.

TO BALANCE PITTA

1. Prefer naturally cooling, soothing foods. Avoid spicy or fermented foods and excess oil. Use cooling spices and condiments such as mint, cilantro, cumin, fennel, and coconut.
2. Prefer naturally sweet, bitter, and astringent tastes.
3. Avoid hot, intense weather.
4. Prefer calming activities, including soothing exercise.
5. Surrender to the moment, and avoid unnecessary competition.
6. Prefer sweet, cool scents like mint, rose, and sandalwood; soothing colors like blue and purple; and sweet music.

TO BALANCE KAPHA

1. Prefer warm, light foods and hot liquids. Use warming spices.
2. Prefer pungent, bitter, and astringent tastes.
3. Avoid oversleeping and daytime naps.
4. Avoid cold, damp weather.
5. Get things moving. Prefer vigorous (but not excessive) exercise, including yoga poses and pranayama.
6. Prefer warm scents like eucalyptus and clove; avoid blue; and prefer active music.

Effects of the Six Tastes on Doshas

	Vata	Pitta	Kapha
Sweet	↓	↓	↑
Sour	↓	↑	↑
Salty	↓	↑	↑
Pungent	↑	↑	↓
Bitter	↑	↓	↓
Astringent	↑	↓	↓

(Lad 2002)

Abhyanga (Massage)

One technique for balancing all three doshas is a daily self-massage, or abhyanga. Assuming there is not a lot of ama, this is traditionally done with warm oil specific to the dosha, such as sesame oil (heating) for vata and kapha, or sunflower oil (cooling) for pitta. Oil carries significant benefits in Ayurveda, including strengthening and toning the tissues and calming the nervous system. In general, use circular motions on the scalp, head, trunk, and joints, and long strokes on the extremities and flanks. This decreases stagnation in the tissues and is also an opportunity for self-nurturing, as the same word (snehan) represents oil and love in Sanskrit.

Topics Specific to Women

PREGNANCY

In an analogy comparing the conception and growth of a child to the germination of a plant from a seed, Ayurveda lists four factors necessary for a healthy pregnancy (Lad 1995):

1. Rtu: "Season." This refers to various timings, including a woman's fertile time of life and of the month and the effect of the seasons. It also includes the proper time for having sex, which is said to be between 9 and 11 PM, as it is thought that daytime sex weakens the kidney; midnight sex weakens the liver; sex at dawn weakens the colon.

2. Kshetra: "Field." This is the body of the woman, and specifically the health of the reproductive organs and the womb.
3. Ambu: "Water." This refers to the woman's ova, proper hormonal balance, and the nutrition the fetus receives. The condition of a woman's egg affects the growth and development of her fetus. Provided her eggs are healthy, the next concern is nutrition. For the mother, a diet rich in fresh, cooked, building foods is recommended, including milk, ghee (clarified butter), wheat, and proteins (assuming mom can digest these). In conjunction with these foods, the mother should also maintain a diet appropriate to her doshic balance. A fetus is also nourished by everything the mother experiences and feels (Slattery 2008).
4. Bija: "Seed." This refers to the health of the sperm. Ovum and sperm carry the doshic balances and imbalances of mother and father. Therefore, Ayurveda recommends that people desiring to become parents should receive cleansing procedures like panchakarma prior to conception.

After birth, the mother is susceptible to vata imbalances in particular and should be given preventative treatments, including massage, abdominal binding, and a nourishing diet. Breast milk is also affected by the doshas. The qualities of the foods that the mother eats, as well as her balanced and imbalanced doshas, affect her milk's qualities. This in combination with the child's own prakruti and vikruti can account for many digestive issues faced by newborns. A simple diet that is appropriate for mom and baby's constitution is best. In other words, if mom or baby have a vata imbalance, and mom consumes a vata-aggravating diet (raw, dry, cold foods), the breast milk will have a vata quality, and could cause more indigestion for the baby. In general, breastfeeding mothers should consume foods that are warm, moist, and nutritious. Examples include ghee, milk, almond milk, rice pudding with almonds and pistachios, sweet potato or yam, pumpkin, dates, tapioca, and mung dal. Of course, this list is general and is recommended with the assumption that it should be followed only if both the mother and baby do not show any intolerance to these foods. The most popular herb for enhancing breast milk production is shatavari (Lad 1995).

THE MENSTRUAL CYCLE

The Vedic tradition, in which Ayurveda is rooted, honors the feminine energy, which brings creativity to fruition. Mother nature works in cycles; it is only natural that the feminine energy also has a cycle that allows for a proliferative, creative phase and a reflective, cleansing phase. Most of the ancient texts of Ayurveda prescribe routines that are appropriate for a healthy menses (Murthy 2005; Sharma 2003, 2004; Tewari 1996), but the gist of all these routines is an inward retreat. It is a monthly reminder to let go of the past and start afresh in the present.

Physically, menses is a taxing experience for the body, as is any cleansing process, and requires rest. However, it is not inherently a painful or disgruntling process. The symptoms of discomfort reflect imbalanced dosha(s), which can be addressed, even with simple measures as discussed above.

Premenstrual Syndrome

While there are over 200 symptoms that have been linked to premenstrual syndrome (PMS) (Dickerson 2003), Ayurveda views the symptoms as one, two, or three imbalanced doshas (Jadhav 2005; Lad 2006).

- Imbalanced vata creates irregularity in cycles, scanty flow, low back pain, cramps, constipation, anxiety, difficulty concentrating, and insomnia.
- Imbalanced pitta manifests as heavy flow, cramps, small clots, irritability, acne, inflammatory conditions, migraines, diarrhea, intense or sharp hunger, excess heat, anger, and judgmental or competitive behavior.
- Imbalanced kapha generates a mucus-like consistency to the menstrual flow, big clots, cramps, water retention and edema, dull aches and cramps, a sense of heaviness, lethargy, desire for "comfort foods," excess sleep, and a depressed mood.

Generally, more than one dosha is involved, often along with ama, and regularity in following the appropriate recommendations is key.

Menopause

The "change of life" is a mind, body, and spirit phenomenon, an evolution into a new stage (Atreya 1999).

The three doshas rule different ages in life. Childhood is dominated by kapha. The child is growing and forming his or her physical and emotional being. Pitta is predominant in early adulthood. This stage is marked by extroverted efforts to establish career and family. Vata prevails in later adulthood, including menopause and beyond. Balanced vata brings creativity, clarity, communication, intuition, and joy. Vata governs elimination, and this is the time to rid oneself of all the old baggage one has accumulated over a lifetime (Svoboda 2000).

Corresponding to this shift in roles, the body also transitions. But menopause does not occur overnight (Grady 2006). If one has arrived at this stage with balanced doshas, one can experience a smooth transition. If one's life experiences thus far have fostered an imbalance in doshas, then the change in hormones is like the loss of a security blanket. One may then feel the intensity of the imbalanced doshas. Vata brings osteoporosis and fractures, osteoarthritis, vaginal dryness, memory loss, and insecurity. Pitta brings sweating, and irritability. Kapha brings weight gain, high cholesterol, and tumors. Certain conditions, such as heart disease, involve multiple doshas, as kapha is necessary for plaque formation, pitta for inflammation, and vata for plaque eruption/movement. Hot flashes can also be related to the heat of pitta and/or the extreme fluctuations of vata.

The intensity of these imbalances is a way for nature to send loud messages. If a woman has not given herself the time and nurturing that she showers on the rest of society, now is the time. And the solution is within reach—rebalance the doshas.

Reintroducing Amy

Now back to Amy again. Her prakruti and vikruti can be determined by interview and physical examination, including pulse examination. Pitta being predominant in her prakruti, she has always been driven, often sacrificing health for work. Her lifestyle and diet all point to one word: irregularity. This aggravates vata dosha, which is composed primarily of space and air and is increased by qualities that match these elements. She travels frequently: movement increases the mobile and light qualities (especially travel by airplane, which goes against gravity and also affects the subtle quality); and being on the go impacts the rough quality (as different roads, vehicles, hotels are "rough" on the body). Her diet does not help ground vata: skipping meals aggravates the light quality; and salads and raw food worsen the rough, dry, cold qualities. Her habits also add to the imbalanced vata: not sleeping because of work aggravates the light quality; and jogging regularly is also rough and drying for joints. And becoming engulfed in the competition at work activates the intensity of pitta. Arriving at a transitional point in her life with imbalanced vata and pitta, she is feeling the results of the imbalance more than ever before: insomnia, flatulence, constipation, osteoarthritis, hot flashes, and insecurity. Her challenge is to ground vata primarily, and secondarily soothe pitta. Routine is key for vata: regular, warm meals; oil massages to ground and calm the nervous system; and less stressful exercise. Eating her largest meal at lunch and choosing warm, cooked foods will also protect her agni, so that she can derive optimal nourishment. Aloe will help pitta and can

Table 8.4. Ayurvedic Herbs Commonly Used in Women's Health (available in the West)

Latin	Sanskrit/English	Dosha Effect**	Traditional Uses in Women's Health	Comments
Aloe indica/ vera/ barbadensis	Kumari/Aloe vera	Gel: VPK = Powder: V+ P− K−	Regulates menses (especially, excess flow), cleanses blood, soothes hot flashes	May inhibit prostaglandins
Asparagus racemosus	Shatavari	V− P− K+	Tones FRO*, regulates menses, helps menopausal symptoms, increases breast milk	
Cyperus rotundus	Musta	V+ P− K−	Regulates menses (especially amenorrhea), improves PMS symptoms (especially bloating, pain, depression), relieves dysmenorrhea	Contains phytoestrogen substance
Glycyrrhiza glabra	Yashti Madhu/ Licorice	V− P− K−/+ in excess	Strengthens FRO*, improves vaginal dryness (improves secretions), can be used in vaginal douche	Avoid in hypertension and electrolyte imbalances
Pueraria tuberosa	Vidari	V− P− K+	Improves quality of FRO*, fertility, increases breast milk production, building/nourishing—good post-partum	
Saraca indica	Ashoka	V+ P− K−	Regulate menses (especially excess flow and congestion), uterine tonic, relieves dysmenorrhea	
Withania somnifera	Ashwagandha	V− P+ K−	Improves sexual (and general) debility, muscle tone, calms stress, and nervous system	Traditionally used to stabilize fetus, but excess may cause abortion

*FRO, Female reproductive organs/artava dhatu.

**Symbols for Dosha effect.

(−) Decreases or pacifies.

(+) Increases or aggravates.

(=) Balances all three doshas.

Sources: Frawley and Lad 2001; Pole 2006; Simon and Chopra 2000; Williamson 2002.

be a support for the menopausal changes, including hormonal changes and hot flashes. And triphala, per Ayurveda, will help cleanse the built up toxins, relieve constipation, and support the immune system. Amy can begin by implementing one recommendation at a time, and even a few simple changes can create a lasting impact on her well-being.

REFERENCES

Atreya. *Ayurvedic Healing for Women*. York Beach: Samuel Weiser, Inc; 1999.

Caldecott T. *Ayurveda: The Divine Science of Life*. Edinburgh, London, New York, Oxford, Philadelphia, St Louis, Sydney, Toronto: Mosby Elsevier; 2006.

Dickerson L, Mazyck P, Hunter M. Premenstrual syndrome. *Am Fam Phys*. 2003;67(8):1743–1752.

Frawley D, Lad V. *The Yoga of Herbs: An Ayurvedic Guide to Herbal Medicine*. 2nd ed. Twin Lakes: Lotus Press; 2001.

Grady D. Management of menopausal symptoms. *N Engl J Med*. 2006;355(22):338–2347.

Jadhav A, Bhutani KK. Ayurveda and gynecological disorders. *J Ethnopharmacol*. 2005;97:151–159.

Lad V. *Ayurveda: The Science of Self-Healing*. Twin Lakes: Lotus Press; 1984.

Lad V. Pregnancy and infant care. *Ayurveda Today*. Winter 1995;8(3):1–6.

Lad V. Female health issues: part one. *Ayurveda Today*. March 2006;18(4):1–6.

Lad V. Female health issues: part two. *Ayurveda Today*. June 2006;18(4):1–5.

Lad V. *Textbook of Ayurveda: A Complete Guide to Clinical Assessment*. Albuquerque: The Ayurvedic Press; 2006.

Lad V. *Textbook of Ayurveda: Fundamental Principles*. Albuquerque: The Ayurvedic Press; 2002.

Lad V. *The Complete Book of Ayurvedic Home Remedies*. New York: Three Rivers Press; 1998.

Miller L. *Ayurvedic Remedies for the Whole Family*. Twin Lakes: Lotus Press; 1999.

Murthy S, trans. *Astanga Samgraha of Vagbhata*. Varanasi: Chaukhambha Orientalia; 2005.

Pole S. *Ayurvedic Medicine: The Principles of Traditional Practice*. Churchill Livingstone Elsevier; 2006.

Sharma PV ed. and trans. *Caraka Samhita*. Varanasi: Chaukhambha Orientalia; 2003.

Sharma PV, ed. and transl. *Susruta-Samhita*. Varanasi: Chaukhambha Visvabharati; 2004.

Simon D, Chopra D. *The Chopra Center Herbal Handbook: Forty Natural Prescriptions for Perfect Health*. New York: Three Rivers Press; 2000.

Slattery DA, Neumann ID. No stress please! Mechanisms of stress hyporesponsiveness of the maternal brain. *J Physiol*. 2008;586(2):377–385.

Svoboda RE. *Ayurveda for Women: A Guide to Vitality and Health*. Rochester: Healing Arts Press; 2000.

Tewari PV, ed., transl., and commen. *Kasyapa-Samhita*. Varanasi: Chaukhambha Visvabharati; 1996.

Williamson EM, ed. *Major Herbs of Ayurveda*. Churchill Livingstone: Dabur Research Foundation and Dabur Ayurvet Limited; 2002.

9

Energy Medicine

ANN MARIE CHIASSON

CASE STUDY

An 80-year-old woman came into my office with severe itching in her lower legs. She was also experiencing grief and worry from a difficult emotional situation with her daughters. Physical examination revealed mild edema and severe excoriations of her lower limbs, with scabbing longitudinally, and areas of hypertrophic skin. She had tried multiple therapies prescribed by her general physician (GP) and dermatologist, including diuretics and topical steroids, with no benefit. My diagnosis was neurodermatitis, either secondary to edema from mild venous stasis or secondary to the stress of her family situation. I prescribed 5 minutes daily of toe tapping, a form of Qi Gong, that moves the energy in the legs, promotes relaxation, and also increases lymphatic flow in the lower limbs. I also prescribed 5 minutes of a heart-centered meditation daily. This meditation stimulates energy in the heart chakra, and will often help with emotional difficulty and reactivity. She came back in 1 month with her symptoms gone and her physical examination much improved. She also felt much more settled about her daughters. She continued to meditate and toe tap for 5 minutes each morning and by her follow up at 2 months, her lower legs were normal and there was no scarring. Two-and-a-half years later, the itching began to return. I suggested she resume the toe tapping and again her symptoms resolved immediately.

This is a dramatic example of healing, and certainly not all patients have remarkable results like this patient. What I found extraordinary was her willingness and ability to complete the prescribed exercise and meditation daily (Figures 9.1 and 9.2).

Toe tapping is a Qi Gong exercise from the Dahn tradition. The patient lies on the floor with legs apart at a comfortable distance. The hips and legs rotate externally and internally, the toes tap at the first toe and metatarsal. It is best done very quickly; playing fast rhythmic music is helpful. It is important the movement comes from rotation of the hips rather than adducting the legs or ankle alone; relaxation of the legs and better rotation of the hips will alleviate most difficulties with the technique. Patients with back problems may do this while lying in bed.

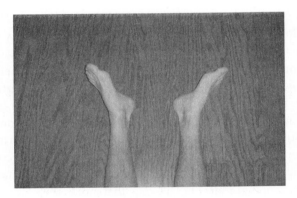

FIGURE 9.1. Legs and feet rotate outward from the hip.

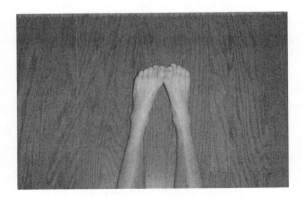

FIGURE 9.2. Legs and feet rotate inward from the hips, toes tap together.

Definition and Prevalence of Energy Medicine Use in the United States

E nergy medicine (EM) is a relatively modern term that attempts to describe those practices that involve the use of energy fields to promote health. The National Center for Complementary and Alternative Medicine (NCCAM) acknowledges that the "concept that human beings are infused with a subtle form of energy" has been around for 2000 years, and has many names, "such as Qi in traditional Chinese medicine (TCM), ki in the Japanese Kampo system, doshas in Ayurvedic medicine, and elsewhere as prana, etheric energy, fohat, orgone, odic force, mana, and homeopathic resonance" (NCCAM 2003). How the energy body and the physical body interact is described differently depending on the tradition but there is general agreement among traditions that this energy system, called the energy body, biofield, or subtle body, is housed within the physical body and is considered fundamental to the functioning of the physical body.

From the perspective of medical history, energy medicine may be seen as a resurgence of the concept of "vitalism" or the belief that an underlying vital force exists and is central to health. This concept predates Hippocrates, who espoused that the vital force was dependent on the balance of four humors. More recently, Franz Mesmer promoted this concept and called it magnetism. This underlying vital energy lost some of its importance when medicine shifted to organ based systems and diagnosis. I think this resurgence is actually an integration of prior views of health and healing with conventional medicine. This may end up augmenting our current views of health and how we treat illness.

The field of EM deals with both measureable and nonmeasurable energies. NCCAM recognizes two types of energy fields, veritable and putative. The veritable energies are those that are measurable (through wavelengths and frequencies) and "employ mechanical vibrations (such as sound) and electromagnetic forces, including visible light, magnetism, monochromatic radiation (such as laser beams), and rays from other parts of the electromagnetic spectrum" (NCCAM 2003). Many medical interventions employ electromagnetic fields including magnetic resonance imaging, cardiac pacemakers, radiation therapy, ultraviolet light for psoriasis, and laser keratoplasty, and more (NCCAM 2003).

Putative energy fields, according to NCCAM, are those that "have defied measurement to date by reproducible methods. Therapists claim that they can work with this subtle energy, see it with their own eyes, and use it to effect changes in the physical body and influence health" (NCCAM 2003). When practitioners and research studies discuss EM, most are referring to therapies that work with the putative field.

Ninety-four cultures have a documented concept, which describes the underlying energy of the body; it is alternately characterized as spiritual healing or energy medicine, and includes aspects of TCM, mind–body medicine, and some manual medicine therapies. Nurses tend to use EM, both in their usual work, and as a separate modality. Healing Touch was developed by a nurse, specifically for nurses as an adjunct therapy for hospitalized patients. Many nurses are also Reiki-trained.

Defining the scope of EM is controversial. Since many EM practitioners postulate that everything is energy, one can place much of complementary and alternative medicine (CAM) within the EM paradigm. This chapter will focus on EM modalities that address the subtle body and do not fall under other CAM paradigms. These modalities include Therapeutic Touch, Healing Touch, Reiki, Joh Rei, Sound Healing, Zero Balancing, Jin Shin Jytsu, Quantum Touch, Barbara Brennan's work, and Rosalyn Bruyere's healing. Spiritual healing, natural healing, and shamanic healing will not be addressed in this chapter (Table 9.1).

Until a method is devised to measure the body's subtle field, confusion about the definition and scope of EM will continue. Currently, gas discharge visualization (GDV), which measures biophoton emissions, superconducting quantum interference devices (SQUID), and low-frequency pulsed electromagnetic field (PEMF), are being used to measure the electromagnetic field of the body (Di Nucci 2005).

Despite the definitional uncertainty, EM modalities are being used in the United States. The 2000 National Health Interview Survey revealed that approximately 1% of adults in the United States use Reiki or another form of EM (CDC 2004). The percentage increases to 45–50% in persons with chronic pain and chronic illness (Rao 1999). Overall, women use EM modalities more than men. Most patients used EM as an adjunct for symptom relief rather than cure (Rao 1999). As of 2002, more than 50 hospitals and clinics in the United States provide some form of EM as an adjunctive therapy (Di Nucci 2005) and new forms of EM techniques and schools are popping up each year.

Table 9.1. A List of Common Energy Medicine Techniques

Technique	Theory
Acupuncture	Uses needles to stimulate energy flow at meridian points on the body.
Healing touch	Transfers energy by laying hands onto the body; based in the chakra system.
Homeopathy	Uses highly diluted substances that would cause symptoms in undiluted quantities.
Joh Rei	Detoxifies the energy body by sending universal energy to the patient from the healers hands across a short distance.
Polarity therapy	A touch therapy that balances positive and negative energy flows in the body.
Qi Gong	Uses movement and laying on of hands to cultivate balanced energy flow throughout the body.
Reiki	Channels universal energy into the patient's body through the hands of the healer.
Sound and light therapies	Use vibration through sound or light to affect the energetic body of the patient.
Tai Chi	A series of movements and postures to stimulate and increase energy flow.
Therapeutic touch	Transfers energy by placing the hands into the patients' electromagnetic field around the body.
Yoga	Philosophy, poses and breathing techniques to promote energy flow and balanced energy.
Zero balancing	A gentle touch and movement therapy that balances energy at the zero-point field of the body.

Source: Adapted from Baggott A. *The Encyclopedia of Energy Healing*. New York, Sterling Publishing; 1999.

Anatomy, Illness, and Healing within the Paradigm of Energy Medicine

The anatomy of the underlying energy field varies according to the tradition. One Qi Gong system (there are multiple of forms of Qi Gong) describes one basic energy center; the Hindu tradition introduced the chakra system with its seven energy centers, while TCM describes energy flows as meridians.

	Energy Fields These are energetic and encompass the body. This model was developed in India and is the most inclusive model.
	Seven Chakras This model is also from India and other cultures as well. These are the main energetic centers of the body responsible for metabolizing and storing specific types of energy.
	Twelve Meridians (or Twelve Energetic Pathways) This model was developed in China. These specialized maps provide us with information about how energy circulates throughout the body.

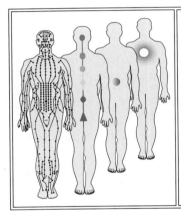

The energy bodies: the **most interior body** represented by a small blue light, is in the chest. On top of that we place the **causal body**, or dan-tien, the small red ball, a few inches in diameter and a few inches below the navel. Over this is the **subtle body**, which contains the seven chakras and the energy field extending to arm's length. Over this is the **physical body** containing the 12 meridians of energy

FIGURE 9.3. A summary of energy anatomy.
Source: Adapted from the University of Arizona, Program in Integrative Medicine Fellowship, 2007.

Conceptually the relationship between these anatomies can be seen as layers. The deepest layer is the primary energy center, the next layer houses the seven chakras, and finally, at the interface with the organs, are the meridians. A simple map of these layers is presented in Figure 9.3.

Different EM techniques work on different layers of the biofield. For example, Zero Balancing is targeted at the deepest layer, Healing Touch works at the chakra layer, while TCM works at the most superficial layer. Healers tend to perceive the energy field of the system they trained in, although some are able to perceive and work in multiple systems and layers.

In the natural history of a disease, the energetic field is thought to go out of balance first, then pathology develops, and finally symptoms appear. Major cellular pathology appears years after a block in the natural flow of energy, although pain, which is considered a form of blocked energy, can occur right away. Factors that contribute to or cause a block include outside insults, genetic or hereditary causes, and physical or emotional trauma. Treatment is based on transferring energy to remove blocks and restore normal energy flow. It is believed that keeping the energy field clear and the energy flowing promotes health and healing.

Energy medicine therapies shift or change the underlying energy field of the body. The most common technique involves laying the hands on, or over, the patient's body. Other techniques employ vibration, light, sound, movement, magnets, or direct current. Movement is extremely important as it promotes energy flow. The patient can continue to "work on themselves" through movement or self administered EM techniques, thus reducing the frequency of visits with an EM practitioner.

Research on Energy Medicine

While there is a paucity of well-done studies on EM, data are emerging. Research on veritable energy fields includes studies on magnet therapy, millimeter wave therapy, sound energy therapy, and light therapy. Unfortunately, the studies on putative energy fields is scant and of poor quality (NCCAM 2003).

Most studies have focused on Therapeutic Touch, developed by Delores Krieger in the 1970s, Healing Touch, a technique developed initially for nurses, and Reiki, a Japanese form of healing. Claims for EM modalities include decreased pain, anxiety, and healing times.

In the 1970s, Dr. Herbert Benson's research demonstrated the effect of relaxation on the body. He documented shifts in blood pressure, heart rate, and brain wave activity as well as improvements in immune system, peristalsis, and kidney function (Benson 1976). Similar physiological changes have been found in studies of EM treatments. For example, two studies demonstrated significant increases in hemoglobin and hematocrit levels in healthy persons learning Reiki (Miles 2003; Movaffaghi et al. 2006). Meehan performed three studies demonstrating that Therapeutic Touch reduces pain after surgery and decreases the time between request for prn analgesic dosing ($p < .01$) (Meehan 1985, Meehan et al. 1990, 1993). Wardell illustrated significant decreases in anxiety and blood pressure (BP), increased salivary IgA, increased skin temperature, and decreased EMG activity during a Reiki treatment (Wardell and Engebretson 2001). Similar findings were demonstrated by Manville with Healing Touch; he reported statistically significant decreases in pretreatment versus posttreatment systolic and diastolic blood pressure, heart rate, skin conductance level, EMG activity, and trait anxiety (Manville et al. 2008).

Placebo effects, relaxation, the effects of human touch, and the healer/ patient relationship are all potentially important factors in EM treatments. EM sessions, which are usually an hour long, can help patients cope more effectively with their illness. Noticeably, the patient's breath shifts during a healing session to slower, deeper, abdominal breathing. Zero Balancing teaches that this breath shift is indicative that the healing is effective.

Systematic reviews of EM in various settings reveal a broad range of rigor; approximately half showed benefit. Jonas et al. (2003) reviewed 19 randomized controlled trials (RCTs), most on TT, and found 11/19 showed statistically significant treatment effects with a mean effect size of 0.60. He concluded that the evidence for EM modalities for relieving pain and anxiety was "level B," or poor to fair. Astin et al. (2000) reported the mean effect of TT was 0.63 in a systematic review of 11 TT studies. He found 7/11 studies showed a positive effect on at least one outcome. When all healing trials (including prayer and distant healing) were reviewed, the mean effect size was 0.40. The mean effect score for distant healing, which included Reiki, was 0.38. A Cochrane review evaluated 24 studies involving 1153 participants. There were 5, 16, and 3 studies on HT, TT, and Reiki, respectively. Participants in these studies had on average of 0.83 units (on a 0 to ten scale) lower pain intensity than unexposed participants (95% Confidence Interval: −1.16 to −0.50). Reiki studies showed greater effects than TT and HT. Two of the five studies evaluating analgesic usage supported the claim that these therapies minimized analgesic usage (So et al. 2008).

Research on Women's Health and EM is limited. Qualitative evidence suggests that EM works well with postpartum women and culturally specific groups such as Hawaiian women (Kiernan 2002; Starn 1998). Brewitt et al. (1997) examined five patients with chronic illness (MS, lupus, fibromyalgia, and goiter) who were given 11 Reiki treatments. They reported a decrease in skin resistance over acupuncture meridians, and the patients reported decreased pain and anxiety. A systematic review of 25 RCTs on nonpharmacological interventions for fibromyalgia syndrome (FS) failed to find evidence of benefit for EM (Sim 2002).

EM may be useful in osteoarthritis. In a review by Ernst, magnet therapy, as measured by PEMF was examined in 75 patients with knee osteoarthritis. While there was no difference overall between the experimental and control group, magnet therapy showed an increase in quality of life (QOL) secondary measures in the intervention group when analyzed by paired analysis (Ernst 2002). Gordon et al. (1998) demonstrated that TT statistically decreased pain and improved function in patients receiving TT vs. mock TT, although there was no difference in the functional disability index. EM has also been used as an adjunct to cancer treatment to help alleviate side effects for over 20 years (Stephen et al. 2007).

Properly used, EM has negligible negative effects. Practitioners report there may be an increase in pain after the first few treatments. This is understood by the practitioners to represent the release of blocked energies and is expected to diminish and dissipate with subsequent treatments.

Consideration for Referral

Patients who are seeking adjunctive therapies for their pain or related symptoms, with a belief, openness, or cultural alignment to EM, may be appropriate for referral. Matching the patients' belief system to the available modalities is useful. Patients with longer duration of illness and more severe pain are good candidates. EM can be a useful adjunct to their medical management, with few side effects. If a patient does not experience positive physical or mental effects within a few visits, it may be more appropriate for the patients to use their resources on another modality.

Most EM modalities have Web sites with certification guidelines and lists of practitioners, i.e., *www.iarp.org*, www.healingtouchinternational.org, www. barbarabrennan.com, and *www.zerobalancing.com*

When choosing a pracitioner for referral, I have a few considerations. I choose practitioners that do not "hex" or put down conventional medicine. I tend to choose practitioners that have more experience, preferably over 3 years. Experience is not equal to expertise, yet I find healers who have been doing it longer are, as a group, better. I try to visit the healer myself prior to referring. I will often do this anonymously so I may have a "standard" session to see what my patients will experience.

Conclusion

EM is based on an ancient concept of a vital force and found in many cultures throughout the world. While research is limited, EM appears to be most helpful for increasing relaxation and decreasing pain and anxiety. It also creates a healing relationship between practitioner and patient which in itself is therapeutic. Women tend to seek out EM practitioners more than men, and EM may be a useful referral for chronic illness or chronic pain.

REFERENCES

Astin, J, Harkness E, Ernst, E. The efficacy of "Distant Healing": a systematic review of randomized trials. *Ann Intern Med.* 2000;132:903–910.

Benson, H. *The Relaxation Response.* New York, Harper Collins, 1976.

Baggott A *The Encyclopedia of Energy Healing.* New York, Sterling Publishing; 1999.

Brewitt B. Hartwell B, Vittetoe T. The efficacy of Reiki: improvements in spleen and nervous system function as qualified by electro-dermal screening. *Alter Ther.* 1997;3:89–97.

CDC. Complementary and Alternative Medicine Use Among Adults in the U.S., 2002. Advance Data: Issue 343; 2004.

Di Nucci, EM. Energy healing: a complementary treatment for orthopaedic and other conditions. *Orthopaedic Nursing.* 2005; 24(4):259–269.

Ernst, E.. Complementary and alternative medicine in rheumatology. *Bailliere's Clin Rheumatol.* 2002:14(4):731–749.

Gordon A, Merenstein JH, D'Amico F, Hudgens D. The effects of therapeutic touch on patients with osteoarthritis of the knee. *J Fam Pract.* 1998; 47(N4):217(7).

Jonas MD, Wayne B, Crawford CC. Science and spiritual healing: a critical review of spiritual healing, "energy" medicine, and intentionality. *Alternat Therap.* 2003;9(2):56–61.

Kiernan J. The experience of therapeutic touch in the lives of five postpartum women. *MCN Am J Matern Child Nurs.* 2002; 27(1):47–53.

Manville JA, Bowen JE, Benham G. Effect of healing touch on stress perception and biological correlates. *Holistic Nurs Pract.* 2008;22(2):103–110.

Meehan TC. *An Abstract of the Effect of Therapeutic Touch on the Experience of Acute Pain in Post-operative Patients* (dissertation). New York University; 1985.

Meehan TC, Mersmann CA, Wiseman M. The effect of therapeutic touch on postoperative pain. *Pain.* 1990;Supplement:149.

Meehan TC. Therapeutic touch and postoperative pain: a Rogerian research study. *Nurs Sci Quart.* 1993;6(2):69–78.

Miles P. Reiki-review of biofield therapy, history, theory, practice and research. *Alternat Therap.* 2003; 9(2):62–72.

Movaffaghi Z, Hsanpoor M, Farsi M, et al.. Effects of therapeutic touch on blood hemoglobin and hematocrit level. *J Holist Nurs.* 2006;24(1):41–48.

National Center for Complementary and Alternative Medicine (NCCAM). *Energy Medicine: An Overview.* Backgrounder, National Institute for Health, 2003.

Rao JK. Use of complementary therapies for arthritis among patients of rheumatologists. *Ann Intern Med.* 1999;131:409–416.

Sim, J, Nicola A. Systematic review of randomized controlled trials of nonpharmacological interventions for fibromyalgia. *Clin J Pain.* 2002;18(5):324–336.

So PS, Jiang Y, Qin Y. Touch therapies for pain relief in adults. *Cochr Database Syst Rev.* 2008; 8;(4):CD006535.

Starn JR. Energy healing with women and children. *J Obstet Gynecol Neonatal Nurs.* 1998; 27(5):576–584.

Stephen JE, Mackenzie G, Sample S, Macdonald J. Twenty years of therapeutic touch in a Canadian cancer agency: lessons learned from a case study of integrative oncology patients. *Supp Care Cancer.* 2007; 15(8):993–998.

Wardell DW, Engebretson J. Biological correlates of Reiki Touch healing. *J Adv Nurs.* 33(4), 439–445.

10

Homeopathy

PAMELA A. PAPPAS AND IRIS R. BELL

CASE STUDY

A 32-year-old woman with history of recurrent genital herpes was 37 weeks into her third pregnancy. Her outbreaks had been mostly controlled with medications over the years, but they would always last for 7 days when they occurred. Presenting with a genital herpes outbreak in the last 24 hours, she had been told by her obstetrician that a C-section would be needed unless this cleared in 48 hours. She did not want a C-section and sought alternatives.

During her first trimester, she had experienced severe nausea and vomiting; recurrent hemorrhoids marked her second trimester. In addition, she described a recurring, intermittent "bearing down" sensation throughout the pregnancy, along with frequent sinus infections. Currently, she experienced labial burning and eruptions similar to her previous outbreaks. She was also quite irritable, having a particular aversion to her husband throughout her pregnancy.

Homeopathic study of the case included the following descriptive rubrics from the Complete 2008 Repertory (van Zandvoort 2008):

FEMALE: Eruptions, Herpetic
STOMACH: Vomiting, Pregnancy in
RECTUM: Hemorrhoids, Pregnancy, in
MIND: Irritability, Pregnancy in

MIND: Husband; Aversion to
FEMALE: Pain; Bearing down

After case analysis, the patient was given one dose of the homeopathic remedy *Sepia*, 200C. Within 8 hours, all signs of herpes resolved. Her OB/GYN repeated the culture, which was negative. The patient went on to have a full-term pregnancy with normal delivery, and the child did well. This case (courtesy of Todd Rowe MD, MD(H), CCH) demonstrates how a remedy prescribed to match the patient's clinical symptoms stimulated her healing responses enough to eliminate a herpes outbreak.

Homeopathic *Sepia* is made from the ink of the Common Cuttlefish, a sea creature belonging to the Cephalopod family such as octopuses and squid. Like its relatives, the cuttlefish can change both the color and texture of its skin, and can escape danger by squirting ink into the water while jetting away in the opposite direction. This remedy has a repertory rubric found nowhere else:

MIND: Dreams; Pursued of being, run backwards, must (van Zandvoort 2008).

Sometimes remedies that heal are found through odd correspondences between patient characteristics and remedy source like this. *Sepia* is known to help many conditions experienced by women, including vaginitis, menopausal hot flushes, depression, and nausea and vomiting in pregnancy. Women responding to *Sepia* for chronic conditions often note irritability, sarcasm followed by remorse, and feeling overwhelmed especially with family responsibilities (Morrison 1993).

Introduction and Background

Classical homeopathy is a controversial 200-year-old system of medicine founded by the German physician Samuel Hahnemann, MD (Lansky 2003; Merrell and Shalts 2002). Like other whole systems of care such as traditional Chinese medicine (TCM) and Ayurveda, homeopathy differs from conventional Western medicine in theoretical foundations, diagnostic approaches, treatments, and outcome assessment (Bell and Koithan 2006; Verhoef et al. 2005) (Table 10.1). Based on the idea that healing is a concerted effort of the entire organism rather than any isolated part, it uses medicines corresponding

Table 10.1. Comparison of Homeopathy and Conventional Medical Models of Disease, Treatment, and Outcome

Feature	Homeopathic Model	Conventional Medical Model
Implicit scientific world view	Holism	Reductionism
Focus of diagnosis	Patient as a unique indivisible dynamical individual	Specific disease entity
Likely mechanism of action for medicines	Unknown. Possibly includes electromagnetic or epitaxic information transfer from the individualized medicine (remedy) to the body water and cells of the person, globally and locally; macro-entanglement hypothesis.	Probably involving specific biochemical ligand-receptor interactions
Goals of treatment	Cure of person's tendency toward disease at any level of organizational scale, mental, emotional, physical	Suppression of expression of disease in each local body part as dysfunctions or lesions develop
Clinical strengths	Chronic diseases with multiple co-morbidities involving dysfunction	Life-threatening emergencies, acute illnesses, and injury/physical trauma
Clinical limitations	Minimal effects on established structural changes	Significant safety risks of side effects and drug–drug interactions

Source: From Bell and Pappas (2008).

precisely to the symptoms experienced in order to stimulate this healing process. Holistic approaches like homeopathy may be particularly useful for women seeking whole-person interventions. Especially when patients present with complex biopsychosocial diagnoses across multiple systems, homeopathy can offer a safe, gentle, and comprehensive approach (Bell and Pappas 2008).

Use of Homeopathy

Homeopathy is one of the most popular forms of complementary and alternative medicine (CAM) in the world, especially in Great Britain, where more than 40% of physicians refer their patients to homeopaths; in France, where 30%–40% of physicians prescribe homeopathic medicines; and in Germany, where 20% of physicians follow this practice (Ullman 2008). Also very popular in Latin America and India, homeopathy leads the list of therapies for 59% of CAM-provider MDs, followed by acupuncture and botanical therapy (WHO 2002).

Use of homeopathy has been limited in the United States (utilization assessed at 3.7% in 1997; Barnes et al. 2004; Eisenberg et al. 1998), due at least partially to the Flexner report in the early 1900s and the rise of pharmaceutical care. Yet this utilization still increased fivefold between Eisenberg's two CAM surveys, with 82% (or 5.5 million) of users self-prescribing rather than consulting homeopathic practitioners (Eisenberg et al. 1998). A 1999 survey found that 17% of Americans were using homeopathy for self-care (Roper Starch Worldwide 1999).

Types of Homeopathic Prescribing

Homeopathy may be used in a variety of ways. This chapter focuses on "classical" homeopathy, which uses one homeopathic medicine ("remedy") at a time, selected for its similarity to the symptoms and state experienced by the patient, and prescribed in the minimum dose necessary to elicit a healing response (Ullman 2008). Thousands of homeopathic remedies are available, many having had clinical "provings" to determine their medicinal and curative properties. "Provings" test the effects of unknown homeopathic remedies on healthy people, similar to Phase 1 drug trials but are often double-blinded. Although Dr. Hahnemann briefly experimented with using multiple remedies simultaneously, this single "proven" remedy approach was the one he strongly recommended (Hahnemann 1843/1996).

Despite Dr. Hahnemann's preferences, there have long been practitioners and pharmacies combining multiple homeopathic remedies in "complexes" or "formulas" to give to a wide variety of people seeking to have the same disease. This is called "complex homeopathy" because multiple remedies, often in different strengths, are contained in the same preparation (Carlston 2003). These prepackaged mixtures are labeled according to condition treated, such as "headaches," "teething," or "menstrual cramps." Although they do not follow the principles of classical homeopathy, there is a research base for their use (Oberbaum et al. 2001; Weiser et al. 1998), suggesting that they provide relief for some people. Combination remedies might be reasonable choices when one cannot figure out which single remedy to give, or when the indicated single remedy is unavailable in the health food store or pharmacy. The needed remedy might be contained in an available "complex," and be a better option than no treatment (Ullman 2008).

While these mixtures have their applications, most experienced homeopaths believe that the symptom relief they afford is usually temporary and that a complete, deep cure is unlikely to be accomplished through them. If a complaint is recurrent, chronic, or keeps returning after the combination or single acute remedy wears off, more in-depth case-taking with a professional homeopath is needed. Some homeopaths also believe that combination remedies may even worsen chronic illnesses if used longer than 10–14 days (Shalts 2004).

Professional homeopathic care for chronic conditions usually focuses on "constitutional" treatment: prescribing a homeopathic medicine ("remedy") based on a woman's genetic inheritance, past health history and medical treatment, plus totality of physical, emotional, and mental/spiritual symptoms (Ullman 2008). This broad assessment is necessary, as the same basic disturbance is expressed on multiple levels. The correct "constitutional" remedy can stimulate healing from chronic diseases, reduce the influence of hereditary diseases, strengthen a woman's emotional and mental state, and reduce the frequency and severity of acute ailments. If acute illness does arise, a dose of one's constitutional remedy may stimulate complete cure.

Unlike herbal or nutritional products, homeopathic remedies are recognized as over-the-counter drugs and undergo regulatory oversight by the Food and Drug Administration (FDA) through the *Homeopathic Pharmacopoeia of the United States*, which standardizes their preparation (Bell and Pappas 2008). This requires homeopathic manufacturers to state the specific condition the homeopathic remedy is indicated to treat—another difference from dietary supplements, for which the FDA does not allow specific disease indications. Homeopathic remedies have many actions on multiple levels, but the FDA-required label might list only one indication. Consumers need to understand this as a feature of FDA regulation rather than the remedies themselves; homeopaths may use a remedy for more complex indications than its label shows.

Women, Healing, and Homeopathy

With a rich tradition in many forms of healing (Achterberg, 1990) ,women have been especially strong proponents of homeopathy (Kirschmann 2004; Ullman 2007). The first woman homeopath was Melanie Hahnemann (Dr. Samuel Hahnemann's second wife) in the 1800s (Winston 1999). Since then, many women have come to homeopathy as patients, to prescribe for their families, and as professional homeopaths.

Historians estimate that two-thirds of homeopathic patients in the nineteenth century were women, possibly seeking safer care than the bleeding, arsenic and mercury treatments conventional physicians favored (Kirschmann 2004). Other reasons may have been homeopathy's success in treating infectious epidemics such as cholera, typhoid, yellow fever, scarlet fever, and others (Ullman 2007).

"Ladies' Physiological Societies" sprang up in the 1840s and 1850s to teach women hygiene principles, including homeopathy; out of these grew the first medical colleges for women (Winston 1999). The women's suffrage movement in the 1840s encouraged this, although it took many years for women to gain admission to male-dominated medical schools. Still, women spread homeopathy's popularity in their communities. At the 1869 meeting of the American Institute of Homeopathy (AIH), one [male] homeopathic physician observed: "Many a woman, armed with her little stack of remedies, had converted an entire community to homeopathy" (Winston 1999, p. 141). The AIH finally opened membership to women in 1870, 5 years before the American Medical Association did.

Beyond treating physical concerns, homeopathy also offered women a way to understand and treat emotional and mental issues. Thus, it was "holistic" before this term ever came into vogue. When suffering a nervous breakdown from Crimean War traumas, the famous nursing pioneer Florence Nightingale (1820–1910) sought care from homeopathic physician Dr. James Gully (Ullman 2007); she referred to him as "a genius" (Jenkins 1972).

Applying Homeopathy in Women's Health

Classical homeopathy has applications in many women's conditions (Steinberg and Beal 2003), including those in pregnancy such as morning sickness, breech presentation, retained placenta (Castro 1993; Moskowitz 1992), and labor induction (Kistin and Newman 2007). Other uses include repeated miscarriage, infertility, postpartum depression (Reichenberg-Ullman 2000), premenstrual syndromes (Jones 2003; Yakir et al. 2001), breast problems including mastitis and nursing issues (Chernin 2006), fibromyalgia (Bell et al. 2004a, 2004b), and menopausal symptoms (Bordet et al. 2008; Jacobs et al. 2005; Relton and Weatherly-Jones 2005). Homeopathy also has applications in psychiatric conditions frequent in women, such as anxiety and mood disorders (Bell and Pappas 2007, 2008), and the aftermath of child sexual abuse (Coll 2002).

Despite these many uses, a big difference exists between prescribing homeopathic remedies for an "acute" or "first aid" condition and for chronic illness (Shalts 2004). Homeopaths distinguish carefully between these types of treatment. The term "first aid" applies to those conditions which are emergent and might be treated with whatever materials are at hand, such as traumatic injury including emotional shock. A true "acute" illness is one that is new, never experienced before, and self-limited. Someone with a single urinary tract infection or episode of diarrhea might meet this definition. However, someone with symptoms that recur monthly or that never really remit has a chronic condition. Successfully prescribing for chronic or repeated illnesses requires much more in-depth interviewing and research through the 4000 to 5000 existing homeopathic remedies for the one that best fits the woman's total state. By comparison, acute illnesses may present more dramatically, have clearer symptom pictures, and respond more readily to the lower potency single remedies available to beginning prescribers. Also as discussed earlier, combination ("complex homeopathy") remedies or mixtures may be helpful for acute conditions as long as their limitations are recognized.

Several women's conditions amenable to homeopathic treatment will be explored in further detail.

MENOPAUSE AND HOMEOPATHY

Menopause can be a challenging transition for many women, bringing uncomfortable symptoms such as poor sleep, hot flushes, and fatigue. When closely tailored to the complete person (in-depth constitutional prescribing), classical homeopathy can offer both lasting relief and improvement in overall health.

An audit of 102 women treated with single remedy, "constitutional" classical homeopathy through a National Health Service menopause clinic (Relton and Weatherly-Jones 2005) found 83 had improvement in their symptoms, including hot flushes, tiredness, anxiety, mood swings, crying, sleep difficulties, headaches, and joint and muscle pains. Bordet et al. (2008) also published an observational study involving 438 patients (average age 55) and 99 homeopathic physicians in 8 countries. Treatment focused on hot flushes, selected through in-depth "constitutional" classical homeopathy, and the most commonly prescribed remedies were *Lachesis*, *Belladonna*, *Sepia*, *Sulphur*, and *Sanguinaria*. Ninety percent of the women reported disappearance or lessening of their symptoms, usually within 15 days of starting homeopathic treatment.

Homeopathic treatment for menopausal symptoms has also been explored in breast cancer survivors. However, results have so far been equivocal. One randomized, double-blind, placebo-controlled study evaluated menopausal symptoms in 57 breast cancer survivors (Thompson and Reilly 2003; Thompson et al. 2005) who showed improvements in symptom scores over the study period. Although 90% of women rated their satisfaction with treatment as 7 or above on a 10-point scale, the study did not clearly show a specific effect of the homeopathic remedy.

Another study (Jacobs et al. 2005) examined the effectiveness of two types of homeopathy for the treatment of breast cancer survivors with menopausal symptoms. Here, 83 such women who had completed all surgery, chemotherapy, and radiation treatment—and who averaged at least three hot flashes per day for the previous month—were randomized to receive an individualized ("constitutional") homeopathic single remedy, a homeopathic combination medicine, or placebo. Seen by homeopathic providers every 2 months for a year, they were evaluated for hot flush frequency and severity, Kupperman Menopausal Index, and a quality of life questionnaire. No statistically significant difference in outcome measure was found, but there was a positive trend in the single remedy group during the first 3 months of the study. Also researchers noted a statistically significant improvement in general health for the single-remedy-treated patients. Alarmingly, evidence of a homeopathic "drug proving" in the subjects receiving the combination homeopathic medicine was also found. A homeopathic drug proving occurs when, after taking a remedy, the patient experiences symptoms that are completely new, or existing symptoms become extremely aggravated. In this case, the suspected symptoms were increased hot flush frequency and severity plus new headaches. The combination medicine contained three remedies, two of which (*Amyl nitrate* and *Sanguinaria*) were in relatively strong crude doses—and the women took these three times daily for a year. Women receiving the combination medicine who had not taken tamoxifen were more likely to experience this intensification of symptoms, but even they noted improved general health test scores compared to the placebo group.

Homeopathic remedies are most effectively prescribed according to the woman's total state rather than to eliminate single symptoms like hot flushes. Remedies such as *Lachesis* (from the Bushmaster snake), *Pulsatilla* (from the wind flower), and *Natrum muriaticum* (from table salt) derive from different kingdoms (animal, plant, and mineral, respectively), have different overall symptom pictures, and yet may all be indicated for menopausal complaints.

PREMENSTRUAL SYNDROMES

Menstrual pain is common in women, often interrupting their work and other life activities. Well-chosen homeopathic remedies can provide rapid relief from pain arising out of acute premenstrual syndrome (PMS). With some study in basic homeopathy courses offered at many homeopathic schools, women can often treat themselves (self-treatment) at least in limited fashion. Even so, they should recognize that while some symptoms may be ameliorated, the remedy selected may not be their overall constitutional one. If symptoms persist after one or two "acute" remedy trials or are recurrent, consultation with a professional homeopath is advised.

One controlled, double-blind study (Yakir 2006) followed 96 women in a university outpatient clinic who were randomized to individualized homeopathic treatment or placebo for menstrual distress. After 3 months, 44% of actively treated women versus 34% of placebo controls perceived themselves as suffering less; 47% versus 22% felt they needed no further treatment. Psychological suggestibility was not correlated with outcomes for either the verum (active remedy) or placebo groups. Jones (2003) also described successfully using remedies such as *Lac caninum* (made from dog milk) and *Natrum muriaticum* to treat women with premenstrual symptoms.

MORNING SICKNESS IN PREGNANCY

As a Consultation-Liaison psychiatrist before homeopathic training, one of us (PP) was frequently asked to see pregnant women with severe nausea and vomiting (hyperemesis gravidarum; Kemker and Gamboa 2006). Often these women did not respond to standard antiemetics. One extremely difficult case involved a 22-year-old single African-American woman, in her fifth month of pregnancy. She had been admitted multiple times for intractable vomiting, inability to eat, and dehydration. She would stay on the Ob-Gyn unit just long enough for IV rehydration and fetal monitoring, before being discharged to home where her abusive boyfriend and mother waited. They never visited her in the hospital. It was a revolving door, and the Maternal-Fetal Medicine team was at its wit's end.

Each time she returned I would see her. She always lay in the dark—irritable and moaning about her belly cramps and headache. The slightest smell of food would evoke new surges of nausea and vomiting, which gave no relief. Crowding her bedside were paper cups filled with the profuse saliva she spat out constantly; seeing me, she would yell, "Get the hell out of here! All you do is torture me!" None of my medicines or manner helped; I also withheld analytic ideas about "oral attempts at abortion" (Chertok 1972) because they seemed both impractical and punitive. In short, my presence was useless.

How enlightening years later to learn about the homeopathic remedy *Ipecacuanha*, which in material doses is a conventional medicine used to induce vomiting (*Ipecac*). Symptoms for which *Ipecacuanha* is known include terrible nausea unrelieved by vomiting; migraine headache; extreme irritability, and profuse salivation with drooling and spitting. Patients are weak and frequently need admission for IV hydration. Were it possible to go back in time, I would have offered this woman a few pellets of *Ipecacuanha* 30C.

Other useful remedies for pregnancy-associated nausea and vomiting (each having a slightly different symptom picture) include *Cocculus*, *Tabacum*, *Sepia*, and *Kreosotum* (Reichenberg-Ullman 2000).

OTHER PREGNANCY-RELATED ISSUES

Appropriately prescribed homeopathic remedies can be helpful for aches and pains during pregnancy. Common ones include *Arnica montana* (from Leopard's bane) whenever there are symptoms of bruising and swelling of muscles, and *Bellis perennis* (from Common Daisy) especially when the uterus and abdominal wall are sore and uncomfortable (Brennan 1999). Breech presentation responds to the remedy *Pulsatilla* up to 40% of the time (Moskowitz 1992). Premature labor can respond to remedies such as *Aconite* (from Monkshood); labor can sometimes be induced with the remedy *Caulophyllum* (from Blue Cohosh; Brennan 1999; Kistin and Newman 2007). As shown by the case study at the start of this chapter, resolution of infections such as herpes in pregnancy is possible as well through homeopathic treatment.

SOMATOFORM AND OTHER PSYCHIATRIC DISORDERS

Fibromyalgia is an idiopathic, chronic nonarticular pain syndrome defined by widespread musculoskeletal pain and generalized tender points. Accompanied by sleep disturbances, fatigue, headache, morning stiffness, depression and anxiety, it is also ~10 times more common in women than men (Chakrabarty and Zoorob 2007). Bell published a 2004 paper in *Rheumatology* describing a double-blind, placebo-controlled trial with 62 fibromyalgia patients randomized to receive an oral daily dose of an individually chosen homeopathic medicine or placebo. Evaluating patients at baseline, 2 months, and 4 months, researchers found that 50% of those given the homeopathic medicine experienced a 25% or greater improvement in tender joint pain, compared to only 15% of those given placebo. After 4 months, the homeopathic patients rated the "helpfulness of treatment" significantly greater than those given placebo (Bell et al. 2004a).

Another feature of Bell's study involved administering the first dose by olfaction (smell) as Hahnemann described in his *Organon* (Hahnemann 1843/1996) with both groups being monitored by an electroencephalogram (EEG). Patients given the "real" homeopathic medicine showed a significant and identifiable difference in EEG patterns compared to those given placebo (Bell et al. 2004b). Combined evidence of clinical improvement with an objective physiological response makes this trial unique. Remedies used included *Rhus toxicodendron* (poison ivy), *Bryonia* (White Bryony, from the gourd family), and *Kalmia* (Mountain Laurel).

Mood and anxiety disorders are approximately twice as common in women as men (Robinson 2006). Mental and emotional symptoms indicate deeper dysfunction of the Vital Force than physical symptoms alone (Vithoulkas 1980). Mood and anxiety complaints are often less specifically described than physical symptoms; this can make finding appropriate homeopathic remedies challenging. Dr. Rajan Sankaran has advanced homeopathic case-taking and prescribing by using such complaints as a starting point, and then allowing patients to progressively describe their experiences. Eventually conversations reach a level deep enough to encompass all mental, emotional, physical, and spiritual symptoms—and the single required remedy can be found (Sankaran 2004; Sankaran 2007). A correctly prescribed remedy catalyzes the self-healing process; consciousness itself shifts to a more free and peaceful state (Sankaran 2007). Extensive reviews of homeopathy's use in psychiatric conditions can be accessed in recent book chapters (Bell and Pappas 2007, 2008).

Childhood sexual abuse, estimated to be present in 25% of adult women in the United States, often leads to the combined physical, emotional, mental, and spiritual symptoms which classical homeopathy excels in treating. Clinical syndromes may include dissociation, depression, extreme rage and anxiety, chronic pain, and so on. The best remedy is determined through case-based research by an experienced homeopath (Coll 2002; Chappel 2008).

ADVERSE EFFECTS OF HOMEOPATHY

Reported rates of adverse effects with homeopathy in large observational studies fall from 2% to 5% (Bell and Pappas 2008). Not only new unexpected adverse symptoms are included in these rates, but also transient "aggravations" (temporary increases in existing symptoms that occur early in treatment and resolve spontaneously). Aggravation rates are reported as up to 24% in the first 2 months of treatment (Thompson et al. 2004). Only a small fraction (0.4%) of patients report prolonged aggravations (Sevar 2005). There are no reports of mortality from unadulterated, properly prepared homeopathic medicines in the clinical literature.

Summary and Recommendations

Despite skeptics who consider it sham or placebo (Lancet 2005) classical homeopathy has a long history of safety and clinical benefits in women's health. Differentiating it from other leading forms of CAM involving natural products, homeopathy has a manufacturing process for its remedies that is standardized and regulated by the Food and Drug Administration (FDA). Basic science, animal, and psychophysiological research (Bell and Pappas 2008) suggest that homeopathically prepared remedies have biological and behavioral effects beyond those of placebo. More research remains to be done.

Qualified homeopathic clinicians can be found through several professional organizations, including the American Institute of Homeopathy (www.homeopathyusa.org) for MDs and DOs, the Homeopathic Academy of Naturopathic Physicians (www.hanp.net) for NDs, the North American Society of Homeopaths (www.homeopathy.org) for professional but medically unlicensed homeopaths, and the National Center for Homeopathy (www.nationalcenterforhomeopathy.org), which is a mixed lay and professional group. For physicians wishing to learn homeopathic prescribing, courses such as those offered through American Medical College of Homeopathy (www.amcofh.org) are helpful. Effective prescribing for first aid and acute illnesses may be learned with 40–50 hours of training and accompanying study, but treating patients with chronic illness is not recommended without full homeopathic training and supervision. Classical homeopathy offers safe, gentle, and effective treatment for many women presenting with complex illnesses.

REFERENCES

Achterberg J. Woman as healer: a panoramic survey of the healing activities of women from prehistoric times to the present. Boston, MA: Shambhala Publications, Inc.; 1990.

Barnes PM, Powel-Griner E, McFann K, Nahin RL. Complementary and alternative medicine use among adults: United States, 2002. In: *Advance Data from Vital and Health Statistics*. CDC; Hyattsville, MD. National Center for Health Statistics; 2004.

Bell IR, Koithan M. Models for the study of whole systems. *Integr Cancer Ther.* 2006;5:294–307.

Bell IR, Lewis DAI, Brooks AJ, et al. Improved clinical status in fibromyalgia patients treated with individualized homeopathic remedies versus placebo. *Rheumatology*. 2004a;43:577–582.

Bell IR, Lewis DAI, Lewis SE, et al. EEG alpha sensitization in individualized homeopathic treatment of fibromyalgia. *Int J Neurosci*. 2004b;114:1195–1220.

Bell IR, Pappas PA. Homeopathy and its applications in psychiatry. In: Mischoulon D, Rosenbaum J, eds. *Natural Medications for Psychiatric Disorders*. 2nd ed., Philadelphia, PA: Lippincott Williams & Wilkins; 2008:303–321.

Bell IR, Pappas PA. Homeopathy. In: Lake JH, Spiegel D, eds. *Complementary and Alternative Treatments in Mental Health Care*. Arlington, VA: American Psychiatric Publishing, Inc.; 2007:195–224.

Bordet MF, Marijnen P, Masson J, Trichard M. Treating hot flushes in menopausal women with homeopathic treatment—results of an observational study. *Homeopathy*. 2008;97:10–15.

Brennan P. Homeopathic remedies in prenatal care. *J Nurse Midwifery*. 1999;44(3):291–299.

Carlston M. Classical homeopathy. Micozzi MS, Series Editor. *Medical Guides to Complementary & Alternative Medicine series*. Philadelphia, PA: Churchill Livingstone; 2003:53–54.

Castro M. *Homeopathy for Pregnancy, Birth, and Your Baby's First Year*. New York: St. Martin's Press; 1993.

CDC. Unintentional poisoning deaths—United States 1999–2004. *MMWR Weekly*. 2007;56:93–95.

Chakrabarty S, Zoorob R. Fibromyalgia. *Am Fam Physician*. 2007;76:247–254.

Chappell P. Post-traumatic stress disorder and the Vital Sensation. Homeopathic Links. 2008, Spring; 21:12–15.

Chernin D. The *Complete Homeopathic Resource for Common Illnesses*. Berkeley, CA: North Atlantic Books; 2006.

Chertok L. The psychopathology of vomiting of pregnancy. In: Howells JG, ed. *Modern Perspectives in Psycho-Obstetrics*. New York: Brunner/Mazel; 1972:283–289.

Coll L. Homeopathy in survivors of childhood sexual abuse. *Homeopathy*. 2002;91:3–9.

Eisenberg D, Davis RB, Ettner SL, et al. Trends in alternative medicine use in the United States, 1990–1997: results of a follow-up national survey. *JAMA*. 1998;280:1569–1575.

Hahnemann S. *Organon of the Medical Art (1843)*. 6th ed. O'Reilly WB, ed., Redmond DS, trans. WA: Birdcage Books; 1996.

Jacobs J, Herman P, Heron K, Olsen S, Vaughters L. Homeopathy for menopausal symptoms in breast cancer survivors: a preliminary randomized controlled trial. *J Alt Comp Med*. 2005;11:21–27.

Jenkins E. Dr. *Gulley's Story*. New York: Coward, McCann & Geoghegan; 1972.

Jones A. Homeopathic treatment for premenstrual symptoms. *J Fam Plann Reprod Health Care*. 2003;29(1):25–28.

Kemker K, Gamboa M. Pregnancy. In: Blumenfield M, Strain JJ, eds. *Psychosomatic Medicine*. Philadelphia, PA: Lippincott Williams & Wilkins, 2006; Chapter 36.

Kirschmann AT. *A Vital Force: Women in American Homeopathy*. Piscataway, NJ: Rutgers University Press; 2004.

Kistin SJ, Newman AD. Induction of labor with homeopathy: a case report. *J Midwifery Womens Health.* 2007;52(3):303–307.

Lansky AL. *Impossible Cure: The Promise of Homeopathy.* Portola Valley, CA: R.L. Ranch Press; 2003.

Merrell WC, Shalts E. Homeopathy. *Med Clin North Am.* 2002;86:47–62.

Morrison R. *Desktop Guide to Keynotes and Confirmatory Symptoms.* Nevada City, CA: Hahnemann Clinic Publishing; 1993.

Moskowitz R. *Homeopathic Medicines for Pregnancy and Childbirth.* Berkeley, CA: North Atlantic Books and Homeopathic Educational Services; 1992.

Oberbaum M, Yaniv I, Ben-Gal Y, et al. A randomized, controlled clinical trial of the homeopathic medication TRAUMEEL S in the treatment of chemotherapy-induced stomatitis in children undergoing stem cell transplantation. *Cancer.* 2001;92(3):684–690.

Reichenberg-Ullman J. *Whole Woman Homeopathy.* Roseville, CA: Prima Publishing; 2000.

Relton C, Weatherly-Jones E. Homeopathy service in a National Health Service community menopause clinic: audit of clinical outcomes. *J British Menopause Soc.* 2005;11(2):72–73.

Robinson GE. Gender differences in depression and anxiety disorders. In: Romans SE, Seeman MV, eds. *Women's Mental Health: A Life-Cycle Approach.* Philadelphia, PA: Lippincott Williams & Wilkins, 2006; Chapter 12.

Roper Starch Worldwide. *The Growing Self-Care Movement.* Washington, DC: Food Marketing Institute; 1999.

Sankaran R. *The Sensation in Homeopathy.* 1st ed. Mumbai, India: Homeopathic Medical Publishers; 2004.

Sankaran R. *Sensation Refined.* 1st ed. Mumbai, India: Homeopathic Medical Publishers; 2007.

Sevar R. Audit of outcome in 455 consecutive patients treatment with homeopathic medicines. *Homeopathy.* 2005;94:215–221.

Shalts E. Homeopathy. In: Kligler B, Lee R, eds. *Integrative Medicine: Principles for Practice.* New York; McGraw-Hill Companies, Inc., 2004; Chapter 12.

Steinberg D, Beal MW. Homeopathy and women's health care. *J Obstet Gynecol Neonatal Nurs.* 2003;32(2):207–214.

The Lancet (editorial). The end of homoeopathy. *Lancet.* 2005;366:690.

Thompson E, Barron S, Spence D. A preliminary audit investigating remedy reactions including adverse events in routine homeopathic practice. *J Am Inst Homeopath.* 2004;93:203–209.

Thompson E, Reilly D. The homeopathic approach to the treatment of symptoms of oestrogen withdrawal in breast cancer patients: a prospective observational study. *Homeopathy.* 2003;92:131–134.

Thompson E, Oxon BA, Montgomery A, Douglas D, Reilly D. A pilot, randomized, double-blinded, placebo-controlled trial of individualized homeopathy for symptoms of estrogen withdrawal in breast-cancer survivors. *J Alt Comp Med.* 2005;11:13–20.

Ullman D. *Homeopathic Family Medicine: Connecting Research to Quality Homeopathic Care.* Berkeley, CA: Homeopathic Educational Services; 2008.

Ullman D. *The Homeopathic Revolution: Why Famous People and Cultural Heroes Choose Homeopathy*. Berkeley, CA: North Atlantic Books; 2007.

Van Zandvoort R. Complete 2008 Repertory. Kent Homeopathic Associates. http://www.kenthomeopathic.com/macrepertory.html#Roger-van-Zandvoort

Verhoef MJ, Lewith G, Ritenbaugh C, Boon H, Fleishman S, Leis A. Complementary and alternative medicine whole systems research: beyond identification of inadequacies of the RCT. *Complement Ther Med*. 2005;13:206–212.

Vithoulkas G. *The Science of Homeopathy*. New York: Grove Press; 1980.

Weiser M, Strosser W., Klein P. Homeopathic vs conventional treatment of vertigo: a randomized double-blind controlled clinical study. *Arch Otolaryngol Head Neck Surg*. 1998;124:879–885.

WHO. The WHO Strategy for Traditional Medicine Review of the Global Situation and Strategy Implementation in the Eastern Mediterranean Region Health and Human Security. Cairo, Egypt, 2002.

Winston J. *The Faces of Homoeopathy: An Illustrated History of the First 200 Years*. Wellington, New Zealand: Great Auk Publishing, 1999.

Yakir M, Kreitler M, Brzesinski A, Vithoukas G, Bentwich P. Women with premenstrual syndrome under homeopathic treatment: improvements in health and quality of life. In Darnell P, Pinder M, Treacy K (eds). *Searching for Evidence: Complementary Therapies Research*. London: Prince of Wales Foundation for Integrated Health; 2006:14–15.

Yakir M, Kreitler S, Brzezinski A, Vithoulkas G, Oberbaum M, Bentwich Z. Effects of homeopathic treatment in women with premenstrual syndrome: a pilot study. *Br Homeopath J*. 2001;90(3):148–153.

11

Manual Medicine

CHERYL HAWK AND RAHELEH KHORSAN

CASE STUDY

Although I had been a chiropractor for many years, my first acquaintance with the effects of manipulation on chronic pelvic pain (CPP) was not through a patient but was shared with me by a friend. Ellen had suffered from CPP since her early twenties. Her gynecological exams were negative, and she was prescribed antidepressants and analgesics, which did not completely manage her symptoms. Her CPP was incapacitating at times. She had been very active in sports in high school and college and had suffered a number of injuries including sprains and strains of her lower back and knees. She had been relatively inactive since college when her symptoms began.

Her CPP symptoms were accompanied by lower back pain (LBP), and during a flare-up of especially bad LBP when she was 31 years old, she went to a chiropractor. The chiropractor manipulated her lower back, sacrum, pelvis, and femur heads, and she was astounded to find that her CPP was gone—permanently! It never came back in the 10 years since that first adjustment.

"You need to do research on this," she told me, since I had just completed my PhD in Preventive Medicine and had begun a career in clinical research. So I did as she suggested, and although I did not find another "miracle cure" like Ellen's, I found manipulation, especially flexion-distraction technique—a low-force technique using a specially designed table—to be a promising conservative approach, often giving a great deal of relief to the women suffering from this complex condition.

Introduction and Background

Spinal manipulation is among the oldest healing methods, and references to its use are recorded in many ancient cultures. In fact, Hippocrates practiced manipulation (Gatterman 2004). For centuries, "bonesetting" was a type of traditional medicine learned through apprenticeship and observation of functional movement of the human body (Meeker and Haldeman 2002). Interestingly, one of the most famous bonesetters in eighteenth century England was a woman, Sarah Mapp, who was so popular that a play was written about her (Gatterman 2004). Osteopathy and chiropractic arose as distinct professions in the late nineteenth century, and both incorporated the tradition of bonesetting as well as the concept of vitalism or life-force that was popular in the 1890s.

Today, "chiropractic" is often considered to be synonymous with "spinal manipulation." However, although chiropractors perform approximately 94% of spinal manipulation in the United States, chiropractic is a profession, not a procedure, and chiropractors provide a broad array of conservative therapies in addition to spinal manipulative therapy (SMT), including soft tissue treatment and counseling on physical activity and other lifestyle factors (Meeker and Haldeman 2002). Some osteopaths, physical therapists, massage therapists, and, in Europe, manual therapists also provide SMT.

"Spinal manipulation" refers to the application of biomechanical force to a spinal joint for the purpose of correcting joint dysfunction. It is believed in both osteopathic and chiropractic theory that such correction enhances function and promotes the body's self-healing capacity (Handoll 2004; Hawk 2007).

SMT has a substantial body of evidence for its effectiveness in relieving musculoskeletal complaints, especially pain that is spine related (Bronfort et al. 2008; Hurwitz et al. 2008). There is much less evidence for its effects on nonmusculoskeletal complaints (Hawk et al. 2007). This chapter will review the evidence on the safety and effectiveness of SMT on conditions commonly experienced by women, both musculoskeletal and nonmusculoskeletal, in order to assist clinicians and their patients in making decisions about appropriate care.

Spinal Manipulation and Conditions Common among Women

The conditions addressed in this chapter are those specific to women, or those that affect women predominantly, for which there is evidence that SMT may

Table 11.1. Women's Health Conditions for Which
Spinal Manipulation May Be of Clinical Benefit

Women's Health Conditions

Disorders of the menstrual cycle
  • Dysmenorrhea
  • Premenstrual syndrome (PMS)

Conditions related to pregnancy
  • Back pain during pregnancy
  • Back pain during labor and delivery
  • Breech presentation

Chronic pelvic pain (CPP)
Conditions with higher prevalence in women
  • Depression
  • Fibromyalgia
  • Migraine and tension headache
  • Multiple sclerosis (MS)

have clinical benefit. Conditions are only included if there is at least some published evidence, ranging from high-level evidences such as systematic reviews and randomized controlled trials (RCTs), to low level, such as case series. If the only available evidence comes from case reports and/or expert opinion articles on theory or technique, the condition is not included. Table 11.1 lists the conditions addressed in this chapter.

BACK PAIN DURING PREGNANCY

There is substantial evidence that SMT is helpful for both acute and chronic LBP in the general adult population (Bronfort et al. 2008). However, due to the physiological, hormonal and biomechanical changes during pregnancy—as well as the "baby on board"—clinicians need to see evidence that these effects may safely be extrapolated to pregnant women.

Although relatively few clinical studies have been conducted among this population, a recent systematic review found that there was limited, but promising, evidence that SMT by chiropractors or osteopaths was of clinical benefit for LBP during pregnancy (Khorsan et al. 2008).

Both chiropractic and osteopathic education include training on appropriate ways to modify manipulative techniques for pregnant patients, and contraindications to manipulation (Borggren 2007; King et al. 2003). Manipulative techniques should be modified to minimize discomfort and the risk of adverse effects. These modifications include avoidance of prone postures and high-force manipulative maneuvers (Borggren 2007). Because of the relaxing of ligaments during pregnancy, the sacroiliac joints become more mobile; thus, manipulation is often indicated not only for the lumbar vertebrae but also the sacroiliac area and pelvis (King et al. 2003).

None of the six published case series, two case-control studies, or one small experimental study reported any adverse effects on patients during their pregnancy or subsequent deliveries. However, one case report described an extremely rare case of a pathological cervical fracture after manipulation performed by a manual therapist in Germany (Schmitz et al. 2005). This illustrates the importance of avoiding high-force manipulation during pregnancy, when routine diagnostic imaging is better not utilized, and using appropriately modified manipulative techniques.

BACK PAIN DURING LABOR AND DELIVERY

There is much less evidence on the effect of manipulation on back pain during labor than during pregnancy. This may be partially explained by the fact that few chiropractors have hospital access to be able to conduct such research, and the number of osteopaths—who do have hospital access—and perform manipulation is relatively small. A 1982 osteopathic study investigated the effect of lumbar pressure applied by the woman's husband, coach or nurse during labor (Guthrie and Martin 1982). They found that requests for pain medication from women during labor were significantly less frequent than those requests from women who did not receive the intervention or received a placebo intervention (pressure applied to the thoracic area). Since this is a very low-risk procedure, and one that can be taught to the birth coach, it is worth a consideration even though the evidence is sparse.

There is somewhat more, but still not substantial, evidence on possible beneficial effects on labor and delivery from manipulation done as part of prenatal care, but not at the actual time of delivery (Diakow et al. 1991; King et al. 2003; Phillips and Meyer 1995). Again, no adverse events during the pregnancy or during labor and delivery were reported related to manipulation.

BREECH PRESENTATION CORRECTION

Although breech presentation occurs in a small proportion of singleton pregnancies, nearly 90% of these births will be by Caesarean section (C-section) (Tiran 2004). The usual medical alternative to a C-section is external cephalic version (ECV), but it has a relatively low success rate (Hutton and Hofmeyr

2006). Since many women and their providers prefer a vaginal birth, for both safety and personal reasons, there is growing interest in complementary and alternative medicine techniques to correct breech presentations (Tiran 2004).

The Webster technique is a manipulative procedure developed by a chiropractor to correct musculoskeletal imbalances believed to contribute to uterine constraint that may result in breech presentation (Ohm 2001; Pistolese 2002). It does not involve an attempt to reposition the fetus as is done in ECV. It involves a low-force manipulation of the sacrum, followed by very light (3 ounces to 6 ounces of pressure) manual trigger point therapy to musculature of the lower abdomen (Kunau 1998; Pistolese 2002).

Only one case series on the Webster technique was identified. It described five cases of successful correction of the breech presentation with no adverse events, which was verified by the women's medical physicians (Kunau 1998). All patients were Amish, a population who generally prefer natural approaches to health care, although all were under medical care also during their pregnancies. In a survey of 1047 chiropractors, out of 187 respondents, 112 reported using the Webster technique, and 102 met with success. No adverse events were reported (Pistolese 2002).

For a patient who desires to avoid a C-section, it may be worthwhile for her provider to locate a chiropractor who is trained and experienced in this technique and determine whether it is possible to evaluate the possible presence of musculoskeletal factors amenable to correction.

DISORDERS OF THE MENSTRUAL CYCLE

Dysmenorrhea

A 2006 Cochrane review of SMT for dysmenorrhea concluded that "there is no evidence to suggest that spinal manipulation is effective for the treatment of primary or secondary dysmenorrhea," but that the risk of adverse effects from SMT are no greater than they are for sham manipulation (Proctor et al. 2006).

However, 2 of the 4 trials analyzed by the Cochrane group used sham manipulations, which were very similar to the high-velocity, low-amplitude (HVLA) manipulation in the active groups, except for the amount of biomechanical force delivered—and there were decreases in pain in both groups. Since many chiropractors and osteopaths use low-force treatments, a maneuver that delivers a lesser amount of biomechanical force is not necessarily "inactive" or a "sham." In fact, the real-world applicability of using a manual placebo or sham procedure has been called into question because there is as yet no definitive evidence on a threshold at which biomechanical force has no effect (Hawk et al. 2005).

An interesting finding in one well-designed RCT (Hondras et al.1999) was that immediate treatment effects were not significant, but that patients showed a tendency to improve over three menstrual cycles. A 2007 systematic review concluded that the evidence was equivocal for chiropractic care for dysmenorrhea and, that the level of biomechanical force that is most appropriate is unclear, but that care extended over at least three menstrual cycles is more likely to be of clinical benefit (Hawk et al. 2007).

Thus, since adverse effects appear minimal, patients with dysmenorrhea who are interested in a therapeutic trial of SMT may benefit, if they are willing to remain under care for several menstrual cycles.

Premenstrual Syndrome

Few studies have investigated the effect of manipulation on premenstrual syndrome (PMS). However, the menstrual distress questionnaire was used in some dysmenorrhea studies, so there is some overlap in findings. One systematic review (Stevinson and Ernst 2001) found evidence insufficient and another (Hawk et al. 2007) found evidence equivocal for the utility of SMT for PMS. It is more likely that SMT would help patients with dysmenorrhea than with PMS symptoms not related to pain.

Chronic Pelvic Pain

Chronic pelvic pain, usually defined as acyclic pain in the pelvis occurring over at least six months, is a common reason for gynecological visits, 40% of laparoscopies, and 10% to 15% of hysterectomies (Tettambel 2005). The majority of women with CPP also experience LBP, and involvement of the musculoskeletal system as a contributing factor to this complex condition is becoming increasingly accepted (Montenegro et al. 2008; Tettambel 2005). Case reports and case series have described the utility of both chiropractic and osteopathic manipulation in managing CPP (Browning 1988, 1989; Tettambel 2005). A single group intervention with 18 women in which chiropractic manipulation, using flexion-distraction technique (a low-force approach not involving rotation of the vertebrae) and manual trigger point therapy, showed significant improvement in CPP after 4 weeks of care (Gay et al. 2005; Hawk et al. 1997).

Integrative approaches to CPP are currently being advocated, and usually include physical therapy (Chou et al. 2007). However, the 2005 Canadian consensus guidelines for management of CPP specifically recommend correction of myofascial dysfunction, postural abnormalities, and immobility of the sacrum (Chou et al. 2007). The addition of SMT, especially the usage of the low-force techniques of osteopathic muscle energy and counterstrain or the chiropractic technique of flexion-distraction—which are unlikely to cause adverse effects—into integrated medical management that includes soft tissue techniques like myofascial release, seems a reasonable approach to care of women with CPP.

DEPRESSION

A 2007 systematic review took an innovative approach to investigating a possible role for SMT in treatment of depression (Williams et al. 2007). This review examined RCTs of SMT for treating back or neck pain that included a measurement of psychological outcomes, such as the mental health subscale of the SF-36 or SF-12, or a depression questionnaire.

In these trials, spinal manipulation or mobilization was performed by, variously, chiropractors, osteopaths, and physical therapists. Although only 12 of 129 RCTs had psychological outcomes that could be analyzed, it did appear that SMT had a modest clinical benefit. Whether this was attributable to pain relief, the positive effect of touch, or the caring effect of the therapist is not clear. However, for individual patients who are interested in an integrative approach to depression or other non-severe psychological disorders such as anxiety, and who have spine-related pain, the combination of established approaches like cognitive behavioral therapy with SMT may be beneficial.

FIBROMYALGIA

Several small controlled studies have been published on both osteopathic and chiropractic manipulation for fibromyalgia (FM), providing some support for a role for SMT in treatment of this complex condition (Blunt et al. 1997; Gamber et al. 2002; Hains and Hains 2000). SMT was combined with soft tissue treatments that included myofascial release, and both low-force manipulation and HVLA manipulation were used in different studies.

A 2004 evidence-based guideline on management of FM stated that there was weak evidence for the efficacy of SMT (Goldenberg et al. 2004). SMT, as part of an integrated medical approach, when combined with appropriate soft tissue treatment, may provide added value above other physical treatments such as exercise or stretching (Gamber et al. 2002). Because of the complexity and individual variation of FM symptoms, it is especially important that, if SMT is recommended by the clinician, the provider of SMT be experienced in a variety of manipulative techniques and be highly responsive to patient needs and preferences.

MIGRAINE AND TENSION HEADACHES

Tension headaches often accompany migraines and therefore are often considered together in clinical studies. A 2004 Cochrane review of noninvasive treatments for headache identified 22 studies with 2628 patients (Bronfort et al. 2004). The authors concluded that SMT may be effective for prophylaxis of migraines, having a similar short-term effect to amitriptyline. However, amitriptyline appears to be more effective than SMT for prophylaxis of chronic tension-type headaches. The review found little risk of adverse effects for either type of headache. Patients who prefer to avoid medications may, therefore, find comparable benefit in a course of SMT without significant risk of harm.

MULTIPLE SCLEROSIS

Only one small pilot study (seven women with multiple sclerosis, MS) that has investigated the effect of SMT on MS has been conducted (Yates et al. 2002). By the end of the study lasting 12 weeks, there was a significant improvement in the strength of the patients and the distance that they were able to walk and no increase in fatigue. Although there no other group existed for a comparison, these findings were still encouraging, especially since no adverse events were noted. Since maintaining functional ability is essential to management of MS, it may be helpful to recommend a course of SMT for patients with low to medium levels of impairment.

SAFETY OF SPINAL MANIPULATION

Serious adverse events caused by SMT are rare, and therefore, it is difficult to estimate risks precisely; serious complications of manipulation of the lumbar spine are estimated to be 1 case per 100 million manipulations (Meeker and Haldeman 2002). The most severe complication of lumbar spine manipulation is cauda equina syndrome.

For cervical spine manipulation, cerebrovascular artery dissection that leads to stroke is the most serious adverse event. This topic has been the subject of a great deal of controversy; estimates of the risk of stroke range from 1 per 400,000 to 3 to 6 per 10 million manipulations. However, all these estimates were based on case reports and unsubstantiated provider surveys (Meeker and Haldeman 2002).

In 2008, a well-designed population-based case-control and case-crossover study found that there was no increased risk of vertebrobasilar artery (VBA) stroke for chiropractic patients, when they are compared to patients of primary care medical physicians (Cassidy et al. 2008). Apparently, patients seek care for headaches and neck pain in the early stages of the VBA dissection, and thus produce an increased association with visits to their health care provider—the increased association was not isolated to chiropractors (Cassidy et al. 2008).

Mild-to-moderate, transient side effects of manipulation are common; they include muscle soreness, stiffness, and increased neck or back pain (Hurwitz et al. 2005). Modifying the manipulative technique—such as using mobilization, which involves slower rotation of the spinal joints than manipulation—may reduce adverse effects (Hurwitz et al. 2005). Use of rotation-type manipulation is a predictor of adverse events—primarily increased headache or neck pain—as is more than 30 days of neck pain in the past year (Rubinstein et al. 2008).

For patients who are considered at risk for an adverse event by the clinician, or who are apprehensive about manipulation, there are many low-force manipulative techniques that do not involve rotation of the spinal joints and do not employ the high-velocity, low-amplitude (HVLA) maneuver, traditionally associated with the term "manipulation." It is important that clinicians become acquainted with local providers who use manipulation so that they know those providers who are skilled at using a variety of manipulative techniques, which they can then tailor to each patient's individual clinical presentation and personal preferences.

Summary and Conclusions

SMT, which is performed by professionals who are trained in its use, has a substantial body of evidence for its utility for musculoskeletal complaints, especially back and neck pain. Because, in most controlled studies, women make up at least half of the patient populations, it is reasonable to assume that their findings are applicable. However, less evidence has been accumulated for its application to special populations like pregnant women.

Similarly, the evidence for the utility of SMT for women with nonmusculoskeletal conditions or complex conditions like MS or FM is in short supply.

Therefore, it is important that interested patients among pregnant women or women with other conditions except common musculoskeletal conditions like back and neck pain be referred to a chiropractor or osteopath who has had success with that condition and with whom the referring clinician has established a relationship of mutual trust and communication.

REFERENCES

Blunt KL, Rajwani MH, Guerriero RC. The effectiveness of chiropractic management of fibromyalgia patients: a pilot study. *J Manipulative Physiol Ther.* 1997;20(6):389–399.

Borggren CL. Pregnancy and chiropractic: a narrative review the literature. *J Chiropractic.* 2007;6(2):70–74.

Bronfort G, Haas M, Evans R, Kawchuk G, Dagenais, S. Evidence-informed management of chronic low back pain with spinal manipulation and mobilization. *Spine J.* 2008;8(1):213–225.

Bronfort G, Nilsson N, Haas M, et al. Noninvasive physical treatments for chronic/recurrent headache. *Cochrane Database Syst Rev.* 2004;3:CD001878.

Browning JE. Chiropractic distractive decompression in the treatment of pelvic pain and organic dysfunction in patients with evidence of lower sacral nerve root compression. *J Manipulative Physiol Ther.* 1988;11(5):426–432.

Browning JE. Chiropractic distractive decompression in treating pelvic pain and multiple system pelvic organic dysfunction. *J Manipulative Physiol Ther.* 1989;12(4):265–274.

Cassidy DJ, Boyle E, Cote P, et al. Risk of vertebrobasilar stroke and chiropractic care. *SPINE.* 2008;33(45):S176–S183.

Chou R, Qaseem A, Snow V, et al. Diagnosis and treatment of low back pain: a joint clinical practice guideline from the American College of Physicians and the American Pain Society. *Ann Intern Med.* 2007;147(7):478–491.

Diakow PR, Gadsby TA, Gadsby JB, Gleddie JG, Leprich DJ, Scales AM. Back pain during pregnancy and labor. *J Manipulativ Physiol Ther.* 1991;14(2):116–118.

Gamber RG, Shores JH, Russo DP, Jimenez C, Rubin BR. Osteopathic manipulative treatment in conjunction with medication relieves pain associated with fibromyalgia syndrome: results of a randomized clinical pilot project. *J Am Osteopath Assoc.* 2002;102(6):321–325.

Gatterman MI. *Chiropractic Management of Spine Related Disorders.* 2nd ed. Baltimore, MD: Lippincott Williams & Wilkins; 2004.

Gay RE, Bronfort G, Evans RL. Distraction manipulation of the lumbar spine: a review of the literature. *J Manipulative Physiol Ther.* 2005;28(4):266–273.

Goldenberg DL, Burckhardt C, Crofford, L. Management of fibromyalgia syndrome. *JAMA.* 2004;292(19):2388–2395.

Guthrie RA, Martin RH. Effect of pressure applied to the upper thoracic (placebo) versus lumbar areas (osteopathic manipulative treatment) for inhibition of lumbar myalgia during labor. *J Am Osteopath Assoc.* 1982;82(4):247–251.

Hains G, Hains, F. A combined ischemic compression and spinal manipulation in the treatment of fibromyalgia: a preliminary estimate of dose and efficacy. *J Manipulative Physiol Ther.* 2000;23(4):225–230.

Handoll, HH. (2004). Energy medicine: an osteopath's personal view. *J Altern Complement Med.* 2004;10(1):87–89.

Hawk, C. (2007). Are we asking the right questions? *Chiropr J Australia.* 2004;37(1):15–18.

Hawk C, Khorsan R, Lisi AJ, Ferrance RJ, Evans MW. Chiropractic care for nonmusculoskeletal conditions: a systematic review with implications for whole systems research. *J Altern Complement Med.* 2007;13(5):491–512.

Hawk C, Long C, Azad A. Chiropractic care for women with chronic pelvic pain: a prospective single-group intervention study. *J Manipulative Physiol Ther.* 1997;20(2):73–79.

Hawk C, Long CR, Rowell RM, Gudavalli MR, Jedlicka, J. A randomized trial investigating a chiropractic manual placebo: a novel design using standardized forces in the delivery of active and control treatments. *J Altern Complement Med.* 2005;11(1):109–117.

Hondras MA, Long CR, Brennan PC. Spina manipulative therapy versus a low force mimic maneuver for women with primary dysmenorrhea: a randomized, observer-blinded, clinical trial. *Pain.* 1999;81(1–2):105–14.

Hurwitz EL, Carragee EJ, van der Velde G, et al. Treatment of neck pain: noninvasive interventions. *Spine.* 2008;33(45):S123–S152.

Hurwitz EL, Morgenstern H, Vassilaki M, Chiang LM. Frequency and clinical predictors of adverse reactions to chiropractic care in the UCLA neck pain study. *Spine.* 2005;30(13):1477–1484.

Hutton EK, Hofmeyr GJ. External cephalic version for breech presentation before term. *Cochrane Database Syst Rev.* 2006;1:CD000084.

Khorsan R, Hawk C, Lisi AJ, & Kizhatkkeveettil A. Spinal manipulative therapy for pregnancy and related conditions: a systematic review. *Obstetr & Gynecol Survey.* 2009;64(6):416–427.

King HH, Tettambel MA, Lockwood MD, Johnson KH, Arsenault DA, Quist, R. Osteopathic manipulative treatment in prenatal care: a retrospective case control design study. *J Am Osteopath Assoc.* 2003;103(12):577–582.

Kunau, P. Application of the Webster in-utero constraint technique: a case series. *J Chiropr Clin Pediatr.* 1998;3(1):211–216.

Meeker WC, Haldeman, S. Chiropractic: a profession at the crossroads of mainstream and alternative medicine. *Ann Intern Med.* 2002;136(3):216–227.

Montenegro ML, Vasconcelos EC, Candido Dos Reis FJ, Nogueira AA, Poli-Neto OB. Physical therapy in the management of women with chronic pelvic pain. *Int J Clin Pract.* 2008;62(2):263–269.

Ohm, J. Chiropractors and midwives: a look at the Webster Technique. *Midwifery Today Int Midwife.* 2001;58:42.

Phillips CJ, Meyer JJ. Chiropractic care, including craniosacral therapy, during pregnancy: a static-group comparison of obstetric interventions during labor and delivery. *J Manipulative Physiol Ther.* 1995;18(8):525–529.

Pistolese RA. The Webster technique: a chiropractic technique with obstetric implications. *J Manipulative Physiol Ther.* 2002;25(6):E1–9.

Proctor ML, Hing W, Johnson TC, Murphy PA. Spinal manipulation for primary and secondary dysmenorrhoea. *Cochrane Database Syst Rev.* 2006;3:CD002119.

Rubinstein SM, Leboeuf-Yde C, Knol DL, de Koekkoek TE, Pfeifle CE, van Tulder MW. Predictors of adverse events following chiropractic care for patients with neck pain. *J Manipulative Physiol Ther.* 2008;31(2):94–103.

Schmitz A, Lutterbey G, von Engelhardt L, von Falkenhausen M, Stoffel, M. Pathological cervical fracture after spinal manipulation in a pregnant patient. *J Manipulative Physiol Ther.* 2005;28(8),633–636.

Stevinson C, Ernst, E. Complementary/alternative therapies for premenstrual syndrome: a systematic review of randomized controlled trials. *Am Obstet Gynecol.* 2001;185(1):227–235.

Tettambel MA. An osteopathic approach to treating women with chronic pelvic pain. *J Am Osteopath Assoc.* 2005;105(9 Suppl 4):S20–22.

Tiran, D. Breech presentation: increasing maternal choice. *Complement Ther Nurs Midwifery.* 2004;10(4):233–238.

Williams NH, Hendry M, Lewis R, Russell I, Westmoreland A, Wilkinson, C. Psychological response in spinal manipulation (PRISM): a systematic review of psychological outcomes in randomised controlled trials. *Complement Ther Med.* 2007;15(4):271–283.

Yates HA, Vardy TC, Kuchera ML, Ripley BD, Johnson JC. Effects of osteopathic manipulative treatment and concentric and eccentric maximal-effort exercise on women with multiple sclerosis: a pilot study. *J Am Osteopath Assoc.* 2002;102(5):267–275.

PART III

Reproductive Health

12

Premenstrual Syndrome

DAPHNE MILLER

CASE STUDY

Every month before my period I get terrible cramping, breast tenderness and mood swings. It's now to the point where I don't want to go to work, and I snarl at my family. My last doctor did not have much to offer me—her only suggestion was that I could start birth control pills or antidepressants. I want to feel better but I don't want to take these medications for a problem that only bothers me for three to four days each month. Plus I am very sensitive to all medication. I have taken different birth control pills in the past and they all give me headaches and make me even more depressed.

Marie M, Age 29

Introduction

Almost every woman of reproductive age experiences some amount of physical or psychological discomfort in the week preceding her menstrual period (Freeman 2003; Halbreich et al. 2007; Johnson 2004). Premenstrual symptoms (Table 12.1), when they are present to a degree that they affect the quality of life, social engagements, and/or the work performance are identified as a "syndrome" (PMS or premenstrual syndrome) or, if more stringent criteria are met, a "disorder" (premenstrual dysphoric disorder). The inclusion criteria for these two diagnoses continue to be debated; yet, it is clear that those premenstrual symptoms, PMS, and PMDD represent a continuum

Table 12.1. Premenstrual Symptoms

Emotional symptoms	Depressed, sad, down or blue
	Anxious, tense, on edge or keyed up
	Angry or irritable
Physical symptoms	Breast tenderness
	Muscle or joint aches
	Stomach bloating or diarrhea
	Carbohydrate craving or increased appetite

of the same entity. In the end, these specific definitions have little relevance for the clinical practitioner (Halbreich et al. 2007). What is important is the degree and nature of symptoms reported by each individual woman and how her experience impacts her quality of life. Therefore, although the term PMS is used throughout this chapter and the research presented primarily includes women with a formal diagnosis PMS or PMDD, the following recommendations will be applicable to anyone wishing to address negative premenstrual symptoms.

Theories abound on the potential causes of PMS, but after 40 years of clinical and epidemiological research, the exact etiology remains unclear. For most women, their symptoms are likely to be a complex interplay of physiological, psychological, and environmental factors. Available pharmacologic and surgical treatments are often considered unacceptable treatments for PMS as they frequently offer disproportionately more side effects than perceived benefits. Community-based studies suggest that over 70% of women seeking to alleviate symptoms first turn to alternative (nonpharmaceutical or nonsurgical) strategies (Pullon et al. 1989). Taking into consideration the heterogeneous nature of PMS, the lack of a single highly effective and widely accepted conventional treatment, and a general preference for alternative therapies, PMS lends itself perfectly to an integrative medical approach.

The Personal and Social Burden of PMS

Most women in developed countries have about 400 to 500 menstrual cycles in their reproductive years, and it is conceivable that a woman could spend 12% of her life suffering from premenstrual symptoms. Severe premenstrual symptoms result in a similar burden of illness (disability-adjusted life years, DALYS) as major dysphoric disorders such as major depression (Halbreich 2002). Compared to women with mild or no premenstrual symptoms, women who suffer moderate to severe PMS miss significantly greater workdays, report lower productivity because of their symptoms, and feel that their personal relationships (especially with spouses) are negatively impacted (Dean and Borenstein 2004; Robinson and Swindle 2000). In one study, women with moderate or worse symptoms had more visits to ambulatory health care providers and incurred higher annual health care costs as compared to women with mild or no PMS (Borenstein et al. 2007). It is also likely that PMS heightens the symptoms of other chronic pain syndromes such as irritable bowel syndrome (IBS), fibromyalgia, and chronic fatigue.

Who Gets PMS?

Accurate prevalence rates are difficult to establish; however, it is estimated that 80% to 90% of women of reproductive age experience at least mild symptoms with each menstrual cycle. Although only 2% to 3% of women have physical and psychological discomfort that is severe enough to meet the criteria for PMDD, over 20% of women have monthly experiences that are so distressing that they warrant treatment (Sternfeld et al. 2002). There are few identified social or biological risk factors for PMS although prevalence studies indicate that younger women tend to have a greater intensity and variety of symptoms (Freeman et al. 1995; Wood et al. 1992). Women of all ethnicities experience premenstrual symptoms, and the negative symptoms related to the premenstrual period appear to transcend sociocultural divides (Sternfeld et al. 2002; Robinson and Swindle 2000). It is interesting to note that women interviewed in areas as different as China and Australia have reported roughly the same constellation of symptoms with irritability and depression emerging as the most frequent complaint in both regions (Gotts et al. 1995; Zhao et al. 1998).

Women are much more likely to underreport premenstrual symptoms if they have the perception that it is not a real health problem or that they should be more stoic (Robinson and Swindle 2000). Therefore, at each clinic visit, remember to ask detailed questions about their symptoms and validate their experience.

Diagnosing PMS

Before diagnosing PMS, it is important to undertake a complete clinical evaluation. One goal of this initial assessment is to rule out other conditions that can be confused with PMS (Table 12.2). A detailed history should include

Table 12.2. Differential Diagnoses of PMS

Psychological Disorders	Medical Conditions
Chronic depression	Dysmenorrhea
Major depressive episode	Endometriosis
Bipolar disorder	Hypothyroidism
Generalized anxiety disorder	Polycystic ovary syndrome
Panic disorder	Migraines
Somatiform disorder	Allergies
Substance abuse	Irritable bowel syndrome
	Perimenopausal symptoms
	Adrenal insufficiency

specific questions about PMS symptoms (Table 12.1) and their significance in a woman's life.

Allowing a woman to explain her symptoms and receive validation can be one of the first steps in treatment. In addition, certain interventions have been shown to be more effective against a particular set of symptoms such as depression, breast pain, or bloating, and therefore, a history can help tailor the intervention. Recording specific symptoms and their severity in a 1 to 10 scale can also help assess effectiveness of treatment. In general, a 50% decrease in symptoms translates into a noticeably improved quality of life for women with PMS (Borenstein et al. 2007).

Diagnosing PMS

The specific diagnosis of PMS or PMDD requires that women use diaries to record symptoms for two consecutive menstrual cycles. Although diaries can be useful for women who are uncertain about the timing or severity of their symptoms, asking them a general question followed up by a more detailed inquiry is often the best approach. The following is an example of the general type of question that I ask to assess for PMS-type symptoms: "Thinking specifically of the week before your period starts, would you describe the level of your symptoms as mild, moderate, strong or severe?"

As part of the initial assessment, every woman should also receive a complete physical and pelvic exam. Laboratory tests to assess for anemia, hypothyroidism, hyperprolactinemia, and cortisol imbalances should be considered.

Approaches to Treating PMS

CONVENTIONAL TREATMENT

In the past 40 years, PMS and PMDD have been the subject of intense biological and epidemiological research in an attempt to identify causes and develop effective treatments. These efforts have uncovered many potentially relevant physiological and environmental explanations including ovarian hormonal dysfunction, abnormal regulation of aldosterone, defects in immunologic response, nutritional deficiencies, and emotional stress. However, there is no consistent link between any of these factors and PMS (Backstrom et al. 2003; Muse 1992).

Conventional treatment strategies have focused on identifying a drug that will interfere with one of these specific processes, be it hormonal, neurohumoral, or inflammatory. This has resulted in the use of a diverse armamentarium of pharmaceuticals including serotonergic antidepressants (SSRIs), nonsteroidal anti-inflammatories (NSAIDS), anxiolytics, spironalactone, and hormones (especially birth control pills). Despite the popularity of these drugs among health care professionals, *SSRIs are the only conventional treatment whose efficacy for PMS has been well supported by clinical trials.* SSRIs, although exceedingly helpful for a select group of women, have a rather large side effect profile and subsequently a high rate of discontinuation (Rapkin 2005). Hormones, including birth control pills, have less compelling evidence and actually seem to exacerbate PMS symptoms in some women. NSAIDS have their own potential side effects; most significant are gastric ulceration and renal dysfunction (see Table 12.3). Given the paucity of data as to the benefits of

Table 12.3. Pharmacological Treatments for PMS

Antidepressants (SSRIs and SNRIs)
Oral contraceptives
Progesterone
Anxiolytics
GnRH analogs
Diuretics

conventional treatments for PMS coupled with a high discontinuation rate due to side effects, first-line treatment with drugs should be reserved for women with severe symptoms (Jarvis et al. 2008).

INTEGRATIVE MODEL FOR PMS TREATMENT

A health practitioner who adopts an integrative approach for treating PMS will focus on the experience of each individual woman and acknowledge that there is likely to be a complex explanation for her symptoms encompassing biophysical, environmental, and/or psychological factors. In addition, the integrative practitioner approaches premenstrual symptoms less as a disorder and more as part of normal woman's cycle. Treatment plans will therefore be multimodal, actively involving the patient and with each recommendation closely matched to her preferences. In each instance, she will begin to address her symptoms with a range of resources be they internal (visualization and biofeedback) or external (herbs, diet, pharmaceuticals) with the goal of giving her the most benefit with the least amount of side effects.

Since pharmaceuticals are discussed in other publications, this chapter focuses principally on alternative treatments. Due to methodological challenges, many of these treatments are not supported by rigorous randomized controlled trials. Nonetheless, all the following interventions have data promising enough to warrant their inclusion. Furthermore, virtually all of these have a wide therapeutic margin and low cost and have been shown to be very acceptable to women with PMS.

PMS Research Challenges

Challenges to assessing the effectiveness of all PMS treatments—both conventional and alternative—include variability in syndrome definition and outcome measures, small sample sizes, problems with blinding, and short treatment periods. In addition, all PMS treatments seem to have a significant placebo effect: a finding that suggests the important role that psychological factors play in PMS symptomotology (Freeman and Rickels 1999; Stevinson and Ernst 2001). Alternative treatments pose their own research challenges because these modalities often rely on personalized or individualized approach that is harder to replicate using the randomized, placebo-controlled double-blinded research model.

Nutrition and PMS

I heard that dietary supplements could make a difference in my symptoms. Can you tell me which ones are most likely to help? I also feel these intense cravings for carbs in the week before each period and find myself binging on cookies and bread. It drives me crazy and I think that is what has led to my slow weight gain.

Marie

Most nutrition studies related to PMS have focused on the effects of nutritional supplements. Nonetheless, there is a mounting body of evidence that dietary choices may contribute to PMS symptoms.

Caffeine

In several observational studies, luteal phase consumption of caffeinated beverages including sodas and coffee has been positively correlated with severity of premenstrual symptoms (Cross et al. 2001; Rossignol and Bonnlander 1990). Caffeine could theoretically exacerbate PMS symptoms by increasing anxiety. To date, however, there has not been an intervention trial to help determine whether these eating patterns are a result of PMS food cravings or whether limiting these foods might actually *improve* PMS symptoms. Furthermore, it is not clear whether it is the caffeine itself or other additives that are also found in caffeinated foods.

Caffeine Holiday

Given the potential benefits and limited risk, I have found that it is worth recommending that women eliminate highly caffeinated foods such as coffee and sodas for two consecutive menstrual cycles in order to see whether this offers them a noticeable improvement.

Carbohydrate Cravings

Women with PMS have been observed to boost their consumption of carbohydrates during the premenstrual phase. One explanation proposed by scientists is that some women are exquisitely sensitive to the natural dips in the neurotransmitter serotonin that occur in the luteal phase. Consequently, they are trying to self-medicate with carbohydrates, which happen to be a rich source of the serotonin precursor tryptophan (Sayegh et al. 1995; Wurtman 1990). Another explanation is that sensitivity to sweetness increases in this phase, thus making carbohydrates more attractive (Farage et al. 2008). Recognizing this cyclical preference for carbohydrates, it is important to counsel women in their selection of starches and steer them toward lower calorie, lower glycemic, more nutritious choices such as tubers, whole grains, and legumes rather than sweets or refined flour products.

High Fiber, Low Fat

Although there are no clinical trials to substantiate this, many women report that diets high in unrefined grains and fermented foods and low in animal fats can alleviate PMS symptoms. Interestingly, there is a biological mechanism to support this observation since estrogen, which is eliminated in the feces in a conjugated form, can be reabsorbed only when it is deconjugated by certain fecal bacteria. These bacteria are present in higher concentration in women who have a diet high in animal fat and refined carbohydrates (Adlercreutz et al. 1984; Orme and Back 1990; Winter and Bokkenheuser 1987). Because estrogen excess is associated with PMS, it could be inferred that a unrefined carbohydrate, low animal fat diet could be beneficial.

Weight Gain and PMS

A subset of women with PMS, do consume an excessive amount of energy in the form of fats and carbohydrates in the premenstrual phase which, over time, leads to weight gain (Cross et al. 2001). This, in turn, may further exacerbate depression, bloating and other negative symptoms of PMS. Therefore, when I discuss diet and weight issues with women, I often focus on premenstrual symptoms and their relationship to eating habits. This can help women pay more attention to food consumption specifically in the luteal phase.

Soy Foods

Soy consumption, both in the form of soy extracts and as whole foods, may play a role in controlling PMS symptoms. It has been hypothesized that the isoflavones in soy (namely, genistein and daidzein) have mixed agonist antagonist effects on estrogen and progesterone receptors. Their role is thought to vary throughout the menstrual cycle, depending on the levels of circulating endogenous hormones (Kurzer 2002; Lu et al. 2001). Transnational epidemiologic studies have shown that women in Asia, where more whole soy foods are consumed, have lower rates of PMS than women in the United States (Takeda et al. 2006). One recent cross-sectional study of 84 Korean women living in the United States showed that dietary soy intake was inversely correlated with PMS symptoms (Kim et al. 2006). Another crossover placebo trial in a diverse group of PMS sufferers reported that 68 mg soy isoflavones had positive effect on PMS-related bloating (Bryant et al. 2005).

Thoughts on Soy

I am most impressed by recent studies suggesting that whole soy foods have a modulating effect on estrogen levels whereas soy extracts have a stronger stimulatory effect (Trock et al. 2006). Whole soy foods (miso, edamame, tempeh, tofu, soy milk, etc.) therefore offer a wider range of nutrients than their more processed counterparts (soy protein extracts, power bars, fake meats, ice creams, etc.), I encourage women with PMS to avoid processed soy products but to include a daily serving of a whole soy food in their diet.

DIETARY SUPPLEMENTS

Many vitamin supplements are promoted for treating PMS symptoms although few have methodologically sound research trials that substantiate their benefits. The exception to this are calcium (as citrate or carbonate) and pyridoxine (vitamin B6), both of which have a number of well-designed randomized controlled trials to suggest that they offer a relatively low-risk, high-reward intervention for women with PMS symptoms (see Table 12.4).

Table 12.4. Nutritional Supplementation for PMS

Vitamin/Mineral	Dose	Level of Evidence
Calcium citrate or carbonate	600 mg twice a day in the luteal phase or daily	b
Vitamin B6	50–100 mg daily	b
Magnesium citrate	400 mg daily	c
Vitamin D	800–1200 IU/day	c

Calcium

Calcium is believed to work by modulating the effect of estrogen and other hormones. In one randomized, multicenter trial, 720 women were given 1200 mg/day of calcium carbonate versus placebo in the week preceding three menstrual cycles. By using a daily standardized PMS rating scale, the study group reported a 48% reduction ($p < 0.001$) in symptoms (Thys-Jacobs 2000; Thys-Jacobs et al. 1998). Since calcium is better absorbed when given in smaller doses, it is best to prescribe calcium carbonate or citrate as 600 mg twice daily to be taken either in the luteal phase or for the entire cycle.

Vitamin B6

Vitamin B6, or pyridoxine, is thought to have positive effects on neurotransmitters such as serotonin, norepinephrine, and dopamine (Ebadi et al. 1982). This has borne out in clinical trials in which pyridoxine has helped to improve the negative mood symptoms associated with PMS (Kashanian et al. 2007). A 1999 review of nine RCTs studying vitamin B6 as a treatment for PMS concluded that a dose of 50 to 100 mg/day was likely to benefit women both in terms of breast pain and depressive symptoms (Wyatt et al. 1999). Because vitamin B6 in excessive doses can cause nerve toxicity resulting in ataxia or neuropathy, the daily dose should not exceed 100 mg/day.

Vitamin D and Magnesium

There are several observational studies linking low serum and/or urine levels of vitamin D and magnesium to PMS symptoms. Furthermore, there are plausible mechanisms for how both of these nutrients could be beneficial in treating PMS as they serve as hormone modulators, smooth muscle relaxants, and inhibitors of prostaglandin synthesis. Unfortunately, to date, there is little evidence that supplementing with either vitamin D or magnesium is truly beneficial as a treatment for premenstrual symptoms (Shamberger 2003; Bertone-Johnson et al. 2005; Girman et al. 2003; Rosenstein et al. 1994). One small, short-term RCT did show that 200 mg of magnesium per day was better than placebo at alleviating the bloating symptoms of PMS (Walker et al. 1998). Another trial found that magnesium 200 mg plus vitamin B6 50 mg compared favorably to magnesium alone for treating the anxiety symptoms associated with the syndrome (De Souza et al. 2000).

Despite the paucity of research, it should be acknowledged that low concentrations of these two nutrients are associated with a myriad of other women's health problems and that they can be safely supplemented at physiologic levels (200 to 400 mg/day magnesium and 800 to 1200 IU/day vitamin D). Therefore, as part of a comprehensive PMS treatment plan, one worthwhile approach would be to recommend supplementation of magnesium and vitamin D to all women with moderate to severe symptoms.

EXERCISE

Elite athletes often develop amenorrhea, and they rarely experience PMS symptoms. One explanation for this phenomenon is that extreme exercise leads to suppression of steroid hormone levels. It has not been demonstrated whether moderate exercise can also reduce hormonal levels. Nonetheless, 30 minutes/day of moderate intensity exercise does seem to help in improving the mood and overall sense of well-being in women with PMS (Stoddard et al. 2007). Like the dietary interventions, a half-hour daily exercise of moderate intensity has so many other proven benefits that it should be considered a first-line treatment for all women with PMS (Steege and Blumenthal 1993).

SMOKING CESSATION

In one observational study of women with PMS, those who smoked experienced increased cramps, required more pain medication and time off from work (Kritz-Silverstein et al. 1999). Smoking correlates with depression and other pain syndromes and therefore, for many women, its link with severe PMS symptoms may be an indirect one. Nonetheless, nicotine has been noted to have a toxic effect directly on the ovaries and eliminating its use may improve symptoms. Smoking cessation is another helpful first-line intervention for women with PMS.

BOTANICALS

Growing up, my grandmother used to give me teas and herbs when I did not feel well. I remember how well they worked. Thanks to the herbs,

I really never needed to take stronger medicines. Are there any safe herbs that I can try for my PMS symptoms?

Marie

Chasteberry

There are at least a dozen botanical supplements that researchers have studied for their potential benefit in treating premenstrual symptoms, and many of these are included in proprietary herbal formulations for women. To date, however, only chasteberry (*Vitex agnus-castus*) has enough scientific evidence to support its use for treatment of negative symptoms associated with menstruation, and in Germany, the herb is used as a first-line treatment for PMS, mastodynia, and menstrual irregularity.

Chasteberry or Vitex, which literally translates into "chaste lamb" in recognition of its presumed libido lowering effects, has a number of potentially active ingredients. In the berry itself are iridoid glycosides and flavonoids whereas the leaves and flowers contain compounds similar to sex hormones. Chasteberry decreases estrogen and prolactin secretion and raises progesterone levels (Roemheld-Hamm 2005). In addition, it may have some mild analgesic effects since methanol extracts of the plant have been noted to activate the mu-opiate receptor (Webster et al. 2006).

One large randomized controlled trial ($n = 170$) of chasteberry reported that after three menstrual cycles, the treatment group had significantly fewer negative premenstrual symptoms than the placebo group ($p < 0.001$). In the active group, 50% of women experienced at least a 50% reduction in symptoms whereas only 7 out of 86 discontinued for side effects (Schellenberg 2001). Another randomized, double-blind, placebo- controlled trial compared chasteberry to fluoxetine as treatments for PMS. The researchers found that both interventions were equally beneficial and significantly better than placebo. Interestingly, the fluoxetine showed a slight advantage in improving psychological symptoms, whereas the chasteberry had a more positive effect on physical symptoms (Atmaca et al. 2003). A third chasteberry trial, which was focused specifically on treating PMS-related mastalgia, also noted a significant improvement in the chasteberry group. However, by the end of the third cycle, this significance had disappeared because of an increasingly positive response noted by the placebo group (Halaska et al. 1999). In summary, chasteberry seems to be a tolerable and effective treatment for PMS.

Caution: Safety of chasteberry in pregnancy is unknown and, due to its inhibitory effect upon prolactin, it should not be used while breastfeeding. In higher doses, chasteberry might also have dopamine agonist activities and could

Chasteberry and Libido

Because of its name, some women worry that chasteberry will cause them to lose their libido. This is not a frequently reported phenomenon when the herb is given in low doses. In fact, many women report to me that the herb has the opposite effect, probably because it helps treat other overwhelming PMS symptoms that can lower sexual drive.

theoretically increase the effects of other dopamine antagonists such as bromocriptine or metoclopramide (Daniele et al. 2005).

Other Botanicals

Three other botanicals warrant mention in this section mainly because they are frequently used for PMS symptoms and may be useful for some women. The first is black cohosh (*Actaea racemosa; Cimicifuga racemosa*), which may modulate luteinizing and follicle stimulating hormones and also act as a mild serotonin reuptake inhibitor. Black cohosh is widely accepted as a treatment for the negative effects of menopause including mood swing, hot flashes, and sleep disturbances. Given its mild SSRI properties, it may have its greatest efficacy as a treatment for negative mood or depression associated with PMS (Low Dog 2001).

St John's Wort (*Hypericum perforatum*), an herb that is widely used for treatment of depression also has some promising pilot data to support its use in treating the depressive symptoms of PMS (Stevinson and Ernst 2000). The standard dose for treatment of mild depression is 300 mg St. John's Wort 3 times a day, standardized to 0.3% hypericin and/or 3% to 5% hyperforin.

Evening primrose oil (*Oenothera biennis*), or EPO, is another popular herbal treatment for PMS symptoms. The seed oil contains essential fatty acids that are necessary to form the anti-inflammatory prostaglandin PGE1. Theoretically, supplementing this oil can help women who are deficient in the enzyme that is needed to endogenously synthesize these prostaglandins. Unfortunately, none of the small trials showed a difference between EPO and placebo, and a systematic review concluded that EPO has little value in treating PMS (Budeiri et al. 1996; Collins et al. 1993; Khoo et al. 1990) (see Table 12.5).

Table 12.5. Herbal Treatment for PMS

Herb	Dose
Chasteberry (*Vitex agnus castus*)	500 mg once a day
Black Cohosh (*Actaea racemosa, Cimicifuga racemosa*)	40–80 mg standardized extract twice a day
St. John's Wort (*Hypericum perforatum*)	300 mg 3 times a day of St. John's Wort standardized to 0.3% hypericin and/or 3%–5% hyperforin
Evening primrose oil	2–3 g/day

Natural Progesterone

Progesterone in the form of pills, pessaries, troches, and creams is a popular treatment for PMS. Its use is based on the theory that women with PMS are experiencing a deficiency in progesterone relative to estrogen and that their symptoms are a result of estrogen dominance. As far back as the 1950s, the British physician Katherine Dalton used high-dose progesterone suppositories (800 mg/day) to treat PMS (Dalton 1990). Although a large portion of her patients reported improvement with this intervention, it appears that her selection criteria would have excluded most women who are currently diagnosed with PMS. Furthermore, there is no laboratory evidence to substantiate this progesterone hypothesis.

A meta-analysis by the Cochrane collaboration of trials of progesterone for PMS identified 2 of 17 studies that merited inclusion in their review. Both studies administered progesterone or placebo from day 14 of the menstrual cycle until the onset of menstruation. One study, using 300 mg oral and 200 mg suppository, concluded that progesterone worked no better than placebo, whereas the other using 400 mg BID of progesterone suppositories suggested that it may be beneficial for a small subgroup of PMS sufferers. Unfortunately, the study paper did not offer criteria to help identify these women. Although progesterone seemed to be a safe therapy, both studies were of limited duration (the longer of the two lasting only four cycles) and had high attrition rates (Ford et al. 2006; Magill 1995; Vaneslow et al. 1996). Side effects of progesterone therapy overlap with many of the symptoms associated with PMS including headache, irregular menses, mood changes, and hypersomnia. Progesterone may also increase fertility, and therefore, women should be advised to use appropriate birth control.

Many alternative practitioners promote "natural," over-the-counter, or compounded progesterone creams as a safer and more physiologic option to prescription formulations of progesterone or progesterone derivatives (progestins) such as medroxyprogesterone and norethindrone . In truth, "natural" may be a misnomer. Although Mexican yams and soy beans are the source of the diosgenin and stigmasterol, the final products are synthesized in a laboratory and are no more natural than oral micronized progesterone. Furthermore, concentrations of progesterone vary widely even within the same product formulation, and most do not seem to achieve a physiologic dose. None of these over-the counter creams have supportive data that has been published in a peer reviewed journal (Boothby and Doering 2008; Cirigliano 2007).

Progesterone therapy may offer symptomatic relief to a subset of women with PMS treatment and might be an appropriate next step when nonpharmacological approaches do not suffice. Given the variability in concentration of over-the-counter creams, it is best to prescribe oral micronized progesterone or progesterone suppositories 200–800 mg/day to be administered at the lowest effective dose from day 14 of the menstrual cycle until the first day of menstrual flow. Long-term safety data for high-dose progesterone therapy is not known.

MIND–BODY

A variety of mind–body techniques have been effective in treating PMS symptoms. These include meditation, breathing, PMR or progressive muscle relaxation, yoga, guided imagery, biofeedback, cognitive-behavioral therapy, and positive reframing. All of these techniques are described in greater detail in other places in this text. Since these are interventions that are tailored for each individual patient, they are hard to study using conventional methodologies. Nonetheless, a growing body of research suggests that when women are given psychological support as well as self-regulatory techniques for dealing with their PMS symptoms, their quality of life and symptom severity improves significantly (Goodale et al. 1990; Rapkin 2005).

In one interesting study, women were taught to use guided imagery as a means to regulate vaginal temperature and subsequently control PMS symptoms. Those women, who managed to raise their vaginal temperature, indicating a rise in progesterone, also experienced an improvement in PMS symptoms (Van Zak 1994). Other forms of guided imagery such as directing women to *fill their pelvis with soft, warm light* or to imagine themselves *floating gently on water* are likely to be just as successful.

Choosing the Most Appropriate Mind–Body Techniques

I usually include a recommendation for at least one kind of mind–body therapy in any PMS treatment plan. These are relatively easy practices that women can do independently without taking a medication or supplement. Since there is insufficient evidence to recommend one treatment over another, I work with each individual woman to decide what best suits her preferences and skills. For example, Marie had some experience with yoga and meditation, and therefore I started with a prescription for deep belly breathing and gave her a restorative yoga pose called viparita kirani (lying on your back with your legs up the wall). Initially, I encouraged her to practice the technique as needed for the duration of her symptoms and to consider incorporating the practice daily throughout the month.

GROUP INTERVENTIONS

Group interventions or group medical visits are a promising and cost-effective way for practitioners to offer women an integrative approach to PMS treatment. In one small study ($n = 28$), women with PMS attended four 2-hour sessions where they learned about the biological, environmental, and psychological causes of PMS as well as nutrition, exercise, and stress reduction tools for treating their symptoms. At the end of the study, attendees reported significant improvement on a PMS symptom rating scale (Morse 1999).

Traditional Chinese Medicine

Traditional Chinese medicine and other oriental medicine systems view PMS primarily as an imbalance of *qi*, or life force, and the principle goal in treatment is to remove the blockage, deficiency, stagnation, or imbalance of *qi*. Studies using traditional Chinese herbs, acupuncture, acupressure, or external *Qigong* therapy, have all been designed to treat specific disharmonies that have led to the imbalance (Chou and Morse 2005). Taking into consideration the heterogeneity of diagnoses and treatments, these studies hardly lend themselves to a randomized controlled design. However, if you look at the literature in its entirety, it suggests that these forms of medicine can have a strong beneficial effect for women with PMS (Chou et al. 2008; Jang et al. 2004; Kimura et al. 2007; Yu et al. 2005).

Manipulative Medicine

One small study with 24 women suffering from PMDD demonstrated that women receiving massage in the later part of the luteal phase experienced fewer symptoms than those assigned to relaxation therapy (Hernandez-Reif et al. 2000). In another study, women with PMS were assigned to real or sham reflexology and those experiencing the true treatment had an improvement in their symptoms score (Oleson and Flocco 1993). One crossover trial to study the benefits of chiropractic manipulation randomized women with PMS to a real treatment or to a placebo. This study showed no difference in benefit for the women who had first experienced the placebo (Walsh and Polus 1999).

Homeopathy

A pilot RCT ($n = 20$) showed that individualized homeopathic therapy offers some benefit for women with PMS symptoms. In this study, 90% of the active treatment group reported more than 30% improvement in symptoms whereas only 37.5% of the controls felt they had experienced this degree of benefit $p = 0.048$ (Yakir et al. 2001). Clearly, further research is needed to test the effectiveness of homeopathy as a PMS treatment.

Marie adopted a number of changes at once. She eliminated coffee and sodas from her diet, cut down on animal fats, increased her consumption of vegetables, and started substituting whole grains for more processed ones. She started a daily breathing practice and tried to take a brisk 30-minute walk on most days. She started taking a number of supplements: a multivitamin, additional calcium, vitamin D, and chasteberry. She also saw an acupuncturist every other week. I saw her again two months after her first visit, and she reported that her bloating and depressive symptoms have been much better during the previous two cycles. Six months later, she returned and told me that she was only going to the acupuncturist once a month, and although some months were better than others, overall her PMS symptoms were relatively mild, and she felt she had the tools to manage things when they got off track.

Table 12.6. Integrative Check-List for Treating PMS

Nutrition	Whole grains, high fiber
	Whole soy
	Limit caffeine
	Limit red meat
Exercise	30 minutes daily moderate intensity
Smoking cessation	
Nutritional supplements	Vitamins B6 and D, calcium, magnesium
Herbals	Chasteberry, Black Cohosh, St. John's Wort
Mind–body	Cognitive-behavioral therapy, group therapy, biofeedback, breathing, yoga
Energy medicine	Acupuncture and Qi Gong
Homeopathy	Individual treatment plans
Pharmaceutical	Assess the need for prescription pharmaceutical when the above modalities do not provide relief or symptoms are very severe

Conclusion

Premenstrual syndrome is a syndrome with many possible etiologies and a variety of manifestations. The integrative approach to PMS takes into to account the individual experience of each woman and seeks to treat her symptoms using a range of modalities that will offer her the maximum amount of relief with a minimum of side effects (Table 12.6). Taking into consideration the wide therapeutic safety and high tolerability of alternative treatments ranging from lifestyle changes to mind–body treatments, these are usually used as first-line therapies by integrative practitioners. In general, conventional treatments such as pharmaceuticals carry a high degree of side effects and therefore are reserved for women who have received no relief with the initial approach or are greatly incapacitated by their PMS symptoms.

REFERENCES

Adlercreutz H, Pulkkinen MO, Hamalainen EK, Korpela JT. Studies on the role of intestinal bacteria in metabolism of synthetic and natural steroid hormones. *J Steroid Biochem.* 1984;20(1):217–229.

Atmaca M, Kumru S, Tezcan E. Fluoxetine versus *Vitex agnus castus* extract in the treatment of premenstrual dysphoric disorder. *Hum Psychopharmacol.* 2003;18(3):191–195.

Backstrom B, Andreen L, Birzniece V, et al. The role of hormones and hormonal treatments in premenstrual syndrome. *CNS Drugs.* 2003;17(5):325–342.

Berger D, Schaffner W, Schrader E, Meier B, Brattstrom A. Efficacy of *Vitex agnus castus* L. extract Ze 440 in patients with pre-menstrual syndrome (PMS). *Arch Gynecol Obstet.* 2000;264(3):150–153.

Bertone-Johnson ER, Hankinson SE, Bendich A, Johnson SR, Willett WC, Manson JE. Calcium and vitamin D intake and risk of incident premenstrual syndrome. *Arch Intern Med.* 2005;165(11):1246–1252.

Boothby LA, Doering PL. Bioidentical hormone therapy: a panacea that lacks supportive evidence. *Curr Opin Obstet Gynecol.* 2008;20(4):400–407.

Borenstein JE, Dean BB, Leifke E, Korner P, Yonkers KA. Differences in symptom scores and health outcomes in premenstrual syndrome. *J Women Health.* 2007;16(8):1139–1144.

Bryant M, Cassidy A, Hill C, Powell J, Talbot D, Dye L. Effect of consumption of soy isoflavones on behavioural, somatic and affective symptoms in women with premenstrual syndrome. *Br J Nutr.* 2005;93(5):731–739.

Bryant M, Truesdale KP, Dye L. Modest changes in dietary intake across the menstrual cycle: implications for food intake research. *Br J Nutr.* 2006;96(5):888–894.

Budeiri D, Li A, Po W, Dornan JC. Is evening primrose oil of value in the treatment of premenstrual syndrome? *Control Clin Trials.* 1996;17(1):60–68.

Chou PB, Morse CA, Xu H. A controlled trial of Chinese herbal medicine for premenstrual syndrome. *J Psychosom Obstet Gynaecol.* 2008;1–8.

Chou P, Morse CA. Understanding premenstrual syndrome from a Chinese medicine perspective. *J Altern Complemen Med.* 2005;11(2):355–361.

Cirigliano M. Bioidentical hormone therapy: a review of the evidence. *J Womens Health.* 2007;16(5):600–631.

Collins A, Cerin A, Coleman G, Landgren BM. Essential fatty acids in the treatment of premenstrual syndrome. *Obstet Gynecol.* 1993;81(1):93–98.

Cross GB, Marley J, Miles H, Willson K. Changes in nutrient intake during the menstrual cycle of overweight women with premenstrual syndrome. *Br J Nutr.* 2001;85(4):475–482.

Dalton K. The aetiology of premenstrual syndrome is the progesterone receptors. *Med Hypothesis.* 1990;31(4):323–327.

Daniele C, Thompson Coon J, Pittler MH, Ernst E. *Vitex agnus castus*: a systematic review of adverse events. *Drug Saf.* 2005;28(4):319–332.

De Souza MC, Walker AF, Robinson PA, Bolland K. A synergistic effect of a daily supplement for 1 month of 200 mg magnesium plus 50 mg vitamin B6 for the relief of anxiety-related premenstrual symptoms: a randomized, double-blind, crossover study. *J Womens Health Gend Based Med.* 2000;9(2):131–139.

Dean BB, Borenstein JE. A prospective assessment investigating the relationship between work productivity and impairment with premenstrual syndrome. *J Occup Environ Med.* 2004;46(7):649–656.

Ebadi M, Gessert CF, Al-Sayegh A. Drug-pyridoxal phosphate interactions. *Q Rev Drug Metab Drug Interact.* 1982;4(4):289–331.

Farage MA, Osborn TW, Maclean AB. Cognitive, sensory, and emotional changes associated with the menstrual cycle: a review. *Arch Gynecol Obstet.* 2008; 278(4):299–307.

Ford O, Lethaby A, Mol B, Roberts H. Progesterone for premenstrual syndrome. *Cochrane Database Syst Rev.* 2006;(4):CD003415.

Freeman EW. Premenstrual syndrome and premenstrual dysphoric disorder: definitions and diagnosis. *Psychoneuroendocrinology.* 2003;(28 Suppl):325–337.

Freeman EW, Rickels K. Characteristics of placebo responses in medical treatment of premenstrual syndrome. *Am J Psychiatry.* 1999;156(9):1403–1408.

Freeman EW, Rickels K, Schweizer E, Ting T. Relationships between age and symptom severity among women seeking medical treatment for premenstrual symptoms. *Psychol Med.* 1995;25(2):309–315.

Girman A, Lee R, Kligler B. An integrative medicine approach to premenstrual syndrome. *Am J Obstet Gynecol.* 2003;188(5 Suppl):S56–65.

Goodale IL, Domar AD, Benson H. Alleviation of premenstrual syndrome symptoms with the relaxation response. *Obstet Gynecol.* 1990;75(4):649–655.

Gotts G, Morse CA, Dennerstein L. Premenstrual complaints: an idiosyncratic syndrome. *J Psychosom Obstet Gynaecol.* 1995;16(1):29–35.

Halaska M, Beles P, Gorkow C, Sieder C. Treatment of cyclical mastalgia with a solution containing a *Vitex agnus castus* extract: results of a placebo-controlled double-blind study. *Breast.* 1999;8(4):175–181.

Halbreich U. The pathophysiologic background for current treatments of premenstrual syndromes. *Curr Psychiatry Rep.* 2002;4(6):429–434.

Halbreich U, Backstrom T, Eriksson E, et al. Clinical diagnostic criteria for premenstrual syndrome and guidelines for their quantification for research studies. *Gynecol Endocrinol.* 2007;23(3):123–130.

Hardy ML. Herbs of special interest to women. *J Am Pharm Assoc (Wash).* 2000;40(2):234–242; quiz 327–329.

Hernandez-Reif M, Martinez A, Field T, Quintero O, Hart S, Burman I. Premenstrual symptoms are relieved by massage therapy. *J Psychosom Obstet Gynaecol.* 2000;21(1):9–15.

Jang HS, Lee MS. Effects of Qi therapy (External Qigong) on premenstrual syndrome: a randomized placebo-controlled study. *J Altern Complemen Med.* 2004;10(3): 456–462.

Jarvis CI, Lynch AM, Morin AK. Management strategies for premenstrual syndrome/ premenstrual dysphoric disorder. *Ann Pharmacother.* 2008;42(7):967–978.

Johnson SR. Premenstrual syndrome, premenstrual dysphoric disorder, and beyond: a clinical primer for practitioners. *Obstet Gynecol.* 2004;104(4):845–859.

Kashanian M, Mazinani R, Jalalmanesh S. Pyridoxine (vitamin B6) therapy for premenstrual syndrome. *Int J Gynaecol Obstet.* 2007;96(1):43–44.

Khoo SK, Munro C, Battistutta D. Evening primrose oil and treatment of premenstrual syndrome. *Med J Aust.* 1990;153(4):189–192.

Kim HW, Kwon MK, Kim NS, Reame NE. Intake of dietary soy isoflavones in relation to perimenstrual symptoms of Korean women living in the USA. *Nurs Health Sci.* 2006;8(2):108–113.

Kimura Y, Takamatsu K, Fujii A, et al. Kampo therapy for premenstrual syndrome: efficacy of Kamishoyosan quantified using the second derivative of the fingertip photoplethysmogram. *J Obstet Gynaecol Res.* 2007;33(3):325–332.

Kritz-Silverstein D, Wingard DL, Garland FC. The association of behavior and lifestyle factors with menstrual symptoms. *J Womens Health Gend Based Med.* 1999;8(9):1185–1193.

Kurzer MS. Hormonal effects of soy in premenopausal women and men. *J Nutr.* 2002;132(3):570S–573S.

Low Dog T. Integrative treatments for premenstrual syndrome. *Altern Ther Health Med.* 2001;7(5):32–39; quiz 40, 139.

Lu LJ, Anderson KE, Grady JJ, Nagamani M. Effects of an isoflavone-free soy diet on ovarian hormones in premenopausal women. *J Clin Endocrinol Metab.* 2001;86(7):3045–3052.

Magill PJ. Investigation of the efficacy of progesterone pessaries in the relief of symptoms of premenstrual syndrome. *Br J Gen Pract.* 1995;45(400):589–593.

Martorano JT, Ahlgrimm M, Colbert T. Differentiating between natural progesterone and synthetic progestins: clinical implications for premenstrual syndrome and perimenopause management. *Compr Ther.* 1998;24(6–7):336–339.

Morse G. Positively reframing perceptions of the menstrual cycle among women with premenstrual syndrome. *J Obstet Gynecol Neonatal Nurs.* 1999;28(2):165–174.

Muse K. Hormonal manipulation in the treatment of premenstrual syndrome. *Clin Obstet Gynecol.* 1992;35(3):658–666.

Oleson T, Flocco W. Randomized controlled study of premenstrual symptoms treated with ear, hand, and foot reflexology. *Obstet Gynecol.* 1993;82(6):906–911.

Orme ML, Back DJ. Factors affecting the enterohepatic circulation of oral contraceptive steroids. *Am J Obstet Gynecol.* 1990;163(6 Pt 2):2146–2152.

Pullon SR, Reinken JA, Sparrow MJ. Treatment of premenstrual symptoms in Wellington women. *N Z Med J.* 1989;102(862):72–74.

Rapkin AJ. New treatment approaches for premenstrual disorders. *Am J Manag Care.* 2005;11(16 Suppl):S480–491.

Robinson RL, Swindle RW. Premenstrual symptom severity: impact on social functioning and treatment-seeking behaviors. *J Womens Health Gend Based Med.* 2000;9(7):757–768.

Roemheld-Hamm B. Chasteberry. *Am Fam Physician.* 2005;72(5):821–824.

Rosenstein DL, Elin RJ, Hosseini JM, Grover G, Rubinow DR. Magnesium measures across the menstrual cycle in premenstrual syndrome. *Biol Psychiatry.* 1994; 35(8):557–561.

Rossignol AM, Bonnlander H. Caffeine-containing beverages, total fluid consumption, and premenstrual syndrome. *Am J Public Health.* 1990;80(9):1106–1110.

Sayegh R, Schiff I, Wurtman J, Spiers P, McDermott J, Wurtman R. The effect of a carbohydrate-rich beverage on mood, appetite, and cognitive function in women with premenstrual syndrome. *Obstet Gynecol.* 1995;86(4 Pt 1):520–528.

Schellenberg R. Treatment for the premenstrual syndrome with agnus castus fruit extract: prospective, randomised, placebo controlled study. *Br Med J.* 2001;322(7279):134–137.

Shamberger RJ. Calcium, magnesium, and other elements in the red blood cells and hair of normals and patients with premenstrual syndrome. *Biol Trace Elem Res.* 2003;94(2):123–129.

Steege JF, Blumenthal JA. The effects of aerobic exercise on premenstrual symptoms in middle-aged women: a preliminary study. *J Psychosom Res.* 1993;37(2):127–133.

Sternfeld B, Swindle R, Chawla A, Long S, Kennedy S. Severity of premenstrual symptoms in a health maintenance organization population. *Obstet Gynecol.* 2002;99(6):1014–1024.

Stevinson C, Ernst E. A pilot study of *Hypericum perforatum* for the treatment of premenstrual syndrome. *BJOG.* 2000;107(7):870–876.

Stevinson C, Ernst E. Complementary/alternative therapies for premenstrual syndrome: a systematic review of randomized controlled trials. *Am J Obstet Gynecol.* 2001;185(1):227–235.

Stoddard JL, Dent CW, Shames L, Bernstein L. Exercise training effects on premenstrual distress and ovarian steroid hormones. *Eur J Appl Physiol.* 2007;99(1):27–37.

Takeda T, Tasaka K, Sakata M, Murata Y. Prevalence of premenstrual syndrome and premenstrual dysphoric disorder in Japanese women. *Arch Womens Ment Health.* 2006;9(4):209–212.

Thys-Jacobs S. Micronutrients and the premenstrual syndrome: the case for calcium. *J Am Coll Nutr.* 2000;19(2):220–227.

Thys-Jacobs S, Starkey P, Bernstein D, Tian J. Calcium carbonate and the premenstrual syndrome: effects on premenstrual and menstrual symptoms. Premenstrual Syndrome Study Group. *Am J Obstet Gynecol.* 1998;179(2):444–452.

Trock BJ, Hilakivi-Clarke L, Clarke R. Meta-analysis of soy intake and breast cancer risk. *J Natl Cancer Inst.* 2006;98(7):459–471.

Vaneslow W, Dennerstein L, Greenwood KM, de Lignieres B. Effect of progesterone and its 5 alpha and 5 beta metabolites on symptoms of premenstrual syndrome according to route of administration. *J Psychosom Obstetr Gynaecol.* 1996;17(1): 29–38.

Van Zak DB. Biofeedback treatments for premenstrual and premenstrual affective syndromes. *Int J Psychosom.* 1994;41(1–4):53–60.

Walker AF, De Souza MC, Vickers MF, Abeyasekera S, Collins ML, Trinca LA. Magnesium supplementation alleviates premenstrual symptoms of fluid retention. *J Womens Health.* 1998;7(9):1157–1165.

Walsh MJ, Polus BI. The frequency of positive common spinal clinical examination findings in a sample of premenstrual syndrome sufferers. *J Manipulative Physiol Ther.* 1999;22(4):216–220.

Webster DE, Lu J, Chen SN, Farnsworth NR, Wang JZ. Activation of the mu-opiate receptor by Vitex agnus-castus methanol extracts: implication for its use in PMS. *J Ethnopharmacol.* 2006;106(2):216–221.

Winter J, Bokkenheuser VD. Bacterial metabolism of natural and synthetic sex hormones undergoing enterohepatic circulation. *J Steroid Biochem.* 1987; 27(4–6):1145–1149.

Wood SH, Mortola JF, Chan YF, Moossazadeh F, Yen SS. Treatment of premenstrual syndrome with fluoxetine: a double-blind, placebo-controlled, crossover study. *Obstet Gynecol.* 1992;80(3 Pt 1):339–344.

Wurtman JJ. Carbohydrate craving. Relationship between carbohydrate intake and disorders of mood. *Drugs.* 1990;39 (Suppl 3):49–52.

Wyatt KM, Dimmock PW, Jones PW, Shaughn O'Brien PM. Efficacy of vitamin B-6 in the treatment of premenstrual syndrome: systematic review. *Br Med J.* 1999;318(7195):1375–1381.

Yakir M, Kreitler S, Brzezinski A, Vithoulkas G, Oberbaum M, Bentwich Z. Effects of homeopathic treatment in women with premenstrual syndrome: a pilot study. *Br Homeopath J.* 2001;90(3):148–153.

Yu JN, Liu BY, Liu ZS, Robinson V. Evaluation of clinical therapeutic effects and safety of acupuncture treatment for premenstrual syndrome. *Zhongguo Zhen Jiu.* 2005;25(6):377–382.

Zhao G, Wang L, Qu C. Prevalence of premenstrual syndrome in reproductive women and its influential factors. *Zhonghua Fu Chan Ke Za Zhi.* 1998;33(4):222–224.

13

Vaginitis

PRISCILLA ABERCROMBIE

CASE STUDY

Tanisha is a 25-year-old African-American woman who suffers from recurrent vaginal infections. She says "I feel like I have an infection every month. Sometimes it's BV (bacterial vaginosis), and sometimes it's yeast." She is embarrassed by the vaginal odor and the amount of vaginal discharge. In addition, she experiences vaginal irritation and itching. She hopes that there is some kind of treatment that will stop this cycle of recurrent vaginal infections. She is particularly interested in using something other than antibiotics; she does not like to take them so often.

Tanisha's story is not unusual. Vaginal symptoms are a common complaint accounting for approximately 10 million office visits a year (Kent 1991). Bacterial vaginosis (BV) is the most common vaginal infection (22% to 50%) followed by vulvovaginal candidiasis (VVC) (17% to 39%) and the sexually transmitted infection trichomoniasis (4% to 35%) (Anderson et al. 2004). The focus of this chapter will be on the integrative management of acute and recurrent VVC and BV.

Although conventional treatments for acute vaginitis have been studied extensively and are highly effective for acute infection, many women suffer from recurrent vaginitis and may choose not to use antibiotics on a long term basis. Other women simply prefer a more "natural" treatment for vaginitis. The evidence that supports some of the alternative treatments for acute vaginitis is not as strong as for conventional medicine, yet the risk is also low. Accepting less compelling evidence may be reasonable in women, who wish to avoid prescription medications. Additionally, some of these treatments may play an important role in the prevention of recurrent vaginitis.

Vaginal Ecosystem

Lactobacilli play a particularly important role in the vaginal ecosystem. At menarche, the ovaries begin to produce estrogen, which causes the vaginal epithelium to become glycogenated; glycogen promotes the growth of lactobacilli. Lactobacilli have a number of roles. They breakdown glucose-producing lactic acid, which helps maintain a normal vaginal pH of 4.0 (3.8 to 4.2). This acidic milieu is hostile to the proliferation of pathogenic organisms. *Lactobacilli* produce hydrogen peroxide that is damaging to anaerobic microflora, such as those found in BV. Finally, the lactobacilli micropili adhere to vaginal epithelial cell receptors and prevent adherence of pathogens.

Many types of lactobacilli exist in the vagina. *L. crispaus, L. iners, L. jensenii,* and *L. gasseri* appear to be the most prevalent (Bolton et al. 2008). Other microfloras that normally exist in the vagina include *Garnerella vaginalis, Mycoplasma hominis,* and *Prevotella bivia.* When the vaginal ecosystem is tipped out of balance, and this second group of microflora proliferates, vaginal conditions such as VVC and BV develop.

Assessment of Vaginal Symptoms

Many women with vaginal symptoms are incorrectly diagnosed. Specialists diagnose vaginitis in about 80% to 90% of cases (Sobel 1990) whereas primary care providers correctly diagnose it in only 50% to 60% of cases (Schaaf et al. 1990). FDA-approved testing kits are available for VVC, BV, and trichomoniasis. These tests are both sensitive and specific and might help providers who do not have access to or expertise in microscopy (Bradshaw et al. 2005).

Women not only endure the physical symptoms of vaginal infections, they also suffer psychosocial ramifications. A prospective study of 44 multiethnic women with vaginitis indicated that they were distressed by their vaginal symptoms and two-thirds felt the symptoms were somewhat moderate to very serious (Karasz and Anderson 2003). Misperceptions about the cause of vaginitis included infidelity, cancer, and past sexual behavior. Although health care providers may view vaginitis as a bothersome condition with few troublesome consequences, women can be quite distressed.

Vulvovaginal Candidiasis

About 75% of women will experience acute VVC in their lifetime; 40% to 50% will have a recurrence (Hurley et al. 1979). The vast majority of VVC infections are caused by *C. Albicans*. Risk factors for VVC include: antibiotics, systemic corticosteroids, allergic rhinitis, high dose oral contraceptives, spermicides, and receptive oral sex (Watson and Calabretto 2007).

The signs and symptoms of VVC include: vaginal itching with thick white "curdy or cottage cheese" discharge, vulvitis, fissures or rash, and normal vaginal pH (<4.5). Microscopy shows the saline field with few white blood cells, rare or no clue cells, and the presence of lactobacilli. The 10% potassium hydroxide (KOH) field will show pseudohyphae, and there will be no amine smell when the KOH is added.

Clinical Pearl

I highly recommend using pH paper for the diagnosis of vaginitis. Women with candida vaginitis will have a normal pH of <4.5. If the pH is >5 then suspect BV or trichomoniasis.

TREATMENT

A Cochrane review found no differences in effectiveness between oral and intravaginal antifungals for the treatment of uncomplicated VVC (Nurbhai et al. 2007). Many women find oral fluconazole easier to use. Although it has excellent efficacy, it can take up to 48 hours before symptoms resolve. Therefore, for women with vulvar irritation and/or inflammation, topical treatment with one of the azole creams may produce more immediate benefit. According to the study made by the Centers for Disease Control and Prevention (CDC) in 2006, " azoles" are effective in 80% to 90% of women who complete therapy (CDC 2006). Topical intravaginal regimens are recommended for 7 days during pregnancy.

Self-medication should only be recommended for women who have been previously diagnosed with VVC and suffer from a recurrence of the same symptoms. One study found that only 34% of 95 symptomatic women who purchased over the counter (OTC) antifungal products actually had yeast (Ferris et al. 2002). Any woman whose symptoms persist after using an OTC preparation should be seen for an examination.

VVC is not a sexually transmitted infection, but partner treatment may be considered in women with recurrent VVC or in partners who are symptomatic (CDC 2006). Women should be informed that the azole creams are oil-based and can weaken latex condoms and diaphragms.

Clinical guidelines for the management of patients with vaginitis are available and updated regularly. **CDC:** http://www.cdc.gov/std/treatment/2006/vaginal-discharge.htm. ACOG Practice Bulletin: Clinical management guidelines for obstetrician–gynecologists, Number 72, May 2006: Vaginitis (ACOG Committee on Practice Bulletins—Gynecology 2006).

Clinical Pearl

Women with debilitating conditions such as uncontrolled diabetes will require a 14-day therapy. In HIV infected women, use of oral agents is associated with colonization of non-albicans species (CDC 2006).

Recurrent VVC

Recurrent VVC is defined as having four or more episodes in one year (CDC 2006). Recurrent VVC affects approximately 5% to 8% of women (Foxman et al. 1998). Vaginal culture can confirm the diagnosis of VVC and identify unusual species of *Candida*. Colonization with non-*albicans* species is rare. One study found that 94% of women ($n = 427$) with recurrent VVC had *C. albicans* (Sobel et al. 2004). The recommended treatment for recurrent VVC is 7 to 14 days of azole therapy followed by maintenance therapy 1 to 2 times weekly for 6 months. Unfortunately, relapse rates after maintenance therapy are as high as 30% to 50% (CDC 2006). Alternatively, oral fluconazole can be used; the dose is 150 mg on days 1, 4, and 7 and then weekly for 6 months (Sobel et al. 2004). This regimen produced a 91% cure at 6 months compared with 36% for placebo. The results at one year were 43% symptom-free in the treatment group versus 22% in the placebo group ($p < 0.0001$).

BORIC ACID

Boric acid has been shown to be an effective treatment for VVC in a few small studies. In a double blinded RCT of 108 women with yeast, the boric acid cure rate was 92% at 7 to 10 days posttreatment and 72% at 30 days and that was significantly more effective than nystatin (Van Slyke 1981). Boric acid also shows promise in the treatment of *non-albicans* species. Cure rates of VVC with *C. glabrata* were 64% in one study (Sobel et al. 2003). In diabetic women with *C. glabrata*, 14 days of boric acid was shown to have a higher mycological cure rate than a single dose of fluconazole although at 3 months the cure rates were similar (Ray et al. 2007a, 2007b).

The usual dose of boric acid is 600 mg in a gelatin capsule inserted in the vagina daily for 2 weeks. A maintenance dose of twice weekly can be used to prevent recurrences. There is little systemic absorption with vaginal administration, but ingestion of large amounts of oral boric acid has been shown to be toxic. Another advantage is its inexpensive price. Boric acid should not be used during pregnancy.

OTHER TREATMENTS FOR VVC

Some small studies suggest that the hormonal contraceptive depot medroxy-progesterone acetate produces a less estrogenic environment in the vagina and leads to a reduction in the colonization of *Candida* (Dennerstein 1986; Toppozada et al. 1979).

Clinical Pearl

Fungal organisms noted on a Pap smear are not necessarily an indicator of a pathologic infection. A confirmatory wet mount and/or clinical symptoms are needed before treatment. "Predominance of coccobacilli consistent with shift in vaginal flora" noted on Pap smear is highly suggestive but not diagnostic of BV (Fitzhugh and Heller 2008).

Bacterial Vaginosis

Bacterial vaginosis (BV) is the most common vaginal infection. BV occurs when *Lactobacilli* in the vagina are replaced with high concentrations of anaerobic bacteria. It is not fully understood why there is a change in vaginal milieu, nor is it clear whether a sexually transmitted pathogen is involved. Risk factors for BV include: multiple sex partners, a new sex partner, douching, and lack of vaginal lactobacilli (CDC 2006). It is beneficial to treat BV in nonpregnant women in order to reduce infections after abortion or hysterectomy, the risk for HIV, and other sexually transmitted infections (CDC 2006). All symptomatic women should be treated.

BV during pregnancy is associated with a number of adverse outcomes including premature rupture of membranes, preterm labor, preterm birth, intraamniotic infection, and postpartum endometritis (CDC 2006). Some studies indicate that treating pregnant women with BV who are at high risk for preterm delivery reduces the risk for prematurity (Hauth et al. 1995; Rosenstein et al. 2000).

The diagnosis of BV is based on clinical exam and microscopic findings. The Amsel criteria for BV are 3 out of 4 of the following: pH≥4.7, positive amine or whiff test, presence of >20% clue cells, or homogeneous grey discharge. The gold standard uses Nugent's criteria, but this is not practical in most clinical settings as it requires a gram stain. A Nugent's score is obtained from evaluating three morphotypes in the vaginal fluid on a score of 1 to 10. A score of 7 or greater is considered diagnostic for BV.

Clinical Pearl

OTC vaginal pH kits such as the Vagisil Screening Kit (Combe Incorporated) can assist women in determining their pH and help them decide whether they should try OTC treatment for VVC (pH < 4.5) or seek medical care (pH ≥ 5.0).

TREATMENT

Several conventional treatment protocols are available for BV. They include oral metronidazole 500 mg twice daily for 7 days, metronidazole gel 0.75%, 5 g intravaginally once daily for 5 days, and clindamycin cream 2%, 5 g intravaginally once daily for 7 days. Oral treatments are recommended in pregnancy and include metronidazole dosed either 500 mg twice daily for 7 days, or 250 mg three times daily for 7 days, or clindamycin 300 mg twice daily for 7 days. Consider a follow-up exam one month after treatment of high-risk pregnant women.

Recurrent BV

BV recurrence rates are high; typical rates are 30% three months after treatment and 80% within nine months (Sobel 1999). Recurrence is associated with past history of BV, regular sex partner, and female sexual partners (Bradshaw et al. 2006). Recurrence is inversely associated with hormonal contraception. The treatment strategies for recurrent BV include: longer treatment period (2 weeks), change to a different antibiotic, or prophylactic maintenance therapy. Examples of maintenance therapies include vaginal metronidazole twice weekly or oral metronidazole 3 times a week. Secondary VVC is common with maintenance therapy (Sobel et al. 2006).

ACIDIFYING AGENTS

A number of research trials have investigated the use of acidifying agents in the treatment and prevention of BV. The goal is to lower vaginal pH in order to support the growth of lactobacilli. In a double blinded RCT (n = 29), an acetic acid-based vaginal gel was not effective in treating BV (Holley et al. 2004). Another RCT showed an acid-buffering gel to be less effective than high dose metronidazole gel for the treatment of symptomatic BV (Simoes et al. 2006). However, when a lactic acid gel was added to metronidazole for the treatment of BV (n = 90), there was a significantly higher growth of lactobacilli (Decena et al. 2006) suggesting that acidifying agents may play a role in the prevention of recurrent BV.

Treatments for VVC and BV

PROBIOTICS

Probiotics containing lactobacilli have been used as an alternative treatment for vaginitis for many years. In BV, there is a clear pathophysiologic relationship between the lack of lactobacilli and the development of vaginitis. Thus, the promoting of the colonization of lactobacilli in the vagina is logical. On the other hand, the role of lactobacilli in the development of VVC is less clear. Lactobacilli can be quite plentiful in the acidic vaginal environment in which fungal organisms thrive. More research is needed to fully elucidate the role, if any, that lactobacilli play in VVC.

Numerous studies have been conducted with lactobacilli in many forms for the treatment or prevention of VVC and BV.

A review of the literature of probiotics for the prevention of recurrent VVC concluded that there was limited evidence to support their use (Falagas et al. 2006). The strains showing the most promise were *L acidophilus*, *L. rhamnosus* GR-1, and *L. fermentum* RC-14. A review of seven RCTs using lactobacilli for the treatment or prevention of BV found that three trials showed efficacy, and four trials showed no beneficial effect (Barrons and Tassone 2008). One trial found that giving oral *L. Rhamnosus* GR-1 and *L. Reuteri* RC-14 after oral metronidazole reduced rates of BV to 30 days when compared with placebo (Anukam et al. 2006). Two other RCT found that yogurt containing *L. acidophilus* was effective in treating BV. One study ($n = 46$) found that the yogurt reduced the rate of recurrent BV and VVC (Shalev et al. 1996), and another study ($n = 84$) showed that a yogurt douche used twice a day was effective in treating BV in the first trimester of pregnancy when compared to tampons with acetic acid or placebo (Neri et al. 1993).

These studies of probiotics have been plagued with methodological issues such as small sample size, lack of culture confirmation of *Candida* or documentation of the colonization of lactobacilli, and no placebo or comparison group. Numerous strains of lactobacilli have been studied in different doses and for various durations and have made it difficult to draw conclusions about the role of lactobacilli in vaginitis.

A myriad of other treatments have been used traditionally for the treatment of vaginitis. The most popular of these botanicals is tea tree oil (*Melaleuca alternifolia*) delivered as a vaginal suppository. It has been shown to have antifungal and antibacterial properties (Hammer et al. 1999). One case study describes successful treatment of BV with tea tree oil suppositories (Blackwell 1991). Most suppositories contain 10% tea tree oil or 200 mg per suppository. Directions are to insert intravaginally for six nights. Rarely, women may experience a hypersensitivity reaction to tea tree oil (Wolner-Hanssen and Sjoberg 1998).

Many botanicals have been tested and found to be effective in vitro against *Candida,* but clinical studies are lacking. When studied in vitro, these botanicals have often been found to be effective against nonalbicans species of *Candida.* See Table 13.1.

Let us come back to Tanisha from our case study at the beginning of the chapter. She has had recurrent mixed vaginal infections; both VVC and BV. She prefers not to take antibiotics. I would start her on 6 days of tea tree oil suppositories because *Melaleuca alternifolia* has both antibacterial and antifungal activity. Then, I would suggest a course of probiotics for about 3 to 6 months to recolonize the vagina with lactobacilli and prevent BV. In addition, I would discuss the risk factors for recurrent vaginal infections including sexual practices and family planning methods as behavioral changes may decrease her risk of recurrence (see Table 13.2).

Table 13.1. Evidence for Botanicals Used for the Treatment of Vaginitis

Botanical	In Vitro C. albicans	In Vitro Non-Albicans speicies	In Vitro Other Vaginitis	Clinical studies
Tea tree oil (Melaleuca alternifolia)	Mondello et al. (2006)	Ergin and Arikan (2002)	For Trich: Mondello et al. (2006)	For BV: Hammer et al., (1999)
Propolis				For BV: Blackwell (1991) and Imhof et al. (2005)
Garlic (Allium sativum)	Santana Perez et al. (1995)	Moore and Atkins (1977)		
Berberine (Berberis aristata)			For Trich: Moore and Atkins (1977)	
Bergamot	Soffar et al. (2001)	Romano et al. (2005)		
Clove oil	Romano et al. (2005)			
Lavender oil (Lavandula augustofolia)	Ahmad et al. (2005)			

Table 13.2. Important Points for Patient Education

- If you have a history of frequent vaginal yeast infections, request an antifungal treatment when you are given a prescription for antibiotics.
- Abstain from vaginal sex during treatment.
- Condoms are at increased risk for breakage when used with vaginal creams.
- Using condoms for one month after treatment may reduce the risk of recurrence.
- Do not insert penis, fingers, or sex toys into the vagina after insertion in the anus.
- Come in for an exam when you are symptomatic.
- Do not douche.

Conclusion

Vaginitis is a common women's health issue. Although conventional treatments have excellent efficacy for acute vaginitis, relapse rates are high. Although many alternative treatments have been used traditionally to treat vaginitis and do show some efficacy in vitro, more clinical research is needed to support their use. Most alternative treatments pose little safety risk, and thus they are good options especially for the prevention of recurrent vaginitis.

REFERENCES

ACOG Committee on Practice Bulletins—Gynecology. ACOG practice bulletin. clinical management guidelines for obstetrician-gynecologists, number 72, Vaginitis. *Obstet Gynecol.* 2006; 107(5):1195–1206.

Ahmad N, Alam MK, Shehbaz A, et al. Antimicrobial activity of clove oil and its potential in the treatment of vaginal candidiasis. *J Drug Target.* 2004;13(10):555–561.

Anderson MR, Klink K, Cohrssen A. Evaluation of vaginal complaints. *JAMA.* 2004;291(11):1368–1379.

Anukam K, Osazuwa E, Ahonkhai I, et al. Augmentation of antimicrobial metronidazole therapy of bacterial vaginosis with oral probiotic lactobacillus rhamnosus GR-1 and lactobacillus reuteri RC-14: randomized, double-blind, placebo controlled trial. *Microbes Infect.* 2006;8(6):1450–1454.

Barrons R., Tassone D. Use of lactobacillus probiotics for bacterial genitourinary infections in women: a review. *Clin Ther.* 2008;30(3):453–468.

Blackwell AL. Tea tree oil and anaerobic (bacterial) vaginosis. *Lancet.* 1991;337(8736):300.

Bolton M, van der Straten A, Cohen, CR. Probiotics: potential to prevent HIV and sexually transmitted infections in women. *Sex Transm Dis.* 2008;35(3):214–225.

Bradshaw CS, Morton AN, Garland SM, Horvath LB, Kuzevska I, Fairley CK. Evaluation of a point-of-care test, BVBlue, and clinical and laboratory criteria for diagnosis of bacterial vaginosis. *J Clin Microbiol.* 2005;43(3):1304–1308.

Bradshaw CS, Morton AN, Hocking J, et al. High recurrence rates of bacterial vaginosis over the course of 12 months after oral metronidazole therapy and factors associated with recurrence. *J Infect Dis.* 2006;193(11):1478–1486.

Centers for Disease Control and Prevention; Workowski KA, Berman SM. Sexually transmitted diseases treatment guidelines. *MMWR.* 2006;55(RR-11):1–94.

D'Auria FD, Tecca M, Strippoli V, Salvatore, G, Battinelli L, Mazzanti G. Antifungal activity of *Lavandula angustifolia* essential oil against *Candida albicans* yeast and mycelial form. *Med Mycol.* 2005;43(5):391–396.

Decena DC, Co JT, Manalastas RM Jr, et al. Metronidazole with lactacyd vaginal gel in bacterial vaginosis. *J Obstet Gynaecol Res.* 2006;32(2):243–251.

Dennerstein GJ. Depo-provera in the treatment of recurrent vulvovaginal candidiasis. *J Reprod Med.* 1986;31(9):801–803.

Ergin A, Arikan S. Comparison of microdilution and disc diffusion methods in assessing the in vitro activity of fluconazole and melaleuca alternifolia (tea tree) oil against vaginal candida isolates. *J Chemother.* 2002;14(5):465–472.

Falagas ME, Betsi, GI, Athanasiou S. Probiotics for prevention of recurrent vulvovaginal candidiasis: a review. *J Antimicrob Chemother.* 2006;58(2):266–272.

Ferris DG, Nyirjesy P, Sobel JD, Soper D, Pavletic A, Litaker MS. Over-the-counter antifungal drug misuse associated with patient-diagnosed vulvovaginal candidiasis. *Obstet Gynecol.* 2002;99(3):419–425.

Fitzhugh VA, Heller DS. Significance of a diagnosis of microorganisms on pap smear. *J Low Genit Tract Dis.* 2008;12(1):40–51.

Foxman B, Marsh JV, Gillespie B, Sobel JD. Frequency and response to vaginal symptoms among white and African American women: results of a random digit dialing survey. *J Womens Health.* 1998;7(9):1167–1174.

Hammer KA, Carson CF, Riley TV. In vitro susceptibilities of lactobacilli and organisms associated with bacterial vaginosis to melaleuca alternifolia (tea tree) oil. *Antimicrob Agents Chemother.* 1999;43(1):196.

Hauth JC, Goldenberg RL, Andrews WW, DuBard MB, Copper RL. Reduced incidence of preterm delivery with metronidazole and erythromycin in women with bacterial vaginosis. *N Engl J Med.* 1995;333(26):1732–1736.

Holley RL, Richter HE, Varner RE, Pair L, Schwebke JR. A randomized, double-blind clinical trial of vaginal acidification versus placebo for the treatment of symptomatic bacterial vaginosis. *Sex Transm Dis.* 2004;31(4):236–238.

Hurley R, De Louvois J. Candida vaginitis. *Postgrad Med J.* 1979;55(647):645–647.

Imhof M, Lipovac M, Kurz C, Barta J, Verhoeven HC, Huber JC. Propolis solution for the treatment of chronic vaginitis. *Int J Gynaecol Obstet.* 2005;89(2):127–132.

Karasz A, Anderson M. The vaginitis monologues: women's experiences of vaginal complaints in a primary care setting. *Soc Sci Med (1982).* 2003;56(5):1013–1021.

Kent HL. Epidemiology of vaginitis. *Am J Obstet Gynecol.* 1991;165(4 Pt 2):1168–1176.

Mondello F, De Bernardis F, Girolamo A, Cassone A, Salvatore G. In vivo activity of terpinen-4-ol, the main bioactive component of melaleuca alternifolia cheel (tea tree) oil against azole-susceptible and -resistant human pathogenic candida species. *BMC Infect Dis.* 2006;6:158.

Moore GS, Atkins RD. The fungicidal and fungistatic effects of an aqueous garlic extract on medically important yeast-like fungi. *Mycologia.* 1977;69(2):341–348.

Neri A, Sabah G, Samra Z. Bacterial vaginosis in pregnancy treated with yoghurt. *Acta Obstet Gynecol Scand.* 1993;72(1):17–19.

Nurbhai M, Grimshaw J, Watson M, Bond C, Mollison J, Ludbrook A. Oral versus intra-vaginal imidazole and triazole anti-fungal treatment of uncomplicated vulvovaginal candidiasis (thrush). *Cochrane Database Syst Rev.* 2007;(4):CD002845.

Ray D, Goswami R, Banerjee U, et al. Prevalence of candida glabrata and its response to boric acid vaginal suppositories in comparison with oral fluconazole in patients with diabetes and vulvovaginal candidiasis. *Diabetes Care.* 2007a;30(2):312–317.

Ray D, Goswami R, Dadhwal V, Goswami D, Banerjee U, Kochupillai N. Prolonged (3-month) mycological cure rate after boric acid suppositories in diabetic women with vulvovaginal candidiasis. *J Infect.* 2007b;55(4):374–377.

Romano L, Battaglia F, Masucci L, et al. In vitro activity of bergamot natural essence and furocoumarin-free and distilled extracts, and their associations with boric acid, against clinical yeast isolates. *J Antimicrob Chemother.* 2005;55(1):110–114.

Rosenstein IJ, Morgan DJ, Lamont RF, et al. Effect of intravaginal clindamycin cream on pregnancy outcome and on abnormal vaginal microbial flora of pregnant women. *Infect Dis Obstet Gynecol.* 2000;8(3–4):158–165.

Santana Perez E, Lugones Botell M, Perez Stuart O, Castillo Brito B. Vaginal parasites and acute cervicitis: local treatment with propolis. preliminary report. [Parasitismo vaginal Y cervicitis agudoi tratamiento local an propoleo. Informe preliminar] *Revista Cubana De Enfermeria.* 1995;11(1):51–56.

Schaaf VM, Perez-Stable EJ, Borchardt K. The limited value of symptoms and signs in the diagnosis of vaginal infections. 1990;150(9):1929–1933.

Shalev E, Battino S, Weiner E, Colodner R, Keness Y. Ingestion of yogurt containing lac-tobacillus acidophilus compared with pasteurized yogurt as prophylaxis for recur-rent candidal vaginitis and bacterial vaginosis. *Arch Fam Med.* 1996;5(10):593–596.

Simoes JA, Bahamondes LG, Camargo RP, et al. A pilot clinical trial comparing an acid-buffering formulation (ACIDFORM gel) with metronidazole gel for the treatment of symptomatic bacterial vaginosis. *Br J Clin Pharmacol.* 2006;61(2):211–217.

Sobel JD. Vaginitis in adult women. *Obstet Gynecol Clin North Am.* 1990;17(4):851–879.

Sobel JD. Vulvovaginitis in healthy women. *Compr Ther.* 1999;25(6–7):335–346.

Sobel JD, Chaim W, Nagappan V, Leaman D. Treatment of vaginitis caused by *Candida glabrata*: use of topical boric acid and flucytosine. *Am J Obstet Gynecol.* 2003;189(5):1297–1300.

Sobel JD, Ferris D, Schwebke J, et al. Suppressive antibacterial therapy with 0.75% met-ronidazole vaginal gel to prevent recurrent bacterial vaginosis. *Am J Obstetr Gynecol.* 2006;194(5):1283–1289.

Sobel JD, Wiesenfeld HC, Martens M, et al. Maintenance fluconazole therapy for recurrent vulvovaginal candidiasis. *N Engl J Med.* 2004;351(9):876–883.

Soffar SA, Metwali DM, Abdel-Aziz SS, el-Wakil HS, Saad GA. Evaluation of the effect of a plant alkaloid (berberine derived from Berberis aristata) on trichomonas vaginalis in vitro. *J Egypt Soc Parasitol.* 2001;31(3):893–904, 1p plate.

Toppozada M, Onsy FA, Fares E, Amir S, Shaala S. The protective influence of progestogen only contraception against vaginal moniliasis. *Contraception.* 1979;20(2):99–103.

Van Slyke KK, Michel VP, Rein MF. Treatment of vulvovaginal candidiasis with boric acid powder. *Am J Obstet Gynecol.* 1981;141(2):145–148.

Watson C, Calabretto H. Comprehensive review of conventional and non-conventional methods of management of recurrent vulvovaginal candidiasis. *Am J Obstet Gynecol.* 2007;47(4):262–272.

Wolner-Hanssen P, Sjoberg I. Warning against a fashionable cure for vulvovaginitis. tea tree oil may substitute candida itching with allergy itching. [Varning for modekur mot vulvovaginit. Tea tree-olja kan ersatta candida-klada med allergiklada]. *Lakartidningen.* 1998;95(30–31):3309–3310.

14

Pregnancy and Lactation

JACQUELYN M. PAYKEL

CASE STUDY

Teresa is a 24-year-old gravida 2, para 1 Hispanic female who presents for her first OB appointment at 8-week gestation. She is complaining of moderate nausea with occasional emesis, constipation, and headaches. Her first pregnancy was complicated by headaches, fetal macrosomia (normal diabetic screening), and induction at 39-week gestation for pregnancy-induced hypertension. Her son was born vaginally weighing 9 pounds 6 ounces and is 13 months old. Teresa's BMI is 32.5, BP 132/78, hematocrit 31%; she is, otherwise, healthy. She has a dedicated spouse and excellent familial support. She states that her most bothersome symptoms include nausea and "feeling tired all the time."

The journey of pregnancy is unique in medicine as it offers health care providers the opportunity to collaborate with women and assist them in maximizing preventive health measures that can last a lifetime. It is our opportunity as integrative clinicians to reinforce healthy lifestyle choices and encourage new self-care practices by engaging the whole person: mind, body, spirit, and community. Most women are motivated during pregnancy to improve their health because they sense that their actions will have a direct impact on the growing life within.

It is important to respect the impact of conventional medicine on the decline of perinatal and maternal morbidity and also mortality over the last century. In the United States, maternal mortality has decreased from 850/100,000 in 1900 to 13.2/100,000 in 1999 (Chang et al. 2003). Engaging women in an *integrative* approach to their pregnancies—combining the best of conventional and the mind-body-spirit-community approach—can result in better maternal/neonatal health and a richer pregnancy experience.

Preconception

PRECONCEPTION COUNSELING

Preconception counseling is intended to open a dialog about a woman's reproductive health and educate her about the importance of pregnancy planning so that she may optimize her health and take actions to optimize her baby's health (American College of Obstetricians and Gynecologists 2005). Collaboration with a trusted health care professional encourages the transition from knowledge acquisition to implementation of a healthy lifestyle. For example, in one study, though 80% of women knew the benefits of folic acid supplementation to prevent birth defects, only 27% regularly consumed multivitamins with at least 400 µg of folic acid prior to pregnancy (Lorenz et al. 2007). Conversely, women who participate in preconception counseling are more likely to change behaviors associated with adverse pregnancy outcomes (e.g., folic acid supplementation and eliminating alcohol consumption) than their counterparts (Elsinga 2008).

Since approximately 50% of all pregnancies are unintended, it is important to offer preconception screening at routine annual exams to all women of reproductive age—not solely to the 15% of women who intentionally seek medical advice in preparation for pregnancy (Henshaw 1998; Lorenz et al. 2007). Currently, only 16% of primary care physicians in the United States offer preconception counseling during routine annual exams (Henderson et al. 2002).

MATERNAL WEIGHT

The abundance of processed foods containing trans fats, saturated fats, and refined sugar, and the simultaneous lack of fresh fruits, vegetables, whole grains, and low-fat meats in the typical American diet contribute not only to the public's health but specifically to pregnancy outcomes. The negative effects are synergized by the sedentary nature of our society. Today, 35% of women of childbearing age in the United States are either overweight or obese (CDC

2007). Obesity during pregnancy increases a woman's risk of miscarriage, fetal malformations (including neural tube defects [NTD]), gestational diabetes, hypertensive disorders of pregnancy, thromboembolism, preterm labor, and intrauterine fetal demise. Delivery complications include an increased rate of labor induction, oxytocin augmentation, longer labors, and instrumental deliveries. Obese women are twice as likely to have a cesarean delivery due to labor dystocia or fetal intolerance as their normal-weight counterparts. If cesarean delivery occurs, they are more likely to experience intraoperative or postoperative complications such as hemorrhage, endometritis, and wound breakdown (ACOG Committee Opinion No. 315, 2005).

In addition, maternal obesity increases the risk of fetal macrosomia, and subsequent risk of birth injury is increased by a factor of 2 when maternal obesity is a factor. Children of obese mothers are three times more likely than their counterparts to be overweight by the age of 7 years and to suffer from a number of health problems including diabetes and its comorbidities.

On the other extreme of the weight spectrum, approximately 13.2% of child-bearing aged women are underweight (CDC 2007). Women with a body mass index of less than 19.7 kg/m^2 at the time of conception are more likely to experience preterm labor and deliver low-birth weight infants—both of which contribute to neonatal morbidity.

The preconception period, when a woman's focus turns to getting pregnant and optimizing her health for her child's welfare, is an opportune time to utilize motivational interviewing (MI) techniques. MI will foster a spirit of collaboration between provider and patient and encourage the mother-to-be to embrace a healthier lifestyle including dietary changes and increased physical activity (ACOG Committee Opinion No. 423, 2009).

DIET

The diet in the preconception period can be thought of as the foundation for a lifetime of healthy choices. Two priorities should be emphasized regarding food choices: (1) improved nutritional value of caloric intake and (2) reduction of chemical load. One example of such a diet is the Mediterranean diet which emphasizes whole grains, fruits and vegetables, iron- and calcium-rich foods, plant protein, animal protein from fish, poultry and dairy, and monounsaturated fats while minimizing red meat, sweets, and processed foods. A recent study demonstrated that children whose mothers consumed a high-quality Mediterranean diet throughout pregnancy experienced an 88% reduction in wheeze and a 45% reduction in allergy in their first 6 years of life (Chatzi et al. 2008).

The chemical load in our food supply is of concern for women anticipating pregnancy and the developing fetus. Decreasing one's exposure to pesticides, preservatives, additives, artificial sweeteners, and processed foods is advised.

If a woman's budget does not allow for an all-organic diet, use the Environmental Working Group's list of "least contaminated" and "most contaminated" foods available at www.ewg.org. Hormone-free foods such as milk, eggs, and meat are also readily available (Fischer-Rasmussen et al. 1991; Roscoe and Matteson 2002).

ALCOHOL CONSUMPTION

Prenatal alcohol consumption, especially binge drinking, is a leading cause of preventable developmental disabilities and mental retardation including fetal alcohol syndrome. Well-woman visits are an optimal time to discuss the effects of alcohol on the developing embryo early in pregnancy—when most women do not know that they are pregnant. Alcohol consumption by women of reproductive age is common; most women change their behavior when they realize they are pregnant. One epidemiologic study in Alberta, Canada consisted of 1042 phone interviews with women who had recently delivered. It was learnt that 80% of women reported consuming alcohol preconceptually, 50% during early pregnancy before they were aware of pregnancy, and 18% after pregnancy awareness. Binge-drinking percentages were 32% during preconception, 11% during early conception, and 0% after pregnancy awareness. Binge drinking was higher among women who smoked, those not planning a pregnancy, and those with low self-esteem (Tough et al. 2006). Women need to be educated about the risks of alcohol consumption during early pregnancy and encouraged to minimize alcohol intake.

SUPPLEMENTS

Theoretically, our food supply should provide all the vitamins and minerals we need. In reality, most of us do not eat well enough to meet the Recommended Dietary Allowances (RDA) published by the Institute of Medicine. In addition, the requirements for folic acid, calcium, iron, and vitamins D, C, and B increase during pregnancy. Supplements should be initiated in the preconception period and continued throughout pregnancy (Gardiner et al. 2008).

Prenatal Vitamins

Debate continues about the necessity of a daily prenatal vitamin during pregnancy. A recent large RCT demonstrated a decreased incidence of NTD, cardiovascular defects, limb defects, cleft palate, and other birth defects in the offspring of mothers who consumed a daily multivitamin (Czeizel 2004). A systematic review of nine trials ($n = 15{,}378$) found a decrease in the number of low birth weight, small-for-gestational-age babies, and maternal anemia when low or middle income women took multivitamins most days during pregnancy (Rumbold et al. 2005). Additional outcomes-based research is needed including a review of side effects and potential overdose (Haider and Bhutta 2006). Current recommendations suggest that, unless contraindicated, all women of reproductive age should take a daily multivitamin containing at least 400 µg of folic acid.

Folic Acid

Folic acid consumption before conception and during the first trimester reduces the incidence of NTD such as spina bifida, anencephaly, as well as certain congenital heart defects (Locksmith and Duff 1998; Lumley et al. 2001). The recommended daily allowance of folic acid for all women of childbearing age was first established by the United States Public Health Service in 1992 as 400 µg (CDC 1992).[18] If a personal or family history of children born with NTD exists, this recommendation is increased to 4000 µg of folic acid. It is estimated that at least 70% of NTD could be prevented if mothers consumed an adequate amount of folic acid (CDC 1992).

Calcium

Most women in the United States do not consume the RDA of calcium prior to or during pregnancy (Harville 2004; Thomas and Weisman 2006). Calcium is important for adequate fetal bone development. High calcium intake during pregnancy has been associated with decreased preterm delivery rates, higher birth weights, and decreased risk of maternal hypertensive illnesses. The current recommendations for calcium intake during the preconception period and throughout pregnancy and lactation is 1000 mg in women aged 19 to 50 years and 1300 mg in women younger than 19 years old (Institute of Medicine 1997).

Elaborating about calcium supplements, calcium citrate is more easily absorbed than calcium carbonate (Reinwald 2008).

Vitamin D

Maternal vitamin D deficiency contributes to bone diseases of the infant including rickets and osteomalacia (Pawley and Bishop 2004). Vitamin D insufficiency has also been associated with asthma, diabetes, autoimmune diseases, and certain cancers (Holick 2007). Populations at highest risk for vitamin D deficiency are African-Americans, women not exposed to enough sunlight, women with inadequate dietary vitamin D intake, and women who wear head covering (Wolpowitz and Gilchrest 2006). The debate continues regarding the recommended daily dosage, safety of higher doses, and benefits that will be realized with vitamin D supplementation. Currently, the RDA is 200 to 400 IU. However, many experts believe that 1000 IU is closer to the amount needed (Pawley and Bishop 2004). More research is needed before definitive recommendations can be made.

Iron

Women experience a dilutional anemia during pregnancy. Normally, the maternal blood supply expands 40% during a singleton pregnancy, and over 40% during multiple gestations. A hematocrit that is less than 34% before 28-week gestation or 32% after 28-week gestation suggests that additional iron is warranted. If that is so, iron supplements should be taken with vitamin C to maximize absorption. Calcium-rich foods should not be consumed simultaneously as calcium impairs iron absorption. A systematic review of forty trials ($n = 12,706$) revealed less postpartum anemia in women who routinely took iron supplementation during pregnancy. However, the effect on maternal and infant outcomes remains uncertain. It was concluded that more studies are needed before a recommendation can be made about routine iron supplementation during pregnancy (Peña-Rosas and Viteri 2006).

Vitamin A

Vitamin A contributes to fetal vision, immunity, skin development, and overall growth. There are two forms of vitamin A. *Preformed vitamin A* comes from animal sources such as liver and whole milk; this form of vitamin A is easily absorbed and is readily converted to retinol—the active form of vitamin A. *Provitamin A carotenoids* (e.g., beta-carotene), found in fruits and vegetables, are more difficult to absorb and less readily converted to retinol. The RDA for retinol is 4300 IU. The tolerable Upper Intake Level (UL) of retinol for pregnant and lactating women is 10,000 IU (Institute of Medicine-Food and Nutrition Board 2001). Higher levels may result in adverse effects such as miscarriage, birth defects, osteoporosis, and central nervous system disorders (Bendich and Langseth 1989). High concentrations of vitamin A naturally occur in liver, which includes cod-liver oil. Vitamin A toxicity, when it occurs, arises from excessive supplementation, rather than the food supply.

ESSENTIAL FATTY ACIDS

The essential fatty acids (EFA), such as omega 6 and omega 3 fatty acids, are essential for cellular function and structure. They are considered *essential* because they cannot be synthesized by the body and must be consumed in the food supply. There are three major types of omega 3 fatty acids ingested in the diet, alpha-linolenic acid (ALA), eicosapentaenoic acid (EPA), and doco-sahexaenoic acid (DHA). Several studies have shown an association between increased DHA from oily fish and enhanced cognitive, motor and visual development in infants (Jacobson et al. 2008). There is also evidence that fish oil taken during pregnancy may increase the length of gestation by 2 to 3 days, slightly increase birth weight, and decrease the number of babies born before 34-week gestation (Facchinetti et al. 2005; Makrides et al. 2006).

In 2005, the FDA and EPA issued a warning that certain fish contain high levels of mercury. Elevated maternal mercury levels can be neurotoxic to the fetus. Therefore, women of childbearing age, especially those who are pregnant or breastfeeding, should limit intake of fish to 12 ounces per week, and avoid consumption of swordfish, king mackerel, shark, and tilefish and consume no more than 6 ounces of albacore tuna per week. Many regions in the United States also have additional local fish consumption advisories. See the U.S. Environmental Protection Agency's website for more details: (http://www.epa.gov/waterscience/fish/advice/index.html). For this reason, fish oil supplements may be the safest source to obtain EPA and DHA. Although there are no current guidelines regarding optimal DHA intake during pregnancy, many experts recommend 200 to 350 mg/day.

PROBIOTICS

Atopy and other allergic conditions are on the rise around the world. It is well known that women with atopic skin disorders are more likely to have an offspring with the same. However, atopy is on the rise in all children, not just those whose mothers are affected. A recent Finnish study demonstrated that women who consume a certain strain of probiotics (*L. rhamnosus*) during pregnancy and while breastfeeding might provide important protection against eczema but not against atopy during their child's first 2 years of life (Kalliomaki et al. 2003). Another RCT confirmed the same and did not show a similar effect by the probiotic B *animalis* spp. *lactis* (Wickens et al. 2008). Probiotics replenish gut flora resulting in a healthier intestinal lining and may decrease the absorption of potential allergens.

Recent studies evaluated the use of probiotics, both orally and vaginally, in the decrease of the rate of preterm delivery. The vaginal application of yogurt with live cultures resulted in an 81% reduction of recurrent bacterial vaginosis during pregnancy, but this was not powered adequately to assess the effect on preterm labor and delivery rates. Larger randomized controlled trials are needed before a formal recommendation can be made (Othman et al. 2007).

Early Pregnancy

NAUSEA AND VOMITING OF PREGNANCY

Roughly 70% to 85% of pregnant women experience nausea and vomiting of pregnancy (NVP) usually starting between 4 and 6 weeks, peaking around 9 weeks, and resolving by 16 weeks (American College of Obstetricians and Gynecologists 2004; Jewell and Young 2003). Up to 2% of women will experience extensive vomiting that requires hospitalization, for example, hyperemesis gravidarum (American College of Obstetricians and Gynecologists 2004). The etiology of NVP is elusive but pregnancy-related hormonal fluctuations and delayed gastric emptying are thought to play a role. Reassurance, dietary changes, lifestyle changes, acupressure wrist bands, ginger (*Zingiber officinale*), vitamin B6, doxylamine, and prescription antiemetics are all useful while supporting a woman through NVP.

DIETARY CHANGES

Sometimes, simple changes in food selections and the manner of consumption may reduce NVP. Typical recommendations include eating small meals or sipping liquids every 2 hours, leaving the stomach neither empty nor full; include bland foods and vitamin B6-rich foods (e.g., chicken, avocados, bananas, whole grains, and corn); avoid spicy and fatty foods, as well as food with strong smells. Prenatal vitamins should be taken before bed or changed to a chewable vitamin

containing 400 μg of folic acid until NVP resolves. However, there is little published evidence that dietary changes affect NVP with the exception of a small
study indicating that meals high in protein were more likely to eliminate NVP
than fatty or carbohydrate-laden meals (American College of Obstetricians and
Gynecologists 2004; Jednak et al. 1999).

ACUPRESSURE OF P6

It is stimulation of the pericardium 6 (P6) acupressure point of the wrist
(approximately two inches above the crease on the volar aspect of the forearm).
Acupressure, acupuncture or nerve stimulation is thought to decrease nausea
and vomiting in pregnancy (Belluomini et al. 1994; O'Brien et al. 1996; Knight
et al. 2001). FDA-approved Sea-Bands are commercially available for this purpose. However, a review of two large RCTs and another standardized review
found equivocal results (see Figure 14.1).

BOTANICALS

Ginger, chamomile (*Matricaria recutita*), peppermint (*Mentha piperita* x)
leaf, and pickled umeboshi (a member of the apricot family) are botanicals
traditionally used to decrease nausea during pregnancy. Only ginger has been

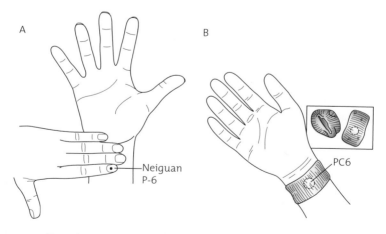

FIGURE 14.1. Demonstration of pericardium 6 acupressure point.
Source: Adapted from Reikel D, *Integrative Medicine*. 2nd ed. Philadelphia, Pennsylvania:
Saunders Elsevier; 2007.

adequately studied during pregnancy; multiple studies support its efficacy for nausea during pregnancy (Borrelli et al. 2005; Fischer-Rasmussen et al. 1991; Vutyavanich et al. 2001). The German Commission E contraindicates ginger during pregnancy; the U.S. Food and Drug Administration lists it as generally regarded as safe (GRAS) as a food additive. Dried ginger is a stronger anti-emetic than fresh. Doses over 4 g/day can theoretically act as an anticoagulant. Standard dosing in RCTs is 1.0 to 1.5 g dried ginger per day taken in 3 to 4 divided doses (Jewell and Young 2003).

VITAMIN B6 (PYRIDOXINE)

Vitamin B6 has also been shown to reduce nausea and vomiting of pregnancy. To prevent adverse neurological effects, the maximum dose is 150 mg/day in divided doses 2 to 4 times/day, although, this dose is much higher than the 40 to 60 mg/day that is typically used for NVP. Combining vitamin B6 with doxylamine (Unisom) is even more effective (ACOG 2004; Thaver et al. 2006).

Homeopathic remedies include Arsenicum, Colchicum, Ipecac, Nux vomica, phosphorus, Pulsatilla, and sepia. There is no compelling evidence that any of these remedies significantly reduce NVP. These should only be prescribed by experienced individuals (DiGaetano 2007).

THREATENED ABORTION

It is 20% of all pregnancies that are affected by bleeding prior to 20-week gestation (i.e., threatened abortion), and 50% of these women will end up miscarrying (Everett 1997). When a woman calls with a complaint of first trimester bleeding, she should be evaluated. Not only will she need psychological and emotional support during this anxiety-provoking time, but a thorough history, physical exam including cervical cultures, a wet prep, and pelvic ultrasound should be performed. A woman can be reassured that if fetal cardiac activity is present on ultrasound, the risk of miscarrying decreases from 50% to 3% (Scroggins et al. 2000). Laboratory evaluation should include complete blood count, Rh typing and serum hCG (Griebel et al. 2005).

Sensitive communication and reassurance for a woman who is experiencing a threatened abortion are vital. Explain your concerns about the potential dangers of early gestational bleeding including spontaneous abortion (SAB), ectopic pregnancy, and the potential for heavy vaginal bleeding. Address any feelings of guilt she might be experiencing regarding herself being the cause of the potential miscarriage. Inform her that 50% of SABs are due to chromosomal abnormalities and that her actions, including recent sexual activity, have not been found to contribute to miscarriage rates. Bed rest has not been adequately studied to recommend it to prevent miscarriage (Aleman et al. 2005). However, low stress activities, a supportive network community, and reliance upon one's spirituality during a potentially stressful time could be of psychological and emotional benefit.

ABDOMINAL CRAMPING

As the uterus grows, women may experience cramping and be concerned about a potential miscarriage. Round ligament pain is typically described as a "cramping" pain that is associated with prolonged standing or sudden twisting movements; the discomfort can usually be recreated on exam. Inquiring about additional symptoms to rule out miscarriage, ectopic pregnancy, constipation, or urinary tract infection is important. Supportive interventions included rest, application of heat, chamomile tea, red raspberry leaf tea, and acetaminophen.

Herbal teas: Chamomile and red raspberry (*Rubus* spp.) leaf tea have been traditionally used to decrease menstrual cramps. No formal studies have been completed to prove efficacy in alleviating uterine cramping during pregnancy. These herbs are listed as Generally Recognized as Safe (GRAS) when used in amounts commonly found in foods by the Natural Medicines Comprehensive Database. Two to four cups of tea per day is probably more than sufficient and carries a low risk of adverse events (Evans and Aronson 2005).

CONSTIPATION, GAS, AND BLOATING

Increased progesterone throughout pregnancy slows down transit in the gastrointestinal tract which can result in constipation, gas, and bloating. (Dietary recommendations include hydration, 30 minutes of exercise per day, consumption of frequent small meals throughout the day, and an increase dietary fiber (i.e., vegetables and fruits like prunes, dates, and raisins). A tablespoon of ground flax seed or wheat germ added to cereal, cottage cheese, yogurt, or salads also serves as an excellent source of fiber.

Limited research has explored these lifestyle interventions. A meta-analysis compared fiber supplements and mild laxatives. The laxatives were more helpful than fiber supplements, but were more likely to cause diarrhea and abdominal pain (Jewell and Young 2001).

Mid and Late Pregnancy

EXERCISE

Exercise transmits an improved sense of well-being and may improve maternal health during pregnancy. Very few high-quality studies have assessed either positive or detrimental effects on maternal or fetal well-being. A systematic review of currently available data is insufficient to make a recommendation regarding the risks or benefits of aerobic exercise for either mother or baby (Kramer and McDonald 2006).

BACK PAIN

Two-thirds of women suffer from back pain during pregnancy. Lifestyle changes frequently recommended include wearing comfortable shoes, correcting one's posture, sitting and standing with support, lifting from bent knees, sleeping with extra pillows, and taking warm baths (Evans and Aronson 2005). Treatment modalities include maternity binders, massage, chiropractic, physical therapy, acupuncture, back exercises, application of hot and cold compresses, and rest. The botanical, valerian (*Valeriana officinalis*), has been recommended for back pain due to its muscle-relaxant qualities. Valerian is generally recognized as safe (GRAS) as a flavoring agent, but it has an unknown safety profile during pregnancy when consumed in medicinal amounts. Very little research has been conducted to prove the efficacy of treatments for back pain during pregnancy. In a systematic review of multiple modalities only water exercises, pelvic-tilt exercises, physiotherapy, and acupuncture were shown to help relieve back pain more than usual prenatal care (Pennick and Young 2007).

HEARTBURN

Gastroesophageal reflux disease (GERD) affects 80% of women in late pregnancy. Current treatment recommendations include dietary changes (elimination of caffeine, spicy, and tomato-based foods), other lifestyle changes, antacids, antihistamines, and proton-pump inhibitors. No studies have been done to assess dietary and lifestyle interventions. A systematic review of three RCTs ($n = 286$) using three medicinal protocols (IM prostigmine, antacid, and antacid plus ranitidine) found favorable results in the treatment groups. More data is needed to make recommendations about treatment of heartburn in pregnancy (Dowswell and Neilson 2008).

STRETCH MARKS

Striae gravidarum (i.e., stretch marks) generally start to appear around the 28th week of pregnancy. They are most commonly seen on the gravid abdomen, thighs, buttocks, and breasts. Over 50% of women will develop this cosmetic concern. Many products are available on the market; most are not helpful. One recent study demonstrated that cocoa butter did not reduce the formation of stretch marks when compared to placebo (Osman et al. 2008). However, another study ($n = 100$) comparing Trofolastin (active ingredient *Centella asiatica* extract) to placebo found that women in the active arm developed fewer stretch marks (Young and Jewell 1996).

VARICOSE VEINS

Increased blood volume, obstructed venous flow, and hormonally mediated relaxation of the vasculature during pregnancy all contribute to the development of varicose veins. Lower extremity elevation may decrease symptoms but does not alleviate varicosities (Jones and Carek 2008). Studies are lacking for treatment of varicose veins during pregnancy.

COMPRESSION STOCKINGS

Compression stockings are frequently offered as a conservative therapy. No studies have been done to prove their efficacy (Bamigboye and Smyth 2007).

BOTANICALS

The botanicals butcher's broom (*Ruscus aculeatus*) and horse chestnut (*Aesculus hippocastanum*) seed extract have both been traditionally used and may be effective in treating chronic venous insufficiency. Although there are several studies addressing the use of a specific horse chestnut extract during pregnancy in the German literature, there is insufficient evidence of safety to recommend its use in pregnancy. The same is true for butcher's broom (Jones and Carek 2008).

HEMORRHOIDS

Dietary modifications (such as increasing fiber and fluids) and topical treatments [such as the application of witch hazel (*Hammamelis virginiana*)] have not been adequately studied during pregnancy (Quijano and Abalos 2005). Though homeopathic arnica gel is recommended by some for application to external hemorrhoids, however, safety is unknown. Non-homeopathic arnica gels should not be used during pregnancy.

PREECLAMPSIA

Preeclampsia affects 2% to 8% of women, most frequently in primagravid, women over the age of 34, obese women, and those with chronic hypertension. By definition, preeclampsia occurs when hypertension and proteinuria exist simultaneously. The hypertension may result in utero-placental insufficiency with decreased blood flow to the fetus. The precise etiology of preeclampsia continues to elude science, which makes prevention difficult. Regular consumption of garlic, salt restriction, antioxidant supplementation, bed rest, and exercise has not been found to decrease the incidence of preeclampsia (Duley and Henderson-Smart 1999; Meher and Duley 2006a, 2006b; Meher et al. 2005; Rumbold et al. 2008).

CALCIUM SUPPLEMENTATION

In a systematic review of 12 trials (n = 15,206), calcium supplementation has been found to decrease the risk of pregnancy induced hypertension and preeclampsia. The effect was greatest in high risk groups (e.g., prior history of preeclampsia) and those with a low baseline calcium intake. Given this data, women should be encouraged to obtain the recommended daily intake for calcium (Hofmeyr et al. 2006).

FETAL MALPRESENTATION AT TERM

Breech presentation occurs in 3% to 4% of term pregnancies (Vetura et al. 1999) The Term Breech Trial (an international, multicentered RCT) demonstrated significantly higher rates of perinatal mortality, neonatal mortality, and serious neonatal morbidity for planned vaginal breech deliveries compared to planned cesarean delivery (ACOG 2006; Hannah et al. 2000). If the fetus remains breech at 36 weeks of gestation, the options in conventional medicine are (1) await spontaneous version; if this does not occur, proceed with cesarean delivery during the 39th week of pregnancy; (2) attempt an external cephalic version (ECV) after 36-week gestation. ECV involves applying pressure to the maternal abdomen to cause the fetus to somersault to vertex presentation. ECV should be performed in a hospital setting and is successful approximately 58% of the time (ACOG 2000).

MOXIBUSTION TO THE BLADDER 67 POINT

Moxibustion entails burning stick of mugwort to warm the Bladder 67 acupuncture point on the lateral aspect of the 5th toes. A systematic review of three trials ($n = 597$) found that moxibustion reduced the need for external cephalic version (RR 0.47, 95% CI 0.33–0.66), though quality of the studies were not considered rigorous (Coyle et al. 2005).

KNEE–CHEST POSITION TO MODIFY OXIPUT-POSTERIOR OR OXIPUT-TRANSVERSE TO OXIPUT-ANTERIOR

In one small trial, women who assumed the knee–chest (compared to sitting upright) position for 10 minutes were more successful in converting an occiput-posterior (OP) or occiput-transverse (OT) presentation to an occiput-anterior (OA) position (RR 0.26, 95% CI 0.18–0.38). However, the recommendation of this same practice for 10 minutes 2 times/day before the onset of labor was not helpful to correct a malpresentation. Assuming this position during labor also reduced backache (Hunter et al. 2007).

ANTEPARTUM PERINEAL MASSAGE

Studies show that 70% of women who deliver babies need some sort of perineal repair after vaginal delivery, which can cause pain, discomfort, and impaired sexual function afterwards. A systematic review of four trials ($n = 2480$) evaluated antepartum perineal massage (APM) and the need for perineal repair after vaginal delivery. APM as little as 2 times/week from the onset of 35 weeks decreased the risk of perineal trauma that required sutures in nulliparous women. One trial involving 376 multiparous women showed a statistical decrease in ongoing perineal pain 3 months after delivery The reviewers recommended that women be informed about the likely benefits of APM and given instructions how to do it (Figure 14.1) (Beckmann and Garrett 2006). This, however, should not be confused with intrapartum perineal massage which has been found to have little value (Stamp et al. 2001).

POST-TERM PREGNANCY AND CERVICAL RIPENING

The rate of post-term pregnancies is 10%. This figure is reduced by labor inductions and cesarean deliveries that occur before 40 complete weeks of gestation. The first trimester ultrasound, the most accurate means of dating a pregnancy, reduces the rate of post-term pregnancy (Neilson 1998). Post-term pregnancies can impact maternal and fetal well-being. Maternal risks include increased risk for fetal macrosomia, prolonged labor, perineal injury, and double the risk of cesarean delivery, and also its associated risks. Fetal risks include perinatal mortality, shoulder dystocia, neurologic injury, meconium-stained amniotic fluid, and altered cord pH. There is evidence to support cervical ripening to decrease maternal and neonatal morbidity and mortality associated with post-term pregnancies (Poma 1999).

ACUPUNCTURE

A 2008 Cochrane Review of three trials ($n = 212$) showed a decreased need for labor induction in women receiving acupuncture as compared to women receiving either placebo or no treatment (Smith and Crowther 2004).

HERBAL SUPPLEMENTS

Commonly prescribed herbs for labor induction include evening primrose (*Oenothera biennis*), black cohosh (*Actaea racemosa*), blue cohosh (*Caulophylum thalictoides*), and red raspberry leaves. Evening primrose oil is generally massaged into the cervix, whereas the others are taken internally. The role of herbs in cervical ripening and labor is still uncertain (Belew 1999). The safety of black and blue cohosh during pregnancy is questionable and probably best avoided.

CASTOR OIL, BATH, AND/OR ENEMA

Castor oil has been used as a labor inducer dating back to ancient Egypt. Only one trial ($n = 100$) assessed castor oil as a labor induction agent as compared to no treatment. The study was of poor quality and had too few participants to define its efficacy. However, 57.7% of women in the treatment arm went into labor within 24 hours versus 4.2% of the control arm. Ingestion of castor oil can cause watery stools and abdominal cramping (Adair 2000; Kelly et al. 2001).

HOMEOPATHY

A systematic review of two double-blind RCTs of moderate quality ($n = 133$) demonstrated no difference between the women who received homeopathic *Caulophyllum* to induce labor and the control groups. There is insufficient evidence to recommend homeopathy for labor induction at this time. However, the hallmark of homeopathy is individualized treatment, and therefore, standardization of the treatment of a particular herb violates classical homeopathic treatment. Rigorous evaluations of individualized homeopathic therapies for labor induction are needed (Smith 2003).

BREAST STIMULATION

Nipple stimulation causes the release of oxytocin from the posterior pituitary gland resulting in increased uterine contractions, the onset of labor, and a decreased risk of post-term pregnancy, and postpartum hemorrhage. Historically, midwives have used nipple stimulation to stimulate labor. However, the safety of this intervention has not been fully evaluated especially in high-risk populations (Kavanagh et al. 2005).

SEXUAL INTERCOURSE

Sexual relations are frequently recommended as a natural method of labor initiation because breast stimulation results in oxytocin secretion and uterine contractions; intercourse may stimulate the lower uterine segment directly resulting in the localized release of prostaglandins. Semen contains prostaglandins, which can induce cervical ripening. Only one small study of 28 women has been published from which no conclusions could be drawn. More research is needed to make sexual intercourse a recommendation for cervical ripening or initiation of labor. There *is* an association between intercourse and preterm labor (Kavanagh, et al. 2001; Summers 1997).

MEMBRANE SWEEPING

A systematic review of 22 trials ($n = 2797$) compares membrane sweeping starting at 38-week gestation to no intervention or to prostaglandin use. Membrane sweeping resulted in a decrease in the duration of pregnancy and the number of women reaching 41-week gestation; it did not result in an increased cesarean rate or an increase in maternal and neonatal infection. However, women in the treatment group experienced more bleeding, irregular contractions, and pain during cervical exam (Boulvain et al. 2005). The number needed to treat to avoid labor induction was 8 (Godberg 2007).

ISOLATED AMNIOTOMY FOR LABOR INDUCTION OR LABOR AUGMENTATION

A systematic review of two trials ($n = 310$) found insufficient data supporting amniotomy alone for labor induction (Bricker and Luckas 2000). Another review published in 2007 (14 studies, $n = 4893$) found that amniotomy to augment spontaneous labor was of no value in shortening the first stage of labor and may actually increase the cesarean delivery rate. Therefore, amniotomy is not recommended for labor induction or labor augmentation in either normally progressing labors or in prolonged labors (Smyth et al. 2007).

Labor and Delivery

NUTRITION DURING LABOR

In the United States, women are generally restricted from ingesting solid food in labor for fear of aspiration (which is very rare). No trials have evaluated the benefit of withholding solid food while a woman labors so that current recommendations are based upon expert opinion. Only "sips and chips" are recommended by the American Society of Anesthesiology Task Force on Obstetrical Anesthesia (American Society of Anesthesiologist Task Force on Obstetrical Anesthesia 1999). In other countries, women are allowed to eat and drink during labor (Berghella et al. 2008).

PAIN CONTROL IN LABOR

Pain modulation during labor is multifaceted. A woman's expectations, preparation for delivery through childbirth classes, and perception of control throughout the delivery experience can all impact her sense of pain control during labor (McCrea and Wright 1999). The physical environment and relationships that she maintains with people present at delivery, including the hospital personnel, can also significantly impact pain control during labor. All these effect her overall level of satisfaction with the entire birth experience. It is recommended that the physical environment be kept as calm as possible and that the laboring woman and her partner be included in the decision-making process.

HOME-LIKE VERSUS INSTITUTIONAL SETTINGS FOR BIRTH

A 2005 systematic review of six trials (n = 8677) found that women who delivered in a home-like setting were more likely to have a spontaneous vaginal delivery, breast-feeding experience, and have a higher satisfaction with their birth experience. They were less likely to need pain medication during labor or to have an episiotomy. However, there was a trend toward higher perinatal mortality in the home-like setting (5 trials, n = 8529; RR 1.83, 95% CI 0.99–3.38) (Hodnett et al. 2005).

DOULAS

In many traditions, birthing women are surrounded by a group of women whom they usually trust and personally select. As birthing moved into the hospital setting, less support was available for women, and many women deliver babies supported only by their partner and the hospital staff. A 2007 systematic review of 14 studies and over 13,000 women found that women who have a continuous labor support person (whether a doula, child birth educator, friend, stranger or family member, other than her partner) had a better birth experience, needed less analgesia, had faster labors, and were more likely to have a vaginal birth (Hodnett et al. 2007).

MIDWIFE-LED CARE

A systematic review of 12,276 women in 11 trials found several benefits and no adverse effects for mothers and their babies who experienced midwife-led care during pregnancy. There was a decreased pregnancy loss rate before 24-week gestation and less regional analgesia in labor; women were more likely to feel in control during the labor process, have a spontaneous vaginal delivery, and initiate breastfeeding after delivery (Hatem et al. 2008).

CAM THERAPIES

A systematic review of 14 trials (n = 1537) evaluated different CAM modalities for pain control in labor. Although shown to personalize and improve the birth experience, there is insufficient evidence to support the benefits of aromatherapy, acupressure, music, massage, relaxation techniques, or white noise. Additional research is needed before recommendations can be made regarding these modalities (Smith et al. 2006). The use of TENS (transcutaneous electrical nerve stimulation) units during labor have also met with mixed results (Goldberg and Zasloff 2007).

ACUPUNCTURE

Multiple systematic reviews have found acupuncture beneficial for pain control in labor. (Lee and Ernst 2004; Smith et al. 2006). One meta-analysis included two studies ($n = 496$) and demonstrated a decrease use of epidural and conventional analgesia in those receiving acupuncture (Goldberg and Zasloff 2007). In one randomized, patient-blinded, placebo-controlled trial, women receiving acupuncture used fewer narcotics during labor and less epidural analgesia (Skilnand et al. 2002).

SELF-HYPNOSIS INSTRUCTION

A total of 288 women in five separate trials experienced a decreased need for analgesia during labor when instructed in self-hypnosis during the antepartum period (Mantle 2000; Smith et al. 2006).

WATER IMMERSION

Water immersion during the first stage of labor significantly reduces a woman's perception of pain and use of epidural, spinal, or paracervical analgesia/anesthesia as reported in a systematic review of eight trials ($n = 2939$). Furthermore, there was no increased risk of Apgar scores of less than 7 at 5 minutes, NICU admissions, instrumental, or cesarean delivery. Only limited data is available for water immersion during the second stage of labor; no recommendations can be made about maternal or neonatal outcomes. No studies have looked at water immersion during the third stage of labor (Cluett et al. 2002).

BOTANICALS AND HOMEOPATHIC REMEDIES

Red raspberry leaf, motherwort, and skullcap are the most commonly used herbs for pain control during labor. Homeopathic remedies include arnica, belladonna, caulophyllum, and cimicifuga. There are insufficient data on the efficacy and safety of these substances to recommend them for use during labor (Goldberg and Zasloff 2007).

EPIDURAL FOR PAIN CONTROL IN LABOR

When compared to non-epidural pain management or no analgesia in labor, epidurals provide better pain relief. Epidurals are associated with a higher rate of operative vaginal delivery, a longer second stage, pitocin augmentation, maternal hypotension, a decrease in mobility after delivery, difficulty when urinating, and increase in the risk of fever. Use of an epidural did not impact the rate of cesarean delivery, long-term backache, or detrimental effects on the newborn (Anim-Somuah et al.). Due to limited space, other conventional pharmaceuticals used for pain control during labor such as antihistamines and narcotics will not be covered here. It is recommended that the reader refer to the ACOG Practice Bulletin No. 36 (*Obstetric Analgesia and Anesthesia* 2002).

Peripartum Perineal Care

PERINEAL SHAVING

Perineal shaving is a routine labor intervention in many countries. Three randomized trials (n = 389) showed there is no evidence to suggest that routine perineal shaving in labor decreases the risk of infection, wound breakdown, or maternal satisfaction with the delivery. Overall, this is an unnecessary practice (Basevi et al. 2000).

Routine episiotomy is no longer recommended. It can lead to more third and fourth degree lacerations, a need for additional suturing, increased pain and other long-term morbidities (Carroli and Belizan 1999; Episiotomy 2006).

SUTURE CHOICE FOR PERINEAL REPAIR AFTER VAGINAL DELIVERY

A recent systematic review of eight trials comparing catgut with synthetic absorbable suture showed that the absorbable suture material for perineal repair caused less short term postpartum perineal pain and less suture dehiscence (Kettle and Johanson 1999). There was no difference in long-term pain or dyspareunia between the two suture types.

COLD PACKS TO PERINEUM POST TRAUMA

A review of seven RCTs (n = 859) supports the use of localized treatment of the perineum with cold packs after vaginal delivery. When compared with no treatment, pain was reduced in the 24 to 72 hours period after delivery (East et al. 2007).

DELIVERY POSITIONING

Two meta-analysis which reviewed 20 trials of variable quality and methodology and included 6135 women found that the upright or lateral positioning during the second stage of labor is preferable to the supine or lithotomy position. The former positions were associated with shorter labors (by 4 minutes), fewer episiotomies and operative deliveries, less pain during and for 3 days after delivery, and less problems with the fetal heartbeat. However, there may be an increased risk of second degree perineal lacerations and increased risk of postpartum hemorrhage of greater than 500 mL (RR 1.63, 95% CI 1.29–2.05). More standardized studies are needed to make recommendations (Gupta and Hofmeyr 2003; Gupta et al. 2004).

Third Stage of Labor and Beyond

CORD CLAMPING

Delayed cord clamping of 30 to 120 seconds resulted in fewer transfusions and less intraventricular hemorrhage in preterm infants but has not been proven to be beneficial for full-term infants (Rabe et al. 2004).

PLACENTAL CORD DRAINAGE

A RCT (n = 147) showed placental cord drainage in the management of the third stage of labor reduces the length of the third stage of labor an average of 5 minutes. Placental cord drainage has also been found to significantly reduce the risk of retained placenta for thirty minutes after birth in a RCT of 477 deliveries (RR 0.28, 95% CI 0.10–0.73) (Soltani et al. 2005).

Uterine massage: In 2004, a joint statement by the International Federation of Gynecologists and Obstetricians and the International Confederation of Midwives indicated that uterine massage after the placenta delivers decreases the risk of postpartum hemorrhage. This statement was supported by a recent RCT (*n* = 200) that compared uterine massage every 10 minutes for 60 minutes following delivery with no massage after the active management of the third stage of labor (i.e., use of oxytocin and cord traction to expeditiously deliver the placenta). Uterine massage decreased the risk of postpartum hemorrhage by 50% and the need for additional utertonics by 80% (Hofmeyr et al. 2008).

BREASTFEEDING

Breast milk is the most complete form of nutrition for infants. In 2003, the World Health Organization recommended that, when possible, children should be exclusively breastfed until 6 months of age. Breast milk digests easily, possesses the right amount of nutrients, protects infants from intestinal infections, increases IQ levels, and decreases the risks of adulthood obesity. Mothers, who breastfeed, experience less postpartum bleeding, more rapid weight loss, and realize an immediate cost savings. Long-term benefits for women include lower risks of breast and ovarian cancer and osteoporosis (*Breastfeeding* U.S. Department of Health and Human Services). More studies are needed to elucidate both short- and long-term benefits of exclusive breastfeeding for a child's first 6 months of life (Kramer and Kakuma 2002). Increased caloric intake of 300 kcal is recommended.

MATERNAL EDUCATION

By engaging women early in the prenatal course, health care providers can significantly increase the number of women who choose to breastfeed (Breastfeeding: Maternal and Infant Aspects 2007a). Postpartum support is also vital to success in breastfeeding. Identifying support personnel in the community and offering this list to women prior to delivery gives them sensitive resources to approach with questions and concerns while breastfeeding. A large meta-analysis of 30,000 women from 14 countries showed that women are much more likely to exclusively breastfeed for 6 months if supported either by lay or professional persons (Britton et al. 2007).

EARLY SKIN-TO-SKIN CONTACT

A meta-analysis of 10 studies ($n = 552$ mother–infant dyads) found that babies who experienced early skin-to-skin contact (babies placed prone on the mother's bare chest at birth and covered with a warm blanket) interacted more with their mothers, cried less, and stayed warmer. They were also more likely to continue breastfeeding for 1 to 4 months after discharge from the hospital (Moore et al. 2007).

METHODS OF BREAST MILK EXPRESSION

For those babies that cannot breastfeed within the first week of life, mothers often use either manual or mechanical methods for breast milk expression. When compared in 12 studies (397 mothers), electric and foot-pedal breast pumps yielded more breast milk than did manual expression. There was no difference in the contamination of the milk supply among the groups. Pumping both breasts simultaneously saved time and did not reduce yield. One study demonstrated that mothers who listened to relaxation tapes while pumping produced a higher volume of breast milk than those who did not (Becker et al. 2008).

LACTOGOGUES

Lactogogues are foods, herbs or medications used to stimulate milk production. Foods that are thought to increase milk production include apricots, asparagus, barley, beer, beet greens, carrots, dandelion greens, green beans, oatmeal, peas, pecans, sweet potatoes, and watercress (Mallory 2008).

Herbs traditionally used to increase milk supply include fenugreek (*Trigonella foenum graecum*), goat's rue (*Galega officinalis*), blessed thistle (*Cnicus benedictus*), borage leaf (*Borago officinalis*), and alfalfa (*Medicago sativa*). Insufficient information is available to recommend herbs as lactogogues. Fenugreek is GRAS (generally regarded as safe) as a food additive the dose is 3 to 6 g/day, and it works within 1 to 3 days. Fenugreek may cause gastrointestinal upset. Though there is insufficient evidence supporting the use of herbs as lactogogues, there is a long history of traditional and historical use suggesting safety and efficacy. However, borage leaves are considered unsafe during lactation as they contain hepatotoxic alkaloids that are excreted in breastmilk and alfalfa may have estrogenic activity in medicinal amounts (Co et al. 2002; Mallory 2008; *Fenugreek*; Swafford and Berens 2000).

MASTITIS

Mastitis is an infection of the breast tissue affecting approximately 2% to 9.5% of breastfeeding women (Breastfeeding: Maternal and Infant Aspects 2007b). It is caused by accumulation of bacteria in the breast tissue compounded by obstructed outlet flow. Symptoms include breast tenderness, edema, erythema, and fever. If a breastfeeding woman calls with symptoms of mastitis, she should be examined to rule out abscess formation. Prescription medications include antibiotics given usually for 10 to 14 days. If an abscess has formed, she may need surgical intervention. If possible, she should be encouraged to breastfeed or pump the affected breast.

Historically, cabbage leaves applied directly to the breast have been used for symptomatic relief of breast engorgement. One meta-analysis of eight studies (*n* = 424) demonstrated that cabbage leaves were as effective as gel packs and cabbage leaf enzymes were similar in efficacy to placebo creams. However, the reviewers found no overall benefit in using cabbage leaves or cabbage leaf extracts to decrease the pain of engorgement (Mangesi and Muzonzini 2008). Sage is a natural anti-inflammatory considered "possibly unsafe" during lactation as it can temporarily decrease milk production (Mastitis: *Natural Medicines Comprehensive Database*). Common homeopathic remedies for mastitis include belladonna, bryonia, silicea, and phytolacca. All except silicea are considered unsafe for use during pregnancy and lactation (Mastitis: *Natural Medicines Comprehensive Database*).

Summary

Pregnancy is a *natural* state that reinforces the importance of the mind-body-spirit-community connection in a woman's life. Whether in anticipation of pregnancy or throughout this journey, women generally seek knowledge desiring the best outcome for their baby. They frequently request "natural" and "safe" therapies for common physiological and psychological changes brought on by the pregnant state. Because of this, an integrative approach to pregnancy can result in a collaboration of wellness that could potentially have a life-long impact on both mother and baby.

REFERENCES

Gupta JK, Hofmeyr GJ. Position for women during second stage of labour. *Cochrane Database Syst Rev.* 2003;(3):CD002006.

Adair CD. Nonparmacologic approaches to cervical priming and labor induction. *Clin Obstet Gynecol.* 2000;43:447–454.

Aleman A, Althabe F, Belizán JM, Bergel E. Bed rest during pregnancy for preventing miscarriage. *Cochrane Database Syst Rev.* 2005;(2):CD003576.

Anim-Somuah M, Smyth R, Howell C. Epidural versus non-epidural or no analgesia in labour. *Cochrane Database Syst Rev.* 2005;(4):CD000331.

Bamigboye AA, Smyth R. Interventions for varicose veins and leg oedema in pregnancy. *Cochrane Database Syst Rev.* 2007;(1):CD001066.

Basevi V, Lavender T, Routine. Perineal shaving on admission in labour. *Cochrane Database Syst Rev.* 2000;(4):CD001236.

Becker GE, McCormick FM, Renfrew MJ. Methods of milk expression for lactating women. *Cochrane Database Syst Rev.* 2008;(4):CD006170.

Beckmann MM, Garrett AJ. Antenatal perineal massage for reducing perineal trauma. *Cochrane Database Syst Rev.* 2006;(1):CD005123.

Belew C. Herbs and the childbearing woman: Guidelines for nurse-midwives. *J Nurse Midwifery.* 1999;44:231–252.

Belluomini J, Litt RC, Lee KA, Katz M. Acupressure for nausea and vomiting in pregnancy: a randomized, blinded study. *Obstet Gynecol.* 1994;84:245–248.

Bendich A, Langseth L. Safety of vitamin A. *Am J Clin Nutr.* 1989;49:358–371.

Berghella V, Baster JK, Chauhan SP. Evidence-based labor and delivery management. *Am J Obstet Gynecol.* 2008;199:445–454.

Borrelli F, Capasso R, Aviello G, Pittler MH, Izzo AA. Effectiveness and safety of ginger in the treatment of pregnancy-induced nausea and vomiting. *Obstet Gynecol.* 2005;105:849.

Boulvain M, Stan C, Irion O. Membrane sweeping for induction of labour. *Cochrane Database Syst Rev.* 2005;(1):CD000451.

Breastfeeding: Maternal and Infant Aspects. ACOG Committee Opinion No. 361. American College of Obstetricians and Gynecologists. *Obstet Gynecol.* 2007a;109:279–280.

Breastfeeding: Maternal and Infant Aspects. Committee on health care for underserved women. Committee on obstetric practice. *ACOG Clin. Rev.* 2007b;12(1)5S(suppl).

Breastfeeding. The National Women's Health Information Center. US Department of Health and Human Services. Office on Women's Health. http://www.womenshealth. gov/breastfeeding/index.cfm?page=227

Bricker L, Luckas M. Amniotomy alone for induction of labour. *Cochrane Database Syst Rev.* 2000;(4):CD002862.

Britton C, McCormick FM, Renfrew MJ, Wade A, King SE. Support for breastfeeding mothers. *Cochrane Database Syst Rev.* 2007;(1):CD001141.

Carroli G, Belizan J. Episiotomy for vaginal birth. *Cochrane Database Syst Rev.* 1999;(3):CD000081.

CDC. Recommendations for the use of folic acid to reduce the number of cases of spina bifida and other neural tube defects. *MMWR*. 1992;41(RR–14):1–7.

CDC. Preconception and Interconception Health Status of Women Who Recently gave birth to a live-born infant—Pregnancy Risk Assessment Monitoring System (PRAMS), United States, 26 Reporting Areas, 2004. Surveillance Summaries, December 14, 2007. *MMWR*. 2007;56(SS–10).

Chang J, Elam-Evans LD, Berg CJ, et al. Pregnancy-related mortality surveillance—United States, 1991–1999. *MMWR Surveillan Sum*. 2003;52(SS02):1–8.

Chatzi L, Torrent M, Romieu I, et al. Mediterranean diet in pregnancy is protective for wheeze and atopy in childhood. *Thorax*. 2008;63:507–513.

Cluett ER, Nikodem VC, McCandlish RE, Burns EE. Immersion in water in pregnancy, labour and birth. *Cochrane Database Syst Rev*. 2002;(2):CD000111.

Co MM, Hernandez EA, Co BG. A comparative study on the efficacy of the different galactogogues among mothers with lactational insufficiency. Abstract, *AAP Section on Breastfeeding*. 2002 NCE, 2002;125.

Coyle ME, Smith CA, Peat B. Cephalic version by moxibustion for breech presentation. *Cochrane Database Syst Rev*. 2005;(2):CD003928.

Czeizel AE. The primary prevention of birth defects: multivitamins or folic acid? *Int J Med Sci*. 2004;1:50–61.

DiGaetano A. Nausea and vomiting in pregnancy. In: Reikl D, ed. *Integrative Medicine*. 2nd ed. Philadelphia, PA: Saunders Elsevier; 2007:Chapter 53.

Dowswell T, Neilson JP. Interventions for heartburn in pregnancy. *Cochrane Database Syst Rev*. 2008;(4):CD007065.

Duley L, Henderson-Smart DJ. Reduced salt intake compared to normal dietary salt, or high intake, in pregnancy. *Cochrane Database Syst Rev*. 1999;(3):CD001687.

East CE, Begg L, Henshall NE, Marchant P, Wallace K. Local cooling for relieving pain from perineal trauma sustained during childbirth. *Cochrane Database Syst Rev*. 2007;(4):CD006304.

Elsinga J. The effect of preconception counseling on lifestyle and other behavior before and during pregnancy. *Womens Health Issues*. 2008;18(6):S117–S125.

Episiotomy. ACOG Practice Bulletin No. 71. American College of Obstetricians and Gynecologists. *Obstet Gynecol*. 2006;107:957–962.

Evans JM, Aronson R. The emotional and physical world of early pregnancy: cramps. In: Joel M Evans ed. *The Whole Pregnancy Handbook—An Obstetrician's Guide to Integrating Conventional and Alternative Medicine Before, During and After Pregnancy*. New York: Penguin Group (USA) Inc; 2005a:Chapter 9.

Evans JM, Aronson R. Pregnancy's effects: back pain. In: *The Whole Pregnancy Handbook—An Obstetrician's Guide to Integrating Conventional and Alternative Medicine Before, During and After Pregnancy*. New York: Penguin Group (USA) Inc: 2005b;Chapter 11.

Everett C. Incidence and outcome of bleeding before the 20th week of pregnancy: prospective study from general practice. *Br Med J*. 1997;315:32–34.

External cephalic version. ACOG Practice Bulletin 2000 No. 13. American College of Obstetricians and Gynecologists. *Obstet Gynecol*. 2000.

Facchinetti F, Fazzio M, Venturini P. Polyunsaturated fatty acids and risk of preterm delivery. *Eur Rev Med Pharmacol Sci.* 2005;9(1):41–48.

Fenugreek. *Natural Medicines Comprehensive Database.* http://www.naturaldatabase. com/(S(x5ausg45unh142vvnwj40455))/nd/Search.aspx?cs=AZ&s=ND&pt=100&fs =ND&id=733&searchid=13503080&ds

Fischer-Rasmussen W, Kjaer SK, Dahl C, Asping U. Ginger treatment of hyperemesis gravidarum. *Eur J Obstet Gynecol Reprod Biol.* 1991;38:19–24.

Gardiner PM, Nelson L, Shellhaas CS, et al. The clinical content of preconception care: nutrition and dietary supplements. *Am J Obstet Gynecol.* 2008;199(6 Suppl 2) S296–S309.

Godberg D. Post-term pregnancy. In: Reikel D, ed. *Integrative Medicine.* 2nd ed. Philadelphia, Pennsylvania: Saunders Elsevier; 2007: Chapter 51.

Goldberg D, Zasloff, E. Labor pain management. In: Reikel D, ed. *Integrative Medicine.* 2nd ed. Philadelphia, Pennsylvania: Saunders Elsevier; 2007: Chapter 52.

Griebel CP, Halvorsen J, Golemon TB, Day AA. Management of spontaneous abortion. *Am Fam Physician.* 2005;72(7):1243–1250.

Gupta JK, Hofmeyr GJ, Smyth R. Position in the second stage of labour for women without epidural anaesthesia. *Cochrane Database Syst Rev.* 2004;(1):CD002006.

Haider BA, Bhutta ZA. Multiple-micronutrient supplementation for women during pregnancy. *Cochrane Database Syst Rev.* 2006;(4):CD004905.

Hannah ME, Hannah WJ, Hewson SA, Hodnett ED, Saigal S, Willan AR. Planned cesarean section versus planned vaginal birth for breech presentation at term: a randomized multicenter trial. Term Breech Trial Collaborative Group. *Lancet.* 2000;356:1375–1383.

Harville EW. Calcium intake during pregnancy among white and African-American pregnant women in the United States. *J Am Coll Nutr.* 2004;23(1):43–50.

Hatem M, Sandall J, Devane D, Soltani H, Gates S. Midwife-led versus other models of care for childbearing women. *Cochrane Database of Syst Rev.* 2008;4:CD004667.

Henshaw SD. Unintended pregnancy in the United States. *Fam Plann Perspect.* 1998;30:24–29,46.

Henderson JT, Weisman CS, Grason H. Are two doctors better than one? Women's physician use and appropriate care. *Womens Health Issues.* 2002;12:139–149.

Hodnett ED, Downe S, Edwards N, Walsh D. Home-like versus conventional institutional settings for birth. *Cochrane Database Syst Rev.* 2005;1:CD000012.

Hodnett ED, Gates S, Hofmeyr GJ, Sakala C. Continuous support for women during childbirth. *Cochrane Database Syst Rev.* 2007;3:CD003766.

Hofmeyr GJ, Abdel-Aleem H, Abdel-Aleem MA. Uterine massage for preventing postpartum haemorrhage. *Cochrane Database Syst Rev.* 2008;3:CD006431.

Hofmeyr GJ, Atallah AN, Duley L. Calcium supplementation during pregnancy for preventing hypertensive disorders and related problems. *Cochrane Database Syst Rev.* 2006;3:CD001059.

Holick MF. Vitamin D Defieciency. *N Engl J Med.* 2007;357:266–281.

Hunter S, Hofmeyr GJ, Kulier R. Hands and knees posture in late pregnancy or labour for fetal malposition (lateral or posterior). *Cochrane Database Syst Rev.* 2007;4:CD001063.

Institute of Medicine. *DRI Dietary Reference Intakes for Calcium, Phosphorus, Magnesium, Vitamin D, and Fluoride.* Washington, DC: National Academy Press; 1997.

Institute of Medicine. *Food and Nutrition Board. Dietary Reference Intakes for Vitamin A, Vitamin K, Arsenic, Boron, Chromium, Copper, Iodine, Iron, Manganese, Molybdenum, Nickel, Silicon, Vanadium, and Zinc.* Washington, DC: National Academy Press; 2001.

Jacobson JL, Jacobson SW, Muckle G, Kaplan-Estrin M, Ayotte P, Dewailly E. Beneficial effects of a polyunsaturated fatty acid on infant development: evidence from the Inuit of arctic Quebec. *J Pediatr.* 2008;152(3):356–364.

Jednak MA, Shadigian EM, Kim MS, et al. Protein meals reduce nausea and gastric slow wave dysrhythmic activity in first trimester pregnancy. *Am J Physiol.* 1999;277:G855–G861.

Jewell D, Young G. Interventions for nausea and vomiting in early pregnancy. *Cochrane Database Syst Rev.* 2003;4:CD000145.

Jewell DJ, Young G. Interventions for treating constipation in pregnancy. *Cochrane Database Syst Rev.* 2001;2:CD001142.

Jones RH, Carek PJ. Management of varicose veins. *Am Fam Physician.* 2008;78(11):1289–1294.

Kalliomaki M, Salminen S, Poussa T, Arvilommi H, Isolauri E. Probiotics and prevention of atopic disease: 4-year follow-up of a randomised placebo-controlled trial. *Lancet.* 2003;361(9372):1869–1871.

Kavanagh J, Kelly AJ, Thomas J. Breast stimulation for cervical ripening and induction of labour. *Cochrane Database Syst Rev.* 2005;3:CD003392.

Kavanagh J, Kelly AJ, Thomas J. Sexual intercourse for cervical ripening and induction of labour. *Cochrane Database Syst Rev.* 2001;2:CD003093.

Kelly AJ, Kavanagh J, Thomas J. Castor oil, bath and/or enema for cervical priming and induction of labour. *Cochrane Database Syst Rev.* 2001;2:CD003099.

Kettle C, Johanson R. Absorbable synthetic versus catgut suture material for perineal repair. *Cochrane Database Syst Rev.* 1999;4:CD000006.

Knight B, Mudge C, Openshaw S, White A, Hart A. Effect of acupuncture on nausea and pregnancy: a randomized, controlled trial. *Obstet Gynecol.* 2001;97:184–188.

Kramer MS, Kakuma R. Optimal duration of exclusive breastfeeding. *Cochrane Database Syst Rev.* 2002;1:CD003517.

Kramer MS, McDonald SW. Aerobic exercise for women during pregnancy. *Cochrane Database Syst Rev.* 2006;3:CD000180.

Lee H, Ernst E. Acupuncture for labor pain management: a systematic review. *Am J Obstet Gynecol.* 2004;191:1573.

Locksmith GJ, Duff P. Preventing neural tube defects: the importance of periconciptional folic acid supplements. *Obstet Gynecol.* 1998;91:1027–1034.

Lorenz D, Lincoln A, Dooley S, et al. Surveillance of preconception health indicators among women delivering live-born infants, Oklahoma, 2000–2003. *MMWR.* 2007:56(25):631–634.

Lumley J, Watson L, Watson M, Bower C. Periconceptional supplementation with folate and/or multivitamins for preventing neural tube defects. *Cochrane Database Syst Rev.* 2001;3:CD001056.

Makrides M, Duley L, Olsen SF. Marine oil, and other prostaglandin precursor, supplementation for pregnancy uncomplicated by pre-eclampsia or intrauterine growth restriction. *Cochrane Database Syst Rev.* 2006;3:CD003402.

Mallory J. Supplement sampler: natural galactogogues. University of Wisconsin Integrative Medicine Department of Family Medicine. 2008. http://www.fammed.wisc.edu/files/webfm-uploads/documents/outreach/im/ss_galactogogues.pdf

Mangesi L, Muzonzini G. Treatments for breast engorgement during lactation (Protocol). *Cochrane Database Syst Rev.* 2008;1:CD006946. Treatment for breast engorgement during lactation. *Cochrane Database Syst Rev.* 2007.

Mastitis. *Natural Medicines Comprehensive Database* http://www.naturaltherapypages.com.au/article/mastitis. Accessed on February 14, 2009

Mantle F. The role of hypnosis in pregnancy and childbirth. In: Tiran D, Mack S, eds. *Complementary Therapies for Pregnancy and Childbirth.* 2nd ed, New York: Balliere Tindall; 2000: Chapter 10.

McCrea BH, Wright ME. Satisfaction in childbirth and perceptions of pain control in pain relief during labour. *J Adv Nurs.* 1999;29:877.

Meher S, Abalos E, Carroli G. Bed rest with or without hospitalisation for hypertension during pregnancy. *Cochrane Database Syst Rev.* 2005;4:CD003514.

Meher S, Duley L. Exercise or other physical activity for preventing pre-eclampsia and its complications. *Cochrane Database Syst Rev.* 2006a;2:CD005942.

Meher S, Duley L. Garlic for preventing pre-eclampsia and its complications. *Cochrane Database Syst Rev.* 2006b;3:CD006065.

Mode of term singleton breech delivery. ACOG Committee Opinion 2006 No. 340. American College of Obstetricians and Gynecologists. *Obstet Gynecol.* 2006;108:235–237.

Moore ER, Anderson GC, Bergman N. Early skin-to-skin contact for mothers and their healthy newborn infants. *Cochrane Database Syst Rev.* 2007;3:CD003519.

Motivational Interviewing: A tool for behavior change. ACOG Committee Opinion No.423. American College of Obstetricians and Gynecologists. *Obstet Gynecol.* 2009;113:243–246.

Nausea and vomiting of pregnancy. ACOG Practice Bulletin No. 52. American College of Obstetricians and Gynecologists. *Obstet Gynecol.* 2004;103:803–815.

Neilson JP. Ultrasound for fetal assessment in early pregnancy. *Cochrane Database Syst Rev.* 1998;4:CD000182.

Obesity in pregnancy. ACOG Committee Opinion No. 315. American College of Obstetricians and Gynecologists. *Obstet Gynecol.* 2005;106:671–675.

Obstetric Analgesia and Anesthesia. ACOG Practice Bulletin No. 36. American College of Obstetricians and Gynecologists. *Obstet Gynecol.* 2002;100:177–191.

O'Brien B, Relyea MJ, Taerun T. Efficacy of P6 acupressure in the treatment of nausea and vomiting during pregnancy. *Am J Obstet Gynecol.* 1996;174:708–715.

Osman H, Usta IM, Rubeiz N, Abu Rustum R, Charara I, Nassar AH. Cocoa butter lotion for prevention of striae gravidarum: a double-blind, randomized and placebo-controlled trial. *BJOG.* 2008;115(9):1138–1142.

Othman M, Neilson JP, Alfirevic Z. Probiotics for preventing preterm labour. *Cochrane Database Syst Rev.* 2007;1:CD005941.

Pawley N, Bishop NJ. Prenatal and infant predictors of bone health: the influence of vitamin D. *Am J Clin Nutr.* 2004;80(6):1748S–1751S.

Peña-Rosas JP, Viteri FE. Effects of routine oral iron supplementation with or without folic acid for women during pregnancy. *Cochrane Database Syst Rev.* 2006;3:CD004736.

Pennick V, Young G. Interventions for preventing and treating pelvic and back pain in pregnancy. *Cochrane Database Syst Rev.* 2007;2:CD001139.

Poma PA. Cervical ripening: a review and recommendations fro clinical practice. *J Reprod Med.* 1999;44:657–668.

Practice guidelines for obstetrical anesthesia: a report by the American Society of Anesthesiologist Task Force on Obstetrical Anesthesia. *Anesthesiology.* 1999;90:600–611.

Quijano CE, Abalos E. Conservative management of symptomatic and/or complicated haemorrhoids in pregnancy and the puerperium. *Cochrane Database Syst Rev.* 2005;3:CD004077.

Rabe H, Reynolds G, Diaz-Rossello J. Early versus delayed umbilical cord clamping in preterm infants. *Cochrane Database Syst Rev.* 2004;4:CD003248.

Reinwald S. The health benefits of calcium citrate malate: a review of the supporting science. *Adv Food Nutr Res.* 2008;54:219–346.

Roscoe JA, Matteson SE. Acupressure and acustimulation bands for control of nausea: a brief review. *Am J Obstet Gynecol.* 2002;186:S244–S247.

Rumbold A, Duley L, Crowther CA, Haslam RR. Antioxidants for preventing pre-eclampsia. *Cochrane Database Syst Rev.* 2008;1:CD004227.

Rumbold A, Middleton P, Crowther CA. Vitamin supplementation for preventing miscarriage. *Cochrane Database Syst Rev.* 2005;2:CD004073.

Scroggins KM, Smucker WD, Krishen AE. Spontaneous pregnancy loss: evaluation, management and follow-up counseling. *Prim Care.* 2000;27:153–167.

Skilnand E, Fossen D, Heiberg E. Acupuncture in the management of pain in labor. *Acta Obstet Gynecol Scand.* 2002;81:943.

Smith CA, Collins CT, Cyna AM, Crowther CA. Complementary and alternative therapies for pain management in labour. *Cochrane Database Syst Rev.* 2006;4:CD003521.

Smith CA, Crowther CA. Acupuncture for induction of labour. *Cochrane Database Syst Rev.* 2004;1:CD002962.

Smith CA. Homoeopathy for induction of labour. *Cochrane Database Syst Rev.* 2003;4:CD003399.

Smyth RMD, Alldred SK, Markham C. Amniotomy for shortening spontaneous labour. *Cochrane Database Syst Rev.* 2007;4:CD006167.

Soltani H, Dickinson F, Symonds I. Placental cord drainage after spontaneous vaginal delivery as part of the management of the third stage of labour. *Cochrane Database Syst Rev.* 2005;4:CD004665.

Stamp G, Kruzins G, Crowther C. Perineal massage in labour and prevention of perineal trauma: randomized controlled trial. *Br Med J.* 2001;322:1277–1280.

Summers L. Methods of cervical ripening and labor induction. *J Nurse Midwifery.* 1997;42:71–85.

Swafford S, Berens P. Effect of fenugreek on breast milk volume. Abstract, *5th International Meeting of the Academy of Breastfeeding Medicine*, Tucson, AZ, September 11–13, 2000.

Thaver D, Saeed MA, Bhutta ZA. Pyridoxine (vitamin B6) supplementation in pregnancy. *Cochrane Database Syst Rev.* 2006;2:CD000179.

The importance of preconception care in the continuum of women's health care. ACOG Committee Opinion No. 313. American College of Obstetricians and Gynecologists. *Obstet Gynecol.* 2005;106:665–666.

Thomas M, Weisman SM. Calcium supplementation during pregnancy and lactation: effects on the mother and the fetus. *Am J Obstet Gynec.* 2006;194(4).

Tough S, Tofflemire K, Clarke M, Newburn-Cook C. Do women change their drinking behaviors while trying to conceive? An opportunity for preconception counseling. *Clin Med Res.* 2006;4(2):97–105.

Vetura SJ, Martin JA, Curtin SC, Mathews TJ. Births: final data for 1997. *Natl Vital Stat Rep.* 1999;47(18):1–96.

Vutyavanich T, Kraisarin T, Ruangsri R. Ginger for nausea and vomiting in pregnancy: randomized, double-masked, placebo-controlled trial. *Obstet Gynecol.* 2001;97:577–582.

Wickens K, Black PN, Stanley TV, et al. A differential effect of 2 probiotics in the prevention of eczema and atopy: a double-blind, randomized, placebo-controlled trial. *J Allergy Clin Immunol.* 2008;122(4):788–794.

Wolpowitz D, Gilchrest BA. The vitamin D questions: how much do you need and how should you get it? *J Am Acad Dermatol.* 2006;54(2):301–317.

Young GL, Jewell D. Crams for preventing stretch marks in pregnancy. *Cochrane Database Syst Rev.* 1996;1:CD000066.

15

Perinatal Depression

MARLENE P. FREEMAN

CASE STUDY

Sandra was a married woman in her mid-thirties, with a graduate degree and worked as a health care provider. She presented for the treatment of a major depressive episode after stopping her medication just prior to conceiving. Despite having had an excellent response to an antidepressant during major depressive episodes previously, Sandra stated that she would not consider restarting medication during her pregnancy. She would, however, be interested in nutritional strategies that might help her manage her mood until she was ready to take an antidepressant after she had her baby and finished breast-feeding. As a health care provider, she could readily understand that complementary and alternative medicine (CAM) therapies did not have a strong evidence base for the treatment of depression, and she understood that restarting an antidepressant was her best strategy for relieving her depression. However, as a pregnant woman with depression, she found herself concerned about possible risks associated with medication.

In my experience...pregnant and postpartum women are often extremely motivated to seek CAM treatments and may feel excessively guilty about using medication. Many women need reassurance that the use of antidepressant medications does not make them less qualified for motherhood. Women may feel guilty about using medication, even when they are suffering from serious depression and have had good previous responses to medication. Pregnant women can be exquisitely motivated to make lifestyle changes and may add exercise to their daily regimen more readily than at other times of life. Postpartum women are often overwhelmed with the care of a new baby, and it is imperative to make sure that treatments are not overly demanding in terms of time and requirement for childcare.

Introduction

Depression during pregnancy and the postpartum (which collectively can be referred to as "perinatal depression") is serious to consider for the mother, baby, and entire family. Perinatal depression is the occurrence of major depressive disorder (MDD) during pregnancy and/or postpartum. Postpartum depression (PPD) is the occurrence of MDD after childbirth. Both prenatal depression and a history of depression in the past increase the risk of PPD (Chaudron et al. 2001).

A major depressive episode consists of least 2 weeks of depressed mood or loss of interest or pleasure, and other symptoms that may include change in sleep, energy or appetite, as well as guilt, suicidal thoughts, and other symptoms. Many of these symptoms are difficult to assess during pregnancy and postpartum. Untreated prenatal depression increases obstetrical risks (Wisner et al. 2000). PPD has a broad negative impact on bonding and child development (Moses-Kolko and Roth, 2004). Therefore, the risks and benefits of both untreated depression and treatment must be considered.

Women use CAM treatments more frequently than men, in general, and in particular for the treatment of depression (Mackenzie et al. 2003; Tindle et al. 2005). In consideration of common utilization and patient preferences, it is important to understand the data regarding the efficacy and safety of CAM treatments for perinatal depression.

Postpartum Depression

Postpartum Depression (PPD) is defined in the *Diagnostic and Statistical Manual* of the American Psychiatric Association (DSM-IV) as a major depressive episode with onset within 4 weeks of delivery, although the literature in this area supports a broader definition that includes a later onset during the postpartum year (American Psychiatric Association 1994; Stowe et al. 2005). It is 10% to 15% of postpartum women who experience the onset of postpartum major depressive episodes (Altshuler et al. 1998; Gavin et al. 2005; Moses-Kolko and Roth, 2004; Pariser et al. 1993). PPD affects the individual and her family, with a negative impact upon children, and noted impairments in attachment, cognitive development, and behavior (Cicchetti et al. 1998; Murray et al. 1996; Newport et al. 2002; Sharp et al. 1995). Women who have suffered from PPD may alter subsequent decisions about whether to have more children due to fear of its recurrence (Peindl et al. 1995).

Once a woman has experienced PPD, she is at increased risk for future episodes. A personal history of mood disorders is a risk factor for PPD (Bloch et al. 2006; O'Hara et al. 1991). Family history of mood disorders and a woman's experience of depression during the pregnancy are also risk factors for PPD (Bloch et al. 2006; Chaudron et al. 2001; Freeman et al. 2005; Halbreich 2004; Robertson et al. 2004).

Many women prefer to minimize or avoid medication during pregnancy and breast-feeding. However, for a woman who has been successfully treated with antidepressants prior to pregnancy, the risk of relapse is increased if she discontinues medication for pregnancy (Cohen et al. 2006). Treatment decisions are complicated by reports of risk from antidepressants, and even more complex as the literature in this area is composed of small, nondefinitive studies that offer conflicting results. Some of the reported risks include cardiac teratogenicity with first trimester paroxetine use; neonatal symptoms associated with antidepressants in late pregnancy, and an association between selective serotonin reuptake inhibitors (SSRIs) in late pregnancy and persistent pulmonary hypertension of the newborn (Chambers et al. 2006; Freeman et al. 2007). Antidepressants are often utilized for PPD, and studies support efficacy (Payne 2007). Most studies demonstrate low levels of medication exposure to infants via breast-feeding, although there are a few case reports of suspected adverse events (Burt et al. 2001). Psychotherapies have been studied for the prevention and acute treatment of PPD and appear effective (Dennis and Hodnett 2007).

Strategies to Prevent PPD

Interpersonal psychotherapy (IPT) approaches appear to decrease PPD in at-risk women when it is provided during pregnancy (Zlotnick et al. 2001). Two randomized placebo-controlled trials have been conducted to determine whether antidepressant medications that have been started immediately after childbirth reduce the recurrence of PPD in women who had experienced PPD in the past. In one trial, sertraline initiated immediately after childbirth was significantly better than placebo, whereas in another study, nortriptyline was not significantly better than placebo (Wisner et al. 2001, 2004).

An Integrated Approach

EXERCISE

The American College of Obstetricians and Gynecologists recommend 30 minutes of daily moderate exercise for pregnant women, unless contraindications exist (Artal et al. 2003). Although exercise is recommended, and most women already know there are health benefits, the symptoms of depression can interfere with a woman's motivation to engage in an exercise regimen, and encouragement from a health care provider may help overcome barriers to implementation.

Regular exercise is associated with decreased prevalence of depressive symptoms (Strawbridge et al. 2002). Treatment studies support antidepressant effects of exercise (Otto et al. 2007; Trivedi et al. 2006). The "dose" and adherence to an exercise program may be particularly relevant to antidepressant effects (Dunn et al. 2001). Except in the rare situation when exercise is contraindicated, exercise is a reasonable addition to treatment for MDD.

In one study, healthy pregnant women were asked to prospectively record information each trimester regarding mood, anxiety, stress, and exercise (Da Cost 2003). More physical activity was associated with significantly lower levels of depressive symptoms in the first and second trimesters, although not sustained in the third trimester. In a randomized controlled trial, 80 postpartum women scoring >10 on the Edinburgh Postnatal Depression Scale (EPDS) at 6 weeks postpartum were randomly assigned either three weekly exercise sessions versus a treatment as usual control (Heh et al. 2008). Women assigned to exercise had significantly greater improvements on depression scores at 5 months postpartum.

In my experience, adding exercise to a treatment regimen can be powerful and empowering for women. Almost all women know the health benefits of exercising, but may not make doing so a priority. Depression can interfere with the motivation, energy, and self-esteem required to start and continue an exercise regimen. Health care providers can discuss the benefits of exercise and make sure that a woman understands that the time it takes to care for herself is essential to her treatment. A "prescription" for exercise can help women understand how important and powerful exercise can be.

Omega-3 Fatty Acids

A substantial amount of evidence supports a role for omega-3 fatty acids in depression. Population studies, animal studies, and laboratory data support a role for omega-3 fatty acids in MDD (Freeman et al. 2006; Parker et al. 2006). Overall, clinical studies demonstrate intriguing results for MDD, especially as an augmentation strategy (Freeman et al. 2006; Parker et al. 2006). Omega-3 fatty acids are especially compelling to consider in the context of childbearing, as they have well-established health benefits, including benefits regarding fetal and infant health and development (Freeman 2006). The typical American diet is composed of a relative deficiency of omega-3 fatty acids compared to other essential fatty acids (Simopoulos 1991). Eicosapentanoic acid (EPA) and docosahexaenoic acid (DHA) are the main omega-3 fatty acids of significance in mood disorders.

Omega-3 fatty acids offer advantages for mother and baby. The maternal omega-3 fatty acid supply in pregnancy is diminished, as the fetal and infant demand is high for optimal brain development (Freeman 2006; McGregor et al. 2001). Insufficient maternal intake in animals is associated with diminished maternal brain DHA (Levant et al. 2006). Despite increased demand, dietary intake is low during pregnancy in the United States, a situation that has worsened since mercury warnings were issued by the U.S. Food and Drug Administration (Benisek et al. 2000; Oken et al. 2003). However, many sources of omega-3 fatty acids (including many commonly consumed species of fish) appear to contain low or negligible amounts of mercury, and encapsulated fish oil undergoes a refining process that removes contaminants (Foran et al. 2003). Omega-3 fatty acid intake is associated with improved obstetrical outcomes and infant development (Dunstan et al. 2008; Hibbeln et al. 2007; McGregor et al. 2001).

PERINATAL DEPRESSION

Hibbeln (2002) demonstrated an association between mothers' fish and seafood intake and prevalence of PPD. Similarly, he demonstrated an inverse relationship between breast milk DHA content and maternal depression. Further study of omega-3 fatty acids as a treatment for perinatal depression was supported by an open study of omega-3 fatty acids for prenatal depression, and a randomized dose-finding study in PPD (Freeman et al. 2006a, 2006b). Three independent placebo-controlled studies were conducted to assess omega-3 fatty acids for the treatment of perinatal depression. In one study, investigators found a significant benefit of omega-3 fatty acids compared with placebo for prenatal depression. In two other studies, there was no observable difference between omega-3 fatty acids and placebo. However, studies included a small number of subjects and, in one study (Freeman et al. in press), all subjects received supportive psychotherapy, and both omega-3 and placebo groups did significantly better after participation. Dose is especially important for future consideration, as the study with the most robust effects utilized the highest dose (Su et al. 2008). Omega-3 fatty acid capsules appear as well tolerated by perinatal women as placebo (Freeman and Sinha 2007).

S-Adenosyl L-Methionine

S-Adenosyl L-methionine (SAMe) occurs naturally in the human body, produced from the amino acid methionine, through a metabolic pathway that requires adequate folate and vitamin B-12 (Mischoulon and Fava 2002). It is most concentrated in the brain and liver and is integral for the methylation of biological compounds with important implications for mood disorders. Meta-analyses and reports support efficacy for MDD (Mischoulon and Fava, 2002). SAMe may also be used in addition to antidepressant medication, as demonstrated by one study (Alpert et al. 2004). SAMe has been demonstrated to be generally well tolerated, and better tolerated than tricyclic antidepressants, with infrequently reported side effects including mild gastrointestinal symptoms, sweating, dizziness, and anxiety; mania has been reported in studies of treatment for bipolar depression (Alpert et al. 2004; Delle Chiaie et al. 2002; Mischoulon and Fava 2002).

PERINATAL DEPRESSION

In a placebo-controlled study of postpartum patients, investigators assessed depressive symptoms (not necessarily MDD) before and after treatment with SAMe. They observed significantly greater improvement in the SAMe group compared to the placebo group after 10 days. No treatment studies have been conducted specifically for prenatal depression. However, SAMe has been studied in cholestasis in pregnancy. It was five of eight of these studies that assessed tolerability and side effects, with no reports of side effects for mothers or newborns (AHRQ, 2002). Therefore, while SAMe has been used in pregnancy for liver disease, systematic study has not yet been conducted for depression during pregnancy, and more rigorous study is needed during pregnancy to evaluate safety outcomes.

There have been no reports of adverse events in breast-fed infants whose mothers used SAMe, although this topic has not received specific study either.

Folic Acid (Folate)

Folate has been studied in terms of its role in MDD. Its role in methylation of homocysteine to SAMe may suggest a mechanism of action for a role in MDD (Botez et al. 1979). Folate levels may predict response to antidepressants, and it may serve as an adjunct to other treatments for MDD. Patients with low folate may be less likely to have a therapeutic response to antidepressant medication (Fava et al. 1997). Low blood folate is associated with poorer and slower response to fluoxetine (Alpert et al. 2003; Papakostas et al. 2004, 2005). Randomized, placebo-controlled trials of folate suggest a role as an augmentation strategy in MDD, even in the presence of normal serum folate (Taylor et al. 2003).

Folate may be especially helpful for women compared to men with MDD (Coppen and Bailey 2000). Women taking fluoxetine were observed to experience a significantly larger decrease in depression scores with the addition of folate compared to placebo, a benefit that is not found for men.

Folate has a low likelihood of adverse effects and important benefits for women. In fact, women who are pregnant or are of reproductive age are advised to take 0.4 to 1 mg of folate daily to decrease the risk of birth defects (McDonald et al. 2003). Although folate does not look to be adequate as a monotherapy for MDD, modest evidence and a good risk/benefit profile supports its use as a part of the treatment of MDD and perinatal depression.

St. John's Wort (*Hypericum perforatum*)

St. John's Wort (usually studied as a standardized extract) is extremely popular in Europe for the treatment of mild to moderate depression, though it has had mixed reviews in the United States (Cott 1995). A recent Cochrane review of 29 studies concluded that St. John's Wort extracts tested in the included trials are superior to placebo in patients with major depression; they are similarly effective as standard antidepressants; and have fewer side effects than standard antidepressants (Linde 2008). Drug interactions are important to consider, as St. John's Wort may affect the metabolism of other drugs via the cytochrome P450 system (notably CYP3A4) and interact with medications such as SSRIs, oral contraceptive pills, and hormones (Roby et al. 2000). Unplanned pregnancy with concomitant use of St. John's Wort, and oral contraception has been reported (Schwarz et al. 2003).

A small amount of data informs the safety profile of St. John's Wort in perinatal depression. In case reports of breast-feeding mothers and their infants (Klier et al. 2002, 2006), the measurement of two active constituents of St. John's Wort (hyperforin and hypericin) have appeared in low levels in breast milk, suggesting low exposure to the breast-fed infant but without observed adverse effects. Safety in pregnancy is not established, and one study suggests caution. In a study following antenatal maternal treatment with St. John's Wort, 5 of 33 newborns exposed to St. John's Wort experienced colic, drowsiness, and lethargy, which is a rate that is more frequent than babies of matched depressed and non-depressed controls (Lee et al. 2003). It is possible that a neonatal syndrome described with antidepressants may also occur after exposure to St. John's Wort during pregnancy, albeit this has not received specific study. An animal study suggests the potential for teratogenic and toxic effects, and human safety during pregnancy and breast-feeding has not received adequate study (Dugoua et al. 2006; Gregoretti et al. 2004).

Acupuncture

Acupuncture is thought to correct energy imbalances from which disease states arise in Traditional Chinese Medicine. Conflicting results have been demonstrated in trials of acupuncture for MDD (Allen et al. 1998; Gallager et al. 2001, Quah-Smith et al. 2005).

PERINATAL DEPRESSION

Consideration of technique is necessary in pregnancy, as stimulation of certain acupuncture points may cause uterine contractions, speeding of labor, and cervical ripening (Rabl et al. 2001). In one preliminary trial in pregnant women, investigators randomized 61 women with MDD to active acupuncture, sham acupuncture, or massage for 8 weeks (Manber et al. 2004). Response rates were higher for active acupuncture (69%) versus the sham acupuncture (47%) or massage (32%).

Light Therapy

Although some studies of light therapy have methodological limitations, more rigorous studies demonstrate a significant benefit in seasonal and non-seasonal

MDD (Golden et al. 2005). There is some evidence that it may speed up antidepressant medication response (Benedetti et al. 2003).

PERINATAL DEPRESSION

In one study, pregnant women with MDD received one hour of bright light
therapy each morning (Oren et al. 2002). Sixteen women completed at least
3 weeks of treatment, and depression scores improved by a mean of 49%. The
scores of seven women who had completed at least two more weeks of treatment decreased by 59%. In another study of prenatal depression ($N = 10$),
women were randomized to either bright light therapy or a dim light placebo,
delivered in a double-blinded fashion (Epperson et al. 2004). One patient experienced hypomania. Bright light resulted in a significant greater antidepressant response than placebo. In a small controlled study of women with PPD,
15 women were randomly assigned to either bright light or a dim light placebo
(Corral et al. 2007). After 6 weeks, there were no significant differences between
groups, with improvement from baseline noted for both (Table 15.1).

Summary

For more mild depression, non-medication treatments may be adequate.
Whether or not medications are utilized, psychotherapy and many other
approaches can be utilized safely in pregnancy and breast-feeding women.
Many of the integrative strategies that would be recommended for perinatal
depression are those that would be seen as important components of disease
prevention, such as exercise and omega-3 fatty acid intake.

For many women, moderate to severe depressive episodes require treatment
with antidepressants. As MDD is a serious disorder, the risks of not treating
it should not be overlooked. Unfortunately, many women care for others better than they care for themselves. Depression adds to this problem. Untreated
depression in a mother negatively impacts the entire family.

There is a general paucity of treatment data in this area, and there are potential
risks of standard pharmacologic treatments in pregnancy and breast-feeding.
We urgently need to study potentially safe, effective, and accessible treatment
options for perinatal depression.

In my experience...sometimes if a mother understands that taking care of
her own health will be good for her children, she will prioritize her own needs
better. Until her depression improves, health care providers can help women
understand that the time and efforts they put into their own well-being benefits those she loves. It is far from selfish, actually the opposite, to take time to

Table 15.1. Commonly used CAM Therapies and Considerations in Perinatal Depression

CAM Treatment	MDD	Postpartum Depression	Antenatal Depression	Other
Exercise	Recommended for general health unless known contraindication	Recommended for general health benefits; reasonable part of a treatment plan for PPD	Safe and recommended for pregnant women unless contraindication exists	difficult to study in terms of adequate placebo control
Omega-3 Fatty Acids	Placebo-controlled studies support adjunctive use in MDD; treatment studies show conflicting evidence for perinatal depression as monotherapy	Maternal demand increased during pregnancy and breastfeeding; needed for optimal neurocognitive development; treatment studies show conflicting evidence for perinatal depression as monotherapy	Greater maternal intake in pregnancy is associated with lower risk of PPD and better neurocognitive development in children; treatment studies show conflicting evidence for perinatal depression as monotherapy	General health benefits and data regarding benefits in mood disorders support omega-3 fatty acids as part of treatment plan
SAMe	Strong support of efficacy in the treatment of MDD	No specific study in PPD and breastfeeding	Insufficient study in pregnancy; studies have assessed SAMe as a treatment for liver disease in pregnancy without reports of adverse effects	A naturally occurring compound in human metabolism; no case reports of adverse events in pregnancy or breastfeeding

Folate	Folate may be especially helpful as an add-on treatment for women with MDD	No known risks; may augment response to antidepressants	Known benefits of prophylaxis of birth defects	Supplementation in usual doses a reasonable addition to treatment for MDD
St. John's Wort	Some placebo-controlled trials support efficacy for mild to moderate depression; less convincing evidence for severe MDD	Inadequately studied in breast-feeding, low exposure via breast milk reported	Inadequate study in pregnancy; safety not established, animal study suggested risk; babies may experience adverse effects after exposure	May decrease efficacy of oral contraceptives and increase risk of unplanned pregnancy
Acupuncture	Mixed findings of efficacy in studies of MDD	Inadequate study for PPD	Some points may stimulate uterine contraction	Difficult to study in terms of adequate placebo control
Bright light therapy	Appears effective for MDD	No specific study in postpartum depression	No evidence of risk in pregnancy	

recover from depression and make sure one's own needs are met. As she feels better, she will gain appreciation for the great gift she is giving herself.

REFERENCES

Allen JJB, Schnyer RN, Hitt SK. The efficacy of acupuncture in the treatment of major depressive disorder in women. *Psychol Sci.* 1998;9:397–401.

Alpert JE, Papakostas G, Mischoulon D, et al. S-adenosyl-L-methionine (SAMe) as an adjunct for resistant major depressive disorder: an open trial following partial or nonresponse to selective serotonin reuptake inhibitors or venlafaxine. *J Clin Psychopharmacol.* 2004;24(6):661–664.

Altshuler LL, Hendrich V, Cohen LS. Course of mood and anxiety disorders during pregnancy and the postpartum period. *J Clin Psychiatry.* 1998;59:29–33.

American Psychiatric Association. *Diagnostic and Statistical Manual of Mental Disorders.* 4th ed. Washington, DC: American Psychiatric Association; 1994.

Artal R, O'Toole M. Guidelines of the American College of Obstetricians and Gynecologists for exercise during pregnancy and the postpartum period. *Br J Sports Med.* 2003;37(1):6–12.

Benedetti F, Colombo C, Pontiggia A, Bernasconi A, Florita M, Smeraldi E. Morning light treatment hastens the antidepressant effect of citalopram: a placebo-controlled trial. *J Clin Psychiatry.* 2003;64(6):648–653.

Benisek D, Shabert J, Skornik R. Dietary intake of polyunsaturated fatty acids by pregnant or lactating women in the United States. *Obstet Gynecol.* 2000;95:77–78.

Bloch M, Rotenberg N, Koren D, Klein E. Risk factors for early postpartum depressive symptoms. *Gen Hosp Psychiatry.* 2006;28(1):3–8.

Botez, MI, Young SN, Bachevalier J, Gauthier S. Folate deficiency decreased brain 5-hydroxytryptamine synthesis in man and rat. *Nature.* 1979;278:182–183.

Bressa GM. S-adenosyl-l-methionine (SAMe) as antidepressant: meta-analysis of clinical studies. *Acta Neurol Scand.* 1994;(Suppl. 154):7–14.

Burt VK, Suri R, Altshuler L, Stowe Z, Hendrick VC, Muntean E. The use of psychotropic medications during breast-feeding. *Am J Psychiatry.* 2001;158(7):1001–1009.

Chambers CD, Hernandez-Diaz S, Van Marter LJ, et al. Selective serotonin-reuptake inhibitors and risk of persistent pulmonary hypertension of the newborn. *N Engl J Med.* 2006;354(6):579–587.

Chaudron LH, Klein MH, Remington P, Palta M, Allen C, Essex MJ. Predictors, prodromes and incidence of postpartum depression. *J Psychosom Obstet Gynaecol.* 2001;22(2):103–112.

Cicchetti D, Rogosch FA, Toth SL. Maternal depressive disorder and contextual risk: contributions to the development of attachment insecurity and behavioral problems in tottlerhood. *Dev Psychopathol.* 1988;10:283–300.

Cohen LS, Altshuler LL, Harlow BL, et al. Relapse of major depression during pregnancy in women who maintain or discontinue antidepressant treatment. *JAMA.* 2006;295(5):499–507.

Coppen A, Bailey J. Enhancement of the antidepressant action of fluoxetine by folic acid: a randomized, placebo-controlled trial. *J Affect Disord.* 2000;60(2):121–130.

Corral M, Wardrop AA, Zhang H, Grewal AK, Patton S. Morning light therapy for postpartum depression. *Arch Womens Ment Health.* 2007;10(5):221–224.

Cott J. Natural product formulations available in Europe for psychotropic indications. *Psychopharmacol Bull.* 1995;31(4):745–751.

Da Cost D, Rippen N, Dritsa M, Ring A. Self-reported leisure-time physical activity during pregnancy and relationship to well-being. *J Psychosom Obstet Gynaecol.* 2003;24(2):111–119.

Dalton K. Progesterone prophylaxis used successfully in postnatal depression. *Practitioner.* 1985;229:507–508.

Davidson et al. Hypericum Depression Trial Study Group. Effect of *Hypericum perforatum* (St. John's Wort) in major depressive disorder. *JAMA.* 2002;287:1807–1814.

Delle Chiaie R, Pancheri P, Scapicchio P. Efficacy and tolerability of oral and intramuscular *S*-adenosyl-*L*-methionine 1,4-butanedisulfonate (SAMe) in the treatment of major depression: comparison with imipramine in 2 multicenter studies. *Am J Clin Nutr.* 2002;76(suppl):1172S–1176S.

Dennis CL, Hodnett E. Psychosocial and psychological interventions for treating postpartum depression. *Cochrane Database Syst Rev.* 2007;(4):CD006116.

Dugoua JJ, Mills E, Perri D, Koren G. Safety and efficacy of St. John's Wort (hypericum) during pregnancy and lactation. *Can J Clin Pharmacol.* 2006;13(3):e268–e276.

Dunn AL, Trivedi MH, Kampert JB, Clark CG and Chambliss, HO. Exercise treatment for depression: efficacy and dose response. *Am J Prev Med.* 2005;28:1–8.

Dunstan JA, Simmer K, Dixon G, Prescott SL. Cognitive assessment at 21/2 years following fish oil supplementation in pregnancy: a randomized controlled trial. *Arch Dis Child Fetal Neonatal Ed.* 2008;93(1):F45–F50.

Epperson CN, Terman M, Terman JS, et al. Randomized clinical trial of bright light therapy for antepartum depression: preliminary findings. *J Clin Psychiatry.* 2004;65(3):421–425.

Fava et al., Folate, vitamin B12, and homocysteine in major depressive disorder. *Am J Psychiatry.* 1997;154(3):426–428.

Foran SE, Flood JG, Lewandrowski KB. Measurement of mercury levels in concentrated over-the-counter fish oil preparations: is fish oil healthier than fish? *Arch Pathol Lab Med.* 2003;127(12):1603–1605.

Freeman MP. Omega-3 fatty acids and perinatal depression: a review of the literature and recommendations for future research. *Prostaglandins Leukot Essent Fatty Acids.* 2006;75:291–297.

Freeman MP. Antenatal depression: navigating the treatment dilemmas. *Am J Psychiatry.* 2007;164(8):1162–1165.

Freeman MP, Davis MF, Sinha P, Wisner KL, Hibbeln JR, Gelenberg AJ. Omega-3 fatty acids and supportive psychotherapy for perinatal depression: a randomized placebo-controlled study. *J Affect Disord.* 2008;110(1–2):142–148.

Freeman MP, Hibbeln JR, Wisner KL, Brumbach BH, Watchman W, Gelenberg AJ. Randomized dose-ranging pilot trial of omega-3 fatty acids for postnatal depression. *Acta Psychiatr Scand.* 2006;113(1):31–35.

Freeman MP, Hibbeln JR, Wisner KL, Watchman M, Gelenberg AJ. An open trial of omega-3 fatty acids for depression in pregnancy. *Acta Neuropsychiat.* 2006;18:21–24.

Freeman MP, Sinha P. Tolerability of omega-3 fatty acid supplements in perinatal women. *Prostaglandins Leukot Essent Fatty Acids.* 2007;77(3–4):203–208.

Freeman MP, Wright R, Watchman M, et al. Postpartum depression assessments at well-baby visits: screening feasibility, prevalence, and risk factors. *J Women Health.* 2005;14(10):929–935.

Gallagher SM, Allen JJ, Schnyer RN, Manber R. Six-month depression relapse rates among women treated with acupuncture. *Complement Ther Med.* 2001;9(4):216–218.

Gavin NL, Gaynes BN, Lohr KN, et al. Perinatal depression: a systematic review of prevalence and incidence. *Obstet Gynecol.* 2005;106(5):1071–1083.

Golden RN, Gaynes BN, Ekstrom RD, et al. The efficacy of light therapy in the treatment of mood disorders: a review and meta-analysis of the evidence. *Am J Psychiatry.* 2005;162(4):656–662.

Gregoretti B, Stebel M, Candussio L, Crivellato E, Bartoli F, Decorti G. Toxicity of *Hypericum perforatum* (St. John's wort) administered during pregnancy and lactation in rats. *Toxicol Appl Pharmacol.* 2004;200(3):201–205.

Halbreich U. Prevalence of mood symptoms and depressions during pregnancy: implications for clinical practice and research. *CNS Spectr.* 2004;9(3):177–184.

Heh SS, Huang LH, Ho SM, Fu YY, Wang LL. Effectiveness of an exercise support program in reducing the severity of postnatal depression in Taiwanese women. *Birth.* 2008;35(1):60–65.

Hibbeln JR. Seafood consumption, the DHA content of mothers' milk and prevalence rates of postpartum depression: a cross-national, ecological analysis. *J Affect Disord.* 2002;69(1–3):15–29.

Hibbeln JR, Davis JM, Steer C, Emmett P, Rogers I, Williams C, Golding J. Maternal seafood consumption in pregnancy and neurodevelopmental outcomes in childhood (ALSPAC study): an observational cohort study. *Lancet.* 2007;369:578–585.

Klier CM, Schaffer MR, Schmid-Siegel B, Lenz G, Mannel M. St. John's wort (*Hypericum perforatum*): is it safe during breastfeeding? *Pharmacopsychiatry.* 2002;35(1):29–30.

Klier CM, Schmid-Siegel B, Schafer MR, Lenz G, Saria A, Lee A, Zernig G. St. John's wort (*Hypericum perforatum*) and breastfeeding: plasma and breast milk concentrations of hyperforin for 5 mothers and 2 infants. *J Clin Psychiatry.* 2006;67(2):305–309.

Lee A, Minhas R, Matsuda N, Lam M, Ito S. The safety of St. John's wort (*Hypericum perforatum*) during breastfeeding. *J Clin Psychiatry.* 2003;64(8):966–968.

Levant B, Radel JD, Carlson SE. Reduced brain DHA content after a single reproductive cycle in female rats fed a diet deficient in N-3 polyunsaturated fatty acids. *Biol Psychiatry.* 2006;60(9):987–990.

Linde K, Berner MM, Kriston L. St John's wort for major depression. *Cochrane Database Syst Rev.* 2008;(4):CD000448.

Luo H, Meng F, Jia Y, Zhao X. Clinical research on the therapeutic effect of the electro-acupuncture treatment in patients with depression. *Psychiatry Clin Neurosci.* 1998;52(S):S338–S340.

Mackenzie ER, Taylor L, Bloom BS, Hufford DJ, Johnson JC. Ethnic minority use of complementary and alternative medicine (CAM): a national probability survey of CAM utilizers. *Altern Ther Health Med.* 2003;9(4):50–56.

McDonald SD, Ferguson S, Tam L, Lougheed J, Walker MC. The prevention of congenital anomalies with periconceptional folic acid supplementation. *J Obstet Gynaecol Can.* 2003;25(2):115–121.

McGregor JA, Allen KG, Harris MA, et al. The omega-3 story: nutritional prevention of preterm birth and other adverse pregnancy outcomes. *Obstet Gynecol Surv.* 2001;56(5 Suppl 1):S1–S13.

Manber R, Schnyer RN, Allen JJ, Rush AJ, Blasey CM. Acupuncture: a promising treatment for depression during pregnancy. *J Affect Disord.* 2004;83(1):89–95.

Mischoulon D, Fava M. Role of S-adenosyl-L-methionine in the treatment of depression: a review of the evidence. *Am J Clin Nutr.* 2002;76 (supp):1158S–61S.

Miyake Y, Sasaki S, Tanaka K, et al.; Osaka Maternal and Child Health Study Group. Dietary folate and vitamins B12, B6, and B2 intake and the risk of postpartum depression in Japan: the Osaka Maternal and Child Health Study. *J Affect Disord.* 2006;96(1–2):133–138.

Moses-Kolko EL, Roth EK. Antepartum and postpartum depression: healthy mom, healthy baby. *J Am Med Womens Assoc.* 2004;59(3):181–191.

Murray L, Fiori-Cowley A, Hooper R, Cooper P. The impact of postnatal depression and associated adversity on early mother-infant interactions and later infant outcome. *Child Dev.* 1996;67:2512–2252.

Newport DJ, Wilcox MM, Stowe ZN. Maternal depression: a child's first adverse life event. *Semin Clin Neuropsychiatry.* 2002;7(2):113–119.

Oken E, Kleinman KP, Berland WE, Simon SR, Rich-Edwards JW, Gillman MW. Decline in fish consumption among pregnant women after a national mercury advisory. *Obstet Gynecol.* 2003;102(2):346–351.

Oren DA, Wisner KL, Spinelli M, et al. An open trial of morning light therapy for treatment of antepartum depression. *Am J Psychiatry.* 2002;159(4):666–669.

Otto MW, Church TS, Craft LL, Greer TL, Smits JA, Trivedi MH. Exercise for mood and anxiety disorders. *J Clin Psychiatry.* 2007;68(5):669–676.

Papakostas GI, Petersen T, Lebowitz BD, et al. The relationship between serum folate, vitamin B12, and homocysteine levels in major depressive disorder and the timing of improvement with fluoxetine. *Int J Neuropsychopharmacol.* 2005;8(4):523–528.

Parker G, Gibson NA, Brotchie H, Heruc G, Rees AM, Hadzi-Pavlovic D. Omega-3 fatty acids and mood disorders. *Am J Psychiatry.* 2006;163(6):969–978.

Pariser S. Women and mood disorders: menarche to menopause. *Ann Clin Psychiatry.* 1993;5:249–254.

Payne JL. Antidepressant use in the postpartum period: practical considerations. *Am J Psychiatry.* 2007;164(9):1329–1332.

Peindl KS, Zolnik EJ, Wisner KL, Hanusa BH. Effects of postpartum psychiatric illnesses on family planning. *Int J Psychiatry Med.* 1995;25(3):291–300.

Quah-Smith JI, Tang WM, Russell J. Laser acupuncture for mild to moderate depression in a primary care setting—a randomised controlled trial. *Acupunct Med.* 2005;23(3):103–111.

Rabl M, Ahner R, Bitschnau M, Zeisler H, Husslein P. Acupuncture for cervical ripening and induction of labor at term—a randomized controlled trial. *Wien Klin Wochenschr.* 2001;113(23–24):942–946.

Rees AM, Austin MP, Parker GB. Omega-3 fatty acids as a treatment for perinatal depression: randomized double-blind placebo-controlled trial. *Aust N Z J Psychiatry.* 2008;42(3):199–205.

Robertson E, Grace S, Wallington T, Stewart DE. Antenatal risk factors for postpartum depression: a synthesis of recent literature. *Gen Hosp Psychiatry.* 2004;26(4):289–295.

Roby CA, Anderson GD, Kantor E, Dryer DA, Burstein AH. St John's Wort: effect on CYP3A4 activity. *Clin Pharmacol Ther.* 2000;67:451–457.

S-Adenosyl-L-Methionine (SAMe) for Depression, Osteoarthritis, and Liver Disease, Structured Abstract. August 2002. Agency for Healthcare Research and Quality, Rockville, MD. http://www.ahrq.gov/clinic/tp/sametp.htm

Schwarz UI, Buschel B, Kirch W. Unwanted pregnancy on self-medication with St John's Wort despite hormonal contraception. *Br J Clin Pharmacol.* 2003;55(1):112–113.

Sharp D, Hay DF, Pawlby S, Schmucker G, Allen H, Kumar R. The impact of postnatal depression on boys' intellectual development. *J Child Psychol Psychiatry.* 1995;36:1315–1133.

Shelton RC, Keller MB, Gelenberg A, et al. Effectiveness of St John's Wort in major depression: a randomized controlled trial. *JAMA.* 2001;285(15):1978–1986.

Sichel DA, Cohen LS, Robertson LM, Ruttenberg A, Rosenbaum JF. Prophylactic estrogen in recurrent postpartum affective disorder. *Biol Psychiatry.* 1995;38(12):814–818.

Simopoulos AP. Omega-3 fatty acids in health and disease and in growth and development. *Am J Clin Nutr* 1991;54:438–463.

Stowe ZN, Hostetter AL, Newport DJ. The onset of postpartum depression: implications for clinical screening in obstetrical and primary care. *Am J Obstet Gynecol.* 2005;192(2):522–526.

Strawbridge WJ, Deleger S, Roberts RE and Kaplan GA. Physical activity reduces the risk of subsequent depression for older adults. *Am J Epidemiol.* 2002;156:328–334.

Su KP, Huang SY, Chiu TH, et al. Omega-3 fatty acids for major depressive disorder during pregnancy: results from a randomized, double-blind, plaeobo-controlled trail. *J Clin Psychiatry* 2008;69:644–651.

Taylor MJ, Carney S, Geddes J, Goodwin G. Folate for depressive disorders. *Cochrane Database Syst Rev.* 2003;(2):CD003390.

Tindle HA, Davis RB, Phillips RS, Eisenberg DM. Trends in use of complementary and alternative medicine by US adults: 1997–2002. *Altern Ther Health Med.* 2005;11(1):42–49.

Trivedi MH, Greer TL, Grannemann BD, Chambliss HO, Jordan AN. Exercise as an augmentation strategy for treatment of major depression. *J Psychiatr Pract.* 2006;12(4):205–213.

Wisner KL, Perel JM, Peindl KS, Hanusa BH, Piontek CM, Findling RL. Prevention of postpartum depression: a pilot randomized clinical trial. *Am J Psychiatry.* 2004;161(7):1290–1292.

Wisner KL, Perel JM, Peindl KS, Hansusa BH, Findling RL, Rapport D. Prevention of recurrent postpartum depression: a randomized clinical trial. *J Clin Psychiatry.* 2001;62(2):82–86.

Wisner KL, Zarin DA, Holmboe ES, et al. Risk-benefit decision making for treatment of depression during pregnancy. *Am J Psychiatry.* 2000;157:1933–1940.

Zlotnick C, Johnson SL, Miller IW, Pearlstein T, Howard M. Postpartum depression in women receiving public assistance: pilot study of an interpersonal-therapy-oriented group intervention. *Am J Psychiatry.* 2001;158(4):638.

16

The Role of Stress in Infertility

BEATE DITZEN, TAMMY L. LOUCKS, AND SARAH L. BERGA

CASE STUDY

Mary is a 25-year-old woman who presents for help with irregular menstrual periods. She reports that she had her first period at age 11 years and regular cycles until she was about 20 years old, and her periods became irregular when she was in college. She was given oral contraceptives to regulate cycle patterns and used them for 4 years. Twelve months ago, she discontinued birth control pills but has had only two episodes of light bleeding since, with the last episode about 4 months ago.

Mary exercises regularly; she runs 2–3 miles a week, takes an occasional cycling class, and recently joined a rowing group on weekends. She is in her second year of law school, is doing extremely well in school, and is at the top of her class. Mary's other pertinent history includes frequent headaches relieved by exercise and rest. (An MRI performed by her primary care physician was normal.) Her weight is stable and she reports no binging or purging. She has many friends and family in the region, and interacts with them regularly. She was in a long-term relationship that ended amicably about a year ago. She reports condom use for birth control. Mary is concerned about the impact of her irregular cycles on her overall health.

On physical examination, she appears healthy. Her height (5'5" inches) and weight (125 lb) (BMI 20.8) are normal. She is Tanner stage 5 with normal gynecoid habitus, distribution of body hair, and presents with no abdominal striae or areas of hyper- or hypopigmentation.

You suspect that she has stress-induced anovulation. The differential diagnosis includes pituitary and other CNS tumors, polycystic ovary syndrome (PCOS), thyroid disorders, eating disorders, psychiatric disorders, substance abuse, and sexual or other abuse. Your initial evaluation includes a pregnancy test and laboratory studies including, LH, FSH, estradiol, progesterone, prolactin, TSH, and thyroxine (T4). An office pregnancy test was negative. Other results appear below.

LH = 3.5 mIU/mL
FSH = 4.2 mIU/mL
Estradiol = 28 pg/mL
Progesterone = 0.5 ng/mL
Prolactin = 8.5 ng/mL
TSH = 2.8 µIU/mL
Thyroxine (T4) = 5.2 µg/dL

The most likely diagnosis is stress-induced anovulation (SIA). A pituitary adenoma is unlikely because the prolactin level is in the low normal range and the MRI findings are normal. Mary's weight and eating habits do not suggest an eating disorder. Further, her history is not suggestive of depression, drug abuse, or social or sexual abuse. Her level of exercise would not likely be sufficient to be the primary cause of functional hypothalamic amenorrhea/stress-induced anovulation (FHA/SIA).

Consistent with SIA is a normal TSH level combined with a low T4 level. This is probably an indicator of stress or hypothalamic hypothyroidism (sick euthyroid syndrome) rather than primary thyroid dysfunction. Resuming oral contraceptives would address the menstrual irregularity but will not interrupt the stress process, reduce elevated cortisol levels, or restore the hypothalamic-pituitary-thyroidal (HPT) axis. Treatment options also include cognitive behavior therapy (CBT) aimed at reducing stress. You recommend this and she agrees. She returns 6 months later and reports that she sought assistance from student mental health services and began seeing a counselor. She also met with a nutritionist and began meditating. She has had menstrual periods the last 2 months and her cycle interval was about 30 days. It has been about 3 weeks since her last period and serum progesterone obtained at the visit is 16 ng/mL, indicating ovulation.

Introduction

Fertility can be viewed from many perspectives. Both unwanted fertility and infertility pose problems for individuals and society. This chapter reviews our understanding of the causes and treatments of infertility and focuses on psychogenic causes of infertility. While we acknowledge many stakeholders, we will primarily consider the perspective of the individual and the couple who are seeking the least technology necessary to achieve their fertility goals.

Reproductive compromise often represents a response to individual and environmental circumstances and may be adaptive. Reduced fertility during nutritional duress and famine is adaptive for both individuals and society. In less extreme circumstances, however, chronic reproductive compromise typically represents lack of adaptation to the commonplace dilemmas inherent to daily living. Chronic reproductive compromise carries acute and chronic negative health consequences for women, offspring, partners, and even extended families.

Both men and women can develop stress-induced reproductive compromise and infertility. The common pathogenetic theme is relatively straightforward. Behaviors that persistently activate the hypothalamic-pituitary-adrenal (HPA) axis and chronically suppress the HP-thyroidal (HPT) activity disrupt hypothalamic-pituitary-gonadal (HPG) functioning. However, the behavioral antecedents that activate the HPA and suppress the HPT axes differ from person to person and there appear to be gender-specific sensitivities to metabolic (nutritional, energetic) and psychogenic stressors. We know from human and animal studies that reproductive capacity exists on a continuum with some individuals having higher rates of fertility and others experiencing subfertility and infertility (Kaplan and Manuck 2004). In women, hypothalamic hypogonadism can be overt and present as amenorrhea or irregular menses or it may be occult, with preserved menstrual interval and reduced or absent estradiol and progesterone secretion from the ovaries that render implantation unlikely. In men, reduced hypothalamic drive is often occult, but it may present as oligoathenospermia during an infertility evaluation and, in severe cases, as diminished libido, muscle mass, and hair growth. This chapter focuses on stress-induced reproductive compromise in women. We will explicate the mechanisms linking stress and reproductive function and review the use of nonpharmacological approaches, particularly cognitive behavior therapy (CBT), to ameliorate stress and restore fertility.

Etiology of Infertility in Women

Infertility has been defined as the inability to conceive following one year of intercourse without the use of contraception (National Institute of Child Health and Human Development, NICHD). Infertility can be classified as primary (never having conceived) or secondary (failure to conceive following a prior pregnancy). The term infertility may also be employed to refer to the failure to support a pregnancy following conception (recurrent miscarriage or spontaneous abortion). In addition, there is the notion of subfertility in which couples may have some factors that make it more difficult to conceive and thus present with a delay in conception. In 2002, more than 7% (about 2.1 million) of married women in the United States were infertile. This rate has remained relatively unchanged since 1995 (Chandra et al. 2005). Infertility affects couples across all socioeconomic, ethnic, and racial groups.

The standard approach to infertility evaluation is to assess both partners to discern if the causes rest with the male or female partner or both. Data obtained from couples seeking assisted reproductive technology (ART) services (CDC 2007) suggest that about half of infertility can be attributed to female factors, about one-fifth to male factors, and in the remaining cases attributable to both partners or remain unexplained (Figure 16.1).

Causes of infertility in women may be divided into four main categories: anatomic, genetic, infectious or inflammatory, and ovulatory dysfunction. Anatomic factors such as developmental anomalies of the reproductive tract

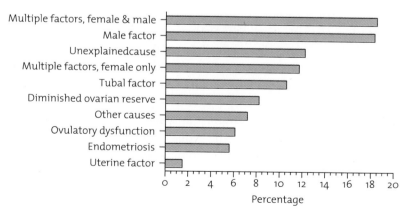

FIGURE 16.1. Causes of infertility among couples who use ART. Adapted from CDC, 2007, *2005 Assisted Reproductive Technology (ART) Report.*

may be diagnosed on physical examination and through imaging procedures. If an anatomic cause, such as tubal blockage, is found, surgical intervention may be helpful or necessary. Genetic causes may present as amenorrhea or menstrual irregularity due to premature oocyte depletion or absence (often termed premature menopause or ovarian failure). In some cases, the genetic abnormality is detectable using chromosomal analysis. Genetic causes may also lead to recurrent miscarriage or male infertility presenting as oligoasthenospermia or azoospermia. There are many infectious agents that can cause pelvic inflammatory disease. Chlamydia is a common infectious agent and the symptoms of the infection may be occult. Endometriosis appears to result from dysregulation of the immune system and may represent an autoimmune disorder in which fertilization, zygote transport, and implantation are impeded rather than prevented.

Disorders of ovulation account for the largest proportion of female infertility. There are many underlying causes. Functional forms of ovarian compromise that present as luteal insufficiency and anovulation are common and theoretically reversible with appropriate milieu and lifestyle alterations. However, to make the diagnosis of functional forms of anovulation, one must first exclude other organic causes such as ovarian failure (oocyte depletion), polycystic ovary syndrome, hyperprolactinemia, adrenal or thyroid disease, autoimmune diseases, and CNS tumors.

Functional Forms of Hypothalamic Hypogonadism

Functional hypothalamic hypogonadism appears to be the underlying cause in about 35% of women seeking evaluation for secondary amenorrhea (Reindollar et al. 1986). Because activation of the HPA appears to be a universal concomitant of functional hypothalamic hypogonadism and functional hypothalamic amenorrhea (FHA), these conditions may be termed SIA. We and others have found that SIA/FHA is characterized by a constellation of neuroendocrine secretory aberrations that includes reduced GnRH drive with low LH and FSH levels, increased circulating and cerebrospinal fluid levels of cortisol (Brundu et al. 2006) reflecting HPA activation, and reduced thyronine and thyroxine with preserved TSH levels that reflect HPT suppression (Berga and Girton 1989).

Acute stress elicits homeostatic responses designed to restore hormonal equilibrium. Chronic stress results in adaptive hormonal alterations that preserve the individual but compromises physiological functioning. Chronic adaptive responses are termed allostatic. Women with SIA or FHA show neuroendocrine allostasis with concomitant alterations in hypothalamic functioning. Specifically, the GnRH/LH/FSH response to reduced ovarian hormone secretion is blunted or absent; CRH secretion does not fall despite elevated cortisol levels and TSH levels do not rise despite a decline in thyroxine and thyroxine levels.

SIA/FHA results when the ovarian suppression is severe enough to result in complete cessation of menses and is both a retrospective diagnosis and diagnosis of exclusion. SIA refers to reduced ovarian activity, that is, reduced or absent folliculogenesis with corresponding reductions in estradiol and progesterone, due to reduced hypothalamic-pituitary (GnRH/LH) input to the gonad and varies in clinical presentation. For purposes of research, we study women with FHA, that is, women with the more severe but more clinically recognizable form. FHA and SIA can be primary (before menarche) or secondary (after menarche). In primary amenorrhea, it is critical to exclude organic conditions such as congenital malformations of the reproductive tract and Kallman's syndrome with anosmia due to failure of GnRH neurons to migrate from the olfactory placode to the hypothalamus. In industrialized countries, FHA/SIA is estimated to affect up to 4% of randomly selected women under the age of 40. This figure may increase to as much as 7% in women younger than 25 (Kaplan and Manuck 2004) and is more common in athletes and those with definable eating disorders and subclinical disordered eating patterns (Laughlin et al. 1998). Most interestingly, FHA is up to three times higher in women with a lifetime history of depression, regardless of age (Bisaga et al. 2002; Harlow et al. 2003).

We studied women with FHA/SIA who did not report excessive exercise, athletic competition, significant weight loss, medical conditions, or known psychiatric conditions including disordered eating. In this group of apparently well women with amenorrhea as the only recognized clinical problem, our studies suggested that metabolic (energetic/nutritional) and psychogenic stressors acted synergistically to induce reproductive compromise (Berga 2003; Berga and Girton 1989; Giles and Berga 1993; Marcus et al. 2001). To confirm the principle of synergism among relatively minor stressors, we developed a cynomolgus monkey model (Williams et al. 2007). In the monkey model, a mild metabolic challenge consisting of running on a treadmill with a 20% calorie reduction had minimal impact on reproductive function. Likewise, a mild psychosocial challenge that involved moving monkeys housed singly in cages to new rooms had little impact on ovarian function. However, combining these metabolic and psychosocial challenges resulted in 70% of the monkeys developing transient anovulation. We suggest that most clinically recognized forms of functional hypothalamic hypogonadism, namely athletic or exercise amenorrhea, disordered eating, and depression develop because of an interaction between psychogenic challenge and energetic imbalance. Although individuals may not readily report high levels of subjective stress, they may nonetheless have at least intermittent activation of the HPA axis, the major hormonal stress signal, and reduced energy intake or increased energy expenditure.

HPA–HPG interactions

An association between HPA activation and HPG suppression is well established and involves suppression of hypothalamic gonadotropin-releasing hormone (GnRH) drive to the pituitary with corresponding reductions in FSH and LH and subsequent gonadal inactivity (Chrousos et al. 1998; Laatikainen 1991). The mechanisms that allow increased HPA activity to reduce HPG output are only partially known. Hypothalamic release of corticotropin-releasing hormone (CRH) drives the HPA axis, but acute increases in exogenously administered cortisol do not seem to be the signal that suppresses GnRH (Samuels et al. 1994). The internal and external determinants of hypothalamic CRH drive are many and the feedback center for regulating CRH drive includes neural centers in the hippocampus and other parts of the limbic lobe. A host of neural factors could mediate the HPA–HPG interaction. In a recent study, Vulliemoz and colleagues (2008) showed that the CRH antagonist astressin B reversed the reproductive compromise initiated by negative energy balance on LH pulse frequency in rhesus monkeys. In rats, ACTH reduced the increase in serum LH following ovariecetomy (Mann et al. 1982), and cortisol directly affected gonadotropins (Ringstrom et al. 1992). Increased cortisol levels may also alter

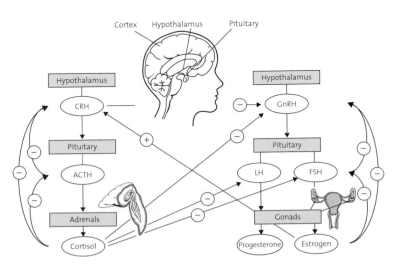

FIGURE 16.2. Interactions of the HPA and the HPG axes on different levels (c.f., Chrousos et al., 1998). (Missing the Thyroid-Maternal Thyroid essential in pregnancy.)

the HPT axis, that, in turn, may independently impair gonadal function (Berga 1989; Daniels et al. 1997; Nepomnaschy et al. 2004). Taken together, available data indicate obligatory interaction between the stress, metabolic, and reproductive axes (Chrousos et al. 1998) (Figure 16.2).

Besides diurnal modulation, HPA axis activity is triggered by a variety of different stressors such as restraint or isolation stress in animals, energy depletion, surgery, and psychosocial stress in humans (Dickerson and Kemeny 2004; Sapolsky et al. 2000). It seems logical to assume that stress-induced activation of the HPA axis might impair reproductive functioning. When stress is defined as the anticipation of an adverse or dangerous situation that exceeds individual coping capacities (Lazarus and Folkman 1984), it would be advantageous to delay reproduction until conditions are more favorable.

Central Mechanisms Mediating HPA and HPG Interactions

The central GnRH pulse generator primarily resides in the arcuate nucleus of the hypothalamus; GnRH release, in the form of GnRH pulses that elicit pituitary LH pulses, drives reproductive function (Berga and Loucks 2007). A decrease in GnRH drive, either in the form of reduced pulse frequency or reduced pulse amplitude, results in a corresponding reduction of pituitary secretion of the gonadotropins LH and FSH and thus reduces the signals for follicle development and ovulation. Understimulated follicles make correspondingly less estradiol and progesterone, which reduces endometrial stimulation. There is also ongoing estrogen deficiency in other tissues, which may heighten the risk for osteoporosis, cardiovascular disease, and psychiatric syndromes. Although a discussion of the long-term impact of stress upon somatic health is beyond the scope of this chapter, we caution against assuming that it is benign.

The GnRH pulse generator is modulated both directly and indirectly by neural and peripheral signals. The exact mechanisms by which the GnRH pulse generator integrates incoming information and then alters its pulsatility, both frequency and amplitude, remains unclear. GnRH neurons form a neural network with one another and signaling is modulated in part by the GnRH cohort size. Neurotransmitter systems and peripheral signals such as insulin and glucose convey information about stress and energy balance to the limbic lobe and hypothalamus (Berga and Yen 2004). Noradrenergic and dopaminergic neurons colocalize with GnRH neurons in the medial preoptic area of the hypothalamus (MPOA) and modulate GnRH activity. GnRH perikarya also are regulated by estradiol and noradrenergic inputs from the brainstem on. GnRH release is affected by opioidergic and GABAergic systems, which in turn are influenced by steroid hormones of the HPA axis (Dobson et al. 2003; Herbison 1998). Galanin-like peptide (GALP) neurons in the arcuate nucleus may transmit neural information from central nuclei to the GnRH pulse generator. GALP neurons are regulated by several hormones involved in the control of energy balance and metabolism, particularly leptin, insulin, and thyroid hormones. Because the role of the hypothalamic neurons is to integrate a vast amount of internal and external information about the individual's circumstance and then to elicit the appropriate neuroendocrine responses to preserve the individual acutely, the complexity and redundancy of signaling inputs is expected and required. Thus, any stressor or combination of stressors of sufficient duration or magnitude have the potential to influence GnRH drive and thereby impact fertility.

Interestingly, we found that women with FHA did not have increased levels in cerebrospinal fluid (CSF) levels of CRH or AVP as compared to eumenorrheic ovulatory women (Berga et al. 2000). However, circulating cortisol levels were 16% higher (Berga et al. 1989, 1997) and CSF cortisol levels were 30% higher in FHA as compared to eumenorrheic women (Brundu et al. 2006). These data suggest resistance to cortisol negative feedback that results in an alteration in the HPA setpoint. This alteration of feedback setpoint of the HPA axis appears to be modulated at least in part by glucocorticoid and mineralocorticoid receptors localized to hippocampal neurons (Brundu et al. 2006; Lupien et al. 1999).

Role of the HPT Axis

There is a constellation of neuroendocrine aberrations that has been described in women with FHA (Berga and Girton 1989; Loucks et al. 1989). The HPT axis responds to psychogenic and metabolic stressors by conserving energy. It does this by reducing TRH drive. This adjustment has been termed functional hypothalamic hypothyroidism or sick euthyroid syndrome. Thyroid-releasing hormone (TRH) secreted from the paraventricular nucleus (PVN) of the hypothalamus stimulate the anterior pituitary to release thyrotropin-stimulating hormone (TSH), which then stimulates thyroidal production of thyroxine (T4) and tri-iodothyronine (T3). Thyroid hormones are involved in the regulation of all major steps of metabolism. In addition to central effects, cortisol inhibits the TSH response to TRH and dampens TSH secretion by the pituitary. Thus, chronic stress might dampen thyroid functioning via elevated glucocorticoid levels, which, in concert with other endocrine factors, such as gonadal steroids, influence weight, appetite, cognitive and emotional functioning (concentration, affect, alertness, libido), bone density, cardiovascular tone, and skin characteristics. Women with FHA have suppressed HPT axis functioning consistent with functional hypothalamic hypothyroidism. Women with FHA display TSH levels in the normal range, but thyroid output is diminished compared to eumenorrheic, ovulatory women (Berga et al. 1989). Spratt and colleagues have characterized the time course of recovery from illness as a model for understanding the endocrine effects of recovery from combined metabolic and psychogenic stress. During convalescence, the HPA axis recovered first followed by recovery of the HPG axis. At 3 weeks, the HPT axis remained unrecovered (Spratt et al. 1993). Our studies of spontaneously recovered women with FHA showed a similar pattern (Berga et al. 1997). Women who spontaneously recovered from FHA displayed circulating cortisol levels identical to ovulatory women and had slightly lower LH pulse frequency. However, TSH levels in recovered FHA were significantly increased compared to eumenorrheic controls and levels of T4 and T3 were intermediate (Berga et al. 1997; Daniels et al. 1997). Taken together, these observations suggest a lag in the recovery of the metabolic axis and indicate ongoing susceptibility to subsequent stress during recovery. The lag in thyroidal axis recovery may explain why full recovery requires more time than would seem necessary. When the HPT is suppressed, the sensitivity of the gonadal and adrenal axes to subsequent stress is likely heightened.

Metabolic Stress and Infertility

Metabolic challenge, defined as energy imbalance due to insufficient calorie intake or excess energy expenditure, is associated with menstrual irregularities, amenorrhea, anovulation, and infertility. Anorectic women display high rates of amenorrhea (Golden and Carlson 2008). A reduction in energy availability sufficient to increase cortisol levels reduced LH pulse frequency and amplitude in eumenorrheic women and produced transient ovarian suppression in some participants (Loucks and Thuma 2003). On a neurophysiological level, nutritional and metabolic signals play a critical role in homeostatic systems. The human brain consumes approximately 25% of the body's available glucose (Leonard and Robertson 1994). Several neural and peripheral systems are involved in maintaining energy production and storage and in conveying information about glucose availability. Circulating glucose and insulin levels provide feedback to the brain regarding fuel availability. Ghrelin is a powerful signal to consume food. Adiponectin and leptin, hormones produced by adipocytes (fat cells), regulate fuel storage. Energy deficiency and unpredictable energy consummation (such as in bulimia nervosa) serves as a potent metabolic stressors and, when of sufficient magnitude, reduce GnRH drive, compromise reproductive function, and increase sensitivity to other stressors.

The current debate focuses on whether metabolic stress should be viewed as a separate entity or independent stressor (Berga 2008). Metabolic stressors elicit psychogenic states and psychogenic states have neuroendocrine concomitants, so technically, to separate metabolic and psychogenic stress is to create a false dichotomy. However, the terms metabolic and psychogenic provide a widely understood vocabulary that facilitates communication, so we continue to use these terms. In experimental human paradigms, LH drive is suppressed when the energetic imbalance is sufficient to drop circulating glucose levels and activate the HPA axis. In the study by Loucks and Thuma, this occurred when they applied a 80% energy restriction (Loucks and Thuma 2003), which is much more than is typically reported by women with FHA (Berga and Girton 1989).

Another signaling system implicated in this process is the thyroid axis, which is responsible for adjusting the basal metabolic rate. The HPT axis works dynamically to adjust energy expenditure and to conserve energy expenditure when there is an energy deficit. Irregular, excess, and insufficient energy intake presents an adaptive challenge. The greater the energy challenge, the more likely is reproductive compromise. Among athletes, the prevalence of amenorrhea is typically 25% or more (Warren and Fried 2001). Human and monkey studies also suggest that energy imbalance sensitizes the brain to subsequent stressors (Petrides et al. 1994), which is why in the clinical setting, women with reproductive compromise rarely report a single stressor (Berga 2006; Bonen 1994; Williams et al. 2007).

Psychosocial Stress and Infertility

In animals, there is convincing evidence that stress causes anovulation, interrupts implantation, and shortens gestation. The association between stress and anovulation is well established in humans (Berga and Girton 1989; Berga and Loucks 2006, 2007; Berga and Yen 2004), but there are fewer data establishing stress as a cause of recurrent miscarriage and preterm labor in humans (Nepomnaschy et al. 2006; Tilbrook et al. 2002). Preterm labor has many determinants and stress is only one, so this makes it difficult to isolate the independent effects of stressors upon pregnancy in humans. However, Hansen et al. (2000) found an increase in fetal anomalies, primarily of neural crest origin, when the mother experienced the highly profound stress of losing a child in early gestation. Several studies have documented elevated basal cortisol levels in women with ovarian dysfunction (e.g., in women with FHA, Berga et al. 1997) and blunted responses of the HPA axis to pharmacological provocation, suggesting involvement of the HPA axis in reproductive impairment (Berga et al. 2000; Kondoh et al. 2001; Meczekalski et al. 2000). Interestingly, women in the process of recovering from FHA showed cortisol levels identical to those of eumenorrheic women before there was complete recovery of GnRH/LH drive (Berga et al. 1997), which suggests that recovery from stress precedes reproductive recovery. To control for the stress of having reproductive compromise, Berga et al. (1997) compared psychometric indices and cortisol levels in women with organic forms of anovulation, women with FHA, and eumenorrheic ovulatory women. Only women with FHA as confirmed by reduced GnRH drive displayed elevated cortisol levels. Further, coping was reduced the most in women with FHA and only modestly reduced in women with organic forms of anovulation (Berga et al. 1997) when compared to ovulatory eumenorrheic women. It is difficult to prospectively apply quantifiable stressors to humans, but when this has been done (Bullen et al. 1985), it appears that acute application of combined psychogenic and metabolic stress elicits transient ovarian compromise. Experimental protocols in animals are guided by humane considerations, but it is easier to know the time course of the stressors and to apply them in a controlled manner. In our monkey study, psychosocial stress alone (moving caged monkeys to new rooms with new neighbors) or exercise and diet alone caused ovarian suppression in 10% of the monkeys whereas combining these stressors lead to abnormal menstrual cycles in 70% of the monkeys (Williams et al. 2007).

Findings from studies of ART practices are inconsistent. There is some evidence that subjective stress, anxiety, or depression impairs ART outcomes, either pregnancy rates or healthy births (Homan et al. 2007). However, other studies did not find stress to be a predictor of ART outcomes (Klonoff-Cohen et al. 2001).

Depression and Infertility

In women with a lifetime diagnosis of major depression, the risk of reproductive impairment is increased (Bisaga et al. 2002; Harlow et al. 2003). In our studies of women with FHA, we found only a minor increase in depressive symptoms compared to healthy controls (Marcus et al. 2001) and the women with FHA did not meet criteria for a diagnosis of depression. However, FHA and major depression are both accompanied by HPA axis alterations. Depression has been found to be accompanied by increased cortisol secretion, resistance to the negative feedback effects of cortisol and dexamethasone, decreased ACTH response to CRH administration, and habitually increased CRH levels (Gold and Chrousos 2002). Antidepressants were shown to decrease CRH hypersecretion in patients with major depression (De Bellis et al. 1993). Thus, one would expect antidepressant use in women with bonafide depression to restore reproductive function, but there are no studies that have definitely investigated this somatic aspect of depression. In addition, serotonin, which plays a key role in the pathogenesis of depression and autonomic stress reactivity, was shown to influence GnRH pulsatility (Gore and Terasawa 2001). Monkeys who were found to be stress-sensitive (i.e., they developed reproductive dysfunction when stressed) also secreted significantly less prolactin and more cortisol than stress-resistant animals following fenfluramine administration (Bethea et al. 2005). The link between central serotonergic function, reproductive compromise, and sensitivity to stress in the female monkey model has been comprehensively summarized (Bethea et al. 2008). Clearly, one mechanism by which stress leads to reproductive compromise is via alteration of central serotonergic function. Further studies are needed to determine if the use of antidepressant medications might help restore reproductive function and improve fertility in women or men with hypothalamic hypogonadism or unexplained infertility.

Personality Factors and Infertility

Personality characteristics have consistently been shown to mediate biological responses to stressors. However, there is no one personality trait that alone promotes infertility per se. High trait anxiety, high levels of neuroticism, an external locus of control possibly as a consequence of learned helplessness, and high perfectionism increase stress susceptibility in humans (e.g., Lovallo and Gerin 2003). In our study comparing women with FHA to women with organic causes of anovulation and ovulatory eumenorrheic women (Marcus et al. 2001), we observed that women with FHA reported a higher "need for approval" (measured by the Dysfunctional Attitude Scale, DAS) and less self-control compared with ovulatory eumenorrheic controls. Women with FHA displayed attitudes about food and body image that were more rigid in the domains concerning "drive for thinness," "ineffectiveness," and "interoceptive awareness" compared to the other groups. They were also more perfectionistic than women in the comparison groups. In a previous study, women with FHA reported greater difficulty in coping with daily stress and tended to endorse greater interpersonal dependence than eumenorrheic controls (Giles and Berga 1993). A prospective observational study found that high school girls who later became amenorrheic when studying abroad were more anxious, stubborn, and perfectionistic prior to departure from home (Shanan et al. 1965). These same girls had higher cortisol levels when abroad, indicating that the move served as a psychological challenge. Based on our studies of the psychological and neuroendocrine profiles of women with FHA and our monkey model showing synergism between metabolic and psychogenic challenge, we developed a targeted program of CBT to address maladaptive cognitions in FHA. We did not ask participants to eat more or differently or to exercise less. We did indicate that diet and exercise were not appropriate ways to cope with psychogenic stressors. We then randomized participants to either observation to be followed by CBT or immediate CBT for 16 sessions to be completed over 20 weeks. CBT restored ovulation and menstrual cyclicity in 80% of the women with FHA whereas only 13% of participants randomized to observation showed recovery of ovarian hormone secretion (Berga et al. 2003). Women treated with CBT showed improvement on subscales of the Dysfunctional Attitudes Survey associated with coping and reduced cortisol levels whereas women with FHA who were only observed showed no improvement. We concluded that CBT promoted stress reduction and ameliorated not only problematic attitudes but also restored neuroendocrine and reproductive functioning (Berga 2003). We consider this sentinel study as a proof of the principle that attitudes do evoke endocrine responses and we concluded that to the extent that attitudes are learned and subject to modification, so too can endocrine functioning be modified and improved. Thus, SIA in the form of FHA is reversible by nonpharmacological measures. We believe that infertility patients should be made aware of the link between stress and infertility when it appears that stress is playing a role. However, we advise clinicians to convey this information in a supportive manner and to be prepared to direct women to appropriate sources of psychological support.

Treatment Considerations

Treatment options for couples wishing to conceive should be based on diagnosis and a consideration of the risks and benefits of the available therapies. These therapies include ovulation induction with clomiphene citrate or exogenous gonadotropin administration for women with anovulation or unexplained infertility, intrauterine insemination for men with oligoasthenospermia or as an aid for timing sperm and egg interaction, in vitro fertilization, and in some cases, surgery to restore reproductive anatomy. Women with FHA or stress-induced reproductive compromise typically have adequate ovarian reserve and the ovaries will typically respond appropriately to ovulation induction with either exogenous GnRH pump or gonadotropins. Due to hypothalamic allostasis and feedback insensitivity to diminished estradiol, the response to clomiphene citrate and other antiestrogens may be impaired and these agents may not elicit ovulation even when there is appropriate ovarian reserve.

Ovulation induction does not correct persistent stress-induced allostatic alterations of the HPA and HPT axes. Further, controlled ovarian hyperstimulation increased metabolic demand with a compensatory rise in TSH and reduction in thyroxine in healthy women (Muller et al. 2000). Women with FHA and stress-induced infertility will be unable to generate a sufficient rise in TSH and thus the metabolic demand of infertility intervention may exacerbate maternal hypothyroxenemia and heighten fetal risk. Likely because of persistent increases in cortisol and reductions in thyroxine, women with FHA who conceive following ovulation induction have an increased risk for preterm labor and intrauterine growth restriction (Challis et al. 2000; McMillan 2004; Wadhwa et al. 2001). In addition, since the mother is the sole source of thyroxine for the fetus during the first and the predominant source during the second and third trimesters of pregnancy and because thyroxine is obligatory for appropriate neural development, the fetuses of women with FHA may be at increased risk for neurodevelopmental disorders, including learning disabilities and autism. Indeed, the offspring of women with subclinical hypothyroidism due to autoimmune thyroiditis have been found to have an increased risk of neurodevelopmental disorders (Haddow et al. 1999; Morreale de Escobar et al. 2000; Pop et al. 2003) and women with FHA have reductions in thyroxine comparable to those of women with subclinical hypothyroidism.

Maternal stress has also been associated with poorer fetal outcomes (Hansen et al. 2000; Lou et al. 1994); it may be that excess cortisol carries risks similar to those seen with hypothyroxinemia. Pharmacological interventions such as gonadotropins only target the reproductive aspects of FHA and stress-induced infertility. Thus, there is a therapeutic need to address the constellation of neuroendocrine aberrations characteristic of FHA. One could consider antidepressants, but they too carry fetal risks. Since psychological interventions, such as cognitive behavioral therapy (CBT) and hypnotherapy, are able to restore ovulation and menstrual cyclicity in women with FHA (Berga et al. 2003; Tschugguel and Berga 2003), nonpharmacological therapies should be considered. Both studies investigating the effect of psychotherapy on reproductive function focused on stress management, attitudes about thinness and eating and body image related cognitions, and both treatments were able to restore menstrual cyclicity in 80% (Berga et al. 2003) and 75% (Tschugguel and Berga 2003) of the participants. However, despite the return of ovarian function, women recently recovered from FHA had lower thyroxine levels (Daniels et al. 1997). Persistent hypothyroxinemia may represent ongoing metabolic stress insufficient to suppress GnRH drive or it may reflect the lag in recovery of the thyroid axis after HPA and HPO recovery.

For individuals without a diagnosis of stress-induced infertility, there is evidence that individual psychological interventions as well as group interventions can increase reproductive success during ART. However, the mechanisms underlying this effect remain unclear. For example, in a randomized controlled trial, Domar and colleagues (2000) compared ART outcomes in 184 women attempting to conceive for 1–2 years. Participants were randomized to CBT, nonspecific support, and observation. There were higher pregnancy rates in both intervention groups (55% and 54%) compared with the control group (20%). In a Turkish study (Terzioglu 2001), counseling provided by a nurse was associated with an increase in ART success rates compared to a standard care group. Both studies suggested a nonspecific benefit of counseling, which might be due to reducing the stress associated with undergoing ART. In a recent meta-analysis, Haemmerli and colleagues (2009) reported that psychological interventions improved fertility outcomes in couples, but this effect was not mediated through the hypothesized psychological mechanisms of improved mood or reduced anxiety. However, based on the FHA studies in monkeys (Williams et al. 2007) and humans (Berga et al. 2003), one could posit that this effect might be mediated through the synergistic effect of targeting multiple treatment foci, rather than one single factor.

Since stress is a common concomitant of infertility treatment, even when stress is not the primary cause of infertility, it would appear that couples would benefit from CBT with an emphasis on stress management.

Summary

Infertility has many causes. Since unexplained infertility and hypothalamic hypogonadism account for a significant proportion of women with infertility, the clinician is advised to consider stress as a concomitant that would benefit from therapeutic attention. To reiterate, stress is one of the most common and most commonly underappreciated causes of infertility. Stress-induced hypothalamic hypogonadism increases the long-term health burden of affected individuals and their offspring (deBoo and Harding 2006; Challis et al. 2000; McEwen 1998, 2002; Sapolsky 2000; 2005). For women and men with functional forms of hypothalamic hypogonadism or for couples with unexplained infertility, we recommend a program of stress reduction such as CBT. However, it is critical that all organic causes be excluded prior to rendering a diagnosis of stress-induced hypothalamic hypogonadism and that the offer of support be communicated in a nonjudgmental manner. If nonpharmacological approaches do not restore fertility and all other causes have been excluded or corrected, then higher technologies can be utilized along with nonpharmacological approaches. Since infertility care is both expensive and carries side effects including high cost, preterm labor, and multiple gestation, it is imperative to aim to achieve treatment goals using the least technology necessary.

REFERENCES

Berga SL. Stress and reproduction: a tale of false dichotomy? *Endocrinology.* 2008;149(3):867–868.

Berga SL, Girton LG. The psychoneuroendocrinology of functional hypothalamic amenorrhea. *Psychiatr Clin North Am.* 1989;12:105–116.

Berga SL, Mortola JF, Girton L, et al. Neuroendocrine aberrations in women with functional hypothalamic amenorrhea. *J Clin Endocrinol Metab.* 1989;68:301–308.

Berga SL, Daniels TL, Giles DE. Women with functional hypothalamic amenorrhea but not other forms of anovulation display amplified cortisol concentrations. *Fertil Steril.* 1997;67(6):1024–1030.

Berga SL, Loucks-Daniels TL, Adler LJ, et al. Cerebrospinal fluid levels of corticotropin-releasing hormone in women with functional hypothalamic amenorrhea. *Am J Obstet Gynecol.* 2000;182(4):776–781; discussion 781–774.

Berga SL, Marcus MD, Loucks TL, Hlastala S, Ringham R, Krohn MA. Recovery of ovarian activity in women with functional hypothalamic amenorrhea who were treated with cognitive behavior therapy. *Fertil Steril.* 2003;80(4):976–981.

Berga SL, Yen SSC. Reproductive failure due to central nervous system-hypothalamic-pituitary dysfunction. In: Strauss JF, Barbieri RL, eds. *Reproductive Endocrinology. Physiology, Pathopysiology, and Clinical Management.*5th edition, Chapter 18. Philadelphia: Elsevier Saunders; 2004:537–594.

Berga SL, Loucks TL. The use of cognitive behavior therapy for functional hypothalamic amenorrhea. In: The 6th Athens congress on women's health and disease. *Ann NY Acad Sci.* 2006;1092:114–129.

Berga SL, Loucks TL. Stress induced anovulation. In: Fink G, ed. *Encyclopedia of Stress.* Vol. 3 Oxford, GB: Oxford Academic Press; 2007:615–631.

Bethea CL, Pau FK, Fox S, Hess DL, Berga SL, Cameron JL. Sensitivity to stress-induced reproductive dysfunction linked to activity of the serotonin system. *Fertil Steril.* 2005;83(1):148–155.

Bethea CL, Centeno ML, Cameron JL. Neurobiology of stress-induced reproductive dysfunction in female macaques. *Mol Neurobiol.* 2008;38(3):199–230.

Bisaga K, Petkova E, Cheng J, Davies M, Feldman JF, Whitaker AH. Menstrual functioning and psychopathology in a county-wide population of high school girls. *J Am Acad Child Adolesc Psychiatry.* 2002;41(10):1197–1204.

Bonen A. Exercise-induced menstrual cycle changes. A functional, temporary adaptation to metabolic stress. *Sports Med.* 1994;17(6):373–392.

Brundu B, Loucks TL, Adler LJ, Cameron JL, Berga SL. Increased cortisol in the cerebrospinal fluid of women with functional hypothalamic amenorrhea. *J Clin Endocrinol Metab.* 2006;91(4):1561–1565.

Bullen BA, Skrinar GS, Beitins IZ, von Mering G, Turnbull BA, McArthur JW. Induction of menstrual disorders by strenuous exercise in untrained women. *N Engl J Med.* 1985;312:1349–1353.

CDC. *2005 Assisted Reproductive Technology (ART) Success Rates: National Summary and Fertility Clinic Reports.* Atlanta, GA; 2007.

Challis J, Sloboda D, Matthews S, et al. Fetal hypothalamic-pituitary-adrenal (HPA) development and activation as a determinant of the timing of birth, and of postnatal disease. *Endocr Res.* 2000;26:489–504.

Chandra A, Martinez GM, Mosher WD, Abma JC, Jones J. Fertility, family planning, and reproductive health of U.S. women: data from the 2002 National Survey of Family Growth. *Vital Health Stat.* 2005;23(25):1–160.

Chrousos GP, Torpy DJ, Gold PW. Interactions between the hypothalamic-pituitary-adrenal axis and the female reproductive system: clinical implications. *Ann Intern Med.* 1998;129(3):229–240.

Daniels TL, Cameron JL, Marcus MD, Berga SL. Recovery from functional hypothalamic amenorrhea (FHA) involves resolution of hypothalamic hypothyroidism. Abstract #P1-378, 79th Annual Meeting of The Endocrine Society, Minneapolis, MN, June 11–14, 1997.

De Bellis MD, Gold PW, Geracioti TD Jr, Listwak SJ, Kling MA. Association of fluoxetine treatment with reductions in CSF concentrations of corticotropin-releasing hormone and arginine vasopressin in patients with major depression. *Am J Psychiatry.* 1993;150(4):656–657.

deBoo HA, Harding JE. The developmental origins of adult disease (Barker) hypothesis. *Aust N Z J Ob Gyneacol.* 2006;46:4–14.

Dickerson SS, Kemeny ME. Acute stressors and cortisol responses: a theoretical integration and synthesis of laboratory research. *Psychol Bull.* 2004;130(3):355–391.

Dobson H, Ghuman S, Prabhakar S, Smith R. A conceptual model of the influence of stress on female reproduction. *Reproduction.* 2003;125(2):151–163.

Domar AD, Clapp D, Slawsby EA, Dusek J, Kessel B, Freizinger M. Impact of group psychological interventions on pregnancy rates in infertile women. *Fertil Steril.* 2000;73(4):805–811.

Giles DE, Berga SL. Cognitive and psychiatric correlates of functional hypothalamic amenorrhea: a controlled comparison. *Fertil Steril.* 1993;60(3):486–492.

Gold PW, Chrousos GP. Organization of the stress system and its dysregulation in melancholic and atypical depression: high vs low CRH/NE states. *Mol Psychiatry.* 2002;7(3):254–275.

Golden NH, Carlson JL. The pathophysiology of amenorrhea in the adolsecent. *Ann NY Acad Sci.* 2008;1135:163–178.

Gore AC, Terasawa E. Neural circuits regulating pulsatile luteinizing hormone release in the female guinea-pig: opioid, adrenergic and serotonergic interactions. *J Neuroendocrinol.* 2001;13(3):239–248.

Haddow JE, Palomaki GE, Allan WC, et al. Maternal thyroid deficiency during pregnancy and subsequent neuropsychological development of the child. *N Engl J Med.* 1999;341(8):549–555.

Haemmerli K, Znoj H, Barth J. The efficacy of psychological interventions for infertile patients: a meta-analysis examining mental health and pregnancy rate. *Hum Reprod Update.* 2009 May–Jun;15(3):279–295.

Hansen D, Lou HC, Olsen J. Serious life events and congenital malformations: a national study with complete follow-up. *Lancet.* 2000;356:875–880.

Harlow BL, Wise LA, Otto MW, Soares CN, Cohen LS. Depression and its influence on reproductive endocrine and menstrual cycle markers associated with perimenopause: the Harvard Study of Moods and Cycles. *Arch Gen Psychiatry.* 2003;60(1):29–36.

Herbison AE. Multimodal influence of estrogen upon gonadotropin-releasing hormone neurons. *Endocr Rev.* 1998;19(3):302–330.

Homan GF, Davies M, Norman R. The impact of lifestyle factors on reproductive performance in the general population and those undergoing infertility treatment: a review. *Hum Reprod Update.* 2007;13(3):209–223.

Kaplan JR, Manuck SB. Ovarian dysfunction, stress, and disease: a primate continuum. *Ilar J.* 2004;45(2):89–115.

Klonoff-Cohen H, Chu E, Natarajan L, Sieber W. A prospective study of stress among women undergoing in vitro fertilization or gamete intrafallopian transfer. *Fertil Steril.* 2001;76(4):675–687.

Kondoh Y, Uemura T, Murase M, Yokoi N, Ishikawa M, Hirahara F. A longitudinal study of disturbances of the hypothalamic-pituitary-adrenal axis in women with progestin-negative functional hypothalamic amenorrhea. *Fertil Steril.* 2001;76(4):748–752.

Laatikainen TJ. Corticotropin-releasing hormone and opioid peptides in reproduction and stress. *Ann Med.* 1991;23(5):489–496.

Laughlin GA, Dominguez CE, Yen SS. Nutritional and endocrine-metabolic aberrations in women with functional hypothalamic amenorrhea. *J Clin Endocrinol Metab.* 1998;83(1):25–32.

Lazarus RS, Folkman S. *Stress, Appraisal, and Coping.* New York: Springer; 1984.

Leonard WR, Robertson ML. Evolutionary perspectives on human nutrition: the influence of brain and body size on diet and metabolism. *Am J Hum Biol.* 1994;6:77–88.

Lou HC, Hansen D, Nordentoft M, Pryds O, Jensen F, Nim J, Hemmingsen R. Prenatal stressors of human life affect fetal brain development. *Dev Med Child Neurol.* 1994;36(9):826–832.

Loucks AB, Mortola JF, Girton L, Yen SS. Alterations in the hypothalamic-pituitary-ovarian and the hypothalamic-pituitary-adrenal axes in athletic women. *J Clin Endocrinol Metab.* 1989;68(2):402–411.

Loucks AB, Thuma JR. Luteinizing hormone pulsatility is disrupted at a threshold of energy availability in regularly menstruating women. *J Clin Endocrinol Metab.* 2003;88(1):297–311.

Lovallo WR, Gerin W. Psychophysiological reactivity: mechanisms and pathways to cardiovascular disease. *Psychosom Med.* 2003;65(1):36–45.

Lupien SJ, Nair NP, Briere S, Maheu F, Tu MT, Lemay M, McEwen BS, Meaney MJ. Increased cortisol levels and impaired cognition in human aging: implication for depression and dementia in later life. *Rev Neurosci.* 1999;10:117–139.

Mann DR, Jackson GG, Blank MS. Influence of adrenocorticotropin and adrenalectomy on gonadotropin secretion in immature rats. *Neuroendocrinology.* 1982;34(1):20–26.

Marcus MD, Loucks TL, Berga SL. Psychological correlates of functional hypothalamic amenorrhea. *Fertil Steril.* 2001;76(2):310–316.

McEwen BS. Protective and damaging effects of stress mediators. *N Engl J Med.* 1998;338:171–179.

McEwen BS. Sex, stress, and the hippocampus: allostasis, allostatic load, and the aging process. *Neurobiol Aging*. 2002;23:921–939.

McMillen IC, Schwartz J, Coulter CL, Edwards LJ. Early embryonic environment, the fetal pituitary-adrenal axis, and the timing of parturition. *Endocr Rev*. 2004;30:845–850.

Meczekalski B, Tonetti A, Monteleone P, et al. Hypothalamic amenorrhea with normal body weight: ACTH, allopregnanolone and cortisol responses to corticotropin-releasing hormone test. *Eur J Endocrinol*. 2000;142(3):280–285.

Morreale de Escobar G, Jesus Obregon M, Escobar del Rey F. Is neuropsychological development related to maternal hypothyroidism or to maternal hypothyroxinemia? *J Clin Endocrinol Metab*. 2000;85(11):3975–3987.

Muller AF, Verhoeff A, Mantel MJ, De Jong FH, Berghout A. Decrease of free thyroxine levels after controlled ovarian hyperstimulation. *J Clin Endocrinol Metab*. 2000;85(2):545–548.

Nepomnaschy PA, Welch K, McConnell D, Strassmann BI, England BG. Stress and female reproductive function: a study of daily variations in cortisol, gonadotrophins, and gonadal steroids in a rural Mayan population. *Am J Hum Biol*. 2004;16(5):523–532.

Nepomnaschy PA, Welch KB, McConnell DS, Low BS, Strassmann BI, England BG. Cortisol levels and very early pregnancy loss in humans. *Proc Natl Acad Sci U S A*. 2006;103(10):3938–3942.

Petrides JS, Mueller GP, Kalogeras KT, Chrousos GP, Gold W, Deuster PA. Exercise-induced activation of the hypothalamic-pituitary-adrenal axis: marked differences in the sensitivity to glucocorticoid suppression. *J Clin Endocrinol Metab*. 1994;79:377–383.

Pop VJ, Brouwers EP, Vader HL, Vulsma T, van Baar AL, de Vijlder JJ. Maternal hypothyroxinaemia during early pregnancy and subsequent child development: a 3-year follow-up study. *Clin Endocrinol (Oxf)*. 2003;59(3):282–288.

Reindollar RH, Novak M, Tho SP, McDonough PG. Adult-onset amenorrhea: a study of 262 patients. *Am J Obstet Gynecol*. 1986;155(3):531–543.

Ringstrom SJ, Suter DE, Hostetler JP, Schwartz NB. Cortisol regulates secretion and pituitary content of the two gonadotropins differentially in female rats: effects of gonadotropin-releasing hormone antagonist. *Endocrinology*. 1992;130(6):3122–3128.

Samuels MH, Luther M, Henry P, Ridgway EC. Effects of hydrocortisone on pulsatile pituitary glycoprotein secretion. *J Clin Endocrinol Metab*. 1994;78(1):211–215.

Sapolsky RM, Romero LM, Munck AU. How do glucocorticoids influence stress responses? Integrating permissive, suppressive, stimulatory, and preparative actions. *Endocr Rev*. 2000;21(1):55–89.

Sapolsky RM. Glucocorticoids and hippocampal atrophy in neuropsychiatric disorders. *Arch Gen Psychiatry*. 2000;57:925–935.

Sapolsky RM. The influence of social hierarchy on primate health. *Science*. 2005;308:648–652.

Shanan J, Brzezinski A, Sulman F, Sharon M. Active coping behavior, anxiety, and cortical steroid excretion in the prediction of transient amenorrhea. *Behav Sci*. 1965;10(4):461–465.

Spratt DL, Cox P, Orav J, Maloney J, Bigos T. Reproductive axis suppression in acute illness is related to disease severity. *J Clin Endocrinol Metab.* 1993;76:1548–1554.

Terzioglu F. Investigation into effectiveness of counseling on assisted reproductive techniques in Turkey. *J Psychosom Obstet Gynaecol.* 2001;22(3):133–141.

Tilbrook AJ, Turner AI, Clarke IJ. Stress and reproduction: central mechanisms and sex differences in non-rodent species. *Stress.* 2002;5(2):83–100.

Tschugguel W, Berga SL. Treatment of functional hypothalamic amenorrhea with hypnotherapy. *Fertil Steril.* 2003;80(4):982–985.

Vulliemoz NR, Xiao E, Xia-Zhang L, Rivier J, Ferin M. Astressin B, a nonselective corticotropin-releasing hormone receptor antagonist, prevents the inhibitory effect of ghrelin on luteinizing hormone pulse frequency in the ovariectomized rhesus monkey. *Endocrinology.* 2008;149(3):869–874.

Wadhwa PD, Sandman CA, Garite TJ. The neurobiology of stress in human pregnancy: implications for prematurity and development of the fetal nervous system. *Prog Brain Res.* 2001;133:131–142.

Warren MP, Fried JL. Hypothalamic amenorrhea. The effects of environmental stresses on the reproductive system: a central effect of the central nervous system. *Endocrinol Metab Clin North Am.* 2001;30(3):611–629.

Williams NI, Berga SL, Cameron JL. Synergism between psychosocial and metabolic stressors: impact on reproductive function in cynomolgus monkeys. *Am J Physiol Endocrinol Metab.* 2007;293(1):E270–276.

17

Polycystic Ovary Syndrome

BRIDGET S. BONGAARD

CASE STUDY

Denise came into my office despondent and desperate. She was
19 years old and increasingly concerned about her erratic menstrual cycles, sometimes going months without having a period.
Denise was embarrassed by the increasing amount of dark hair
that was growing on her chin, upper lip, and now around her nip-
ples. She admitted that she was also feeling somewhat depressed
about her weight, as she had gained roughly 40 pounds in the
last 3 years. After taking a good personal and family history and
ordering a few laboratory tests, I explained that she had a condition known as polycystic ovary syndrome and that together we
would create a plan that would help her lose weight, regulate her
menstrual cycle, and slow the growth of unwanted hair.

Introduction

Polycystic ovary syndrome (PCOS) is the most common premenopausal
endocrine disorder in women, affecting 5% to 10% of all women of reproductive age. It generally starts at puberty with an increased incidence of
menstrual abnormalities, hirsutism, acne, and infertility. If left unmanaged, it
can lead to miscarriage, cardiovascular complications, endometrial cancer, and
a sevenfold greater risk of type 2 diabetes (Avery and Braunack-Mayer 2007).
The presentation at the time of diagnosis varies with the symptom complex and
the age of the patient. Some women might present with complaints of excessive

central adiposity or signs of androgen excess, while others might only present with menstrual irregularities or problems in conceiving and have a thin body habitus. The clinical practitioner must therefore be keenly aware of the variance, and launch a thorough diagnostic workup.

While once considered a "benign nuisance" disorder of irregular menses, obesity, and hirsutism, PCOS should be regarded as a real threat to the woman's health due to the increased risk of cancer, diabetes, and coronary artery disease (Sheehan 2004).

Pathophysiology

The ovary responds to the pituitary gland's secretion of follicle stimulating hormone (FSH) to make and mature ova; it releases them on the command of luteinizing hormone (LH). Without the correct cycling of FSH and LH, disturbances in ovulation and menstruation develop. If the pituitary chronically secretes more LH than FSH, the ova will neither mature nor release, and the woman will not have a menstrual cycle. In addition to ova, the ovary is composed of fibrous supportive tissue containing specialized thecal cells. These cells are responsible for making and secreting testosterone. While testosterone is important for women's healthy sexual libido and hair growth, in excess amounts, it can cause unwanted hair growth on the chin, upper lip, back, breasts, abdomen, and buttocks. In susceptible individuals it also can stimulate the production of acne and development of male pattern balding.

There is no single cause of PCOS, but is rather a complicated admixture of endocrine and metabolic abnormalities. First, there is excessive thecal cell proliferation in the ovary with subsequent increased androgen production in response to elevated gonadotropins, hyperinsulinemia and production of oxidative stress (Kodaman and Duleba 2008). Roughly 80% of women with PCOS suffer from anovulation. This may present as oligomenorrhea (light menstrual flow), amenorrhea (no flow), dysfunctional uterine bleeding (erratic flow), and/or infertility (Sheehan 2004). The prolonged exposure to estrogen, progesterone deficiency, and androgen excess increase the risk of gynecologic cancers later on in life (Karadeniz et al. 2007). Prolonged anovulation can also predispose women to the development of uterine fibroids (Wise et al. 2007). Fertility is also impaired in many PCOS patients. If and when pregnancies do occur, the first trimester rate of miscarriage is as high as 30% to 50% (Sheehan 2004).

Insulin resistance has been noted in women with PCOS. Hyperinsulinemia is a major contributor to the excessive production of androgen by the thecal and stromal cells of the ovary (Kodaman and Duleba 2008). Elevated insulin levels also inhibit the production of sex hormone binding globulin (SHBG) in the liver. This hepatic protein normally binds circulating androgens and lowers serum levels. Dimunition in the hepatic manufacture of SHBG thereby allows this increased free (serum) androgen bioavailability to affect target tissues. Androgen excess not only creates problems with the development of hirsutism and acne, but also increases the risk of cardiovascular disease by adversely altering lipid parameters: lowering HDL and increasing LDL, triglycerides, and VLDL (Kodaman and Duleba 2008). Insulin resistance is independent of obesity, although obesity plays an amplifying role (Corbould and Dunaif 2007). Simply said, women with PCOS may have insulin resistance whether or not they are obese. Defects in glucose metabolism observed in adipose cells in women with PCOS are acquired secondary to the hormonal milieu rather than due to intrinsic defects in the adipocyte (Corbould and Dunaif 2007).

How Related Diseases Increase Risk?

Increased cardiovascular mortality in women with PCOS has not been conclusively demonstrated. Some studies suggest increased cardiac events while other studies reveal no increase compared with normal cycling women (Cho et al. 2007). Hyperinsulinemia stimulates the release of insulin growth factor-1 (IGF-1) that then contributes to the development of hypertension by causing vascular smooth muscle hypertrophy. Interestingly, hyperandrogenism also contributes to vascular endothelial dysfunction associated with the development of atherosclerosis. Abnormally elevated insulin levels further complicate cardiovascular problems by enhancing sodium retention, stimulating the sympathetic nervous system (which enhances the production of vasoconstricting agents such as angiotensin II), and hence precipitating the development or worsening of hypertension. Elevated angiotensin II levels also independently further aggravate insulin resistance. Finally, hyperinsulinemia also contributes to a prothrombotic state by elevating plasminogen activator inhibitor (PAI-1) and reducing fibrinolysis.

PCOS patients are also predisposed to an increased state of inflammation. Fat cells are metabolically active and secrete inflammatory agents such as tumor necrosis factor (TNF), interleukin 6 (IL-6), PAI-1, leptin, resistin, adiponectin, and angiotensinogen (Cho et al. 2007). TNF stimulates the production of C-reactive protein and IL-6. The latter increases the liver's production of triglycerides, thereby increasing cardiovascular risk. These inflammatory compounds produce increased oxidative stress even in lean women with PCOS (Cho et al. 2007).

Diabetes alone is a well-known risk factor for cardiovascular disease. At the onset of diagnosis of PCOS, one study found that 31% of patients had impaired glucose tolerance, while 7.5% met the criterion for type 2 diabetes mellitus regardless of obesity or lean body mass (Sheehan 2004). By the age of 40, up to 40% of women with PCOS will have type 2 diabetes, or impaired glucose tolerance (Lord et al. 2003) due to long-standing insulin resistance and hyperinsulinemia. The risk of gestational diabetes is increased 10-fold, compared to the general population (Sheehan 2004).

Screening and Diagnosis of PCOS

The clinical features of PCOS include oligo or amenorrhea, infertility or first trimester miscarriage, truncal or central obesity, hirsutism, acne acanthosis nigricans, and male pattern balding. Excluding other diagnoses that can mimic PCOS is the first priority. Congenital adrenal hyperplasia, Cushing's disease, and androgen-secreting tumors of the ovary or adrenal gland must be ruled out (Cho et al. 2007).

> The diagnostic criteria for metabolic syndrome includes three or more of the following: Waist circumference >88 cm (35 inches), triglycerides ≥150 mg/dL, HDL-cholesterol <50 mg/dL, blood pressure ≥130/85, and a fasting glucose ≥110 mg/dL (Sheehan 2004).

Even in the early stages of PCOS, 30% to 40% of women are unable to regulate their glucose levels. It is recommended that women at risk be screened with a 2-hour glucose tolerance test (Lau 2007). Other recommended laboratory evaluation includes a cholesterol panel and free and total testosterone levels (should less than 200 ng/dL). The LH/FSH ratio is also measured. A ratio of ≥2.0 is suggestive of PCOS, but is not highly sensitive or specific, and can be affected by the use of oral contraceptives (Sheehan 2004). Ovarian ultrasound can be helpful in identifying women with PCOS, but is not 100% reliable as 20% of women have the ultrasound features, yet not the disease. Ultrasound criteria for PCOS are increased ovarian area (>5.5 cm²) or volume (11 mL), and/or presence of ≥12 follicles measuring 2–9 mm in diameter (mean of both ovaries) when present, the diagnosis of PCOS can be made with 99% specificity and a 75% sensitivity (Sheehan 2004).

Integrative Treatment Options

The goals of treatment should be directed toward the immediate reduction of hyperinsulinemia/insulin resistance/abnormal glucose control and central visceral obesity, treatment of ovulation and fertility issues, management of dyslipidemia and hypertension, and treatment for androgen excess symptoms such as hirsutism and acne. Due to the complex endocrine and metabolic nature of PCOS, the treatment plan requires a multipronged approach.

INSULIN SENSITIZERS—METFORMIN AND THE THIAZOLIDINEDIONES

Metformin is effective in the treatment of the metabolic syndrome and may improve hirsutism by improving insulin resistance and hyperandrogenism (Cho et al. 2007). In one study, normalization of menstrual cycles and ovulation occurred in 40% of women taking metformin, with 79% of these women becoming pregnant within 3 months of starting the medication (Sheehan 2004). The addition of clomophene to induce ovulation increased that rate to 89%. Metformin also reduces the rate of first trimester pregnancy miscarriages. Metformin does not change waist-to-hip ratio or reduce BMI, and therefore is weight neutral. It does not have a significant effect on total cholesterol levels, triglycerides or HDL, though it does modestly lower LDL as well as both systolic and diastolic blood pressure (Lord et al. 2003). Metformin can cause gastric upset, nausea, and diarrhea in some patients. To avoid this, the drug should be started slowly and gradually increased. Metformin should not be used by those with creatinine clearance below 30 mL/min.

Thiazolidinediones (TZDs) are a class of insulin-sensitizing drugs that have shown positive cardiometabolic effects, reduction of hyperandrogenism and hirsutism, and improvement in menstrual cycle regulation in patients with PCOS. The insulin-sensitizing function occurs via increase in the number and function of the glucose transport receptors in skeletal muscle and the liver. It also may stimulate the beneficial release of adiponectin (Skov et al. 2008) by the adipose tissue cells, which then downregulates the insulin resistance and inflammatory effects. This allows the more effective disposal of the circulating glucose insulin complex, thereby lowering blood sugar and insulin levels. Rosaglitazone, one of the TZD drug class members, was studied in PCOS patients who had failed clomophene induction of ovulation. Ovulation occurred in 33% those taking Rosaglitazone (4 mg twice daily) alone, versus 77% in the combination group of clomophene and rosaglitazone. The resulting pregnancy rate was 8% for the TZD alone and 15% for the combination treatment (Sheehan 2004). Side effects of TZD include modest weight gain, development of edema, and liver enzymes elevation.

STATIN DRUGS

Statins inhibit the synthesis of mevalonate, the key precursor to cholesterol production; statins may decrease maturation of insulin receptors, inhibit steroidogenesis, and alter the signal transduction pathways that mediate cellular proliferation (Kodaman and Duleba 2008). Statins also have intrinsic antioxidant properties and anti-inflammatory properties as they improve nitric oxide–mediated endothelial function and antiproliferative actions on vascular smooth muscle. In PCOS patients, the increased oxidative stress and systemic inflammation overcomes the antioxidant reserves even in lean PCOS patients (Kodaman and Duleba 2008). The effects of statin drugs inhibit both oxidative stress pathways as well as that of cellular proliferation, cholesterol synthesis, and ovarian androgen production, improving not only the cholesterol abnormalities but also the effects of hyperandrogenemia in PCOS patients.

BIRTH CONTROL PILLS

The mainstay of treatment for decades has been oral contraceptive pills (OCPs) because of their ability to regulate unpredictable menstrual periods. OCPs also increase sex hormone-binding globulin, thereby increasing the binding of free testosterone and decreasing hyperandrogenemia. The most effective OCPs in PCOS are those that contain both an estrogen, and an antiandrogen/weak progestinal agent such as cyproterone acetate. OCPs should not be used in patients with hypercoagulable state, those who have a history of deep venous thrombosis, or in women older than 35 years who smoke (Sheehan 2004).

Other Antiandrogen Strategies

Drugs such as spironolactone confer a mild antiandrogen effect, may have an additive benefit when combined with OCP agents, however, they can take a significant time (months) to work and may increase serum potassium levels. Creams such as eflornithine hydrochloride 13.9% (Vaniqa) can act as a mild depilatory agent in PCOS patients with hirsutism, while plucking/shaving and electrolysis can further diminish unsightly hair.

Diet and Exercise

Although obesity is not the cause of PCOS, it may aggravate the dysfunction. Significant weight loss reduces hyperinsulinemia and subsequently hyperandrogenemia (Sheehan, 2004) by increasing sex hormone–binding globulin and reducing basal levels of insulin (Cho et al. 2007). In one study, women who lost

5% of their initial body weight with caloric restriction achieved spontaneous pregnancy (Kiddy et al. 1992). An exercise program consisting of a brisk walk 20 minutes a day was shown to achieve a 7% weight loss (Sheehan 2004).

A 3- to 6-month aggressive lifestyle modification program may be a prudent first step before considering insulin sensitizers. On the other hand, asking obese women to lose weight before treatment may increase the stigmatization (Balen et al. 2006). In the study by Balen, women's weight loss generally does not exceed a mean of 5–15 kg, and is typically closer to 3 kg, after 2 years of diet and exercise treatment, which is close to placebo rate. It is argued, therefore, that obese women with PCOS should be offered treatment to improve ovulatory dysfunction rather than awaiting the effects of a prescribed diet and exercise program. When metformin therapy is added to intensive lifestyle modification, the risk of diabetes was reduced by 58% versus 31% for lifestyle change alone (Cho et al. 2007).

Good dietary patterns are essential for the prevention of type 2 diabetes, insulin resistance, and the resulting associated endocrine, metabolic, endothelial dysfunction, and inflammatory disease outcomes. See Chapter 2 on Nutrition for anti-inflammatory diet recommendations.

The effect of alcohol consumption on the development of type 2 diabetes is variable, depending on the amount ingested. Mild to moderate alcohol consumption lowers insulin resistance by precipitating a 44% increase in insulin-stimulated glucose disposal. Excessive alcohol consumption (≥ 360 mL/day) increases the risk of diabetes.

The consumption of tea and coffee also affects the inflammatory milieu in PCOS patients. Moderate doses of caffeine results in reduced insulin sensitivity. Both coffee and tea possess antioxidants that afford protection against diabetes, cardiovascular disease, and cancer. Drinking 6 cups of green tea or 3 or more cups of coffee per day had a 33% and 42% lowering of risk for the development of type II diabetes unrelated to their caffeine content (Hayes 2008).

Insulin sensitizers

CHROMIUM, CINNAMON, GINSENG, AND ALPHA-LIPOIC ACID

Accumulating evidence suggests that chromium enhances glucose metabolism, decreases cardiovascular risk, and may benefit atypical depression (Pattar et al. 2006). It enhances the metabolic action of insulin and decreases total cholesterol and LDL, which then decreases the amount of cholesterol in cell membranes of skeletal and fat cells. It has the greatest benefit on obese, insulin-resistant individuals. The typical dose is 200–1000 µg/day of chromium picolinate.

Cinnamon (*Cinnamomum verum*) is another insulin-sensitizing agent that can be added to the diet. It stimulates glucose uptake and synthesis by fat cells (lowering glucose and insulin levels), lowers blood pressure, and improves abnormal lipid profiles. Use of cinnamon extract in one study increased lean body mass even after controlling for smoking, physical activity, dietary habits, blood pressure, glucose, and lipid levels (Zeigenfuss et al. 2006). A small study of 15 women with PCOS and an average BMI of 28.8 found that 1 g of cinnamon extract was superior to placebo in reducing fasting glucose and insulin resistance (Wang 2007). Other studies have used doses ranging from 1 to 6 g of cinnamon and shown dose-dependent decreases in fasting blood glucose and lipid levels (Zeigenfuss et al. 2006). This inexpensive spice can certainly be added to the tool bag to treat the metabolic syndrome in PCOS patients.

Ginseng (*Panax ginseng, Panax quinquefolius*) demonstrates antidiabetic effects as well. A 3-g dose of ginseng extract administered prior to an oral glucose tolerance test resulted in a decrease of blood sugar in both diabetic and nondiabetic patients (Hayes 2008). However, it is difficult to offer specific recommendations, as a meta-analysis of ginseng studies reveals variability depending on the species and plant parts (root, leaf, stem) used (Dey et al. 2003; Seivenpiper et al. 2003, 2004).

Alpha-lipoic acid, also known as thioctic acid, is an antioxidant associated with improving skeletal muscle glucose transport activity, thereby reducing insulin resistance and oxidative stress. Typical doses of alpha-lipoic acid range from 200 to 400 mg tid. Side effects include nausea and skin rashes.

There are other potent therapies that can be used to decrease the inflammatory response and improve altered lipid profiles in PCOS patients. Please refer to the Chapter 35 on cardiovascular health for information on the use of statin drugs red yeast rice, plant stanols and sterol preparations, and bulk fiber agents.

Acupuncture

Patients with metabolic syndrome appear to have a higher sympathetic nervous system tone. Clinically this presents as diastolic hypertension from enhanced adrenal stimulation. This increased sympathetic outpouring decreases blood flow to the ovaries, which some hypothesize decreases a woman's ability to ovulate. In one small study of 24 PCOS patients, the women were treated with low-frequency (2 Hertz) electroacupuncture (EA) and had successful induction of regular ovulation in one-third of the cohort (Stenor-Victorin et al. 2000). The women with the best results were those with a less hyperandrogenic hormonal profile before treatment. It is postulated that EA induces ovulation by decreasing sympathetic stimulation of the ovary.

Mind–Body Medicine

While there are studies on mind–body approaches for cardiovascular risk reduction and diabetes, there are none that specifically address PCOS. It is reasonable to include mind–body approaches in the treatment of PCOS as they are known to reduce inflammation, anxiety, and help balance the autonomic nervous system by downregulating the sympathetic nervous system and stimulating the parasympathetic response. The resulting reduction in stress hormones (which activate the inflammatory cascade in the body) would decrease blood pressure as well as blood sugar levels. Mind–body therapies such as yoga, guided visualization, hypnosis, biofeedback, and aromatherapy can be utilized by women to achieve these goals and to improve body image concerns.

Summary

PCOS patients are challenged from many different directions both physically and emotionally. There is not one simple treatment strategy to recommend to all comers as each patient presents with her own unique combination of symptoms and disease manifestation. PCOS affected women may reside anywhere on the spectrum from having only menstrual irregularities to Denise's full-blown presentation of abnormal menses, hirsutism, and metabolic syndrome. It is best to try and understand the underlying pathophysiology, and craft a more effective comprehensive treatment plan with the addition of integrative strategies. Women should be taught as much as possible about their pathophysiology so that they can be champions for their healing. Sharing these strategy options with the patient can empower her to participate more fully in her care and improve the overall outcome when she is then educated and committed.

Recommendations

Any woman suspected of having PCOS should undergo a complete history and physical, and if presenting with hirsutism and acne, be screened for other causes of hyperandrogenism (with a free testosterone, DHEA, 17-OH progesterone, and 24-hour urine for cortisol) before the diagnosis of PCOS is made. Screening tests for LH:FSH ratio and an ovarian ultrasound are also important.

The diagnosis requires that two of the following three be present:

1. Oligoanovulation
2. Hyperandrogenism
3. Polycystic ovaries on ultrasonography

For those women presenting primarily with ovarian dysfunction (infertility or irregular menses, or anovulation) and insulin resistance without central obesity, birth control pills may be a good choice if there are not contraindications. Acupuncture also may help restore ovulation by increasing ovarian blood flow. A low glycemic index diet and routine exercise program should also be recommended.

In women with more advanced symptoms, including infertility or amenorrhea, hyperandrogenemia, and increasing insulin resistance in the form of metabolic syndrome, it is imperative that a more extensive treatment plan be initiated. This patient is at high risk of developing diabetes, inflammatory cardiovascular disease, nonalcoholic steatohepatitis, and endometrial cancer. An exercise program confers significant benefit in this population and should strongly be encouraged and monitored. Beginning first with simply encouraging the patient to increase her physical activity and flexibility in any healthy way possible, the physician then proceeds to collaborate to develop a creative fitness regimen adding strength, then endurance training. In addition to the measures above, the patient would be advised to start insulin sensitizers (cinnamon, tea, coffee, alpha-lipoic acid, ginseng, and chromium), start metformin, and/or TZD therapy. The exercise and dietary recommendations should be more stringent as this boosts the effectiveness of the drugs in reversing the symptoms. Fish oil supplements should also be added to decrease cardiovascular risk, as should one aspirin a day.

Electrolysis or topical creams can be added to decrease the distressing appearance of the hirsutism. Spironolactone can be initiated. Acupuncture may also be helpful in this group to improve ovarian function. Birth control pills may be initiated however one must be aware of the contraindications of hypertension, hypertriglyceridemia, hypercoagulable state, or smoking habit in a woman age >35 or more. The patient should undergo screening with a 2-hour glucose tolerance test and blood lipid panel. If lipid abnormalities are found, additional therapy in the form of a statin drug, or red yeast rice should be initiated, and the lipid panel followed carefully.

Never forgetting the integrative concept of treating the whole person, the emotional and spiritual needs of the patient must be acknowledged as these crucially affect the physical body and outcome of treatment. Evidence-based integrative therapies such as yoga, massage, acupuncture, guided visualization or hypnosis, biofeedback, aromatherapy, and energy medicine can lead to rebalancing the individual. A comprehensive treatment plan that impacts all parameters of being: emotional health, physical health, and spiritual well being, vastly improves the quality of life for these patients and amplifies their participation in the healing process.

REFERENCES

Avery JC, Braunack-Mayer AJ. The information needs of women diagnosed with polycystic ovarian syndrome-implications for treatment and health outcomes. *BMC Women Health.* 2007;7:1–10.

Balen AH, Dresner M, Scott EM, Drife JO. Should obese women with polycystic ovary syndrome receive treatment for infertility? *BMJ.* 2006;332:434–435.

Cho LW, Randeva HS, Atkin SL. Cardiometabolic aspects of polycystic ovarian syndrome. *Vascular Health Risk Manag.* 2007;3(1) 55–63.

Corbould A, Dunaif A. The adipose cell lineage is not intrinsically insulin resistant in polycystic ovary syndrome. *Metabolism.* 2007;56(5):716–722.

Dey L, Xie JT, Wang A, Wu J, Maleckar SA, Yuan CS. Anti-hyperglycemic effects of ginseng: comparison between root and berry. *Phytomedicine.* 2003;10:600–605.

Karadeniz M, Erdongan M, Gerdeli A, et al. The progesterone receptor PROGINS polymorphism is not related to oxidative stress factors in women with polycystic ovary syndrome. *Cardiovasc Diabetol.* 2007;6:29.

Kiddy DS, Hamilton-Fairley D, Bush A, et al. Improvement in endocrine and ovarian function during dietary treatment of obese women with polycystic ovary syndrome. *Clin Endocrinol (Oxf).* 1992;36:105–111.

Hayes NP, Galasetti PR, Coker RH. Prevention and treatment of type 2 diabetes: current role of lifestyle, natural product, and Pharmacological interventions. *Pharmacol Ther.* 2008;118(2):181–191

Kodaman PH, Duleba AJ. Statins in the treatment of polycystic ovary syndrome. *Semin Reprod Med.* 2008;26(1):127–138.

Lau DCW. Screening for diabetes in women with polycystic ovary syndrome. *CMAJ.* 2007;176(7):951.

Lord JM, Flight IHK, Norman RJ. Metformin in polycystic ovary syndrome: systematic review and meta-analysis. *Br Med J.* 2003;1–6.

Pattar GR, Tackett L, Liu P, Elmendorf JS. Chromium picolinate positively influences the glucose transporter system via affecting cholesterol homeostasis in adipocytes cultured under hyperglycemic conditions. *Mutat Res.* 2006;610(1–2):93–100.

Sheehan MT. Polycystic ovarian syndrome: diagnosis and management. *Clin Med Res.* 2004;2(1):13–27.

Sievenpiper JL, Arnason JT, Leiter LA, Vuksan V. Variable effects of American ginseng; a batch of American ginseng (Panax quinquefolius L.) with a depressed ginsenoside profile does not affect postprandial glycemia. *Eur J Clin Nutr.* 2003;57;243–248.

Sievenpiper JL, Arnason JT, Leiter LA, Vuksan V. Decreasing, null and increasing effects of eight popular types of ginseng on acute postprandial glycemic indices in healthy humans: the role of ginsenosides. *J Am Coll Nutr.* 2004;23:248–258.

Skov V, Glintborg D, Knudsen S, et al. Pioglitazone enhances mitochondrial biogenesis and ribosomal protein biosynthesis in skeletal muscle in polycystic ovary syndrome. *Plos One.* 2008;3(6):e2466, 1–9.

Stenor-Victorin E, Waldenstrom U, Tagnfors U, et al. Effects of electro-acupuncture on anovulation in women with polycystic ovary syndrome. *Acta Obstet Gynecol Scand.* 2000;79:180–188.

Wang JG, Anderson RA, Graham GM, et al. The effect of cinnamon extract on insulin resistance parameters in polycystic ovary syndrome: a pilot study. *Fertil Steril.* 2007;88(1):240–243.

Wise LA, Palmer JR, Stewart EA, Rosenberg L. Polycystic ovary syndrome and risk of uterine leiomyomata. *Fertil Steril.* 2007;87(5):1108–1115.

Zeigenfuss TN, Hofheins JE, Mendel RW, et al. Effects of a water-soluble cinnamon extract on body composition and features of the metabolic syndrome in pre-diabetic men and women. *J Int Soc Sports Nutr.* 2006;3(2):45–53.

18

Endometriosis

MARGEVA MORRIS COLE

CASE STUDY

Ellen is a 28-year-old magazine editor who is eager to conceive. She and her husband have tried for more than 1 year without success. She has predictable monthly menses and her testing for ovulation has been normal. Her husband, Tom, just received results documenting a normal semen analysis. Ellen has no history of sexually transmitted diseases and her hysterosalpingogram showed a normal uterine cavity and patent tubes.

Further discussion with Ellen reveals that she has had severe cramping with her menses since she was a teen. She requires large doses of ibuprofen for control. Her cramping has been better during the years she was on oral contraceptives (OCs). Ellen is active physically but admits to eating whatever is available due to her busy schedule. Her stress at work and the concern over possible infertility has caused her great anxiety. Her tension and irritability is starting to put a strain on her emotional and sexual relationship with her husband, Tom.

After discussion with the couple, Ellen opts to undergo a diagnostic laparoscopy at which multiple endometriosis implants are noted throughout the pelvis. The visible implants are excised or ablated using laser and cautery. She recovers well. When the surgical findings are reviewed with the couple, Ellen's physician explains the impact of endometriosis on fertility. Ellen has several choices: to suppress the endometriosis with a GnRH agonist for several months, to proceed with infertility therapy such as in vitro fertilization with a specialist, or to continue to try on their own for several more months.

Ellen is eager to continue to try on her own for 6 more months. She does not want the delay that Lupron would require and is not ready yet to move on to assisted reproductive interventions. Her physician discusses with her an approach to suppression of inflammation in her body through a healthy diet with fresh fruits and vegetables, whole grains, and healthy oils. Preconception nutrition with supplementation of folic acid, vitamin D, and omega-3 fatty acids is also reviewed. Herbal therapies are not encouraged at this time due to lack of data on efficacy and safety in early pregnancy. The physical and psychological benefits of stress reduction through yoga and mindfulness-based stress reduction techniques are emphasized. Options for couples counseling and group forums to explore the stresses of and responses to infertility are also offered. Ellen's physician makes her confident that whenever she is ready to return to discuss other avenues, the door will be open.

Introduction

Endometriosis is a common but enigmatic condition, affecting up to 50% of asymptomatic reproductive age women (Fauconnier and Chapron 2005) (Table 18.1).

Its diagnosis and management are hampered by poor correlation between the degree of symptoms and the extent of disease (Fedele et al. 1990; Vercellini et al. 1996).

Table 18.1. How Many Women Have Endometriosis?

1% of women undergoing major surgery for all gynecologic indications

1%–7% of women undergoing tubal sterilization

12%–32% of women of reproductive age undergoing laparoscopy for pelvic pain

9%–50% of women undergoing laparoscopy for infertility

50% of teenagers undergoing laparoscopy for evaluation of chronic pelvic pain or dysmenorrhea

Sources: Chatman and Ward (1982); Sangi-Haghpeykar and Poindexter (1995); Missmer, Hankinson et al. (2004).

Pathogenesis

Endometriosis can be defined as the presence of ectopic implants of endometrial glands and stroma outside the uterus. Several theories of pathogenesis attempt to explain its variable presentations (Schenken 1989) (Table 18.2).

Endometriosis most commonly affects the pelvic peritoneal surfaces and the external surfaces of the ovary, fallopian tubes, and uterus (Jenkins et al. 1986) (Figure 18.1). More severe disease can involve invasion into the bowel and bladder or distant metastases to other organs such as the lungs (Fauconnier et al. 2002). Endometriosis can also develop in the abdominal wall, most often in the incision following Cesarean section (Minaglia et al. 2007).

The cause of endometriosis is still unclear but many factors may influence its development in a given individual (Hadfield et al. 1997; Hediger et al. 2005; Houston 1984; Olive and Henderson 1987; Sangi-Haghpeykar and Poindexter 1995; Simpson et al. 1980) (Table 18.3).

One study has suggested a higher prevalence of endometriosis in women with other autoimmune inflammatory diseases such as hypothyroidism, asthma, allergies, chronic fatigue syndrome, and fibromyalgia (Sinaii et al. 2002). Another study suggests the possible role of environmental factors such as exposure to dioxins and PCBs (Foster and Agarwal 2002).

Table 18.2. Theories of Pathogenesis

Name	Theory	Supporting Evidence
Retrograde menstruation	Implantation of endometrial cells onto peritoneum due to retrograde flow of menses through the fallopian tube	Increased incidence of endometriosis in women with congenital obstruction of the reproductive tract
Coelomic metaplasia	Transformation of multipotential peritoneal cells into endometrial glands	Development of endometriosis in women with uterine agenesis
Hematologic or lymphatic spread	Transport of endometrial glands through the vascular and lymphatic systems	Presence of endometriosis in sites outside the abdominal cavity
Direct transplantation	Iatrogenic displacement of cells into the body wall at the time of surgery	Endometriosis implants in scars from Cesarean sections and episiotomies

Source: Schenken RS. *Endometriosis: Contemporary Concepts in Clinical Management*. Philadelphia, PA: Lippincott; 1989.

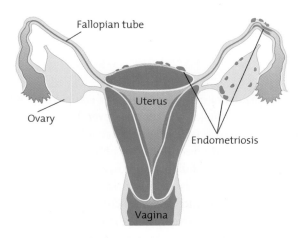

FIGURE 18.1. Common locations for endometriosis implants in the pelvis.

Table 18.3. Risk Factors for Endometriosis

Nulliparity [1]

Delayed childbearing [1]

Family history/genetic factors [1, 2]

Decreased BMI [3]

Increased height [3]

Caucasian race [4, 5]

Congenital anatomic variations that obstruct menstrual flow – (blind uterine horn, cervical agenesis, transverse vaginal septum) [6]

Sources:

1. Simpson JL, Elias S, Malinak LR, Buttram VC Jr. Heritable aspects of endometriosis. I. Genetic studies. *Am J Obstet Gynecol.* 1980;137(3):327–331.

2. Hadfield RM, Mardon HJ, Barlow DH, Kennedy SH. Endometriosis in monozygotic twins. *Fertil Steril.* 1997;68(5):941–942.

3. Hediger ML, Hartnett HJ, Louis GM Association of endometriosis with body size and figure. *Fertil Steril.* 2005;84(5):1366–1374.

4. Sangi-Haghpeykar H, Poindexter AN III. Epidemiology of endometriosis among parous women. *Obstet Gynecol.* 1995; 85(6):983–992.

5. Houston DE. Evidence for the risk of pelvic endometriosis by age, race and socioeconomic status. *Epidemiol Rev.* 1984;6:167–191.

6. Olive DL, Henderson DY. Endometriosis and mullerian anomalies. *Obstet Gynecol.* 1987;69(3 Pt 1):412–415.

Symptoms/Diagnosis

Symptoms of endometriosis vary in intensity, confounding attempts at diagnosis. Cyclic severe dysmenorrhea may be the most common presenting symptom but chronic pelvic pain, dyspareunia, delayed fertility, and abnormal bleeding can also be associated with endometriosis (Kennedy et al. 2005; Sinaii et al. 2008). Overlapping symptoms such as cyclic bowel and bladder symptoms, and sharp pelvic pain can complicate the differentiation of endometriosis from irritable bowel syndrome, inflammatory bowel disease, interstitial cystitis, and pelvic inflammatory disease (Husby et al. 2003).

Pain from endometriosis appears to arise from release of proinflammatory substances such as cytokines and prostaglandins as well as direct infiltration of local nerves (Harada et al. 2001; Lebovic et al. 2001; Ryan et al. 1995; Van Langendonckt et al. 2002).

Though certain physical examination findings can be suggestive of endometriosis, the physical examination is often entirely unremarkable (Vercellini et al. 1996) (Table 18.4). Radiologic imaging is generally not sensitive enough to detect endometriosis unless an endometrioma is present on one or both ovaries (Abrao et al. 2007; Guerriero et al. 1996; Kinkel et al. 2006; Moore et al. 2002).

Definitive diagnosis is made by biopsy at laparoscopy (Stratton et al. 2002; Walter et al. 2001). Sensitivity and accuracy of diagnosis at the time of laparoscopy depends on the experience and diligence of the surgeon. Implants can be subtle and variable in appearance. They can hide behind ovaries and other structures or under the peritoneal surface, or involve less obvious locations such as the surface of the appendix (Gustofson et al. 2006). Careful surveillance and multiple biopsies increase the rate of detection (Wykes et al. 2004). If extensive implants are visible, diagnosis by photography and biopsy can be straightforward and conclusive (Marchino et al. 2005). Despite careful evaluation, the extent of findings at laparoscopy does not always correlate well with

Table 18.4. Physical Examination Findings in Endometriosis

Adnexal mass

Fixed, retroverted uterus

Nodularity of uterosacral ligaments, rectovaginal septum, or posterior cul-de-sac

Shortening of cardinal ligament

Pain with palpation of uterus, cul-de-sac, or uterosacral ligaments the magnitude of the patient's symptoms or chances for fertility (Fedele et al. 1990).

Psychological Effects

Endometriosis can have a dramatic effect on a woman's well-being. Aside from the impact of cyclic or chronic pelvic pain, sexual relationships and enjoyment can also be affected by deep dyspareunia. In addition, approximately 30%–50% of patients with endometriosis may have difficulty conceiving (Winkel 2003). These difficulties can affect a woman's sense of wholeness and her ability to cope with stress, resulting in increased rates of depression (Lorencatto et al. 2006).

Management

Management of endometriosis focuses on both the reduction of symptoms and improvement in the quality of life. These approaches may also minimize the extent of disease.

MEDICAL INTERVENTION

Medical management of endometriosis offers a variety of options for treatment. Nonsteroid anti-inflammatory drugs (NSAIDs) are often the first-line therapy for dysmenorrhea (Allen et al. 2005). Hormonal treatments can be offered to those not currently seeking pregnancy. Most commonly, OCs are used in either a cyclic or continuous fashion. They induce a progestin-dominant hormonal state that causes decidualization and atrophy of endometrial tissue. OCs are more effective in reducing dysmenorrhea than dyspareunia (Harada et al. 2008; Winkel 2003).

Other sources of progestins can have a similar effect with varying side effect profiles. Oral progestins such as medroxyprogesterone and norethindrone have been used continuously for suppression of endometriosis with good success (Prentice et al. 2000). Injectable depot medroxyprogesterone acetate (DMPA or DepoProvera) reduced dysmenorrhea and pelvic pain significantly in one study (Crosignani et al. 2006). Several studies now also point to the successful use of the levonorgestrel IUD for reduction of pelvic pain and dysmenorrhea (Lockhat et al. 2005; Petta et al. 2005; Vercellini et al. 1999, 2003).

Danazol is another oral agent used with great success for suppression of symptoms associated with endometriosis. Its use in recent years has decreased

I have found that the Mirena levonorgestrel IUD is invaluable in women looking for long-term relief from dysmenorrhea who are not interested in hysterectomy. It is equally effective in cases of primary dysmenorrhea, endometriosis, and adenomyosis, thus avoiding the need for laparoscopy if the IUD gives relief. The Mirena can simply be replaced every 5 years until the woman is menopausal.

due to its extensive side effect profile, including hirsutism, acne, weight gain, and depression (Selak et al. 2007).

Gonadotropin-releasing hormone (GnRH) agonists have become the mainstay of medical therapy for patients with moderate to severe pain. The medication induces a hypoestrogenic state, mimicking menopause. The removal of estrogenic stimulation then induces atrophy of active endometriosis lesions (Ling 1999; Prentice et al. 2000). A 6-month course of intramuscular or intranasal therapy can lead to 85%–100% improvement in symptoms (Winkel and Scialli 2001). The side effects of the medication also mimic menopause (hot flashes, vaginal dryness, bone loss) and are eliminated by hormonal "add-back" therapy without loss in GnRH efficacy (Surrey 1999).

Newer medications used in endometriosis therapy include progesterone antagonists, selective progesterone receptor modulators, and aromatase inhibitors (Prentice et al. 2000). All are being used effectively in early pilot studies (Attar and Bulun 2006; Chwalisz et al. 2005; Patwardhan et al. 2008). Ovarian suppression with GnRH agonists should be considered when using aromatase inhibitors due to their potential for causing development of painful ovarian cysts in ovulatory women (Remorgida et al. 2007).

SURGICAL MANAGEMENT

Surgical management allows definitive diagnosis but also incurs surgical risk. It is often the preferred path of therapy for those wishing to conceive as soon as possible, since the medical therapies either preclude or are contraindicated in pregnancy. Surgery can be definitive or conservative. Definitive surgery involves hysterectomy with or without removal of the ovaries. This route is often pursued by women with severe unrelenting disease who do not wish future childbearing. In most instances, hysterectomy should be discouraged in young women who may later choose to have children (MacDonald et al. 1999). Recurrence of endometriosis is rare after hysterectomy (Namnoum et al. 1995).

Conservative surgery usually involves laparoscopy to investigate the pelvis and treat as much of the endometriosis as possible while leaving the pelvic organs in place (Crosignani et al. 1996). Endometriosis lesions can be excised sharply or ablated with laser or electrosurgery. The extent of treatment can be limited by the proximity of implants to important pelvic structures such as ureters and pelvic vessels and nerves.

When present, endometriomas may require only excision of the cyst or partial/total oophorectomy. Interruption of the presacral or uterosacral nerve pathways at the time of laparoscopy has not been found to increase the success rate after surgery (Proctor et al. 2005). Follow-up after conservative surgery suggests good short-term relief at 6 months but significant recurrence of symptoms at 1–2 years (Sutton et al. 1994; Jacobson et al. 2001). A significant number of women will require repeat surgery over time (Shakiba et al. 2008). Postoperative therapy with GnRH agonists or levonorgestrel IUD appears to delay recurrence of symptoms (Hornstein et al. 1997; Vercellini et al. 2003).

Integrative Approaches

Integrative approaches to endometriosis often focus on reducing the inflammatory response that fosters the pain experienced by the patient as well as moderating the psychological and emotional stress engendered by chronic pain.

As in other areas of medicine, one of the primary areas of emphasis should be education about the role of the anti-inflammatory diet. Simple interventions such as reducing intake of processed foods and red meat and increasing intake of fresh fruits, green vegetables, and omega-3 fatty acids can help ameliorate a patient's symptoms (Fjerbaek and Knudsen 2007; Fugh-Berman and Kronenberg 2003; Parazzini et al. 2004). For more information on the anti-inflammatory diet, see Chapter 3 on nutrition in women's health.

The experience of pain and dysmenorrhea has a significant effect on a woman's psychological and emotional well-being. Similarly, significant social stressors and weak social networks can aggravate the intensity of dysmenorrhea (Alonso and Coe 2001). Mind–body techniques such as mindfulness-based stress reduction, cognitive behavioral therapy, hypnosis, guided imagery, and biofeedback have been used for decades to reduce stress and increase coping skills. Research on the use of these techniques for the management of different types of chronic pain is ongoing and the results have been mixed (Astin 2004). Symptoms of dysmenorrhea and pelvic pain may be reduced with these behavioral interventions, which can reduce the body's responsiveness to the stress of pain (Proctor et al. 2007). In the setting of endometriosis, these techniques offer the woman a measure of self-control as she learns to cope with her symptoms. The ability to relax, to alleviate accumulated stress, and to allay anxiety can be powerful tools while other interventions begin to take effect. The woman

> Patients with chronic pain often develop a panicky response to each episode of pain or to new stimuli such a pelvic examination. Teaching them coping skills such as breathing exercises or imagery can help them weather each experience with less fear and tension.

may feel more whole when she gains more control over her body's response to stress.

Chronic tension in the muscles of the abdomen, legs, and pelvic floor may result from years of conditioned response to pelvic pain. Regular exercise can decrease the amount of pain experienced (Fugh-Berman and Kronenberg 2003). Stretching and yoga may increase the patient's day-to-day functioning and sense of well-being. Targeted pelvic floor physical therapy with a specially trained therapist can reduce pain scores, especially in chronic pelvic pain and dyspareunia. Massage can also be a relaxing adjunctive therapy. There are no clinical trials of the use of these modalities with endometriosis. Research on frequently utilized spinal manipulation techniques has not been shown to be effective in cases of primary or secondary dysmenorrhea (Proctor et al. 2006).

> In patients who have years of pelvic pain due to endometriosis, pain may persist after effective treatment due to "trigger points" or "knots" in the muscles of the abdominal wall due to years of guarding against the pain. I have found that these patients are often best served with a referral to a skilled physical therapist with specialized training in techniques focused on the pelvis. Other excellent referral options include experienced acupuncturists or practitioners skilled in manual interventions such as the counterstrain technique.

Acupuncture has been posited as a possible effective treatment for endometriosis-related pelvic pain and dysmenorrhea due to its descending pain inhibition and possible reduction in cytokine release (Lundeberg and Lund 2008; Wayne et al. 2008). At this time, no large studies have been completed to examine this treatment approach. Two small pilot studies suggest that acupuncture may be a safe, well-accepted and possible effective treatment for endometriosis in adolescents (Highfield et al. 2006; Wayne et al. 2008). Several other smaller studies have focused on the relief of dysmenorrhea not specific to endometriosis. These have found that acupuncture reduces the intensity of both dysmenorrhea up to 6 months after treatment, although secondary dysmenorrhea may be less responsive than primary (Helms 1987; Iorno et al. 2008; Witt et al. 2008).

Botanical therapies have been used for centuries to reduce pain in the pelvis as well as elsewhere in the body. Studies suggest that these herbs and their multiple constituent bioactive compounds may work through COX-2 inhibition, suppression of cytokines, antioxidant effects, and direct sedative and antinociceptive properties (Wieser et al. 2007) (Table 18.5).

Table 18.5. Medicinal Herbs and Natural Compounds Used in the Treatment of Endometriosis and Their Anti-inflammatory Effects

| Herbs | Antiproliferative | Antinociceptive, Sedative | Anti-inflammatory Action | | |
| | | | Antioxidant | Suppression | |
				COX-2	Cytokines	NF-KappaB
Bupleurum	+				+	+
Chinese angelica	+	+	+		+	
Dahurian angelica root	+	+		+	+	+
Cattail pollen					+	
Cinnamon twigs		+		+		
Cnidium fruit	+	+				
Corydalis		+			+	
Curcuma (turmeric)	+	+	+	+	+	+
Cyperus	+		+			
Frankincense	+	+			+	+
Licorice root	+	+		+	+	+

(continued)

Herbs	Antiproliferative	Antinociceptive, Sedative	Anti-inflammatory Action			
			Antioxidant	Suppression		
				COX-2	Cytokines	NF-KappaB
Myrrh		+	+		+	
Persica					+	
Poria	+	+		+	+	
Red peony root			+			
Rhubarb	+	+			+	+
Salvia root		+	+			+
Scutellaria	+			+	+	
Sparganium		+			+	
Tortoise shell						+
White peony root				+	+	

Source: Wieser F, Cohen M, Gaeddert A, et al. Evolution of medical treatment for endometriosis: back to the roots? *Hum Reprod Update*. 2007;13(5):487–499, by permission of Oxford University Press.

At this time, there are few high-quality evidence-based studies that examine the efficacy, side effects, and interactions of these medicinal herbal compounds in women, although protocols are currently underway (Flower et al. 2007; Zhu et al. 2008). Commonly used herbs with a benign safety profile include chaste tree berry, black cohosh, black haw, cramp bark, dong quai, and ginger. No studies exist to assess their efficacy in endometriosis and dysmenorrhea (Low Dog and Micozzi 2005) (Table 18.6).

Small studies have evaluated pycnogenol and the traditional Japanese herbal formula Toki-shakuyaku-san and found them to be helpful in reducing dysmenorrhea (Kohama et al. 2007; Suzuki et al. 2008; Tanaka 2003). Traditional Chinese medicine has used many herbal compounds alone and in combination to battle dysmenorrhea through a reduction of Qi stasis in the liver (Table 18.7).

Early research data on these compounds exists in a few Chinese language studies (Jia et al. 2006). The primary side effects of these compounds seem to be interaction with anticoagulant medications (Wieser et al. 2007).

Table 18.6. Commonly Used Herbs

Common Name	Scientific Name	Effect	Side Effects	Contraindications
Chaste tree berry	Vitex agnus castus	Enhances progesterone activity/binding		
Black cohosh	Cimicifuga racemosa	Antispasmodic, Anti-inflammatory		Pregnancy, lactation
Black haw	Viburnum prunifolium	Uterine relaxant		Active oxalate-containing kidney stones
Cramp bark	Viburnum opulus	Uterine Relaxant		
Dong quai	Angelica sinensis	Uterine relaxation and stimulation, anti-inflammatory, analgesic	Prolongation of prothrombin time	Pregnancy, warfarin use
Ginger	Zingiber officinale	antispasmodic		Active gallstone disease
Kava	Piper methysticum	Muscle relaxant, sedative	CNS depression, possible hepatotoxicity	Pregnancy, lactation, depression
Pulsatilla	Anemone pulsatilla	Antispasmodic, sedative, analgesic		Pregnancy, lactation
Cotton root bark	Gossypium spp.	Atrophy of endometrial tissue (possibly antiprogestational)	Hypokalemia	Pregnancy, lactation
Yellow vine	Tripterygium wilfordii	Anti-inflammatory, immunosuppressive	Menstrual irregularities	Pregnancy. lactation

Source: Low Dog T, Micozzi MS. Women's Health in Complementary and Integrative Medicine: A Clinical Guide. St. Louis, MO: Elsevier Churchill Livingstone; 2005.

Table 18.7. TCM Herbs Commonly Used for Dysmenorrhea

Pharmacopia Name	Binomial Name
Caulis Sargentodoxae	*Sargentodoxa cuneata*
Cortex Cinnamomi Cassiae	*Cinnamomum cassia*
Cortex Moutan	*Paeonia suffruticosa*
Faeces Trogopterorum	*Trogopterus xanthipes* or *Pteromys volans*
Flos Carthami	*Carthamus tinctorius*
Flos Rosae Chinensis	*Rosa chinensis*
Fructus Akebiae	*Akebia quinata*
Fructus Foeniculi	*Foeniculum vulgare*
Fructus Jujubae	*Ziziphus jujuba*
Herba Leonuri and Fructus Leonuri	*Leonurus heterophyllus*
Herba Selaginellae	*Selaginella tamariscina*
Herba Lycopi	*Lycopus lucidus*
Herba Verbenae	*Verbena officinalis*
Lignum Sappan	*Lignum sappan*
Pollen Typhae	*Typha angustifolia*
Radix Angelicae Sinensis	*Angelicae sinensis*
Radix Astragali	*Astragalus membranaceus*
Radix Curcumae	*Aromaticae Curcuma aromatica*
Radix Linderae	*Lindera strychnifolia*
Radix Paeoniae Alba and Radix Paeoniae Rubra	*Paeonia veitchii and Paeoni lactiflora*
Radix Rehmanniae	*Rehmannia glutinosa*
Radix Salviae Miltiorrhizae	*Salvia miltiorrhiza*
Rhizoma Chuanxiong	*Ligusticum chuanxiong*
Rhizoma Corydalis	*Corydalis yanhusuo*
Rhizoma Curcumae Longae	*Curcuma longa*
Rhizoma Cyperi	*Cyperus rotundus*
Semen Persicae	*Prunus persica*
Semen Vaccariae	*Vaccaria segetalis*

Source: Jia W, Wang X, Xu D, et al. Common traditional Chinese medicinal herbs for dysmenorrhea. *Phytother Res.* 2006;20(10):819–24.

My approach with a woman with severe dysmenorrhea Thorough history including

- Menstrual and sexual history including age of onset of menses, age of onset of dysmenorrhea, frequency of menses, age of first coitus, pain throughout menstrual cycle, and dyspareunia
- General medical history of other inflammatory conditions, depression, and pain syndromes
- Surgical history of prior abdominal procedures
- Family history of endometriosis, fibroids, early hysterectomy
- Social history (diet, stressors)
- Current medications and supplements

Careful physical examination to evaluate for abnormalities as noted in Table 18.4.

If abnormalities of uterus or ovaries are noted on physical examination, then I will order imaging by ultrasound. Significant evidence of scarring and nodularity will prompt me to consider laparoscopy earlier in the evaluation.

Initial therapy usually involves prescription-strength NSAIDs such as Naproxen and oral contraceptives unless there is a medical contraindication to estrogen. I usually start with cyclic OCs and then move to continuous OCs after 3 months if the cyclic therapy has not been sufficient. Some patients will do well with Depo-Provera or oral norethindrone.

We also discuss the anti-inflammatory diet, stress reduction, stretching, exercise, and application of heat. Referrals for physical therapy, acupuncture or other complementary modalities are offered to the patient according to her needs and interests.

If continuous OCs do not control the patient's dysmenorrhea or if the patient declines OC therapy, we discuss laparoscopy or empiric GnRH agonist therapy.

At the time of laparoscopy, all evident lesions are ablated or excised. Postoperative suppression of endometriosis follows with continuous OCs, oral or injectable progestin, GnRH agonist injections, or levonorgestrel IUD. GnRH agonist therapy usually lasts 6 months. I use add-back with either norethindrone acetate 5 mg/day or low-dose ethinyl estradiol 1mg/norethindrone acetate 5 mg/day (femhrt Warner Chilcott). If started at the time of the first GnRH agonist injection, patients rarely experience the classic hot flashes associated with GnRH therapy.

After the 6-month course, the patient then chooses suppression with OCs, progestins, or levonorgestrel IUD long-term unless she wishes to try for pregnancy.

Most patients will have several years of relief before recurrence of symptoms.

Summary

Endometriosis is a medical condition with unclear etiology and aggravating factors. Currently, the most well-studied approaches involve surgery, nonsteroidal use, and hormonal therapies. Alternative therapies offer a less-invasive approach focused on reducing the pain associated with endometriosis implants, but, as yet, there is minimal scientific evidence to support its efficacy.

REFERENCES

Abrao MS, Gonçalves MO, Dias JA Jr, Podgaec S, Chamie LP, Blasbalg R. Comparison between clinical examination, transvaginal sonography and magnetic resonance imaging for the diagnosis of deep endometriosis. *Hum Reprod.* 2007;22(12):3092–3097.

Allen C, Hopewell S, Prentice A, Gregory D. Non-steroidal anti-inflammatory drugs for pain in women with endometriosis. *Cochrane Database Syst Rev.* 2005;(4):CD004753.

Alonso C, Coe CL. Disruptions of social relationships accentuate the association between emotional distress and menstrual pain in young women. *Health Psychol.* 2001;20(6):411–416.

Astin JA. Mind-body therapies for the management of pain. *Clin J Pain.* 2004;20(1):27–32.

Attar E, Bulun SE. Aromatase inhibitors: the next generation of therapeutics for endometriosis? *Fertil Steril.* 2006;85(5):1307–1318.

Chatman, DL, Ward AB. (1982). Endometriosis in adolescents. *J Reprod Med.* 27(3):156–160.

Chwalisz K, Perez MC, Demanno D, Winkel C, Schubert G, Elger W. Selective progesterone receptor modulator development and use in the treatment of leiomyomata and endometriosis. *Endocr Rev.* 2005;26(3):423–438.

Crosignani PG, Luciano A, Ray A, Bergqvist A. Subcutaneous depot medroxyprogesterone acetate versus leuprolide acetate in the treatment of endometriosis-associated pain. *Hum Reprod.* 2006;21(1):248–256.

Crosignani PG, Vercellini P, Biffignandi F, Costantini W, Cortesi I, Imparato E. Laparoscopy versus laparotomy in conservative surgical treatment for severe endometriosis. *Fertil Steril.* 1996;66(5):706–711.

Fauconnier A, Chapron C. Endometriosis and pelvic pain: epidemiological evidence of the relationship and implications. *Hum Reprod Update.* 2005;11(6):595–606.

Fauconnier A, Chapron C, Dubuisson JB, Vieira M, Dousset B, Bréart G. Relation between pain symptoms and the anatomic location of deep infiltrating endometriosis. *Fertil Steril.* 2002;78(4):719–726.

Fedele L, Parazzini F, Bianchi S, Arcaini L, Candiani GB. Stage and localization of pelvic endometriosis and pain. *Fertil Steril.* 1990;53(1):155–158.

Fjerbaek A, Knudsen UB. Endometriosis, dysmenorrhea and diet—what is the evidence? *Eur J Obstet Gynecol Reprod Biol.* 2007;132(2):140–147.

Flower A, Lewith GT, Little P. Seeking an oracle: using the Delphi process to develop practice guidelines for the treatment of endometriosis with Chinese herbal medicine. *J Altern Complement Med.* 2007;13(9):969–976.

Foster WG, Agarwal SK. Environmental contaminants and dietary factors in endometriosis. *Ann N Y Acad Sci.* 2002;955:213–229; discussion 230–232, 396–406.

Fugh-Berman A, Kronenberg F. Complementary and alternative medicine (CAM) in reproductive-age women: a review of randomized controlled trials. *Reprod Toxicol.* 2003;17(2):137–152.

Guerriero S, Mais V, Ajossa S, Paoletti AM, Angiolucci M, Melis GB. Transvaginal ultrasonography combined with CA-125 plasma levels in the diagnosis of endometrioma. *Fertil Steril.* 1996;65(2):293–298.

Gustofson RL, Kim N, Liu S, Stratton P. Endometriosis and the appendix: a case series and comprehensive review of the literature. *Fertil Steril.* 2006;86(2):298–303.

Hadfield RM, Mardon HJ, Barlow DH, Kennedy SH. Endometriosis in monozygotic twins. *Fertil Steril.* 1997;68(5):941–942.

Harada T, Iwabe T, Terakawa N. Role of cytokines in endometriosis. *Fertil Steril.* 2001;76(1):1–10.

Harada T, Momoeda M, Taketani H, Hoshiai H, Terakawa N. Low-dose oral contraceptive pill for dysmenorrhea associated with endometriosis: a placebo-controlled, double-blind, randomized trial. *Fertil Steril.* 2008;90(5):1583–1588.

Hediger ML, Hartnett HJ, Louis GM. Association of endometriosis with body size and figure. *Fertil Steril.* 2005;84(5):1366–1374.

Helms JM. Acupuncture for the management of primary dysmenorrhea. *Obstet Gynecol.* 1987;69(1):51–56.

Highfield ES, Laufer MR, Schnyer RN, Kerr CE, Thomas P, Wayne PM. Adolescent endometriosis-related pelvic pain treated with acupuncture: two case reports. *J Altern Complement Med.* 2006;12(3):317–322.

Hornstein MD, Hemmings R, Yuzpe AA, Heinrichs WL. Use of nafarelin versus placebo after reductive laparoscopic surgery for endometriosis. *Fertil Steril.* 1997;68(5):860–864.

Houston DE. Evidence for the risk of pelvic endometriosis by age, race and socioeconomic status. *Epidemiol Rev.* 1984;6:167–191.

Husby, GK, Haugen RS, Moen MH. Diagnostic delay in women with pain and endometriosis. *Acta Obstet Gynecol Scand.* 2003;82(7):649–653.

Iorno V, Burani R, Bianchini B, Minelli E, Martinelli F, Ciatto S. Acupuncture Treatment of dysmenorrhea resistant to conventional medical treatment. *Evid Based Complement Alternat Med.* 2008;5(2):227–230.

Jacobson TZ, Barlow DH, Garry R, Koninckx P. Laparoscopic surgery for pelvic pain associated with endometriosis. *Cochrane Database Syst Rev.* 2001;(4):CD001300.

Jenkins S, Olive DL, Haney AF. Endometriosis: pathogenetic implications of the anatomic distribution. *Obstet Gynecol.* 1986;67(3):335–338.

Jia W, Wang X, Xu D, Zhao A, Zhang Y. Common traditional Chinese medicinal herbs for dysmenorrhea. *Phytother Res.* 2006;20(10):819–824.

Kennedy S, Bergqvist A, Chapron C, et al. ESHRE guideline for the diagnosis and treatment of endometriosis. *Hum Reprod.* 2005;20(10):2698–2704.

Kinkel K, Frei KA, Balleyguier C, Chapron C. Diagnosis of endometriosis with imaging: a review. *Eur Radiol.* 2006;16(2):285–298.

Kohama T, Herai K, Inoue M. Effect of French maritime pine bark extract on endometriosis as compared with leuprorelin acetate. *J Reprod Med.* 2007;52(8):703–708.

Lebovic DI, Mueller MD, Taylor RN. Immunobiology of endometriosis. *Fertil Steril.* 2001;75(1):1–10.

Ling FW. Randomized controlled trial of depot leuprolide in patients with chronic pelvic pain and clinically suspected endometriosis. Pelvic Pain Study Group. *Obstet Gynecol.* 1999;93(1):51–58.

Lockhat FB, Emembolu JO, Konje JC. The efficacy, side-effects and continuation rates in women with symptomatic endometriosis undergoing treatment with an intrauterine administered progestogen (levonorgestrel): a 3 year follow-up. *Hum Reprod.* 2005;20(3):789–793.

Lorencatto C, Petta CA, Navarro MJ, Bahamondes L, Matos A. Depression in women with endometriosis with and without chronic pelvic pain. *Acta Obstet Gynecol Scand.* 2006;85(1):88–92.

Low Dog T, Micozzi MS. *Women's Health in Complementary and Integrative Medicine: A Clinical Guide.* St. Louis, MO: Elsevier Churchill Livingstone; 2005.

Lundeberg T, Lund I. Is there a role for acupuncture in endometriosis pain, or 'endometrialgia'? *Acupunct Med.* 2008;26(2):94–110.

MacDonald SR, Klock SC, Milad MP. Long-term outcome of nonconservative surgery (hysterectomy) for endometriosis-associated pain in women <30 years old. *Am J Obstet Gynecol.* 1999;180(6 Pt 1):1360–1363.

Marchino GL, Gennarelli G, Enria R, Bongioanni F, Lipari G, Massobrio M. Diagnosis of pelvic endometriosis with use of macroscopic versus histologic findings. *Fertil Steril.* 2005;84(1):12–15.

Minaglia S, Mishell DR Jr, Ballard CA. Incisional endometriomas after Cesarean section: a case series. *J Reprod Med.* 2007;52(7):630–634.

Missmer SA, Hankinson SE, et al. (2004). Incidence of laparoscopically confirmed endometriosis by demographic, anthropometric, and lifestyle factors. *Am J Epidemiol.* 160(8):784–796.

Moore J, Copley S, Morris J, Lindsell D, Golding S, Kennedy S. A systematic review of the accuracy of ultrasound in the diagnosis of endometriosis. *Ultrasound Obstet Gynecol.* 2002;20(6):630–634.

Namnoum AB, Hickman TN, Goodman SB, Gehlbach DL, Rock JA. Incidence of symptom recurrence after hysterectomy for endometriosis. *Fertil Steril.* 1995;64(5):898–902.

Olive, DL, Henderson DY. Endometriosis and mullerian anomalies. *Obstet Gynecol.* 1987;69(3 Pt 1):412–415.

Parazzini F, Chiaffarino F, Surace M, et al. Selected food intake and risk of endometriosis. *Hum Reprod.* 2004;19(8):1755–1759.

Patwardhan S, Nawathe A, et al. Systematic review of the effects of aromatase inhibitors on pain associated with endometriosis. *BJOG*. 2008;115(7):818–822.

Petta CA, Ferriani RA, Abrao MS, et al. Randomized clinical trial of a levonorgestrel-releasing intrauterine system and a depot GnRH analogue for the treatment of chronic pelvic pain in women with endometriosis. *Hum Reprod*. 2005;20(7):1993–1998.

Prentice A, Deary AJ, Bland E. Progestagens and anti-progestagens for pain associated with endometriosis. *Cochrane Database Syst Rev*. 2000;(2):CD002122.

Prentice A, Deary AJ, et al. Gonadotrophin-releasing hormone analogues for pain associated with endometriosis. *Cochrane Database Syst Rev*. 2000;(2):CD000346.

Proctor ML, Hing W, Johnson TC, Murphy PA. Spinal manipulation for primary and secondary dysmenorrhoea. *Cochrane Database Syst Rev*. 2006;3:CD002119.

Proctor ML, Latthe PM, Farquhar CM, Khan KS, Johnson NP. Surgical interruption of pelvic nerve pathways for primary and secondary dysmenorrhoea. *Cochrane Database Syst Rev*. 2005;(4):CD001896.

Proctor ML, Murphy PA, Pattison HM, Suckling J, Farquhar CM. Behavioural interventions for primary and secondary dysmenorrhoea. *Cochrane Database Syst Rev*. 2007;(3):CD002248.

Remorgida V, Abbamonte LH, Ragni N, Fulcheri E, Ferrero S. Letrozole and desogestrel-only contraceptive pill for the treatment of stage IV endometriosis. *Aust N Z J Obstet Gynaecol*. 2007;47(3):222–225.

Ryan IP, Tseng JF, Schriock ED, Khorram O, Landers DV, Taylor RN. Interleukin-8 concentrations are elevated in peritoneal fluid of women with endometriosis. *Fertil Steril*. 1995;63(4):929–932.

Sangi-Haghpeykar H, Poindexter AN III. Epidemiology of endometriosis among parous women. *Obstet Gynecol*. 1995;85(6):983–992.

Schenken RS. *Endometriosis: Contemporary Concepts in Clinical Management*. Philadelphia, PA: Lippincott; 1989.

Selak V, Farquhar C, Prentice A, Singla A. Danazol for pelvic pain associated with endometriosis. *Cochrane Database Syst Rev*. 2007;(4):CD000068.

Shakiba K, Bena JF, McGill KM, Minger J, Falcone T. Surgical treatment of endometriosis: a 7-year follow-up on the requirement for further surgery. *Obstet Gynecol*. 2008;111(6):1285–1292.

Simpson JL, Elias S, Malinak LR, Buttram VC Jr. Heritable aspects of endometriosis. I. Genetic studies. *Am J Obstet Gynecol*. 1980;137(3):327–331.

Sinaii N, Cleary SD, Ballweg ML, Nieman LK, Stratton P. High rates of autoimmune and endocrine disorders, fibromyalgia, chronic fatigue syndrome and atopic diseases among women with endometriosis: a survey analysis. *Hum Reprod*. 2002;17(10):2715–2724.

Sinaii N, Plumb K, Cotton L, et al. Differences in characteristics among 1,000 women with endometriosis based on extent of disease. *Fertil Steril*. 2008;89(3):538–545.

Stratton P, Winkel CA, Sinaii N, Merino MJ, Zimmer C, Nieman LK. Location, color, size, depth, and volume may predict endometriosis in lesions resected at surgery. *Fertil Steril*. 2002;78(4):743–749.

Surrey ES. Add-back therapy and gonadotropin-releasing hormone agonists in the treatment of patients with endometriosis: can a consensus be reached? Add-Back Consensus Working Group. *Fertil Steril*. 1999;71(3):420–424.

Sutton CJ, Ewen SP, Whitelaw N, Haines P. Prospective, randomized, double-blind, controlled trial of laser laparoscopy in the treatment of pelvic pain associated with minimal, mild, and moderate endometriosis. *Fertil Steril*. 1994;62(4):696–700.

Suzuki NK, Uebaba K, Kohama T, Moniwa N, Kanayama N, Koike K. French maritime pine bark extract significantly lowers the requirement for analgesic medication in dysmenorrhea: a multicenter, randomized, double-blind, placebo-controlled study. *J Reprod Med*. 2008;53(5):338–346.

Tanaka T. A novel anti-dysmenorrhea therapy with cyclic administration of two Japanese herbal medicines. *Clin Exp Obstet Gynecol*. 2003;30(2–3):95–98.

Van Langendonckt A, Casanas-Roux F, Donnez J. Oxidative stress and peritoneal endometriosis. *Fertil Steril*. 2002;77(5):861–870.

Vercellini P, Aimi G, Panazza S, De Giorgi O, Pesole A, Crosignani PG. A levonorgestrel-releasing intrauterine system for the treatment of dysmenorrhea associated with endometriosis: a pilot study. *Fertil Steril*. 1999;72(3):505–508.

Vercellini P, Frontino G, De Giorgi O, Aimi G, Zaina B, Crosignani PG. Comparison of a levonorgestrel-releasing intrauterine device versus expectant management after conservative surgery for symptomatic endometriosis: a pilot study. *Fertil Steril*. 2003;80(2):305–309.

Vercellini P, Trespidi L, De Giorgi O, Cortesi I, Parazzini F, Crosignani PG. Endometriosis and pelvic pain: relation to disease stage and localization. *Fertil Steril*. 1996;65(2):299–304.

Walter AJ, Hentz JG, Magtibay PM, Cornella JL, Magrina JF. Endometriosis: correlation between histologic and visual findings at laparoscopy. *Am J Obstet Gynecol*. 2001;184(7):1407–1411; discussion 1411–1413.

Wayne PM, Kerr CE, Schnyer RN, et al. Japanese-style acupuncture for endometriosis-related pelvic pain in adolescents and young women: results of a randomized sham-controlled trial. *J Pediatr Adolesc Gynecol*. 2008;21(5):247–257.

Wieser F, Cohen M, Gaeddert A, et al. Evolution of medical treatment for endometriosis: back to the roots? *Hum Reprod Update*. 2007;13(5):487–499.

Winkel CA. Evaluation and management of women with endometriosis. *Obstet Gynecol*. 2003;102(2):397–408.

Winkel CA, Scialli AR. Medical and surgical therapies for pain associated with endometriosis. *J Womens Health Gend Based Med*. 2001;10(2):137–162.

Witt CM, Reinhold T, Brinkhaus B, Roll S, Jena S, Willich SN. Acupuncture in patients with dysmenorrhea: a randomized study on clinical effectiveness and cost-effectiveness in usual care. *Am J Obstet Gynecol*. 2008;198(2):166 e1–8.

Wykes CB, Clark TJ, Khan KS. Accuracy of laparoscopy in the diagnosis of endometriosis: a systematic quantitative review. *BJOG*. 2004;111(11):1204–1212.

Zhu X, Proctor M, Bensoussan A, Smith CA, Wu E. Chinese herbal medicine for primary dysmenorrhoea. *Cochrane Database Syst Rev*. 2008;(2):CD005288.

19

Chronic Pelvic Pain

BETTINA HERBERT

C hronic pelvic pain (CPP), the subject of whispered complaints and misplaced shame, diminishes the quality of life and overall well-being for almost one in four women (Zondervan et al. 1999). It is the second most common gynecological complaint and accounts for 13%–20% of gynecological consultations and up to 52% of diagnostic laparoscopy (Ghaly and Chien 2000).

The "disease with 20 names" has many, often overlapping, physical, functional, and psychological etiologies (Hahn 2001). It can be challenging to elucidate the pain generators (Anderson 2006). For many women, despite enduring multiple interrogations and procedures, there will be no definitive diagnosis (Mathias et al. 1996). Often symptom relief, rather than resolution, is the treatment goal. After a brief respite, pain may return, treatment side effects may become intolerable, and the woman is forced back into the medical maze—or to resign herself to living her life in pain (McGowan et al. 2007).

This is not a comprehensive overview of CPP. Rather it is a look at the difficult journeys of three women that illustrate, in part, the oft-overlooked role of nonphysiologic changes in body mechanics impacting somatic structures (muscle, fascia, ligament, tendon). Such imbalances can, over time, be the cause of considerable pain and discomfort; the effects can multiply as the body accumulates layers of compensation. The result may be hard to identify and treat unless malalignment or somatic dysfunction is included in the differential diagnosis.

Another often under-deduced contributor to chronic pain is past or present abuse: physical, sexual, and emotional, including neglect. This is by far the most delicate part of a patient's history to explore and yet, it may be as important to address as the physiologic changes. In fact, abuse can impact physiology and anatomy through the effects of a chronically overactive, hypervigilant sympathetic nervous system (Van der Kolk 1994).

Perhaps these additional approaches, or others they inspire, can expand our diagnostic and therapeutic options and help diminish the disappointment and inadequacy we experience when we are unable to ease our patients' suffering. The third case is presented in significantly more detail than the first two as it covers more ground, in prevalence, time, and complexity.

Case Study I

DYSMENORRHEA: IT'S JUST A SPRAINED ANKLE

Pamela's gynecologist referred her for recent onset dysmenorrhea. Up until 8 months prior, she had been free of premenstrual and menstrual morbidities. At age 38, her cramps became so severe that she started to miss work. Lab results and imaging studies failed to reveal any abnormalities. A detailed history that included questions about trauma and injury uncovered a traumatic sprained ankle about 18 months prior. It had taken weeks to heal; the only therapy had been ice and rest.

Physical examination revealed tenderness at both sacroiliac joints. The ankle had normal range of motion and no residual talofibular ligamentous laxity. A twitch response in the inferior rectus abdominis identified a trigger point. Osteopathic palpatory diagnosis revealed tenderness at the superior aspect of the pubic symphysis and a "listening" (restriction) of the right broad and round ligaments.

Utilizing osteopathic manipulative treatment (OMT) and viscerofascial techniques, Pamela was treated three times over 6 weeks for alignment of the pelvic bowl and sacrum, rebalancing the pelvic floor muscles and pelvic organs using external maneuvers. A short course of physical therapy corrected a lack of proprioception at the ankle (common after sprains and a source of chronic reinjury), and Pamela's dysmenorrhea was resolved.

Discussion

Malalignment of anatomical structures can have a dramatic effect on physiology (Korr 1997; Schamberger 2002). Once there is a disruption in the biomechanical relationships within the body, all surrounding and supported structures compensate (Alexander 2006). Changes include asymmetries in muscle length, power, and weight-bearing and can affect circulation and neurophysiology as well as entire organ systems (Prendergast and Weiss 2003).

In Pamela's case, the ankle was abruptly inverted past its physiologic limit, transmitting a traumatic force through the femur to the pelvic floor muscles, pelvis, and fascia (sidebar). The resulting malalignment affected not only the connective tissue and organs, but also the circulatory and neural elements within the connective tissue (Smutney 1997). The "ligaments" of the pelvis, unlike most in the body, contain blood vessels and nerves, therefore acting more like mesenteries. Over time and amplified by many movements, somatic dysfunction (sidebar) developed. Untreated, this positive feedback cycle could also, over time, impact autonomic innervation as well as induce vasoconstriction and visceral spasm with a concomitant slowing of venolymphatic flow (Barral 1993). The "ripple effect" can transmit even further and often leads to a reorganization of structures that results in pain far removed in time and location from the initial injury.

Musculoskeletal dysfunction can affect internal organs that are innervated at the same spinal cord segment (Holtzman et al. 2008). Similarly, visceral afferents can create somatic dysfunction (Kuchera and Kuchera 1994a) that may also include active trigger points that are often present in women with CPP, irrespective of the presence or type of the underlying pathology (Ling and Slocumb 1993). They may be of autonomic reflexive origin or the result of muscles being either too long or too short. While treatment with injection (Slocumb 1984), dry needling and OMT such as positional release and muscle energy is very useful (Kuchera and Kuchera 1994b; Travell and Simons 1983, 1992; Holtzman 2008), sometimes it does not result in permanent relief. Both structural and visceral elements need to be evaluated.

> *Fascia*—More than just fibroelastic connective tissue, fascia is a mobius strip in the body. The fibers of supportive structures, such as ligaments and tendons, peritonea and pleura, periosteum and dura, interdigitate with each other, forming a continuous web throughout the body. Thus a disruption in one area can affect not only immediately surrounding structures, but also those distal (Brous 1997).

> *Somatic dysfunction*: Impaired or altered function of related components of the somatic (body framework) system: skeletal, arthrodial, and myofascial structures as well as related vascular, lymphatic, and neural elements. Somatic dysfunction is identified using: tissue texture abnormality (effusions, laxity, stability, tone of soft tissue); asymmetry (misalignment, defects, masses, crepitation); and restriction of motion. Often there is a fourth criterion: tenderness. The mnemonic is TART.

These are diagnosed using observation, e.g., shoulder height discrepancy (Schiowitz 1997), and skilled palpation—a tension in muscles, ligaments, fascia, and other connective tissue. The abnormal feel of tissue is often due to muscle hypertonicity, second to increased alpha motor neuron stimulation. The altered activity of skin may be due to altered pilomotor, vasomotor, and sudomotor functions under the control of the sympathetic nervous system.

ICD-9 codes for somatic dysfunction are separated into 10 anatomic regions including abdomen, pelvis, cervical spine, etc.

Case Study II

POSTPARTUM PAIN AND STRESS INCONTINENCE—BUT THE BONE SCAN WAS NEGATIVE!

Since the birth of her son 6 months prior, Susie continued to have low back and pelvic pain. She had experienced an uneventful pregnancy and delivery with some mild low back pain after the 32nd week. Raising a leg to get her son strapped into his car seat, getting dressed, and climbing stairs hurt the most. Her pain was 5/10, with climbing stairs being "just about unbearable." Clearly upset, Susie also reported ongoing stress incontinence and a mood that grew darker daily. She was increasingly distraught about the future, about not being able to keep up with her son when he started crawling and walking. No significant stressors or contributory past traumas were elicited.

Imaging: Lumbar spine and pelvic X-rays were unremarkable; bone scan, normal.

Physical examination revealed tenderness to palpation at the right quadratus lumborum, anterior inferior iliac spine, posterior superior iliac spine, and ischial tuberosity and decreased one-legged balance. Osteopathic examination revealed tenderness at the symphysis pubis and asymmetry of the pubic tubercles (left tubercle cephalad). Sacral sulci were asymmetric. The left medial umbilical ligament was shortened and a restriction noted over the right pubovesicular (PV) ligament. After reassurance and explaining what had happened and the treatment approach, Susie was treated using OMT myofascial techniques including musle energy that utilized adductor activation while realigning the pubic tubercles. The inguinal ligament was gently released; sacral torsion was treated using a balanced ligamentous tension approach.

To address the stress incontinence, the left medial umbilical ligament was restored to normal length using external viscero-fascial manipulation. Tension over the right PV ligament had already resolved. Finally, a short course of acupuncture helped release any remaining muscle tension as well as help restore Susie's normally sunny disposition. In short order, she was back to celebrating and giving a mother's special love.

Discussion

Somatic dysfunction frequently occurs in the context of normal imaging. While there was no disruption of the symphysis pubis and despite the absence of radiological evidence of osteitis pubis, there were both connective tissue and myofascial pain generators (Costello 1998).

The body may not regain its previous physiologic relationships after the profound changes of pregnancy (Tettambel 2005). In this case, nonphysiologic alignment affected the symphysis pubis—and therefore the pelvic bowl—as well as suspensory structures of the bladder. The slight change in the fibro-cartilaginous pubic symphysis altered the muscle length and power of certain hip flexors that, in turn, exacerbated the already irritated symphysis. This relatively small deviation also affected the alignment of the sacrum between the ilia (Lee 2004). Each step over the past 6 months had increased the discomfort and inflammation and, reinforced the altered, painful alignment of structures.

Stress incontinence may affect up to 10% of women at 3 months postpartum (Torrisi et al. 2007). In this case, the shortened medial umbilical ligament plus the pelvic floor disruption lessened the acute angle of the bladder neck, leading to decreased inhibition of urine flow during valsalva maneuvers. Realigning both specific cystic fascia as well as the supporting structures of the pelvis resolved the stress incontinence (Barral 1993).

Visceral dysfunction from many etiologies—childbirth, surgery, infection and trauma (both physical and emotional)—can affect the soma (Nelson 2007a, 2007b, 2007c, 2007d). Adding this approach to a treatment plan has helped relieve many chronic pelvic pain syndromes (Barral and Mercier 1988).

Case Study III

THE INVISIBLE PANDEMIC—ABUSE

CAN I TRUST YOU?

Katherine had suffered for 30 years with debilitating back and right leg pain and ulcerative colitis. She had broken several vertebrae in two severe automobile crashes, often lost her balance and fell, sometimes from spinal "lightning strikes." Despite this, Katherine had excelled in an international career, combating the pain until finally, at 52, she could no longer work.

Imaging: CT—old anterior-posterior compression fracture of pelvis; complex fracture posterior pelvis; flexion/distraction fractures T5–T8; transverse process fractures L2–L5.

Physical examination revealed a thin woman with kyphosis, missing spinous processes of T5–T8 with numerous well-healed scars over her entire body. The right anterior superior iliac spine was painful to palpation and her right iliopsoas was in spasm. She demonstrated decreased one-legged balance, no right great toe or ankle proprioception, and right-sided myoclonic jerks.

Despite the CT findings and somatic guarding of her pelvis, Katherine complained only of leg and spine pain. Although it was clear that she had pelvic pain, her wishes were respected and her pelvis was treated only indirectly (from surrounding areas), until the time she could say more.

After 6 months of weekly treatment yielding steady but slow progress, one day Katherine was unable to lie on the treatment table, arching her pelvis into the air. Looking away, she hesitatingly confessed to previously unspoken of pain "shooting from the right hip across to my left," that today was "louder than the beast in my spine."

Several months earlier, well into the therapy—work she had agreed could be lengthy due to the complex nature of her injuries—to questions about trauma (physical, emotional, sexual, and spiritual) and, other than the vehicle crashes, had been negative on all counts. It was not until that day she described the childhood beatings and vertebrae broken long before her accidents.

With Katherine's consent and her psychologist's active involvement, monthly 4-handed sessions were added using somatoemotional release (SER) (a body-centered therapy for uncovering and resolving residual effects of trauma) to address the pelvic pain. In that "understanding, safe room" she was able to allow images and associations to develop with gentle palpation, positional support and a few open-ended questions at appropriate times.

The sessions allowed a controlled, safe return to key traumatic events. Skilled palpation revealed parts of her body that were "holding"—the expression of the sentient overload of her tissue. With the subtle pressure of "listening" hands, Katherine began to revisit certain traumas, the effects of which were stored in her body. Unfortunately, it came as no surprise that she had been a victim of severe emotional and sexual abuse, as well as relentless beatings. Based on her physical expression and dramatic body movements, the nonverbal periods took her to a hell where only brutality had existed. Often her body was just silently supported as it moved seemingly of its own volition into various postures.

During the third SER session, a child's tremulous voice emerged during Katherine's semitrance state asking, "Can I trust you?" She was greeted, and told, "I can't answer that. You will have to decide for yourself." One month later she returned, identifying herself as Katherine's inner healer who had decided she could trust and, proceeded to guide both the therapy and her healing. That dialogue blossomed over the ensuing sessions into the purest expression of inner healer, patient and physician working in partnership.

At first, Katherine could only access this innate healing knowledge during the sessions. As her inner healer grew stronger and matured, Katherine started being able to "hear" her without going into a trance-like state. In this way, she learned self-care that had not been demonstrated in her childhood. Gradually she made significant lifestyle changes: terminated an abusive relationship, started an anti-inflammatory diet, added supplements, botanicals, and key nutrients, and started to meditate.

Her analgesic regimen of Kadian 1800 mg/day and Valium 10 mg three times daily changed to buprenorphine 28 mg/day in divided doses with devil's claw (*Harpagophytum procumbens*) (Low Dog 2008), as well as hops (*Humulus lupulus*) and wild yam (*Dioscorea villosa*) for the cramping of her ulcerative colitis. Valerian (*Valeriana officinalis*), passionflower (*Passiflora incarnata*), kava kava (*Piper methysticum*) (Pittler and Ernst 2003), and ashwaghanda (*Withania somniferum*) were also added. As her pain subsided, so did her myoclonic jerks.

Other providers added to her team included an endocrinologist for the hormonal changes caused by long-term opioid use and the effects of chronic trauma (Heim et al. 2001), a specialist in post-traumatic stress disorder who used eye movement desensitization therapy (EMDR) and a physical therapist for balance training.

Nine months into this intensive multidisciplinary approach, Katherine started being able to access memories while wide awake and identify and lessen the effects of triggers in the environment. Over time, this ability became integrated into her conscious awareness and behavior. The "beast" in her spine and pelvis, miraculously, became an ally, a harbinger of dangerous emotions, to be heeded, not battled.

Discussion

Chronic Pain and Abuse

The Centers for Disease Control's 2005 report on Adverse Childhood Events reveals that in the general population women suffer childhood physical, sexual, and emotional abuse at rates of 27%, 24.7%, and 13.1%, respectively. In the chronic pain population, those percentages range as high as 50% (Goldberg et al. 1999; Goldberg and Goldstein 2000; Davis et al. 2005) and in chronic pelvic pain up to 64% (Fry et al. 1997; Collett et al. 1998). While abuse may or may not be causal, it can affect coping with pain and recovery (Jarrell et al. 2005). Invisible trauma such as sexual and emotional abuse may often have a direct effect on the body (Drossman et al. 1990; Lesserman 2005; Lory 2008). Concomitant depression (Goldberg 1994; Fillingim et al. 1999; Lampe et al. 2003) and anxiety along with hypervigilance (Gunter 2008), a facilitated sympathetic nervous system and alterations in the hypothalamic-pituitary-adrenal axis may contribute to the distress (Heim et al. 1998, 2001).

Eliciting and treating this level of trauma call for a primary therapeutic relationship of trust with a health care professional. For people who have been abused, trusting is difficult, betrayal always looms. Often emotional distress and not being taken seriously may lead patients to keep silent, especially during the initial visits (Price et al. 2006). It takes time, patience, and a consistently nonjudgmental demeanor to gain a patient's trust (Rubin 2005).

Studies encourage practitioners to inquire about abuse and that is often the case in clinical practice (Walker et al. 1992; Hurst et al. 2003; Read et al. 2006). However, some women would rather not be asked (Pikarinen et al. 2007). If they are in states of denial, fear, or repression (Thomas et al. 2006), one hopes to create a bond of trust and nonjudgment (shame is frequently the overarching emotion) while remaining patient.

Another option for asking about abuse might be using normalization (Lesserman 2005) to help remove the stigma, sense of isolation, and shame so many feel about a history of violence and the devastating footprint it leaves behind (Dubowitz and DePanfilis 2000). A segue to asking about abuse, therefore, might be "in about half of women with pain similar to yours, we have found that people treated them badly, sometimes years earlier, even in childhood."

Chronic pelvic pain as a pain syndrome responds to a multidisciplinary team (Peters et al. 1991; Gunter 2007) that ideally includes a mental health specialist who is willing to work openly and collaboratively (Sharp and Keefe 2005). Over 30% of women referred to a chronic pelvic pain clinic had a positive screen for PTSD (Meltzer-Brody et al. 2007). The clinician may consider some of the mind–body therapies that are useful in other pain syndromes, such as progressive relaxation, mindfulness-based stress reduction (Grossman et al. 2007), hypnosis (Axelrad et al. 2009), biofeedback, and guided imagery or approaches such as cognitive behavioral therapy (Robertson 2004) and EMDR (Bisson et al. 2007) that may be useful in PTSD as well.

Body-centered therapies such as OMT, massage, gentle chiropractic, Feldenkrais, Alexander, myofascial release (Madore and Kahn 2008), and trigger point therapy may be appropriate, as long as the practitioner is experienced and vigilant for signs of remembered or reexperienced trauma. These cases should include the active involvement of a mental health professional for addressing emotions and memories that may arise.

Nutritional changes including, at times, an elimination diet, play a key role in ameliorating both gastrointestinal as well as inflammatory contributors to CPP (Sulindro-Ma 2008; Parcell 2008). Educating the patient in ways of self-nourishment that contribute to healing can have positive effects in both physical and emotional arenas. Often a little improvement from implementing small changes, such as adding one vegetable portion daily, sipping chamomile tea, or eliminating refined sugar, can be the catalyst for embracing the long-term attitudinal changes about self-care.

Because of the intricate interweaving of abuse into every aspect of a woman's life, and the lack of high-quality evidence for targeted treatments for specific patient subgroups, the clinician needs to use great delicacy, intuition, and understanding to be able to engage the woman and embark upon a healing journey (Selfe 1998). In presenting the possibility of a psychological component, the physical reality must still be validated, or the woman who is already bathed in shame and fear, may misinterpret and blame herself. Our challenge is to gently explain how psychophysiology may affect CPP (Elliott 2004). Mind and body are a unity, despite our medical model of separate specialties (Grace 1998; Steege 1998).

What You Can Do

1. Watch how your patient walks: in the waiting room, in the hallway, paying special attention to asymmetry of pelvic movement, side-to-side, if one hip flares more than the other, or the time spent on one leg is shorter than on the other. Any of these may indicate somatic dysfunction or "guarding" of an injured area.

2. Take a full history of trauma: physical, emotional, and sexual, including neglect. Be vigilant for changes in posture, eye contact, and vocal inflection and, redirecting the question.

3. Take a careful dietary history. Sometimes food intolerances and proinflammatory foods may aggravate an existing condition. An elimination diet is an inexpensive way to test. Add antiinflammatory and anxiolytic teas, herbs, and supplements as needed.

4. Evaluate the pelvic bowl—check for asymmetry and/or tenderness (often both) at the superior aspect of the pubic symphysis or at the posterior part of the bowl, at the sacral sulci. Sometimes, there can be symmetry but tenderness on both sides of the sacrum, common after childbirth.

5. Check the posterior superior iliac spines using the Gillet, also called the stork test. A thumb on the ipsilateral PSIS should move caudad while the knee is being raised to marching position (thigh parallel to the floor). If one PSIS does not move, there is dysfunction.

6. Forge partnerships with skilled providers in mental health, mind–body, and other medical paradigms, such as acupuncture and osteopathy. You will create a referral network as well as a virtual "team approach" for each patient.

7. Consider referral to a physiatrist well-trained in neuromusculoskeletal medicine to create and coordinate a treatment plan.

8. Offer a mind–body therapy such as MBSR, qi gong, or hypnosis as part of a treatment plan.

9. Manage expectations. It may take weeks or months to notice significant change. Patient education about time frames and recognizing incremental change can reduce frustration and increase self-observation skills.

Summary

Though there are myriad etiologies of CPP, common therapeutic targets include inflammation, somatic dysfunction, and psychological disturbances. Inflammation may be addressed not only with dietary changes including nutritional and botanical supplements but also with mind–body therapies. Somatic dysfunction may respond to manipulative therapies provided by osteopaths (Greenman 2003), naturopaths, chiropractors, and some physical therapists. Therapists may also offer visceral, craniosacral, myofascial, and other whole-body therapies, as can highly trained massage therapists and bodyworkers. Mental health care may be key in many cases.

Integrative medicine heralds the return to a sense of the human being's intrinsic capacity for healing, incorporating the vitalism of many of the therapies' origins (traditional Chinese medicine, indigenous medicine, ayurveda, osteopathy, chiropractic, etc.) with the gains made by a more reductionistic tradition. Given the complexity and wide variation of etiologies and symptoms of CPP, using an integrative approach may offer expanded therapeutic solutions (Bailey 2008). We must expand our capacity to listen to each patient—with ears, eyes, mind, heart, and hands (Milne 1995). Each treatment plan may then be tailored to the unique history and perspective that lie within the individual. Doing so requires the essential elements of time, skill, and love.

Resources

While the best sources for referrals are in your own network and community and from patients and colleagues, the following Web sites are available for practitioners of the work described above. This is only a partial list of therapeutic approaches that may be useful for chronic pelvic pain:

American Academy of Medical Acupuncture
  http://www.medicalacupuncture.org/
American Academy of Osteopathy
  http://www.academyofosteopathy.org
American Academy of Physical Medicine and Rehabilitation (physiatrists)
  http://www.aapmr.org/
American Association of Acupuncture and Oriental Medicine
  http://www.aaaomonline.org/
American Association of Naturopathic Physicians
  http://www.naturopathic.org/

American Botanical Council (membership required)
  http://abc.herbalgram.org/site/PageServer
American Physical Therapy Association
  http://www.apta.org/ Select "women's health" under expertise. (Infertility clinics may also employ physical therapists who specialize in pelvic manipulation)
American Society of Clinical Hypnosis
  http://www.asch.net/
Biodynamics of Osteopathy (physicians trained in biodynamic cranial osteopathy)
  www.biodo.com/
Center for Mindfulness in Medicine, Health Care and Society
  http://www.umassmed.edu/cfm/mbsr/
EMDR International Association
  http://www.emdria.org/
Milne Institute (craniosacral therapists)
  www.milneinstitute.com/
National Association of Myofascial Trigger Point Therapists
  http://www.namtpt.shuttlepod.org/ Note: Many physicians, especially physiatrists, work with trigger points as well.
Natural Standard: The Authority on Integrative Medicine (membership required)
  http://www.naturalstandard.com/
The Alexander Technique
  http://www.alexandertechnique.com/
The Barral Institute (for visceral manipulation)
  http://www.barralinstitute.com/
The Cranial Academy (physicians trained in cranial osteopathy)
  http://www.cranialacademy.com/
The Feldenkrais Method of Somatic Education
  http://www.feldenkrais.com
The Upledger Institute
  http://www.iahp.com/pages/search/index.php Note: Search for therapists with many classes and experience in visceral, craniosacral, lymphatic, and/or somatoemotional release techniques.

REFERENCES

Alexander J. Trauma. In:Jones DS, ed. *Textbook of Functional Medicine.* Gig Harbor, WA: Institute for Functional Medicine; 2006:140–147.
Anderson RU. Traditional therapy for chronic pelvic pain does not work: what do we do now? *Nat Clin Pract Urol.* 2006;3(3):145–156.

Axelrad DA, Brown D, Wain H. Hypnosi. In: Sadock BJ, Sadock VA, Ruiz P, eds. *(9th edition)* Philadelphia PA: Lippincott Williams & Wilkins; 2009, Ch 30.4.

Bailey A, Stein M. Integrative pain medicine models: women's health programs. In: Audette JF, Bailey B, eds. *Integrative Pain Management: The Science and Practice of Complementary and Alternative Medicine in Pain Management.* Totowa NJ: Humana Press; 2008:497–545.

Baker PK. Musculoskeletal problems. In: Steege JF, Metzger DA, Levy BS, eds. *Chronic Pelvic Pain: An Integrated Approach.* Philadelphia PA: W.B. Saunders; 1998:215–240.

Barral JP. *Urogenital Manipulation.* Seattle WA: Eastland Press; 1993:39–108.

Barral JP, Mercier P. *Visceral Manipulation.* Seattle WA: Eastland Press; 1988:216–231.

Bisson JI, Ehlers A, Matthews R, Pilling S, Richards D, Turner S. Psychological treatments for chronic post-traumatic stress disorder. Systematic review and meta-analysis . *Br J Psychiatry.* 2007;190:97–104.

Brous N. Fascia. In: DiGiovanna EL, Schiowitz S, eds. *An Osteopathic Approach to Diagnosis and Treatment.* 2nd ed. Philadelphia, PA: Lippincott-Raven; 1997: 19–20.

Centers for Disease Control and Prevention. ACE study: adverse childhood experiences. Available at: http://www.cdc.gov/NCCDPHP/ACE/prevalence.htm. Accessed November 1, 2008.

Collett BJ, Cordle CJ, Stewart CR, Jagger C. A comparative study of women with chronic pelvic pain, chronic nonpelvic pain and those with no history of pain attending general practitioners. *Br J Obstet Gynaecol.* 1998;105(1):87–92.

Costello K. Myofascial syndromes. In: Steege JF, Metztger DA, Levy BS, eds. *Chronic Pelvic pain: An Integrated Approach.* Philadelphia: W.B. Saunders; 1998:251–266.

Davis DA, Luecken LJ, Zautra AJ. Are reports of childhood abuse related to the experience of chronic pain in adulthood? A meta-analytic review of the literature. *Clin J Pain.* 2005;21(5):398–405.

Drossman DA, Leserman, Nachman G, et al. Sexual and physical abuse in women with functional or organic gastrointestinal disorders. *Ann Intern Med.* 1990;113:828–833.

Dubowitz H, DePanfilis D.eds. *Handbook for Child Protection Practice.* Thousand Oaks, CA: Sage; 2000:76–77.

Elliott ML. Treating the patient with pelvic pain. In: Turk DC, Gatchel RJ, eds. *Psychological approaches to pain management: a practitioner's handbook, 2nd ed.* New York: Guilford Press; 2002:455–469.

Fillingim RB, Wilkinson CS, Powell T. Self-reported abuse history and pain complaints among young adults. *Clin J Pain.* 1999;15:75–76.

Fry RPW, Crisp AH, Beard RW. Sociopsychological factors in chronic pelvic pain: a review. *J Psychosom Res.* 1997;42:1–15.

Ghaly AFF, Chien PFW. Chronic pelvic pain: clinical dilemma or clinician's nightmare. *Sex Trans Infect.* 2000;76:419–425.

Goldberg RT. Childhood abuse, depression, and chronic pain. *Clin J Pain.* 1994;10:277–281.

Goldberg RT, Goldstein R. A comparison of chronic pain patients and controls on traumatic events in childhood. *Disabil Rehabil.* 2000;22(17):756–763.

Goldberg RT, Pachas WN, Keith D. Relationship between traumatic events in childhood and chronic pain. *Disabil Rehabil.* 1999;21(1):23–30.

Grace VM. Mind/body dualism in medicine: the case of chronic pelvic pain without organic pathology: a critical review of the literature. [Review] [73 refs] *Int J Health Ser.* 1998;28(1):127–151.

Greenman PE. The manipulative prescription. In Greenman PE *Principles of Manual Medicine.* 3rd ed. Philadelphia: Lippincott Williams & Wilkins; 2003: 45–52.

Grossman P, Tiefenthaler-Gilmer U, Raysc A, Kesper U. Mindfulness training as an intervention for fibromyalgia: evidence of postintervention and 3-year follow-up benefits in well-being. *Psychotherapy and Psychosomatics.* 76(4): 226–233. 2007

Gunter J. Chronic pelvic pain: an integrated approach to diagnosis and treatment. *Obstet Gynecolog Surv.* 2003;58(9):615–623.

Gunter J. The neurobiology of chronic pelvic pain. In Potts JM, ed. *Genitourinary Pain and Inflammation: Diagnosis and Management.* Totowa, NJ: Humana Press; 2008:3–17.

Gutke A. Ostgaard HC, Oberg B. Association between muscle function and low back pain in relation to pregnancy. *J Rehabil Med.* 2008;40(4):304–311.

Hahn L. Chronic pelvic pain in women. A condition difficult to diagnose—more than 70 different diagnoses can be considered. Lakartidningen 2001;98:1780–1785.

Heim C, Ehlert U, Hanker JP, Hellhammer DH. Abuse-related posttraumatic stress disorder and alterations of the hypothalamic-pituitary-adrenal axis in women with chronic pelvic pain. *Psychosom Med.* 1998;60(3):309–318.

Heim C, Newport DJ, Bonsall R, Miller AH, Nemeroff CB. Altered pituitary-adrenal axis responses to provocative challenge tests in adult survivors of childhood abuse. *Am J Psychiatry.* 2001;158(4):575–581.

Holtzman DA, Petrocco-Napuli KL, Burke JR. Prospective case series on the effects of lumbosacral manipulation on dysmenorrhea. *J Manipulative Physiol Ther.* 2008;31(3):237–246.

Hurst C, MacDonald J, Say J, Read J. Routine questioning about nonconsenting sex: a survey of practice in Australasian sexual health clinics. *Int J STD AIDS.* 2003;14(5):329–333.

Jarrell JF, Vilos GA, Allaire LC, et al. Chronic pelvic pain working group. SOGC. Consensus guidelines for the management of chronic pelvic pain. *Journal of Obstretrics & Gynaecology (Canada: JOGC).* 2005;27(8):781–826.

Korr IM. Hyperactivity of sympathetic innervation: a common factor in disease. In: King HH, ed. *The Collected Papers of Irvin M.* Korr. Vol 2. Ann Arbor MI: American Academy of Osteopathy; 1997:70–76.

Kuchera ML, Kuchera WA. *Osteopathic Principles in Practice.* 2nd ed. Columbus, OH: Greyden Press; 1994a:74

Kuchera ML, Kuchera WA. *Osteopathic Principles in Practice.* 2nd ed. Columbus, OH: Greyden Press; 1994b:131–151.

Lampe A, Doering S, Rumpold G, et al. Chronic pain syndromes and their relation to childhood abuse and stressful life events. *J Psychosom Res.* 2003;54(4):361–367.

Lee D. *The Pelvic Girdle: An Approach to the Examination and Treatment of the Lumbopelvic-Hip Region.* Elsevier Philadelphia: Churchill Livingstone; 2004.160–161, 163–177.

Leserman, J. Sexual abuse history: prevalence, health effects, mediators, and psychological treatment. *Psychosom Med.* 2005;67(6):906–915.

Ling FW, Slocumb JC. Use of trigger point injections in chronic pelvic pain. *Obstet Gynecol Clin North Am.* 1993;20(4):809–815.

Lovy A. The psychiatric patient. In: Nelson KE, Glonek T, eds. *Somatic Dysfunction in Osteopathic Family Medicine.* Philadelphia, PA: Lippincott, Williams and Wilkins; 2007:73–86.

Low Dog T. Botanicals in the management of pain. In: Audette JF, Bailey B, eds. *Integrative Pain Management: The Science and Practice of Complementary and Alternative Medicine in Pain Management.* Totowa NJ; Humana Press; 2008:447–470.

Madore A, Kahn JR. Therapeutic massage and bodywork in integrative pain management. In: Audette JF, Bailey B, eds. *Integrative Pain Management: The Science and Practice of Complementary and Alternative Medicine in Pain Management.* Totowa, NJ: Humana Press; 2008:353–378.

Mathias SD, Kuppermann M, Liberman RF, Lipschutz RC, Steege JF. Chronic pelvic pain: prevalence, health-related quality of life, and economic correlates. *Obstet Gynecol.* 1996;87(3):321–327.

McGowan L, Luker K, Creed F, Chew-Graham CA. How do you explain a pain that can't be seen?: The narratives of women with chronic pelvic pain and their disengagement with the diagnostic cycle. *Br J Health Psychol.* May 2007;12(Pt 2):261–274.

Meltzer-Brody S, Leserman J, Zolnoun D, Steege J, Green E, Teich A. Trauma and posttraumatic stress disorder in women with chronic pelvic pain. *Obstet Gynecol.* 2007;109(4):902–908.

Milne H. *The Heart of Listening: A Visionary Approach to Craniosacral Work.* Berkeley, CA: North Atlantic Books; 1995:44–66;78–101;131–142.

Nelson KE. Diagnosing somatic dysfunction. In: Nelson KE, Glonek T, eds. *Somatic Dysfunction in Osteopathic Family Medicine.* Philadelphia, PA: Lippincott, Williams and Wilkins; 2007a:12–26.

Nelson KE. The manipulative prescription. In: Nelson KE, Glonek T. eds. *Somatic Dysfunction in Osteopathic Family Medicine.* Philadelphia, PA: Lippincott, Williams and Wilkins; 2007b;27–32.

Nelson KE. Viscerosomatic and somatovisceral reflexes. In: Nelson KE, Glonek T, eds. *Somatic Dysfunction in Osteopathic Family Medicine.* Philadelphia, PA: Lippincott, Williams and Wilkins; 2007c:33–55.

Nelson KE, Rottman J. The female patient. In: Nelson KE, Glonek T, eds. *Somatic Dysfunction in Osteopathic Family Medicine.* Philadelphia, PA: Lippincott, Williams and Wilkins; 2007d:105–126.

Parcell S. Biochemical and nutritional influences on pain. In: Audette JF, Bailey B, eds. *Integrative Pain Management: The Science and Practice of Complementary and Alternative Medicine in Pain Management.* Totowa, NJ: Humana Press; 2008:133–172.

Peters AA, van Dorst E, Jellis B, et al. A randomized clinical trial to compare two different approaches in women with chronic pelvic pain. *Obstet Gynecol.* 1991;77:740–744.

Pikarinen U, Saisto T, Schei B, Swahnberg K, Halmesmaki E. Experiences of physical and sexual abuse and their implications for current health. *Obstet Gynecol.* 2007;109:1116–1122.

Pittler MH, Ernst E. Kava extract for treating anxiety. *Cochrane Database Systemic Rev.* 2003;(2):CD003383.

Prendergast SA, Weiss JM. Screening for musculoskeletal causes of pelvic pain. *Clin Obstet Gynecol.* 2003;46(4):773–782.

Price J, Farmer G, Harris J, Hope T, Kennedy S, Mayou R. Attitudes of women with chronic pelvic pain to the gynaecological consultation: a qualitative study. *BJOG.* 2006; 113(4): 446–452.

Read J, McGregor K, Coggan C, Thomas DR. Mental health services and sexual abuse: the need for staff training. *J Trauma Dissociation.* 2006;7(1):33–50.

Robertson MF, Humphreys L, Ray R. Psychological treatments for posttraumatic stress disorders: recommendations for the clinician based on a review of literature. *Journal of Psychiatric Practice.* 2004;10(2):106–118.

Rubin JJ. MD psychosomatic pain: new insights and management strategies. *South Med J.* 2005;98(11):1099–1110.

Schamberger W. *The Malalignment Syndrome: Implicatons for Medicine and Sport.* London UK. Churchill Livingstone. 2002:231–240.

Schiowitz S. Static symmetry. In: DiGiovanna EL, Schiowitz S, eds. *An Osteopathic Approach to Diagnosis and Treatment.* 2nd ed. Philadelphia PA: Lippincott-Raven; 1997:37–47.

Selfe SA, Matthews Z, Stones RW. Factors influencing outcome in consultations for chronic pelvic pain. *J Womens Health.* 1998;7(8):1041–1048.

Sharp J. Keefe B. Psychiatry in chronic pain: a review and update. *Curr Psychiatr Rep.* 2005;7(3):213–219.

Slocumb JC. Neurological factors in chronic pelvic pain: trigger points and the abdominal pelvic pain syndrome. *Am J Obstet Gynecol.* 1984;149(5):536–543.

Smutney CJ, Hitchcock ME. Dysmenorrhea and premenstrual syndrome. In: DiGiovanna EL, Schiowitz S, eds. *An Osteopathic Approach to Diagnosis and Treatment.* 2nd ed. Philadelphia, PA: Lippincott-Raven; 1997:455–459.

Steege JF. Philosophy of the integrated approach: overcoming the mind-body split. In: Steege JF, Metztger DA, Levy BS, eds. *Chronic Pelvic Pain: An Integrated Approach.* Philadelphia, PA: W.B. Saunders; 1998:5–12.

Sulindro-Ma M, Ivy CL, Isenhart AC. Nutrition and supplements for pain management. In: Audette JF, Bailey B, eds. *Integrative Pain Management: The Science and Practice of Complementary and Alternative Medicine in Pain Management.* Totowa NJ: Humana Press; 2008;417–446.

Tettambel MA. An osteopathic approach to treating women with chronic pelvic pain. *JAOA.* 2005;105(suppl 4):20–22.

Thomas E, Moss-Morris R, Faquhar C. Coping with emotions and abuse history in women with chronic pelvic pain. *J Psychosom Res.* 2006 Jan;60(1):109–112.

Torrisi G, Sampugnaro EG, Pappalardo EM, D'Urso E, Vecchio M, Mazza A. Postpartum urinary stress incontinence: analysis of the associated risk factors and neurophysiological tests. *Minerva Ginecologica.* 2007;59(5):491–498.

Travell JG, Simons DG. *Myofascial Pain and Dysfunction: The Trigger Point Manual.* Baltimore: Williams & Wilkins; 1983.

Travell J, Simons D. *Myofascial Pain and Dysfunction: The Trigger Point Manual.* Vol. 1. Baltimore: Williams & Wilkins; 1992.

Van der Kolk BA. The body keeps the score: memory and the evolving psychobiology of posttraumatic stress. *Harv Rev Psychiatry*. 1994;1:253–265.

Walker EA, Katon WJ, Hansom J, et al. Medical and psychiatric symptoms in women with childhood sexual abuse. *Psychosom Med*. 1992;54(6):658–664.

Zondervan KT, Yudkin PL, Vessey MP, et al. The community prevalence of chronic pelvic pain in women and associated illness behaviour. *Br J Gen Pract*. 2001;51(468):541–547.

OTHER SUGGESTED READING

Barral JP, *Urogenital Manipulation*. Seattle WA: Easland Press; 1993.

Barral JP. *Visceral Manipulation II*. Seattle WA: Eastland Press; 1989.

Barral JP, Croibier A. *Trauma: An Osteopathic Approach*. Seattle WA: Eastland Press; 1999.

Dong M, Anda RF, Dube SR, Giles WH, Felitti VJ. The relationship of exposure to childhood sexual abuse to other forms of abuse, neglect, and household dysfunction during childhood. *Child Abuse Negl*. 2003;27:625–639.

Henk W, Voorham-van der Zalm PJ, Pelger, RCM. How reliable is a self-administered questionnaire in detecting sexual abuse: a retrospective study in patients with pelvic-floor complaints and a review of literature. *J Sex Med*. 2007;4(4, Part I):956–963.

Korr IM. *Neurobiological Mechanisms of Manipulative Therapy*. New York: Plenum Press; 1978.

Kuchera ML, Kuchera WA. *Osteopathuc Considerations in Systemic Dysfunction*. Columbus, OH: Greyden Press; 1994.

Latthe P, Mignini L, Gray, R Hills R, Khan K. Factors predisposing women to chronic pelvic pain: systematic review. *BMJ*. 2006;332:749–755.

Leserman J. Identification of diagnostic subtypes of chronic pelvic pain and how subtypes differ in health status and trauma history. *Am J Obstet Gynecol*. 2006;195(2):554–560; discussion 560–561.

Poleshuck EL, Dworkin RH, Howard FM, et al. Contributions of physical and sexual abuse to women's experiences with chronic pelvic pain. *J Reprod Med*. 2005;50(2):91–100.

Sutherland WG, Wales AL, eds. *Teachings in the Science of Osteopathy*. Fort Worth, TX: Sutherland Cranial Teaching Foundation; 1990.

Taylor GJ. The challenge of chronic pain: a psychoanalytic approach. *J Am Acad Psychoanal Dyn Psychiatr*. 2008;36(1):49–68.

Walsh CA, Jamieson E, Macmillan H, Boyle M. Child abuse and chronic pain in a community survey of women. *J Interpers Violence*. 2007;22(12):1536–1554.

20

Uterine Fibroids

JOANNE L. PERRON

CASE STUDY

Louisa H. presented to me for an evaluation of abnormal uterine bleeding (AUB), pelvic pressure, and urinary frequency over a 15-month duration. She is a 46-year-old, Caucasian female, Gravida 1 Para 1, with contraception provided by tubal sterilization. She is a busy manufacturing executive who travels constantly for her company's business needs and has been inconvenienced and embarrassed by the erratic AUB and heavy menstruation, often soaking her clothes. The pelvic pressure and AUB have interfered with her ability to participate in marathon training and mountain climbing. She is an avid yoga practitioner, eats healthy when at home, but succumbs to fast food when traveling.

When she was on a business trip to Thailand, she underwent evaluation at a prominent Bangkok hospital for a heavier than normal bleeding episode. A vaginal probe ultrasound revealed three fibroids, two intramural and one suspicious for submucosal involvement, the largest measuring 5 cm. Laboratory testing was significant for hemoglobin of 10.4 g/dL and a normal urinalysis. Louisa was advised to seek gynecological care upon her return to the United States. Louisa first decided to consult with a traditional Chinese medicine (TCM) practitioner. After four months of treatment with Chinese herbal formulations and acupuncture, the AUB had improved and her menstrual cycle lightened while her pelvic pressure remained unchanged. Despite her satisfaction with the improvement in bleeding, she found the herbal regimen distasteful and overly onerous, especially with her busy schedule, and thus discontinued it. She had a regular bleeding pattern for another 2 months, but then had resumption of AUB.

When she presented to me, she reported having one episode of AUB that lasted 10 days. The remainder of her past medical history was unremarkable. Physical examination was remarkable for a 14-week-sized bulky, nontender uterus on pelvic examination. There was no pelvic floor laxity or uterine decensus. An endometrial biopsy showed benign endometrium with the cavity sounding to 10 cm. Saline infusion sonogram exhibited a multifibroid uterus, the largest measuring 7 cm and was also remarkable for a 4-cm submucous fibroid.

Management options were discussed with the patient. She declined uterine artery embolization and elected to undergo total abdominal hysterectomy (TAH). Two weeks prior to surgery, the patient began listening to guided imagery tapes designed to assist her in visualizing relaxation, healing, and an optimal surgical outcome. Louisa underwent an uncomplicated TAH with an estimated blood loss of less than 50 mL. Her postoperative course went smoothly and within 2 weeks, she began a walking regimen. At 2 months after surgery, she was running 5 miles four times per week and practicing yoga daily. She expressed great satisfaction with her decision and began to plan a mountain climbing trip to South America.

Introduction

Fibroids are the most common of female pelvic tumors and are composed of monoclonal uterine smooth muscle and connective tissue. An epidemiological study screening for leiomyomata, or uterine fibroids, found the estimated cumulative incidence of fibroid tumors by age 50 years was >80% for black women and nearly 70% for white women (DayBaird et al. 2003). Fibroids cause considerable morbidity, reducing the quality of life for women, as well as substantially impacting the U.S. health care system. From 2000 through 2004, an estimated 3.1 million U.S. women had a hysterectomy for uterine fibroids, accounting for 38.7% of hysterectomies performed in 2004 (Whiteman et al. 2008). In 2000 alone, $2.6 billion in surgical and nonsurgical hospitalizations were attributed to uterine fibroids (AHRQ 2005). Because of the increased resource use and work loss cost, women with fibroids spent 2.6 times more on health care costs than women without fibroids (Hartmann et al. 2006).

The most common symptoms related to fibroids are abnormal uterine bleeding, variants of pelvic pain or mass effect, and infertility. Many variables are taken into consideration before determining the course of fibroid management. The individualized treatment options are dependent on an evaluation of symptomatology, fibroid characteristics, patient age, and desire for future fertility or uterine preservation.

Conventional surgical management is either hysterectomy or myomectomy. The past 15 years have brought some innovative and less invasive options to standard hysterectomy and myomectomy, including laparoscopic assisted removal of the uterus or the fibroids, hysteroscopic resection of submucous fibroids with ablation of the uterine cavity, uterine artery embolization (UAE), and magnetic resonance–guided focused ultrasound surgery (MRgFUS).

From a public health perspective, uterine fibroids are a common and costly problem and there is substantial uncertainty and disagreement among physicians and patients regarding optimal management. According to a recent Agency for Healthcare Quality and Research (AHRQ) report, there is a lack of rigorous evidence supporting the long-term effectiveness of most conventional medical interventions, including surgical procedures, medical therapy, and watchful waiting (AHRQ 2007). Perhaps due to their nonmalignant nature, fibroid research is underfunded and therapeutic treatments have much room for improvement (Walker and Stewart 2005). It is understandable that women and their health care providers yearn for less expensive and invasive, but safe and effective options for fibroid management. Proven strategies to prevent, limit growth, and treat fibroids nonsurgically are needed especially for women in their childbearing years. Unfortunately, for clinicians trying to provide an integrative approach to fibroid management, there is also a paucity of quality research studying alternative options (Ausk and Reed 2004). Current complementary and alternative medicine (CAM) therapies can offer relief from fibroid symptomatology such as AUB or pain, but are unlikely to significantly decrease fibroid size (Hudson 2008). An integrative approach to fibroids does not eschew conventional medicine nor does it blindly embrace CAM. Rather, it blends the best from both to devise an evidence-based and patient-centered treatment plan that has been developed after mindful listening and understanding of the unique woman's needs.

Risk Factors

Despite their frequency, over 50% of women with fibroids are asymptomatic and thus require no intervention. Presentation commonly occurs when a women is in her thirties or forties. The growth of uterine fibroids is subject to hormonal stimuli of estrogen and progesterone, with most fibroids presenting after menarche, having a growth spurt in the few years before menopause, and becoming quiescent after menopause. There is considerable racial disparity with African-American women suffering disproportionately (Kjerulff et al. 1996). A higher fibroid incidence is associated with early menarche, nulliparity, having first degree relatives with fibroids, and obesity. There is an inverse relationship between smoking and presence of fibroids (Flake et al. 2003). Use of birth control pills or menopausal hormone replacement therapy generally does not stimulate significant fibroid growth. Increased physical activity and consumption of a plant-based dietary choices are probably protective, but the exact mechanisms are poorly understood (Flake et al. 2003).

Etiology

The precise mechanism for fibroid development is not understood. It appears to be a complex interplay of genetics, hormone (endogenous and foreign) promoters, and growth factors found in smooth muscle cells and fibroblasts. Fibroids strongly respond to estrogen and have elevated levels of estrogen and progesterone receptors. Estrogen metabolism is altered in fibroids, resulting in elevated aromatase levels (Walker and Stewart 2005). Fibroid growth factors affecting angiogenesis are posited to lead to vascular abnormalities, causing women with fibroids to experience excessive bleeding (Stewart and Nowak 1996).

Although uterine fibroids are proliferative, they are not undifferentiated, unlike uterine sarcomas, which show complex chromosomal rearrangements and aneuploidy. Fibroids can be associated with a rare syndrome, hereditary leiomyomatosis and renal cell carcinoma (HLRCC) caused by a fumarate hydratase mutation with affected females having an increased risk of premenopausal uterine sarcomas. In general, it is rare for benign fibroids to progress to leiomyosarcomas because of these cytogenetic differences (Stewart and Morton 2006). However, the fibroid's size, location, and risk of recurrence after myomectomy are influenced by the karyotype (Stewart et al. 2002).

There is emerging research and growing evidence in the field of environmental health that xenoestrogens such as pesticides, heavy metals, pharmaceuticals, plasticizers, and even phytoestrogens act as endocrine disrupting chemicals in vertebrates via changes in gene expression without DNA sequence changes. This epigenetic change can become persistent and inherited, causing long-term effects and possibly impacting subsequent generations (McLachlan et al. 2006).

Presentation and Manifestations

Symptomatic uterine fibroids can be responsible for a menagerie of problems, which usually correlate to their location, size, and number. The three most common fibroids make their uterine home on the surface (subserosal), in the wall (intramural), or in the lining (submucous), and when grossly enlarged can make the nonpregnant uterus appear the size of a term pregnancy (Herbst et al. 1992).

The direction of growth can determine if the fibroid will become externally pedunculated (subserosal) and even parasitic or move laterally into the broad ligament and mimic an ovarian neoplasm. Intramural fibroids may compress the fallopian tubes if their location is near the cornua. Less commonly occurring submucous fibroids can be the most troublesome clinically as they can cause AUB (menstrual and intermenstrual), distortion of the uterine cavity frequently contributing to miscarriage and infertility, and internal pedunculation, often leading to an aborting myoma (Herbst et al. 1992).

Menorrhagia is the most frequent type of AUB associated with fibroids, but not all AUB is caused by fibroids; therefore, other causes of abnormal bleeding should be ruled out, such as coagulopathies, endometrial hyperplasia, carcinoma, or polyps.

Pressure, bulk symptoms, and increasing abdominal girth are frequent manifestations of uterine fibroids and can result in dyspareunia, urinary tract dysfunction, including urgency, frequency, and obstruction of the ureter; or gastrointestinal disturbances from pressure on the intestinal viscera. Secondary dysmenorrhea, while sometimes attributed to fibroids, may rather be due to the concomitance of adenomyosis. In the case of acute pain, fibroid degenerative changes, torsion of a peduncluated fibroid, or cervical dilatation from an aborting myoma are the most common etiologies (Wallach and Vlahos 2004).

During pregnancy, most fibroids do not increase in size significantly. If growth does occur it generally happens early, sometimes causing a size to gestational age discrepancy and usually returning to prepregnancy size during the postpartum period. Pregnancy-related complications from fibroids include degeneration of the fibroid with subsequent pain as the blood supply diverts to the growing fetus and increased Caesarean section rate due to lower uterine segment obstruction or fetal malpresentation (Parker 2007). The risk of preterm labor is slightly elevated in patients with fibroids (Klatsky et al. 2008). The research is conflicting when examining other obstetrical complications such as premature rupture of membranes and placental complications (Parker 2007).

Neonatal outcomes do not differ in women with fibroids when compared to controls (Klatsky et al. 2008).

> Give reassurance to pregnant patients with fibroids and a cephalic presentation that vaginal delivery is the most likely outcome.

Diagnosis and Evaluation

A frequent scenario at the annual well-woman examination finds asymptomatic women surprised by the clinician's finding of a fibroid uterus. The pelvic examination will reveal an enlarged, irregularly shaped, firm and nontender uterus. Transvaginal ultrasound (TVS) is a readily available and economical technique to confirm the physical findings and also evaluate the adnexa. Transabdominal ultrasound or magnetic resonance imaging (MRI) is recommended for large fibroids. Confirmation of a suspected submucosal fibroid requires saline infusion sonography (SIS), hysteroscopy (HSC), or an MRI. Both SIS and HSC can be performed in the office setting with minimal or local anesthesia.

> Avoid hesitating to obtain a SIS or HSC for a patient with fibroids and AUB. The diagnosis of a submucous fibroid is expedited and the patient can then be counseled appropriately, as operative removal generally brings more patient satisfaction than the less interventional options.

An MRI is more sensitive and specific when compared to the other modalities in identifying submucous fibroids and is superior for precise delineation of submucous fibroid penetration into the wall of the uterus (Parker 2007). If there is suspicion that the fibroid impinges on and compromises the ureter, then an IVP or renal ultrasound should be part of the evaluation for hydronephrosis (Wallach and Vlahos 2004).

A predominant complaint of heavy AUB warrants evaluation of a woman's hemoglobin and hematocrit. Additional laboratory testing may include pregnancy testing, complete metabolic panel, prolactin (PRL) level, or thyroid testing to rule out other causes of AUB. An office endometrial biopsy may also be prudent if the clinician is suspicious that hyperplasia, carcinoma, or sarcoma is the etiology of the AUB. Rapid fibroid growth was traditionally felt to be an indication of uterine sarcoma; however, this association has not been substantiated (ACOG 2008). Leiomyosarcoma may be diagnosed preoperatively with total serum lactic acid dehydrogenase (LDH), LDH isoenzyme 3, and gadolinium-enhanced MRI (Parker 2007).

An Integrative Approach

The conventional treatment spectrum includes various medications, extirpative surgery, and more recently noninvasive, uterine-sparing procedures. It is beyond the scope of this chapter to do a thorough review of the topic. A review of current practice guidelines can be found in American College of Obstetricians and Gynecologists (ACOG) Practice Bulletin, Alternatives to Hysterectomy in the Management of Leiomyomas, Number 96, August 2008. This section will focus on treatment approaches that generally fall outside conventional gynecological practice.

Lifestyle: Nutrition, Diet, and Supplements

A thorough discussion of lifestyle habits that contribute to an elevated estrogen milieu should be undertaken by the clinician. There is an association between obesity and increased risk of fibroids due to conversion of androgens to estrogens in adipose tissue via aromatase (Flake et al. 2003). A comparison of former college athletes to nonathletes revealed that nonathletes were slightly more likely to develop fibroid tumors (Wyshak et al. 1986). A recent study showed that women in the highest category of physical activity were significantly less likely to have fibroids (Baird et al. 2007). As with other diseases related to obesity, clearly there is a benefit to regular exercise.

> Motivating patients to increase physical activity and select healthier foods can be facilitated by connecting them to their vision of health and wellness (e.g. less bothersome symptoms from fibroids), helping them to set achievable goals, and thus increasing their self-efficacy by that success.

Dietary choices influence estrogen excretion. Vegetarian women have a threefold increase in fecal excretion of estrogen and 15–20% lower serum estrogen levels (Gorbach and Goldin 1987). An Italian study found a moderate association between the risk of uterine myomas and the consumption of red meat, with a high intake of green vegetables demonstrating a protective effect (Chiaffarino et al. 1999). The most likely explanations include: high-fiber and low-fat diets which shield estrogen absorption, or reduce enterohepatic estrogen recirculation; and/or ingested phytoestrogens which compete with endogenous estrogens at the receptor level or alter fibroid aromatase activity (Flake et al. 2003).

Isoflavones and lignans are the two main classes of phytoestrogens. Findings suggest a modest inverse association between urinary excretion of the mammalian lignans enterodiol and enterolactone and the development of uterine fibroids. Lignan consumption, found in flaxseed and whole grains, may be a viable dietary strategy for reducing the risk of uterine fibroids (Atkinson et al. 2006). The isoflavones, daidzein and genistein, are found predominately in soy foods. In vitro, genistein has variable effects on leiomyomata cells, with low concentrations eliciting proliferative effects and high concentrations inhibiting growth (Moore et al. 2007). However, in a recent report of three cases, women consuming a high daily intake of soy products had worsening of their gynecological disorders (including fibroids). When the soy products were discontinued, their symptoms resolved (Chandrareddy et al. 2008). The variable effects of soy products on the female reproductive system merit patient counseling regarding concentrated and/or processed soy products and recommending prudent consumption of whole soy foods.

The phytochemical, indole-3-carbinol (I3C), found in cruciferous vegetables (broccoli, brussels sprouts, cabbage, and cauliflower) alters estrogen metabolism by promoting the formation less potent estrogen metabolites (Minich and Bland 2007). This lends additional support to the consumption of a plant-based diet in women with uterine fibroids.

The type of fat consumed may play a role in fibroid promotion. A recent study concluded that the primary in vivo aromatase promoter in leiomyomata tissues in non-Asian U.S. women is the PGE2/cyclic adenosine monophosphate (cAMP)-responsive 1.3/II region (Imir et al. 2007). Encouraging women with fibroids to consume a higher intake of antiinflammatory omega 3 fatty acids, and reduce their consumption of omega 6 fatty acids, would theoretically curb fibroid growth along with the other known benefits of these fatty acids.

High caffeine and coffee intake ($\geq$500 mg/day) may increase early follicular phase estradiol (E2) levels compared to those with lower levels of consumption ($\leq$100 mg/day) independent of alcohol consumption or tobacco use (Lucero et al. 2001). Therefore a moderate consumption of caffeine products would be recommended for women with fibroids. Limiting alcohol consumption to <1 serving per day seems prudent in view of alcohol's effects on the liver and hence estrogen metabolism.

Recently, there has been some intriguing research showing significant growth-inhibiting effects of physiologic vitamin D on leiomyomata cells that are mediated predominately through a G1/S phase block of the cell cycle. Hypovitaminosis D may play an important role in fibroid growth (Blauer et al. 2009).

If heavy AUB and secondary iron deficiency anemia are a concern, then iron-rich foods, taken with vitamin C to enhance absorption, are recommended. Vitamin C and bioflavonoids significantly strengthen blood vessel walls in women with menorrhagia (Cohen 1960). Depending on the class of bioflavonoid, antiinflammatory, antioxidant, and antiproliferative properties have been described.

BOTANICAL RECOMMENDATIONS

In addition to advising a woman with fibroids to eat a more plant-based, spice-enhanced diet and assuring adequate vitamin D levels, it would be prudent to recommend consumption of pesticide-free foodstuffs, since it has been shown that organochlorine pesticides stimulate proliferation of leiomyomata cells in animal models (Hodges et al. 2000). If the postulations of environmental causes from xenoestrogens hold true, then fibroids will continue to be a substantial public health concern for women despite medical innovations.

There are several botanicals that might assist in the symptomatic management of fibroids. While there are few rigorous studies supporting their use, many plants have been used over the centuries in traditional herbal formulations to reduce uterine hemorrhage and pain. It may take several months to achieve significant benefit, fibroids are likely not to shrink, but the herbal therapies may inhibit further growth and subdue symptoms of AUB or secondary dysmenorrhea until natural menopause occurs (Hudson 2008).

Chaste tree berry (*Vitex agnus castus*) is often recommended for women with AUB because of its progesterogenic effect, especially on the endometrial lining (Low Dog and Micozzi 2005). It increases luteinizing hormone (LH) and inhibits follicle-stimulating hormone (FSH). Chaste tree also has dopaminergic properties, giving it an ability to inhibit PRL release (Hudson 2008). Using it with hormonal contraception or replacement therapy, dopamine-related medications are theoretically contraindicated. It is not advised in women with breast cancer (NCCAM/NIH 2008). Minimal, reversible side effects have included itching or rash, headache, gastrointestinal disturbance, menstrual disorders, acne, and diminished libido. The usual daily dose is 240–500 mg crude herb, 215 mg extract standardized to 0.6% aucubin, or 175 mg extract standardized to 0.75% agnuside (Hudson 2008).

Ginger and turmeric may be beneficial to women with fibroids, given their antiinflammatory activity. Ginger (*Zingiber officinale*) and curcumin, an active compound in turmeric (*Curcuma longa*), are dual inhibitors of cyclooxygenase (PGE biosynthesis) and lipoxygenase (leukotriene biosynthesis) (Grzanna et al. 2005; Roa 2007). A recent in vitro study demonstrated curcumin's

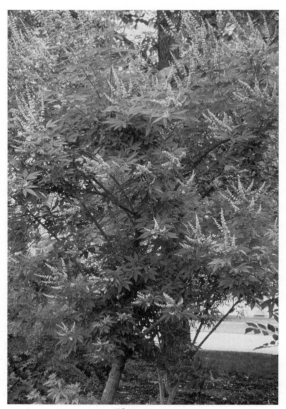

Chaste tree

antiproliferative effect on leiomyoma cell lines (Malik et al. 2008). Ginger is useful in reducing the flow from heavy and protracted menses. The dose for menorrhagia is 1–4 g/day dried powder or ginger root extract (5% gingerols) 100 mg/day, as needed (Hudson 2008). The dose should not exceed 4 g/day. Ginger is often used for dysmenorrhea as well.

Shepherd's purse (*Capsella bursa-pastoris*), an astringent herb, has hemostatic properties, making it useful for reducing heavy menstrual flow (Low Dog and Micozzi 2005). It has been approved for internal use in Germany for the symptomatic treatment of mild menorrhagia and metrorrhagia (German Commission 1998). The dose for tincture (1:5) is 3 mL four to six times per day. The tincture should not be more than 6 months old—it loses its styptic properties with age (Low Dog and Micozzi 2005). There are no known contraindications or side effects (German Commission 1998).

Yarrow (*Achillea millefolium*) has been valued since ancient times for its ability to staunch the flow of bleeding (Low Dog and Micozzi 2005). Traditional herbalists often recommended it for excessive AUB. The dose is 2–4 g dried herb in capsules, three times per day. There are no reports in the scientific literature that yarrow interacts with known conventional medications. Pregnant women should avoid using yarrow, as should persons allergic to plants in the Asteraceae family (Ehrlich 2007).

Red raspberry leaf (*Rubus idaeus*) is best known for use during pregnancy to tone the uterus and facilitate labor, but can also be used for pain relief and excessive bleeding during menstruation (Hobbs 1998). The recommended dosage is one to two cups of tea, two to three times daily (Hobbs 1998) beginning with onset of menstruation.

This is just a sampling of the various botanicals used for managing the symptoms of fibroids. The clinician is referred to textbooks of botanical and naturopathic medicine for additional information. While serious side effects and contraindications are uncommon, they do occur, so the expertise of an experienced naturopath or herbalist should be enlisted for consultation if the clinician is unsure of herbal management for fibroids.

Mind–Body Medicine

Stress is not a known cause of fibroids, but having symptomatic fibroids can cause enormous stress, especially if conservative management is proving ineffective in treating the fibroids. Management of stress should be individualized to harmonize with the patient's belief system, and there are numerous mind–body approaches that can be recommended, including mantra meditation, breath meditation, yoga (moving meditation), guided imagery, hypnosis, martial arts, Tai Chi, and Qi Gong, as well as physical activity performed while in "the zone." Evidence from randomized controlled trials and systematic reviews of the literature suggests that these practices have a beneficial impact on health (NCCAM/NIH 2008).

> During surgical procedures, allow the patient to choose the music in the operating room during preparation and when she is waking from anesthesia.

> Yoga is this author's personal preference for stress management as it combines breath connection with strength and flexibility asanas (postures). Yoga teaches adaptability to uncertainty which, when taken off the yoga mat, brings a sense of peace and freedom in dealing with life's difficulties. Many of the asanas increase blood flow to the pelvis by working the hip and groin

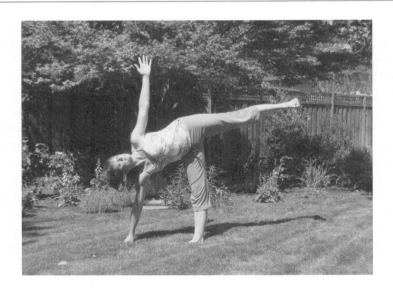

areas and are stated to be beneficial for heavy menstruation, such as half-moon pose (Ardha Chandrasana). Inversions such as Headstand (Sirsasana) are contraindicated during menstrual bleeding (Sparrowe 2002). Registered Yoga teachers (RYT), who have completed a 200-hour minimum training and complied with minimum educational standards established by Yoga Alliance, can be located on that organization's website (www.yogaalliance.org).

TRADITIONAL CHINESE MEDICINE

First depicted in approximately 100 B.C., uterine fibroids can arise from imbalances in other bodily systems and so choice in treatment (herbal formulas or acupuncture points) may vary depending on the clinician's specific findings. Until recently, pelvic examinations were not practiced in China so fibroids were not distinguished from other abdominal masses. The three primary causes of abdominal masses are: mental depression with qi and blood stagnation, improper diet with production of turbid phlegm, and finally, the attack and retention of pathogenic factors such as cold, dampness, heat, or toxins (Dharmananda 2003). According to TCM, uterine bleeding may have several etiologies, such as heat in the blood, blood stasis, or spleen qi deficiency (Dharmananda 2008).

Chinese herbal remedies are chosen on the basis of ability to circulate and replenish qi, remove blood stasis, soothe the liver, resolve phlegm, or invigorate the spleen depending upon the examiner's evaluation of the patient. A sentinel uterine fibroid therapy first described in approximately 220 A.D., Guizhi Fuling Wan (Keishi-bukuryo-gan in Japan) and now called Cinnamon and Hoelen formula is often used, with and without minor variations on the original formulation (Dharmananda 2003). Its pharmacological effects were investigated in 110 premenopausal patients with fibroids less than 10 cm in an uncontrolled study, which found that hypermenorrhea and dysmenorrhea were improved in over 90% of the cases and fibroids shrank in approximately 60% of the cases. The authors had previously reported that the herbal remedy might act as a LH-releasing hormone antagonist and a weak antiestrogen in uterine DNA synthesis in immature rats (Sakamoto et al. 1992). Another uncontrolled study compared two TCM remedies and found that Kangfu Xiaozheng tablet was more effective than Guizhi Fuling pill for shrinking fibroids with improvement of irregular menstruation and pain (Sang 2004). Unfortunately, many Chinese herbal studies are poorly constructed, side effects underreported, and not easily accessible to the Western-trained clinician (Dharmananda 2008).

Because of the complexity and variability in treatment, consultation with an experienced TCM practitioner is recommended if the patient desires this type of management for her fibroids.

AYURVEDA

Ayurvedic recommendations and treatment for a woman with fibroids would be specific to her doshic imbalance. One Ayurvedic compound that has prominent usage for fibroid associated uterine bleeding is derived from the bark of the sacred Ashoka tree (*Saraca indica*). Traditional usage recognizes its astringent effects, which may decrease uterine bleeding. Usually the bark is boiled in either milk or water, and then removed. Most often, Saraca is found in formulation with numerous herbs (Dharmananda 2004) (see chapter on Ayurveda for more information).

Conclusion

When determining the optimal course of action for a woman with fibroids, a clinician must take into account the variability and complexity of the problem, along with the necessity for individualization of management. At present, conventional medicine offers no ideal option in the treatment of fibroids, so many women are exploring CAM approaches that are perceived to be safer, less costly, and at least as efficacious as conventional approaches. While CAM management of fibroids may ameliorate the more common symptoms of fibroids, delaying intervention until menopause arrives, significant diminishment or banishment of problematic fibroids generally requires more powerful conventional intervention. Integrative treatment can be on a continuum over time, readjusted as necessary, and reflective of the severity of the symptoms taking into account the unique needs of the woman . Integrative management of fibroids can happen when the clinician looks into a patient's eyes, holds her hand and, synchronizes the breath with the patient as she releases into anesthetic sleep for a surgical intervention.

REFERENCES

Atkinson C, Lampe J, Scholes D, et al. Lignan and isoflavones excretion in relation to uterine fibroids: a case-control study of young to middle-aged women in the United States. *Am J Clin Nutr.* September 2006;84(3):587–593.

Ausk, K, Reed, S. Alternative approaches for treatment of uterine fibroids. *Alternative Therapies in Women's Health.* September 2004;6(9):65–72.

Baird DD, Dunson DB, Hill MC, et al. Association of physical activity with the development of uterine leiomyoma. *Am J Epidemiol.* January 15, 2007;165(2):157–163.

Blauer M, Rovio PH, Ylikomi T, Heinonen PK. Vitamin D inhibits myometrial and leiomyoma cell proliferation in vitro. *Fertility and Sterility.* May 2009;91(5):1919–1925.

Chandrareddy A, Muneyyirci-Delale O, McFarlane S, Murad O. Adverse effects of phytoestrogens on reproductive health: a report of three cases. *Complementary Therapies in Clinical Practice.* 2008:14:132–135.

Chiaffarino F, Parazzini F, La Vecchia C, et al. Diet and uterine fibroids. *Obstet Gynecol.* 1999;94;395–398.

Cohen JD, Rubin HW. Functional *menorrhagia*: treat- ment with *bioflavonoids* and *vitamin C. Curr Ther Res.* 1960;2:539–544.

Day Baird D, Dunson DB, Hill MC, et al. High cumulative incidence of uterine leiomyoma in black and white women: ultrasound evidence. *Am J Obstet Gynecol.* January 2003;188(1):100–107.

Dharmananda S. September 2003. Chinese Herbal Therapy for Uterine Fibroids. http://www.itmonline.org/arts/fibroids.htm. Accessed on 8/25/08.

Dharmananda S. August 2008. Director, Institute for Traditional Medicine, Portland Oregon, personal correspondence 8/27/08.

Dharmananda S. September 2004. Excessive Uterine Bleeding Treated With Saraca, An Ayurvedic Herb. http://www.itmonline.org/arts/saraca.htm. Accessed on 8/25/08.

Ehrlich SD, Yarrow, May 2007. http://www.umm.edu/altmed/articles/yarrow-000282.htm, Accessed on 7/18/09.

Elizabeth A, Stewart MD. Clinical management guidelines for obstetrician-gynecologists, alternatives to hysterectomy in the management of leiomyomas. *ACOG Practice Bulletin.* August 2008;96:387–400.

Flake G, Andersen J, Dixon D. Etiology and pathogenesis of uterine leiomyomas: a review. *Environ Health Perspect.* June 2003;111(8): 1037–1054.

Gorbach SL, Goldin BR. Diet and the excretion and enterohepatic cycling of estrogens. *Prev Med.* July 1987;16(4):525–531.

Grzanna R, Lindmark L, Frondoza CG. Ginger—an herbal medicinal product with broad anti-inflammatory actions. *J Med Food.* Summer 2005;8(2):125–132.

Hartmann KE, Birnbaum H, Ben-Hamadi R, et al., Annual costs associated with diagnosis of leiomyomata. *Obstet Gynecol.* 2006;108:930–937.

Herbst AL, Mishell DR Jr, Stenchever MA, Droegemueller W. *Comprehensive Gynecology.* St. Louis, Missouri: Mosby Year Book; 1992.

Hobbs C, Keville K, *Women's Herbs, Women's Health.* Loveland, Colorado: Interweave Press; July 1998:61–62.

Hodges LC, Bergerson JS, Hunter DS, Walker CL. 2000 Estrogenic effects of organochlorine pesticides in uterine leiomyoma cells in vitro. *Toxicol Sci.* 54;355–364.

http://nccam.nih.gov/health/acupuncture/#status. Accessed on 8/25/08.

http://nccam.nih.gov/health/backgrounds/mindbody.htm#meditation. Accessed on 8/29/08.

http://nccam.nih.gov/health/chasteberry/#science. Accessed on 8/28/08.

http://www.nlm.nih.gov/medlineplus/druginfo/natural/patient-turmeric.html. Accessed on 8/28/08.

Hudson T. *Women's Encyclopedia of Natural Medicine, Alternative Therapies and Integrative Medicine for Total Health and Wellness.* New York: McGraw-Hill; 2008.

Imir AG, Lin Z, Yin P, et al. Aromatase expression in uterine leiomyomata is regulated primarily by proximal promoters 1.3/II/. *J Clin Endocrinol Metab.* May 2007;92(5):1979–1982.

Kjerulff KH, Langenberg P, Seidman JD, et al. Uterine leiomyomas: racial differences in severity, symptoms, and age at diagnosis. *J Reprod Med.* 1996;41:483–490.

Klatsky PC, Tran ND, Caughey AB, et al. Fibroids and reproductive outcomes: a systematic literature review from conception to delivery. *Am J Obstet Gynecol.* April 2008;198(4):357–366.

Low Dog T, Micozzi M. *Women's Health in Complementary and Integrative Medicine, A Clinical Guide.* St. Louis, Missouri: Elsevier Inc.; 2005.

Lucero J, Harlow BL, Barbieri RL, Sluss P, Cramer DW. Early follicular phase hormone levels in relation to patterns of alcohol, tobacco, and coffee use. *Fertil Steril.* October 2001;76(4):723–729.

lik M, Mendoza M, Payson M, Catherino WH. Curcumin, a nutritional supplement with antineoplastic activity, enhances leiomyoma cell apoptosis and decrease fibronectin expression. *Fertil Steril.* June 12, 2008 [Epub ahead of print].

Management of uterine fibroids: An update of the Evidence Structured Abstract. AHRQ publication no. 07-E011 July 2007. Agency for Healthcare Research and Quality, Rockville, MD. http://www.ahrq.gov/clinic/tp/uteruptp.htm. Accessed on 6/26/08.

McLachlan JA, Simpson E, Martin M. Endocrine disrupters and female reproductive health, Best Practice & Research. *Clin Endocrinol Metab.* 2006;20(1):63–75.

Minich DM, Bland JS. A Review of the clinical efficacy and safety of cruciferous vegetable phytochemicals. *Nutrition Reviews*. June 2007;65(6):259–267.

Moore AB, Castro L, Yu L, Zheng X, et al. Stimulatory and inhibitory effects of genistein on human uterine leiomyoma cell proliferation are influenced by the concentration. *Hum Reprod*. 2007;22(10):2623–2632.

Parker WH. Etiology, symptomatology, and diagnosis of uterine myomas. *Fertil Steril*. April 2007a;87(4).

Roa CV. Regulation of COX and LOX by curcumin. *Adv Exp Med Biol*. 2007;595:213–226.

Sakamoto S, Yoshino H, Shirahata Y, et al. Pharmacotherapeutic effects of kuei-chih-fu-ling-wan (keishi-bukuryo-gan) on human uterine myomas. *Am J Chin Med*. 1992;20(3–4):313–317.

Sang H. clinical and experimental research into treatment of hysteromyoma with promoting qi flow and blood circulation, softening and resolving hard lump. *J Trad Chin Med*. December 2004; 24(4):274–279.

Sparrowe L, Walden P. *The Woman's Book of Yoga and Health, A Lifelog Guide To Wellness*. Boston & London: Shambhala; 2002:8, 93.

Stewart EA, Morton CC. The Genetics of Leiomyomata—What clinicians need to know. *Obstet Gynecol*. 2006;107:917–921.

Stewart EA, Faur AV, Wise LA, et al. Predictors of subsequent surgery for uterine leiomyomata after abdominal myomectomy. *Obstet Gynecol*. 2002;99:426–432.

Stewart EA, Nowak RA. Leiomyoma-related bleeding: a classic hypothesis updated for the molecular era. *Hum Reprod Update*. July–August 996;2(4):295–306.

The Complete German Comission E Monographs, Therapeutic Guide to Herbal Medicines. Blumenthal M, senior editor, 1998 American Botanical Council, Integrative Medicine Communications, Boston, Massachusetts.

The FIBROID Registry: Report of Structure, Methods, and Initial Results. AHRQ Publication No. 05(06)-RG008, October 2005. Agency for Healthcare Research and Quality, Rockville, MD. http://www.ahrq.gov/research/fibroid/. Accessed on 6/18/08.

Walker CL, Stewart EA Uterine fibroids: the elephant in the room. *Science*. June 10, 2005;308.

Wallach EE, Vlahos NF, Uterine myomas: an overview of development, clinical features, and management. *Obstet Gynecol*. 2004;104:393–406.

Whiteman MK, Hillis SD, Jamieson DJ, et al. Inpatient hysterectomy surveillance in the United States, 2000–2004. *Am J Obstet Gynecol*. 2008;198(1):34.e1–e7.

Wyshak G, Frisch RE, Albright TE, Schiff I. Lower prevalence of benign diseases of the breast and benign tumors of the reproductive system among former college athletes compared to non-athletes. *Br J Cancer*. 1986;54:841–845.

21

Cervical Cancer

LISE ALSCHULER

CASE STUDY

Sylvia was a healthy 35-year-old mother of two. She had been happily and monogamously married for 10 years. Sylvia did not smoke or drink alcohol, was a healthy weight and her only health issue was long-standing psoriasis. At Sylvia's routine gynecological examination, she was told that her cervix looked a little suspicious. The results of her subsequent Pap smear revealed cervical atypia. She was shocked. She was also panicked as she was supporting her father who was dying from lung cancer and was worried about this being a precancerous condition. Her gynecologist told her not to worry and that any necessary treatment would be determined after a repeat Pap in 3 months. Sylvia could not sleep and realized that she could not simply wait for 3 more months. She sought my consultation. I recommended a comprehensive supplement dietary and stress management program. Sylvia adhered to the program with enthusiasm, experiencing a sense of wellness she had not realized that she was missing. In 3 months, her repeat Pap came back normal. Sylvia breathed a sigh of relief and vowed to continue to promote her health and wellness.

Introduction

Cervical cancer is the second most common cancer in women worldwide, and is the most common female cancer in many developing countries (Rock et al. 2000). Just a century ago, cervical cancer was the leading cause of death among women in the United States (Trimble et al. 2008). Over the past 30 years, widespread adoption of screening with Pap smears along with effective treatments for precancerous cervical conditions has cut the death rate from cervical cancer in half. The recent development of vaccines against the causative human papilloma virus (HPV) may reduce the prevalence of cervical cancer even further in the decades to come. Of significance too is the growing awareness of the role that certain lifestyle behaviors, diet, selected nutrients, and certain botanicals play in the prevention and treatment of cervical cancer.

Epidemiology

The worldwide incidence of cervical cancer is about 440,000 cases annually. In the United States, there are an estimated 15,000 cases of cervical cancer each year, representing an annual incidence of 8.7 per 100,000 women. However, these numbers represent a fraction of the total number of cervical abnormalities, which are considered risk factors for cervical cancer (Table 21.1). The mortality rate for cervical cancer among non-Hispanic white women in the United States is 2.6 per 100,000 and 4.9 per 100,000 for African American women (Trimble et al. 2008). In the United States, cervical cancer is most prevalent and more deadly in socioeconomically disadvantaged black and Hispanic women.

Significant to the epidemiology of cervical cancer is the rate of HPV infection among women, some strains of which are considered causal agents. The incidence of HPV in women is alarmingly high. In the United States, it is estimated that close to 25 million women between the ages of 14 and 59 years are infected

Table 21.1. Prevalence of Cervical Atypia

Cervical Atypica	Number of Cases per Year
Atypical squamous cells of uncertain significance (ASCUS)	2,000,000
Low-grade squamous intraepithelial lesions (LGSIL)	1,250,000
High-grade squamous intraepithelial lesions (HGSIL)	300,000

Source: Rock et al. (2000).

with HPV (Huh and Roden, 2008) Furthermore, it is predicted that 80% of all women will acquire genital HPV infection by 50 years of age (Huh and Roden 2008). Genital HPV, particularly HPV 16 and 18, and to a lesser extent HPV 6 and 11, are thought to cause two-thirds of all cervical cancers. Fortunately, the road from viral infection to cancer is not a one-way trajectory. Other factors such as dietary habits, smoking, sexual partners, and nutrient status play a role in viral virulence, thus creating a window for a multifaceted integrative approach to prevention and treatment.

> Declaring that cervical cancer should be eradicated is now a rational statement. Effective and low-cost screening, prevention vaccines and targeted lifestyle practices can make cervical cancer a disease of the past. I hope that in my time as a physician, the day will come when I will no longer witness anyone dying from cervical cancer.

PATHOPHYSIOLOGY AND DIAGNOSIS

There are three major histological types of cervical cancer. Squamous cell carcinoma is the most common type, followed by adenocarcinoma and then small cell carcinoma. Small cell carcinoma is a very rare form of cervical cancer and is associated with a worse prognosis and increased tendency for distant metastases (Chen et al. 2008). Cervical cancer is often asymptomatic in early stages. When symptoms do occur, it is often when the cancer is more advanced. These symptoms may include abnormal vaginal bleeding, heavy discharge, dyspareunia, dysuria, and pelvic pain. Advanced cervical cancer is characterized by metastases to the abdomen and lung primarily. Cervical cancer is diagnosed with cervical cytology (Pap smear) followed by biopsy and staged according to the International Federation of Gynecology and Obstetrics (FIGO) classification system (Table 21.2).

Cervical cancer is considered to be the result of infection with HPV, particularly types 16 and 18 (Munoz et al. 2003). The virus is introduced through sexual contact and proliferates in the basal cells of squamous epithelium. Host infection with HPV involves HPV early genes, namely E1, E2, E5, E6, and E7, the expression of which contributes to viral replication and abnormal proliferation. HPV-infected cells do not fully differentiate and thus do not express many viral proteins on their surfaces. This allows for immune evasion. In addition, the infected cell matures in the deeper epithelial layers, which are located further away from the highest concentration of T-cells. Thus, the more mature (still not fully differentiated) cervical cells avoid contact with the cellular arm of our immune system. Individuals with defects in T-cell-mediated immunity, such as

Table 21.2. Abbreviated FIGO Staging of Cervical Cancer

Stage I is carcinoma strictly confined to the cervix. The diagnosis of both Stages IA1 and IA2 should be based on microscopic examination of removed tissue, preferably a cone, which must include the entire lesion.

Stage II is carcinoma that extends beyond the cervix, but does not extend into the pelvic wall. The carcinoma involves the vagina, but not as far as the lower third.

Stage III is carcinoma that has extended into the pelvic sidewall. The tumor involves the lower third of the vagina.

Stage IV is carcinoma that has extended beyond the true pelvis or has clinically involved the mucosa of the bladder and/or rectum and includes spread to distant organs.

Source: TNM Classification of malignant tumours. In: Sobin L, Wittekind Ch, eds. *UICC International Union against Cancer*. 6th ed. Geneva, Switzerland; 2002:155–157.

women with HIV, are especially vulnerable to HPV-associated cancer as there is little chance at any point for mounting a cytotoxic attack. Despite the adeptness of immune evasion, HPV infection does not necessarily lead to the development of cervical cancer. In fact, the majority of women infected with HPV are able to eradicate this infection or prevent the pathogenicity of the virus. This is the primary opportunity for disease prevention and control in HSV-infected women and is influenced by several behavioral and nutritional factors.

Influencing the Pathogenicity of HSV Infection

There are well-established behavioral influences on HSV pathogenicity. Women with later sexual experiences, fewer sexual partners, female sexual partners, male sexual partners who use condoms, and women who are nonsmokers are all at decreased risk of developing cervical cancer if infected with HPV (Rock et al. 2000). HPV is transmitted sexually and increased sexual activity increases this exposure. Smoking is a direct carcinogen and cervical cells seem particularly vulnerable to the genotoxic effects of cigarettes. Counseling women about all of these factors should be the basis of a comprehensive integrative approach.

In addition, dietary intake and serum concentrations of carotenoids, vitamin C, vitamin E, and folate are inversely correlated with persistence of cervical HPV infection and development of cervical cancer (Rock et al. 2000). A unifying theory for the protective role of these nutrients against the development of cervical cancer in HPV-infected women centers around the role of peroxidation and DNA mutations. Reactive oxygen species (ROS) are considered to be involved in the initiation and progression of carcinogenesis. Low antioxidant activity has been observed in women with cervical cancer along with increased lipid peroxidation and suppressed cellular immunity compared to healthy controls ($n = 94$) (Kazbariene et al. 2004). Carcinogenesis is initiated by ROS-induced damage to oncogenes, the fragile genes in the DNA particularly susceptible to viral and oxidative damage. Women with cervical cancer have lower levels of endogenous antioxidants, such as glutathione, vitamin E, vitamin C, and coenzyme Q10 (Palan et al. 2003). It has been postulated that this low antioxidative status results from depletion due to lipid peroxide scavenging (Manju et al. 2002). Over time, impaired antioxidation will allow virally and oxidatively induced carcinogenesis to persist.

In addition to providing general antioxidation, carotenoids, vitamin C, vitamin E, and folate possess antineoplastic activity against cervical cancer cells. Carotenes induce apoptosis of dysplastic cells by downregulating epidermal growth factor receptor (EGFR) (Muto et al. 1995). Vitamin C stimulates phagocytosis, protects DNA against ROS damage, and may inhibit oncogene formation (Potischman et al. 1996). Vitamin E enhances cell-mediated immunity and phagocytosis (Meydani et al. 1997). Folate supports DNA methylation, particularly of HPV 16 oncogenes, thus silencing neoplastic formation (Hublarova et al. 2008). Additionally, adequate folate may protect against the incorporation of HPV DNA at folate-sensitive fragile sites (Butterworth et al. 1992).

Integrative Prevention Strategies

The role of individual nutrients in the pathogenesis of cervical cancer has been well elucidated and has given rise to specific lifestyle-based prevention strategies. A number of well-designed studies have demonstrated the protective link between certain nutrients and the development of cervical cancer. High intakes of vegetables, fruits, fiber, beta-carotenes, folic acid, retinols, vitamin E, and vitamin C are associated with up to 60% risk reduction for development of cervical cancer in HPV-positive women (Table 21.3).

It is important to note that the inverse relationship between these nutrients and cervical cancer has been specifically observed from food intake. This data does not directly support the use of individual dietary supplements for prevention.

Any discussion of prevention of cervical cancer would be incomplete without mention of HPV vaccination. HPV 16 and 18 are responsible for causing 70% of all cases of cervical cancer (Hoops and Twiggs 2008). The development

Table 21.3. Protective Effects of Dietary Components against Development of Cervical Cancer

Dietary Nutrients Studied	Study Design	Outcome	Citation
Vegetables, fruits, beta-carotene, vitamins C, E, fiber	Matched case control, $n = 170$	22%–44% lower risk of developing cervical cancer	Atalah et al. (2001)
Vitamin A, retinol	Matched cohort study, $n = 184$	Reduced risk of both in situ disease and invasive disease	Shannon et al. (2002)
Fiber, vitamins C, E, A, α-carotene, β-carotene, lutein, folate, total fruit and vegetable intake	Hospital-based, case–control study, $n = 239$	Risk reduction of 40%–60% was observed for women in the highest versus lowest tertiles of dietary intake of each nutrient	Ghosh et al. (2008)

of a vaccine that could protect a majority of women against pathogenic HSV infection, and thus cervical cancer, has led to widespread efforts to make this vaccine universally available. In addition to the obvious positive impact on human suffering, cost–benefit analysis demonstrates significant cost savings in the next several decades when the total cost of managing cervical cancer is considered (Prasad and Hill 2008). However, caution is warranted as HPV vaccination has not been in use long enough to fully determine long-term adverse effects.

Two vaccines are available which contain virus-like particles derived in one from HPV 16 and 18 (Cervarix) and the other from HPV 6,11, 16, and 18 (Gardasil). In a Phase 3 study, Cervarix showed 84% (97.9% CI, 73.5%–91.1%) efficacy against 6-month persistent infections with HSV type 16 and 74% (97.9% CI, 49.1%–87.8%) efficacy against HSV type 18. Gardasil has been shown to be 98% effective in preventing CIN 2+ lesions associated with HSV types 16 and 18 (Huh and Roden 2008) Clinical efficacy has been measured up to 5.5 years and is predicted to provide lifelong protection in the majority of people. In the United States, the Advisory Committee on Immunization Practices recommends HPV vaccination for females aged 11–12 years—ideally before they become sexually active. "Catch up" vaccination in females aged 13–26 is also recommended as this is the group with the highest prevalence of HPV infection (Wright et al. 2008). It is important for women to know that even with the cervical cancer vaccine, they must come in for their annual gynecological examination.

Integrative Treatment

It is simply beyond the scope of this chapter to delve extensively into the conventional treatment for cervical cancer. I would refer you to appropriate texts and articles on the topic. For this chapter, I want to stress that the bulk of integrative therapies in the management of cervical carcinoma lies within the realm of preventing HPV-induced dysplasia from becoming carcinoma. The impact of several nutrients as chemopreventive agents has already been discussed.

A woman with cervical dysplasia is a prime candidate for lifestyle modification, dietary medication, and supplementation. We can assume that women with cervical dysplasia have some degree of immunosuppression given the presence of a viral pathology. It is well-established that stress and chronic negative emotions (anger, anxiety, depression) disrupt immunity. Conversely, positive emotional states (happiness, joy, optimism) support immunity. Thus, counseling women with cervical dysplasia about stress management and their emotional well-being is critical. In many ways, cervical dysplasia can be viewed as a wake-up call for these women and can help motivate them to assess their emotional well-being. I am a strong proponent of giving women explicit permission to be happy and joyful (it astounds me how many women don't feel that they deserve to be happy) and will utilize the diagnosis of this precancerous condition to create this dialogue. A natural sequel to this conversation is a conversation about specific stress management practices. Helping a woman discover effective stress management techniques such as exercise, meditation, yoga, cooking, artwork, and so on will improve her immune function and will add wellness to her life. In addition to these important benefits, a lifestyle-based wellness program will also encourage her interest in, and compliance with, a supplement program.

It is common naturopathic practice to provide an aggressive dietary and supplement recommendations in order to reverse the dysplasia. Dietary recommendations constellate around a whole foods diet replete with colorful (antioxidant rich) fruits and vegetables. Excessive consumption of refined sugar and alcohol should be avoided due to their immunosuppressant effects. I have personally observed the benefits of additional supplementation. Along with my naturopathic colleagues, I routinely recommend several supplements. Folic acid, typically at 10 mg/day, can reverse cervical dysplasia (Butterworth et al. 1982). In addition, given the association between vitamins C and E and cervical cancer protection, combined with the fact that many Americans are functionally deficient in these antioxidants, their supplementation is indicated. I typically recommend vitamin C at 500 mg at least three times daily and vitamin E (d-alpha-tocopherol) at 400 IU twice daily. In addition to these supplements, there is compelling preclinical data that supports the use of green tea to reverse cervical dysplasia and prevent progression to cancer.

Several botanicals are indicated for women with cervical dysplasia. Green tea polyphenols, particularly polyphenon E, induce apoptosis, arrest the cell cycle, and decrease the production of epidermal growth factor receptor (EGFR), which is necessary for cervical cancer progression (Ahn et al. 2003). Green tea also supports hepatic detoxification (all phases) and provides antioxidation effects. I recommend daily consumption of at least 8 cups of good quality green tea or consumption of 600–1200 mg standardized extract of green tea (standardized to 80% polyphenols, of which at least 50% is EGCG) taken in divided doses and always taken with food. If a woman is willing, I will also recommend a retention vaginal douche with cooled green tea. Topical treatment with green tea has demonstrated benefit for cervical dysplasia (Ahn et al. 2003).

A naturopathic alternative to LEEP, conization or cryotherapy for precancerous cervical lesions, when there is a satisfactory colposcopy, is herbal escharotics treatment. This involves repeated application of enzyme and botanical agents in a sequential manner to the cervical tissue. I have used this treatment and, while more labor- and time-intensive, it is effective and offers the patient weekly opportunities for focused healing sessions in a supportive and safe environment. Naturopathic escharotic treatments involve twice weekly applications of ablative agents to the cervix. Agents used in naturopathic escharotics treatments are sequentiallly painted on the cervix and consist of bromelain, compounded zinc chloride, blood root (*Sanguinaria canadensis*) tincture and calendula (*Calendula officinalis*) succus tincture, followed by vaginal depletion packs, which are essentially tampons coated with a mixture of thuja oil, golden seal root (*Hydrastis canadensis*) tincture, tea tree essential oil, bitter orange essential oil, vitamin A, and ferrous sulfate. The agents used in escharotics treatments debride the cervical tissue, reduce inflammation, support local immunity, and induce apoptosis of virally infected cells. A full course of naturopathic escharotics treatments requires at least one-and-a-half months to be effective.

Indole-3-carbinol (I3C) and its gastric breakdown product, diindolylmethane (DIM) also available as a supplement, are useful natural agents for cervical dysplasia. I3C and DIM induce apoptosis of human cervical cancer cells and HPV-16 infected cervical cells (Chen et al. 2001). DIM also induces 2-hydroxylation of estrogen over 16-hydroxylation, whereas I3C induces both 2-hyrdoxylation and 4-hydroxylation. Women with CIN 2 and 3 have a higher 16-hydroxylation to 2-hydroxylation ratio, which is problematic in that 16-hyroxylated estrogen metabolites are strongly estrogenic and carcinogenic. In contrast, 2-hydroxylated estrogen metabolites are weakly estrogenic and not carcinogenic. Of note, 4-hydroxylated estrogen metabolites are strongly estrogenic and carcinogenic, raising concern about long-term upregulation of 4-hydroxylation with substances such as I3C. Administration of 200–400 mg of I3C can reverse CIN as demonstrated in a randomized control trial ($n = 30$) of women with CIN 2 or 3 (Bell et al. 2000).

Curcuma longa, or turmeric, is an Indian culinary herb. The past decade has seen an outpouring of preclinical and some clinical studies regarding *Curcuma longa* and one of its main constituents, curcumin (diferuloylmethane), as an antineoplastic agent. One such in vitro study demonstrated that curcumin induces apoptosis of cervical cancer cells in a concentration-dependent manner. Curcumin also selectively inhibits expression of viral oncogenes E6 and E7. Finally, curcumin downregulates NFkappaB, thus decreasing inflammation, a known potentiator of carcinogenesis (Divya and Pillai 2006). A phase I clinical trial of curcumin included four patients with cervical intraepithelial neoplasia (CIN). These patients, along with the other 21 patients in the study, tolerated doses of up to 8 g/day of curcumin doses without adverse effect. In addition, one of the four CIN patients demonstrated histological improvement and one of the four CIN patients proceeded to develop frank malignancy (Cheng et al. 2001). Of note, this was a phase I study and therefore not powered or designed to assess clinical effect.

Curcuma longa may also be beneficial for those patients undergoing chemoradiation. In one in vitro study, curcuminoids were found to decrease MDR-1 gene expression in multidrug-resistant human cervical carcinoma cells (Limtrakul et al. 2004). This result suggests that curcuminoids may reduce MDR-1 production of P-glycoprotein, a major cell membrane protein involved in cellular efflux of, and therefore resistance to, chemotherapy agents. Another in vitro study demonstrated cervical cancer cell sensitization to the cytotoxic effects of Taxol when these cells were simultaneously exposed to curcumin. This sensitization effect was not observed in normal cervical cells (Bava et al. 2005). Finally, pretreatment of cervical cancer cells with curcumin resulted in significant dose-dependent radiosensitization of these cells. Normal cells were not radiosensitized (Javvadi et al. 2008). Preclinical data indicates that curcumin may have potential as a synergistic agent with chemoradiation treatment for cervical carcinoma. When recommending turmeric, I encourage women to use turmeric generously in their cooking and will also recommend supplementation with 4000 mg *Curcuma longa* extracts standardized to 95% curcuminoids.

Other potentially useful integrative natural agents include ascorbic acid and *Agaricus blazei* (Brazilian sun mushroom) and acupuncture. One of the mechanisms of HPV carcinogenesis involves the viral degradation of p53 in cervical cancer cells, thereby interfering with the cell's apoptotic ability. An in vitro study demonstrated that ascorbic acid stabilized p53, restoring apoptosis. Intact apoptosis is necessary for successful chemotherapeutic response (Reddy et al. 2001). Thus, ascorbic acid may contribute to decreased tumor burden, particularly in conjunction with some chemotherapeutic agents. Of note, ascorbic acid has no known or theoretical interference with cisplatin, the standard first-line chemotherapy agent, and, in effect, may be synergistic with platin chemotherapy.

A small randomized placebo-controlled trial of 100 gynecologic patients, which included 61 cervical cancer patients, stages Ia–IIIb received with either carboplatin and etoposide or carboplatin and Taxol every 3 weeks with or without daily oral *Agaricus blazei* (3 packs daily of *A. blazei* Muril). Parameters of immune function and tolerance to treatment were observed. Those patients who received *A. blazei* had improved natural killer cell activity and improved appetite, less alopecia, better emotional stability, and less general weakness (Ahn et al. 2004). Of note, this study did not assess whether the *A. blazei* might have interacted with the chemotherapy in such a way as to decrease its efficacy (along with the decreased side effects as observed).

One of the adverse effects of radiation therapy for cervical cancer can be radiation rectitis. In an open trial of 44 patients with cervical cancer, receiving radiation therapy and with radiation rectitis, acupuncture was done once daily for up to 1 week. Of the patients, 72.73% of them experienced complete resolution of their radiation rectitis symptoms, 9.09% experienced marked improvement of their symptoms, 18.18% experienced somewhat improved symptoms, and no patients reported no benefit from acupuncture (Zaohua 1987). Acupuncture is also helpful in reducing radiation-induced fatigue and malaise. Acupuncture is a complementary therapy that should always be considered given its low risk and high potential benefit.

Some natural agents have preliminary data that suggests direct antineoplastic action against cervical cancer cells. A mixture containing lysine, proline, arginine, ascorbic acid, and green tea demonstrated significant antiproliferative effects on human cervical cancer cells via inhibition of matrix metalloproteinases (Roomi et al. 2006). Whether this antimetastatic action occurs *in vivo* remains to be determined. Finally, another natural substance, coenzyme Q10, has been shown to inhibit the cell growth and induce apoptosis of human cervical cancer cells (Gorelick et al. 2004). Although this effect has not yet been studied in humans, the preliminary data, combined with the minimal toxicity profile of coenzyme Q10, should be given consideration in an integrative treatment plan.

Conclusions

The key to successful integrative management of cervical cancer is prevention and early diagnosis. Lifestyle adjustments, which are heavily reliant upon dietary modifications, form the cornerstone of an integrative approach. Supplementation of selected nutrients and herbs also has a place in prevention and quite possibly in the management of established cervical carcinoma. Ultimately, with the adoption of prevention-oriented lifestyles, the advent of preventive vaccinations and continued screening practices, cervical cancer will be a disease of the past and this chapter will become obsolete to the integrative health care practitioner.

REFERENCES

Ahn WS, Huh SW, Bae SM, et al. A major constituent of green tea, EGCG, inhibits the growth of a human cervical cancer cell line, CaSki Cells, through apoptosis, G(1) arrest, and regulation of expression. *DNA Cell Biol.* 2003 Mar;22(3):217–224.

Ahn W.S, Kim DJ, Chae GT, et al. Natural killer cell activity and quality of life were improved by consumption of a mushroom extract, *Agaricus blazei* Murill Kyowa, in gynecological cancer patients undergoing chemotherapy. *Int J Gynecol Cancer.* 2004;14:589–594.

Atalah E, Urteaga C, Rebolledo A, et al. [Diet, smoking and reproductive history as risk factor for cervical cancer] (in Spanish). *Rev Med Child.* 2001;129(6):597–603.

Bava S, Puliappadamba V, Deepti A, et al. Sensitization of taxol-induced apoptosis by curcumin involves down-regulation of nuclear factor-kappaB and the serine/threonine kinase Akt and is independent of tubulin polymerization. *J Biol Chem.* 2005;280(8):6301–6308.

Bell MC, Crowley-Nowick P, Bradlow HL, et al. Placebo-controlled trial of indole-3-carbinol in the treatment of CIN. *Gynecol Oncol.* 2000;78(2):123–129.

Butterworth C. Effect of folate on cervical cancer: synergism among risk factors. *Acad NY Acad Sci.* 1992;669:293–299.

Butterworth CE, Hatch KD, Gore H, Krumdieck CL. Improvement in cervical dysplasia associated with folic acid therapy in users of oral contraceptives. *Am J Clin Nutr.* 1982 Jan;35(1):73–82.

Chen D, Qi M, Auborn KJ, et al. Indole-3-carbinol and diindolylmethane induce apoptosis of human cervical cancer cells and in murine HPV 16-transgenic preneoplastic cervical epithelium. *J Nutr.* 2001;131(12):3294–3302.

Chen J, Macdonald O, Gaffney D. Incidence, mortality, and prognostic factors of small cell carcinoma of the cervix. *Obstet Gynecol.* 2008;111(6):1394–1402.

Cheng A, Hsu C, Lin J, et al. Phase I clinical trial of curcumin, a chemopreventive agent, in patients with high-risk or pre-malignant lesions. *Anticancer Res.* 2001;21:2895–2900.

Davelaar E, van de Lande J, von Mensdorff-Pouilly S, Blankenstein M, et al. Combination of serum tumor markers identifies high-risk patients with early-stage squamous cervical cancer. *Tumour Biol.* 2008;29(1):9–17.

Divya C, Pillai M. Antitumor action of curcumin in human papillomavirus associated cells involves downregulation of viral oncogenes, prevention of NFkB and AP-1 translocation, and modulation of apoptosis. *Mol Carcinog.* 2006;45(5):320–332.

Garcia-Closas R, Castellsague X, Bosch X, et al. The role of diet and nutrition in cervical carcinogenesis: a review of recent evidence. *Int J Cancer.* 2005;117:629–637.

Ghosh C, Baker J, Moysich K, et al. Dietary intakes of selected nutrients and food groups and risk of cervical cancer. *Nutrition Cancer.* 2008;60(3):331–341.

Gorelick C, Lopez-Jones M, Goldberg G, et al. Coenzyme Q10 and lipid-related gene induction in HeLa cells. *Am J Obstet Gynecol.* 2004;190(5):1432–1434.

Haie-Meder C, Morice P, Castiglione M. Cervical cancer: ESMO clinical recommendations for diagnosis, treatment and follow-up. *Ann Oncol.* 2008;19(Suppl. 2):ii17–Sii18.

Hoops K, Twiggs L. Human papillomavirus vaccination: the policy debate over the prevention of cervical cancer—a commentary. *J Low Genit Tract Dis.* 2008; 12(3):181–S184.

Hublarova P, Hrstka R, Vojtesek B. [The significance of methylation in HPV16 genome to cervix carcinogenesis] (in Czech). *Ceska Gynekol.* 2008;73(2):87–92.

Huh W, Roden R. The future of vaccines for cervical cancer. *Gyn Oncol.* 2008;109:S48–SS56.

Javvadi P, Segan A, Tuttle S, et al. The chemopreventive agent curcumin is a potent radiosensitizer of human cervical tumor cells via increased reactive oxygen species production and overactivation of the mitogen-activated protein kinase pathway. *Mol Pharmacol.* 2008;73(5):1491–S14501.

Kazbariene B, Prasmickiene G, Krikstaponiene A, et al. [Changes in the parameters of immune and antioxidant systems in patients with cervical cancer] (in Lithuanian). *Medicina* (Kaunas). 2004;40(12):1158–1164.

Limtrakul P, Anuchapreeda S, Buddhasukh D. Modulation of human multidrug-resistance MDR-1 gene by natural curcuminoids. *BMC Cancer.* 2004;17;4:13.

Manju V, Sailaja K, Nalini N. Circulating lipid peroxidation and antioxidant status in cervical cancer patients: a case-control study. *Clin Biochem.* 2002;35:621–625.

Meydani S, Meydani M, Blumberg B. Vitamin E supplementation and in vivo immune response in healthy elderly subjects: a randomized controlled trial. *JAMA.* 1997;277:1380–1386.

Munoz N, Bosch X, Sanjose S, et al. Epidemiologic classification of human papillomavirus types associated with cervical cancer. *NEJM.* 2003;348:518–527.

Muto Y, Fujii J, Shidoji Y. Growth retardation in human cervical dysplasia-derived cell lines by beta-carotene through down-regulation of epidermal growth factor receptor. *Am J Clin Nutr.* 1995;62:6S.

Palan P, Mikhail M, Shaban D, et al. Plasma concentrations of coenzyme Q10 and tocopherols in cervical intraepithelial neoplasia and cervical cancer. *Eur J Cancer Prev.* 2003;12:321–326.

Potischmann N, Brinton L. Nutrition and cervical neoplasia. *Cancer Cases Control.* 1996;7:113–126.

Prasad S, Hill R. A cost-benefit analysis on the HPV vaccine in Medicaid-enrolled females of the Appalachian region of Kentucky. *J Ky Med Assoc.* 2008;106(6):271–276.

Reddy V, Khanna N, Singh N. Vitamin C augments chemotherapeutic response of cervical carcinoma HeLa cells by stabilizing p53. *Biochem Biophys Res Commun.* 2001;282(2):409–415.

Rock C, Michael C, Reynolds R, Ruffin M. Prevention of cervix cancer. *Crit Rev Oncol/Hematol.* 2000;33:169–185.

Roomi M, Ivanov V, Kalinovsky T, et al. Suppression of human cervical cancer cell lines HeLa and DoTc2 by a mixture of lysine, proline, ascorbic acid, and green tea extract. *Int J Gynecol Cancer.* 2006;16(3):1241–1247.

Shannon J, Thomas D, Ray R, et al. Risk factors for invasive and in-situ cervical carcinoma in Bangkok, Thailand. *Cancer Causes Control.* 2002;13(8):691–699.

Trimble E, Harlan L, Gius D, et al. Patterns of care for women with cervical cancer in the United States. *Cancer.* 2008:9.

Wright T, Huh W, Monk B, et al. Age considerations when vaccinating against HPV. 2008;109:S40–S47.

Zaohua Z. Effect of acupuncture on 44 cases of radiation rectitis following radiation therapy for carcinoma of the cervix uteri. *J Trad Chin Med.* 1987;792:139–140.

22

Breast Cancer

SUSAN LOVE AND DIXIE J. MILLS

CASE STUDY

Debra, a perimenopausal woman, has an abnormal mammogram. She is referred to a surgeon who reviews the films with her and shows her the abnormality—a cluster of microcalcifications with a small irregular distortion. Given the suspicious nature of the films, she is referred for a stereotactic biopsy, which returns positive for an invasive cancer.

Although Debra's mother had breast cancer at 60 and had a mastectomy, Debra prefers to have a lumpectomy, sentinel node to be followed by radiation. Her nodes are negative and her tumor is sent for Oncotype DX testing, which shows a low reoccurrence score. Initially, she is concerned about radiation and drugs and wants to spend some time doing some personal healing. She then decides to have the radiation and to start on tamoxifen; however, it increases her perimenopausal symptoms. She cuts back on her tamoxifen while she is referred to a nutritionist and an exercise program. She is able to lose a few pounds by eliminating snack foods and substituting healthier alternatives such as nuts and vegetables. The exercise routine is also helping her sleep patterns. After a few months, she is back on her full dose of tamoxifen and having fewer side effects.

Overview

Breast cancer remains the most common cancer in women both in the United States and around the globe. An estimated 182,000 new breast cancer cases are expected to be diagnosed in the United States in 2008 (Ries et al. 2008). While the etiology of the steady increase in cases since the 1960s is not totally apparent, an affluent Western lifestyle and delayed child-bearing practices appear to be contributing factors. Mortality rates from breast cancer have decreased slightly in the last several years and since 2003, the number of estrogen positive cancers in postmenopausal women has also decreased (Ravdin et al. 2007). This decline appears to be directly attributable to the abrupt stoppage of hormone replacement after the results of the Women's Health Initiative (WHI) study (Rossouw 2002). While the incidence is highest among white women, African-Americans have a higher mortality rate, and Hispanics have the lowest incidence and mortality. Breast cancer in men is rare, accounting for only 1% of all breast cancers.

Cancer begins in the lining of the ducts and lobules of the breast (Wellings et al. 1973). Historically, breast cancer types were primarily distinguished histologically by whether they were ductal or lobular in origin. It is now recognized that there is a greater range of diversity based on genetic and molecular changes starting with progenitor cells. More attention is now being given to the importance of the breast stroma and microenvironment with its growth factors and the host immune status in cancer initiation and progression (Fournier et al. 2006).

Risk

Breast cancer risk appears to be correlated with high levels of endogenous estrogen at certain lifetime periods, including in utero, puberty, and menopause. Increasing age is a risk factor in the Western world as is a maternal or paternal family history. Other risk factors include childhood or adolescent exposure to ionizing radiation, exogenous estrogens, and possibly chemicals and viruses. Table 22.1 illustrates the risk factors that have been identified in numerous epidemiological studies. However, most women who develop breast cancer have few if any of these known risk factors, while some women who have all of them may never develop the disease. Mammographic density is a newly identified risk factor that implicates the role of the breast stroma, which accounts for much of the density reading. Two large tumor suppressor genes, BRCA1 and 2, located on chromosomes 17 and 13, account for approximately 5% of all breast cancers. Women who carry one of these mutations have a lifetime breast cancer risk of 40%–80%, depending on mutation, penetrance, and other host factors. No recommendations exist at this time for population screening for these mutations. Women interested in testing should be counseled and evaluated at a high risk or genetic counseling center.

Table 22.1. Factors that Increase the Relative Risk for Breast Cancer in Women

Relative Risk	Factor
>4.0	Female
	Increasing age
	Genetic mutations (BRCA1 and or BRCA2)
	Two or more first-degree relatives diagnosed at an early age
	Personal history of breast cancer
2.1–4.0	One first-degree relative with breast cancer
	Biopsy confirmed atypical hyperplasia
	High-dose radiation to chest
	High bone density (postmenopausal)
	Late age at first full-term pregnancy (>30 years)
	Early menarche (<12 years)
	Late menopause (>55 years)
	No full-term pregnancies
	Never breastfed a child
	Recent oral contraceptive use
1.1–2.0	Recent and long-term use of hormone replacement therapy
	Obesity (postmenopausal)
	Personal history of endometrium, ovary or colon cancer
	Alcohol consumption
	Height (tall)
	High socioeconomic status
	Jewish heritage

American Cancer Society, Breast Cancer Facts & Figures 2005–2006 assessed on line www.cancer.org

Conventional Prevention Strategies

The selective estrogen receptor modulator (SERM) Tamoxifen was approved by the Food and Drug Administration (FDA) for the prevention of breast cancer in high-risk women in the early 1990s (Wolmark and Dunn 2001). While Tamoxifen has been shown to reduce risk by almost 50%, its use has not been widely adopted by doctors and women, largely because of the potential side effects such as uterine cancer and pulmonary emboli and the inability to identify which women clearly benefit. The FDA recently approved the use of raloxifene (Evista), a SERM used for osteoporosis prevention, for breast cancer risk reduction in postmenopausal women (Vogel et al. 2006). Other SERMs, aromatase inhibitors, and COX-2 inhibitors are in clinical trials. Due to time and costs, there may never be a large randomized controlled trial (RCT) of any functional food or exercise program as prevention.

Surgery, usually in the form of prophylactic skin-sparing mastectomies, is becoming more popular perhaps because of better reconstruction (Singletary 1996; Tuttle et al. 2007). The success rate of this strategy may be over 90% if no cancer is detected in the breast tissue; but it comes at an obvious cost especially as most women overestimate their risk (Geiger et al. 2005). Nipple sparing procedures are currently being evaluated. Bilateral oophrectomy reduces breast cancer risk by 50% in BRCA1 and 2 carriers (Mokbel 2003).

Population Screening

Annual mammograms are the currently accepted imaging technique beginning at age 40, unless high risk. Breast self-examination (BSE) has not been shown to decrease mortality; however, women are still encouraged to get to know their breasts and report any changes. Clinical breast examinations are a routine part of an annual examination, yet many primary care providers are not sufficiently trained in this technique (Saslow et al. 2004). An updated Cochrane Review (Kösters and Gøtzsche 2008) found no benefit from screening by BSE and instead suggested that it leads to increased harm due to the number of benign lesions identified and an increased number of biopsies performed. At present, they did not recommend screening by BSE or physical examination.

Newer imaging methods are available, such as magnetic resonance imaging (MRI), ultrasound, and breast PET scans, but are all relatively expensive as well as time-consuming for the woman and the radiologist. This limits their potential for routine or widespread, global use. Newer thermography cameras and light source imaging are still investigational and should not be substituted for mammography at this time. Studies are underway to identify markers in blood, nipple aspirate fluid, urine, or saliva that could indicate the presence of cancer or increased risk but none have been validated at this time (Fabian 2007). While estrogen is implicated in breast cancer promotion, there is no recommendation for estrogen blood level testing at this time. Estrogen metabolite ratio testing is available in some laboratories but has not been standardized or validated (Greenlee et al. 2007).

Diagnosis and Treatment

Women usually first present with a lump or an abnormal mammogram. Tissue diagnosis is obtained with a needle biopsy performed as an outpatient procedure with ultrasound or mammographic guidance or by palpation. Despite popular concern, there is no evidence that needles spread viable cancer cells (Chagpar et al. 2005). Breast cancer treatment is a multidisciplinary field that includes surgery, radiation, and oncology with an integrative component. Standard treatment guidelines are shown in Figure 22.1. Most women are offered a choice of surgery options. The overall survival from lumpectomy and mastectomy has been shown to be equivalent and breast conservation has been preferable since the Consensus Statement of 1990 (Jacobson et al. 1995). The sentinel lymph node procedure is now standard of care and saves the morbidity of a full axillary dissection for many women. Sentinel node pathology has led to an increased finding of micrometastasis and isolated tumor cells on immunohistochemistry. The significance of these remains controversial. Newer FDA-approved molecular and genetic tests are available (Oncotype Dx, Mammoprint) and can be ordered on the tumor for prognostic information that can guide decisions about systemic therapy. This is a step toward a more personalized medicine from the prior one-size-fits-all approach. Herceptin is the first directed molecular antibody used to treat women whose tumors are her-2-neu positive and is given along with chemotherapy. Future therapies will most likely be based on these more targeted approaches.

CLINICAL TIP: PATIENT EMPOWERMENT

- In our experience, most women will benefit from being seen at a center that offers a multidisciplinary team approach. Breast cancer treatment regimes work best if they can be individualized for each woman. Women should be included in the decision-making, although some may defer to their providers. The adjuvantonline.com program is

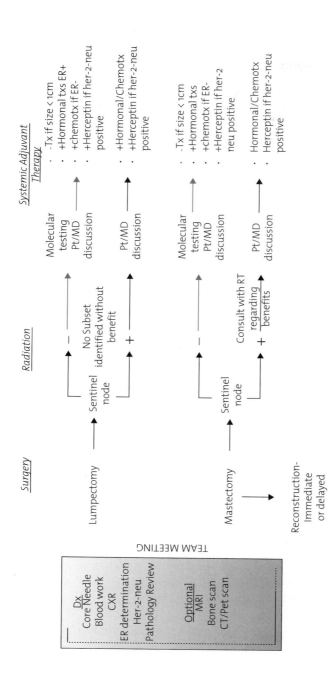

FIGURE 22.1. Guidelines for multidisciplinary treatment for invasive breast cancer.

useful in helping understand the statistical benefits of systemic treatments. Many women want to partner with their providers and take an active, empowered role.

Special Cases: DCIS

The number of cases of ductal carcinoma in situ (DCIS) has been growing in recent years, most likely due to better mammographic detection. Treatment for DCIS remains based on an invasive cancer model. As a result, surgery, radiation, and hormonal treatments are advocated for this noninvasive, nonlife-threatening disease. It is important for patients to know that less than 1% of women die from DCIS and that they have time to gather all of the information they need before making treatment decisions. Clinical trials now underway are exploring the potential of treating the affected duct through the nipple as well as looking to distinguish molecular signatures of aggressive types of DCIS from those that do not progress.

INTEGRATIVE APPROACHES

Awareness of and interest in complementary therapies is increasing among patients with cancer in general and in women with breast cancer in particular (Navo et al. 2004). Integrative therapies are clearly available and can be utilized at many times in a woman's life, including during treatment, after and before (Table 22.2).

Individuals with cancer have access to a vast amount of information. Most patients feel empowered by being able to access this information. However, not all will know how to assess which sources are providing evidence-based recommendations and could benefit from some guidance. We recommend the following Web sites:

- www.cancer.gov
- www.dslrf.org
- www.clinicaltrials.gov
- www.breastcancertrials.org
- www.adjuvantonline.com
- www.mskcc.org (source for reviews of studies on herbs)
- www.mdanderson.org (source for integrative oncology program resources)
- www.naturalstandard.com (database for evidence-based studies on complementary treatments)

Table 22.2. Integrative Therapies for Breast Cancer Prevention, Treatment and Survivorship

Types of therapies	During traditional treatment	After	Prevention
NUTRITION			
Weight control	*	**	**
Healthy diet	*	*	*
Soy, phytoestrogens	* in diet	*in diet	**
Alcohol	–	** less than 2 drinks/day	** less than 2 drinks/day
Low glycemic		*	*
Green tea	*	*	*
Garlic	*	*	*
SUPPLEMENTS			
Antioxidants	↓	*	*
Vitamin D	*	**	**
Omega-3-fatty acids/fish oil	*	**	*
Curcumin	*	**	*
Melatonin	*	*	
Ginger	*	*	*
Medicinal mushrooms—maitake		*	
CoQ-10	*	*	
Mistletoe	*	*	
PHYSICAL ACTIVITY			
Exercise	**	**	*
Yoga	**	**	*
MIND–BODY			
Stress reduction techniques	**	**	*
Social support	**	**	*
Spirituality/faith/prayer	*	*	*

(continued)

Table 22.2. (Continued)

Types of therapies	During traditional treatment	After	Prevention
MANIPULATIVE			
Acupuncture	**	**	
Massage	**	*	

* – small RCTs or other studies of varying quality
** – large, methodologically sound RCTs or positive systematic reviews.
↓– not recommended

Physical Activity

There is now convincing evidence that physical activity can reduce breast cancer risk by about 20%–30% (Friedenreich and Cust 2008). While recreational activity appears to offer the most benefit, with a dose–response seen with moderate to vigorous intensity activity, walking, household and occupational activity have been found to confer benefits as well. Risk reductions have been observed for activities performed at all age periods with lifetime activity of at least 3 hours a week most consistently associated with a decrease in risk. One study found that patient preference for a type of exercise during chemotherapy played an important part in quality of life outcomes and that benefits were maximized when training programs were matched to a patient's personal, demographic, and medical factors (Courneya et al. 2008). It is not yet fully understood why and how exercise affects breast cancer risk. Proposed biological mechanisms include a reduction in circulating estrogens and exposure to sex steroid hormones with concurrent changes in metabolism pathways, changes to insulin-related factors, and the modulation of the inflammatory response. Although further research is needed to tease out the critical factors, it is now widely recognized that physical activity has a role to play in breast cancer prevention and treatment. Other forms of exercise such as yoga, qigong, and tai chi have also been shown to be useful during and after breast cancer treatments.

Nutrition

The effect of diet on breast cancer risk remains not completely clear. Caloric restriction, energy balance, and weight control play important roles in maintaining overall health. Although obesity is a risk factor for postmenopausal women, it does not appear to increase breast cancer risk in premenopausal women. One study found that weight loss in menopause resulted in a 40% reduction in risk (Eliassen et al. 2006).

The evidence is mixed about which foods are protective and which are promoting of breast cancer. Elements of the Mediterranean-style diet with high intake of whole grains, fruits, and vegetables and olive oil are recommended for overall good health but no one component stands out as a magic bullet. Meta-analysis of the role of dairy foods does not support any compelling association between consumption and risk (Parodi 2005). Evidence for risk related to high fat intake is mixed. While international epidemiological studies seemed to link high fat to risk of breast cancer, several recent prospective studies show little association between total fat intake and breast cancer incidence or reoccurrence (Michels et al. 2008). On the other hand, WINS showed that a low fat diet might be particularly important for women with ER negative breast cancer where it reduced the risk of recurrence by 42% (Chlebowski et al. 2006). Studies on glycemic load, index, and carbohydrate and sugar intake are mixed with positive links focusing on weight gain, suggesting insulin-related effects (Lajous et al. 2008).

Alcohol intake of two or more drinks per day is known to be associated with an increased risk of breast cancer with a dose–response effect in both premenopausal and postmenopausal women. Use of folate may neutralize this effect. Estrogen and androgen levels increase in women consuming alcohol and the effect appears to be additive with hormone replacement therapy (HRT) (Suzuki et al. 2005). Consumption of well-done red meat is associated with increased risk, probably relating to the chemicals created by high-heat cooking.

The role of phytoestrogens in the diet remains controversial; there is conflicting evidence as to whether eating isoflavones-rich foods during adulthood can reduce breast cancer risk. However there is evidence that early exposure to isoflavones is protective for most sex-hormone-related cancers (Duffy et al. 2007). Because soy, an excellent nonanimal protein source contains estrogen-like compounds, many patients and providers alike have questioned what role it should play in the diet of breast cancer survivors. Several NCI and NCCAM sponsored clinical trials (Fleming 2002) are currently exploring whether soy intake can improve quality of life and reduce treatment-related menopausal symptoms in women with breast cancer. Phytoestrogen consumption for postmenopausal women with breast cancer is considered controversial; women taking Tamoxifen are advised to avoid soy food consumption. The role of flaxseed, an excellent source of lignans, omega 3, and fiber, in breast cancer prevention and treatment is now being studied.

Grapefruit has been shown in one study to increase the incidence of breast cancer in postmenopausal women (Monroe et al. 2008). It has been theorized that grapefruit increases endogenous hormone levels. Until further studies are done on this topic, it may be advisable for older women to limit their grapefruit consumption.

A recent review found that neither coffee nor tea usage increased breast cancer risk in the Nurses Health Study (Ganmaa et al. 2008).

CLINICAL TIP

- It has been our experience that many women view their breast cancer diagnosis as a wake-up call and want to make lifestyle changes. They can often benefit from the nutritional counseling offered by a registered dietitian with knowledge of integrative medicine. At this time, there is no evidence that any particular dietary regime can substitute for traditional cancer care. However, patients may be drawn to certain diets they believe will help them fight their cancer and need the supervision of a qualified provider to ensure nutritional adequacy.

Supplements

While nutrition in the form of food is always preferable, multivitamin and mineral supplements are used by a majority of Americans and cancer survivors. Physicians are usually unaware of what supplements their patients use and at this time, there are no evidence-based guidelines for supplement use among breast cancer survivors (Velicer et al. 2008).

ANTIOXIDANTS

The use of antioxidant supplements during chemotherapy and/or radiation therapy is controversial. A recent overview concluded that their use should be discouraged because of the possibility of tumor protection and reduced survival (Lawenda et al. 2008). Antioxidants found in food, usually fruits and vegetables, are considered safe (Norman 2003).

VITAMIN D

There is growing evidence that vitamin D deficiency is surprisingly common and that vitamin D3 may play a significant role in breast cancer prevention (Gissel et al. 2008). It is safe to supplement with at least the daily recommended intake of 400 IU with an upper limit of 2000 IU. Levels can be monitored by checking 25-hydroxy-vitamin D and then dosing accordingly to get within the therapeutic range of 35–50 ng/mL as an excess, though rare, may lead to hypercalcemia.

COENZYME Q10

It has been suggested that the antioxidant coenzyme Q10 can decrease toxicity to the myocardial muscle, especially during chemotherapy. Although a few studies have confirmed this, a recent Cochrane review found no benefit (van Dalen et al. 2008).

MELATONIN

Melatonin is an OTC hormone generally used for sleep disorders. Because it is an antioxidant, antiinflammatory, antiangiogenic, apoptotic, and hormone modulator, it may have benefits for cancer patients and a role in breast cancer prevention. Disrupted sleep has been shown to be a potential risk factor for breast cancer and nighttime shift workers appear to be at higher risk. It has been theorized that this is because light exposure at night suppresses melatonin (Hansen 2001). The common dose is 3 µg–3 mg at bedtime; however, doses of 20–40 mg/day have been studied in patients with solid, metastatic tumors (Mills et al. 2005). Women taking it should be cautioned that dramatic dreams are a common side effect.

INDOLE-3-CARBINOL

Indole-3-carbinol (I3C), a phytochemical found in cruciferous vegetables, has been shown to be a potent antiproliferative agent in human breast cancer cells (Brew et al. 2005). When taken in pill form, it appears to be well tolerated and to have the same effect on estrogen metabolites as eating cruciferous vegetables. The dose typically used in studies is 400 mg/day. Diindolylmethane (DIM), a biologically active congener of I3C, has also been shown to be a promising agent for the prevention of estrogen-sensitive cancers (Mulvey et al. 2007).

Botanicals and Herbs

BLACK COHOSH (ACTAEA RACEMOSA)

Extracts of the rhizome of the herb black cohosh, a native North American plant used by American Indians for gynecological problems, has been studied in Germany for decades as a nonestrogenic treatment for menopausal symptoms. Studies have confirmed that it does not have estrogenic effects on breast tissue (Ruhlen et al. 2007) and can be safely used for treatment of menopausal symptoms, although its success is limited. A small number of case reports suggesting liver toxicity in women taking black cohosh products led the regulatory bodies of Australia, Canada, and a number of European countries to mandate a cautionary statement on the label, advising women to discontinue using the product if symptoms of liver disease develop.

Immune Modulators

MISTLETOE

The German health authorities approve mistletoe injections as a palliative therapy for malignant tumors. It is believed to boost the immune system and reduce stress. The most common commercial preparations used in Europe are sold under the trade names Iscador and Helixor. Mistletoe is not FDA-approved or readily available in the United States. Mistletoe is used in addition to standard treatments and has not been studied as a sole primary treatment.

Medicinal mushrooms, that is, shiitake, maitake, reishi, are believed to be immune-modulating and can be used as complementary treatments. Doses vary by product.

ANTIINFLAMMATORIES

Green tea (Camellia sinensis)

Compounds in green tea have been shown to exert potent antioxidant activity and preliminary research suggests it may be a chemopreventive agent. A meta-analysis of four epidemiological studies found a 20% reduction in breast cancer cases in women who drank at least 5 cups of green tea a day (Sun et al. 2006). Women should be mindful of the caffeine content.

Turmeric (Curcuma longa)

This is used widely as a tea, spice, or condiment. It is also available as an herbal supplement, often standardized to concentrated levels of curcumin, the highly active yellow pigment found in turmeric rhizome. Laboratory studies have found that it can induce apoptosis (Ramachandran 2005). It is also a strong aromatase inhibitor with antiinflammatory and antioxidant properties. Although few clinical studies have been done, it would appear safe given its use over centuries in India and Asia. Standardized extracts providing 1–2 g of curcuminoids per day are typically used for inflammatory conditions.

Ginger (Zingiber officinale)

Ginger used as a spice or tea has shown to be effective in reducing nausea associated with chemotherapy. Antiemetic doses generally range from 1 to 2 g/day.

Stress Reduction

MIND–BODY TECHNIQUES

The most common stress reduction methods are breathing and meditation. These simple techniques have been found to be effective in reducing hot flashes in breast cancer patients on Tamoxifen treatment (Domar et al. 1997). Mind–body techniques have also been shown to be effective in presurgical programs to reduce pain levels, anxiety, drug requirements, and days in the hospital (Astin et al. 2003). These techniques have recently been shown to change gene expression (Dusek et al. 2008).

It is recommended that women be offered group or individual support. The sharing of stories, whether in a group or by keeping a journal, has been shown to improve psychoneuroimmunological markers. Many women use the diagnosis of breast cancer as an opportunity to make sense, search for meaning, or reaffirm their spiritual faith. Studies have not found a relationship between personality type and breast cancer risk (Lillberg et al. 2002).

ACUPUNCTURE OR ACUPRESSURE

These have both been shown to be effective in relieving the nausea and fatigue that often accompany chemotherapy and radiation therapy (Ezzo et al. 2007). A growing body of research supports the use of acupuncture for hot flashes and neuropathy (Deng et al. 2007; Frisk et al. 2008; Walker et al. 2007; Visovsky et al. 2007; Wong and Sagar 2006).

MASSAGE

Massage therapy and therapeutic touch programs have been shown to reduce distress, pain, physical and emotional discomfort levels, and fatigue in hospitalized and out-patients (Menefee and Monti 2005). Lymphatic massage is helpful in the prevention and treatment of lymphedema.

CLINICAL TIPS

- The term "chemobrain" is often used to describe the symptoms that many women experience after the completion of chemotherapy. It typically manifests as moderate cognitive impairment with some memory loss, difficulty finding words, decreased speed in performing routine activities, and an inability to multitask. After ruling out organic causes, most women find it helpful to know that it typically dissipates over time. Aerobic exercise, regular sleep, mind stretching "games," and learning new tasks also help.
- The class of hormone treatments called aromatase inhibitors often result in muscle and joint pain. We have found that a combination of nonsteroidal antiinflammatory OTC drugs, fish-oil supplements, and yoga may be helpful. Reducing the drug dose to every other day and then gradually increasing it to every day may help as well.

REFERENCES

Astin JA, Shapiro SL, Eisenberg DM, Forys KL. Mind-body medicine: state of the science, implications for practice. *J Am Board Fam Pract*. 2003;16:131–147.

Brew CT, Aronchik I, Hsu JC, et al. Indole-3-carbinol activates the ATM signaling pathway independent of DNA damage to stabilize p53 and induce G1 arrest of human mammary epithelial cells. *Int J Cancer*. 2005. 2006 Feb 15;118(4):857–868.

Chagpar AB, Martin RC, Scoggins CR, et al. Factors predicting failure to identify a sentinel node in breast cancer. *Surgery*. 2005;138:56–63.

Chlebowski RT, Blackburn GL, Thomson CA, et al. Dietary fat reduction and breast cancer outcome: interim efficacy results from the Women's Intervention Nutrition Study. *J Natl Cancer Instit*. 2006;98(24):1767–1776.

Courneya K, McKenzie D, Mackey J, et al. Moderators of the effects of exercise training in breast cancer patients receiving chemotherapy: a randomized controlled trial. *Cancer*. 2008;112(8):1845–1853.

Deng G, Vickers A, Yeung S, et al. Randomized, controlled trial of acupuncture for the treatment of hot flashes in breast cancer patients. *J Clin Oncol*. 2007;25(35):5584–5590.

Domar A, Irvin J, Mills D. Use of relaxation training to reduce the frequency and intensity of tamoxifen-induced hot flashes. *Mind/Body Med*. 1997;2(2):82–86.

Duffy C, Perez K, Partridge A. Implications of phytoestrogen intake for breast cancer. *CA Cancer J Clin*. 2007;57:260–277.

Dusek JA, Otu HH, Wohlhueter AL, et al. Genomic counter-stress changes induced by the relaxation response. *PLoS One*. 2008;3(7):e2576.

Eliassen AH, Colditz GA, Rosner B, Willett WC, Hankinson SE. Adult weight change and risk of postmenopausal breast cancer. *JAMA*. 2006;296(2):193–201.

Ezzo JM, Richardson MA, Vickers A, et al. Acupuncture-point stimulation for chemotherapy-induced nausea or vomiting. *Cochrane Database Syst Rev.* 2006;(2):CD002285.

Fabian CJ. Is there a future for ductal lavage? *Clin Cancer Res.* 2007;13(16):4655–4656.

Fleming G. Soy protein supplement in treating hot flashes in postmenopausal women receiving Tamoxifen for breast disease. 2002. Retrieved June 23, 2008, from http://clinicaltrials.gov.

Fournier MV, Martin KJ, Kenny PA, et al. Gene expression signature in organized and growth-arrested mammary acini predicts good outcome in breast cancer. *Cancer Res.* 2006;66(14):7095–7102.

Friedenreich CM, Cust AE. Physical activity and breast cancer risk: impact of timing, type and dose of activity and population subgroup effects. *Br J Sports Med.* 2008;42(8):636–647.

Frisk J, Carlhall S, Kallstrom AC, et al. Long-term follow-up of acupuncture and hormone therapy on hot flushes in women with breast cancer: a prospective, randomized, controlled multicenter trial. *Climacteric.* 2008;11(2):166–174.

Ganmaa D, Willett WC, Li TY, et al. Coffee, tea, caffeine and risk of breast cancer: a 22-year follow-up. *Int J Cancer.* 2008;122(9):2071–2076.

Geiger AM, Yu O, Herrinton LJ, et al. A population-based study of bilateral prophylactic mastectomy efficacy in women at elevated risk for breast cancer in community practices. *Arch Intern Med.* 2005;165(5):516–520.

Gissel T, Rejnmark L, Mosekilde L, et al. Intake of vitamin D and risk of breast cancer—A meta-analysis. *J Steroid Biochem Mol Biol.* 2008;111(3–5):195–199.

Greenlee H, Chen Y, Kabat GC, et al. Variants in estrogen metabolism and biosynthesis genes and urinary estrogen metabolites in women with a family history of breast cancer. *Breast Cancer Res Treat.* 2007;102(1):111–117.

Hansen J. Light at night, shiftwork, and breast cancer risk. *J Natl Cancer Inst.* 2001;93:1513–1515.

Jacobson JA, Danforth, DN, Cowan KH, et al. Ten-year results of a comparison of conservation with mastectomy in the treatment of stage I and II breast cancer. *Engl J Med.* 1995;332:907–911.

Kösters JP, Gøtzsche PC. Regular self-examination or clinical examination for early detection of breast cancer. *Cochrane Database of Syst Rev.* 2008;(2):CD003373, 1–24.

Lajous M, Boutron-Ruault M, Fabre A, et al. Carbohydrate intake, glycemic index, glycemic load, and risk of postmenopausal breast cancer in a prospective study of French women. *Am J Clin Nutr.* 2008;87:1384–1391.

Lawenda BD, Kelly KM, Ladas EJ, et al. Should supplemental antioxidant administration be avoided during chemotherapy and radiation therapy? *J Natl Cancer Instit.* Advance Access published on June 4, 2008; *J Natl Cancer Inst.* 100:773–783.

Lillberg K, Verkasalo PK, Kaprio J, et al. Personality characteristics and the risk of breast cancer: a prospective cohort study. *Int J Cancer.* 2002;100;361–366.

Menefee LA, Monti DA. Nonpharmacologic and complementary approaches to cancer pain management. *J Am Osteopath Assoc.* 2005;105:S15–S20.

Michels K, Mohllajee A, Roset-Bahmanyar E, Moysick K. Diet and breast cancer: a review of the prospective observational studies. *Cancer.* 2007;109(12 Suppl):2712–2749.

Mills E, Wu P, Seely D, et al. Melatonin in the treatment of cancer: a systematic review of randomized controlled trials and meta-analysis. *J Pineal Res.* 2005;39:360–366.

Mokbel K. Risk-reducing strategies for breast cancer—a review of recent literature. *Int J Fertil Womens Med.* 2003;48(6):274–277.

Monroe KR, Murphy SP, Kolonel LN, et al. Prospective study of grapefruit intake and risk of breast cancer in postmenopausal women: the Multiethnic Cohort Study. *Br J Cancer.* 2008;98(1):240–241.

Mulvey L, Chandrasekaran A, Liu K, et al. Interplay of genes regulated by estrogen and diindolylmethane in breast cancer cell lines. *Mol Med.* 2007;13(1–2):69–78.

Navo MA, Phan J, Vaughan C, et al. An assessment of the utilization of complementary and alternative medication in women with gynecologic or breast malignancies. *J Clin Oncol.* 2004;22:671–677.

Parodi PW. Dairy product consumption and the risk of breast cancer. *J Am Coll Nutr.* 2005;24:556S–568S.

Ravdin PM, Cronin KA, Howlader N, et al. The decrease in breast-cancer incidence in 2003 in the United States. *N Engl J Med.* 2007;356:1670–1674.

Ries LAG, Melbert D, Krapcho M, et al. SEER Cancer Statistics Review, 1975–2005, *National Cancer Institute.* Bethesda, MD, http://seer.cancer.gov/csr/1975_2005/, based on November 2007 SEER data submission, posted to the SEER web site, 2008.

Rossouw JE. Risks and benefits of estrogen plus progestin in healthy postmenopausal women: principal results from the Women's Health Initiative randomized controlled trial. *JAMA.* 2002;288(3):321–333.

Ruhlen RL, Haubner J, Tracy JK, et al. Black cohosh does not exert an estrogenic effect on the breast. *Nutr Cancer.* 2007;59(2):269–277.

Saslow D, Hannan J, Osuch J, et al. Clinical breast examination: practical recommendations for optimizing performance and reporting. *CA Cancer J Clin.* 2004;54:327–344.

Singletary SE. Skin-sparing mastectomy with immediate breast reconstruction: the M. D. Anderson Cancer Center experience. *Ann Surg Oncol.* 1996;3:411–416.

Sun C-L, Yuan J-M, Koh W-P, et al. Green tea, black tea and breast cancer risk: a meta-analysis of epidemiological studies. *Carcinogenesis.* 2006;27(7):1310–1315.

Suzuki R, Suzuki R, Ye W, et al. Alcohol intake and ER-PR-defined Breast cancer among postmenopausal women in Sweden. *J Natl Cancer Instit.* 2005;97:1601–1608.

Tuttle TM, Habermann EB, Grund EH, et al. Increasing use of contralateral prophylactic mastectomy for breast cancer patients: A trend toward more aggressive surgical treatment. *J Clin Oncol.* 2007;0:JCO.2007.12. 5203–5209.

van Dalen EC, Caron HN, Dickinson HO, Kremer LC. Cardioprotective interventions for cancer patients receiving anthracyclines. *Cochrane Database Syst Rev.* 2008;(2):CD003917.

Velicer CM, Ulrich CM. Vitamin and mineral supplement use among US adults after cancer diagnosis: a systematic review. *J Clin Oncol.* 2008;26:665–673.

Visovsky C, Collins M, Abbott L, et al. Putting evidence into practice: evidence-based interventions for chemotherapy-induced peripheral neuropathy. *Clin J Oncol Nurs.* 2007;11(6):901–913.

Vogel VG, Costantino JP, Wickerham DL, et al. for the National Surgical Adjuvant Breast and Bowel Project (NSABP). Effects of Tamoxifen vs Raloxifene on the risk of developing invasive breast cancer and other disease outcomes: the NSABP Study of Tamoxifen and Raloxifene (STAR) P-2 trial. *JAMA.* 2006;295(23):2727–2741.

Walker G, de Valois B, Davies R, et al. Ear acupuncture for hot flushes—the perceptions of women with breast cancer. *Complement Ther Clin Pract.* 2007;13(4):250–257.

Wellings RR, Jensen HM. On the origin and progression of ductal carcinoma in the human breast. *J Natl Cancer Inst.* 1973;50:1111–1118.

Wolmark N, Dunn BK. The role of tamoxifen in breast cancer prevention: issues sparked by the NSABP breast cancer prevention trial (P-1) *Ann NY Acad Sci.* 2001;949:99–108.

Wong R, Sagar S. Acupuncture treatment for chemotherapy-induced peripheral neuropathy—a case series. *Acupunct Med.* 2006;24(2):87–91.

23

Menopause

TORI HUDSON

CASE STUDY

Martha is a 49-year-old woman who is seeking information about treatment options to relieve her menopausal symptoms. She has been experiencing vaginal dryness, hot flashes, night sweats, and problems with sleep. She has been otherwise healthy, with normal lipids, glucose, thyroid, pap smears, and mammograms, although she has gained 10 pounds in the last year. She is very interested in a "natural approach" to addressing her menopausal symptoms. Finally, she is interested in learning if she is at risk for osteoporosis, and if so, what options might be available to her outside of taking hormonal replacement therapy (HRT).

The goals of an integrative medicine approach to menopause are to provide relief from common menopausal symptoms and to prevent and/or treat osteoporosis, heart disease, and other diseases of aging while minimizing the risk of breast cancer, blood clots, strokes, or gallbladder disease. The evaluation reveals a woman's symptoms, health habits, mental/emotional stressors, and risks for future diseases. The integrative provider then uses a spectrum of interventions including diet, exercise, stress management, nutritional supplements, herbal therapies, hormones, and prescription and over-the-counter (OTC) pharmaceuticals.

The changes associated with menopause can be mild, moderate, or severe. Some women have very few symptoms, while others have progressive and problematic symptoms for many years. The most common symptoms are vasomotor (hot flashes and nightsweats), sleep disturbances, and vaginal dryness. This chapter will focus primarily on menopausal symptom relief.

Menopause Evaluation

Tests to determine ovarian function are not routinely done because the diagnosis of menopause is largely made by the medical history. Practitioners can use hormone testing on an individual basis, mostly to differentiate menopause from thyroid problems, abnormal causes of amenorrhea, or premature ovarian failure.

The follicle-stimulating hormone (FSH) test is not as accurate as we would like; if consistently elevated above 30 mIU/mL, a diagnosis of menopause can be established. Unfortunately, FSH tests fluctuate and are frequently normal in the perimenopause. While very popular, salivary testing is not yet a validated method for testing sex hormone levels; they are only approved for cortisol and DHEA levels.

Serum testing can be done to determine estrogen, progesterone, and testosterone levels; however, there is often little reason to check levels. Hormone activity is erratic in many women leaving the tests of little value. For women taking HRT, it is tempting to think that we could test the blood or saliva to determine the optimal dose. While a popular recommendation in some consumer menopause books, there is no grid comparing values of estrogen, progesterone, or testosterone levels and how that would translate to a certain dose of a hormone. The majority of the time, it requires the practitioner's experience, and careful listening to the patient, to determine the dose and form of hormones that may work best. Testing to evaluate other aspects of a woman's health and determine her risks for cardiovascular disease, osteoporosis, and diabetes may be warranted.

The Integrative Medicine Approach

Once symptoms have been pinpointed and disease risks have been identified, the following treatment categories are recommended:

1. Diet, exercise, lifestyle, stress management
2. Nutritional supplementation
3. Botanical supplementation

4. Compounded bioidentical hormone preparations
5. Bioidentical conventional HRT
6. Nonbioidentical conventional HRT
7. Nonhormonal OTC and prescription medications

Diet, exercise, lifestyle, and/or nutritional supplements and botanical therapies will be effective for the management of menopause symptoms in the majority of women. When these are not adequate, hormone therapy or other medications can be recommended.

Diet, Exercise, and Stress Management

NUTRITION

Nutrition plays a fundamental role in integrative medicine. While dietary advice should be individualized, common themes include a diet rich in whole "natural" and unprocessed foods, with an emphasis on vegetables, whole grains, beans, seeds, nuts, fruits, lean low fat proteins, healthy fats, and low in saturated fats, fried foods, simple carbohydrates, alcohol, sugar, and salt. Some foods, such as soy and flax, have been studied for their beneficial effects on menopause related symptoms. Refer to the chapters on Nutrition, Heart Disease, and Osteoporosis for more specific details.

Soy

Soy foods may be useful in menopause primarily for its potential benefits for bone, cholesterol, blood pressure, and coronary artery disease. There are hundreds of studies on soy for health conditions and dozens on soy for hot flashes, some showing effect and others not, making it difficult to make any definitive conclusion. Two systematic reviews of isoflavones (from soy and red clover [*Trifolium pratense*]) and menopausal symptoms, and one consensus opinion from the North American Menopause Society offer a good summary of the research. The first systematic review evaluated the literature of randomized controlled clinical trials on soy and perimenopausal symptoms (Huntley and Ernst 2004). Only four out of 10 trials showed benefit. In the second systematic review, 25 trials of soy and red clover isoflavones involving approximately 2300 women met the study criteria (Krebs et al. 2004).

Only one soy food trial and two soy extract trials were shown to reduce hot flashes. The final report comes from a consensus opinion of the North American

Menopause Society (Consensus Opinion, 2000). They concluded the evidence for isoflavones and hot flashes are contradictory and that there was insufficient data to evaluate the effect of isoflavones on breast and other cancers, bone mass, and vaginal dryness, but there was convincing evidence that isoflavones reduce low-density lipoproteins and triglycerides, and increase high-density lipoproteins. In reviewing traditional Asian diets, the average adult daily intake is somewhere between 50 and 150 mg of soy isoflavones per day. The isoflavone content of soy foods varies with the form.

Flaxseeds

Another significant dietary source of phytoestrogens is flaxseeds (*Linum usitatissimum*). Flaxseed contains the lignans, matairesinol, and secoisolariciresinol, which are known to have estrogenic activity, as well as other lignans that are modified by intestinal bacteria to form estrogenic compounds. Lignans are absorbed in the circulation and have both estrogenic and antiestrogenic activity (Thompson et al. 1991). Not much research has been done in the area of flaxseeds and hot flashes. One small but encouraging study, in 2007, showed that women who consumed two tablespoons of flaxseed twice per day halved their number of hot flashes within 6 weeks and reduced the intensity of their hot flashes by 57% (Pruthi et al. 2007).

EXERCISE

The benefits of exercise for peri- and postmenopausal women are wide and deep. Women can achieve substantial reductions in cardiovascular disease (Manson et al. 2002), breast cancer risk (McTiernan et al. 2003), increase in bone density (Kemmler et al. 2003), and lower body fat and body mass index, as well experience an improved sense of well-being (Fitzpatrick and Santen 2002). Whether exercise can reduce hot flashes during menopause is not clear. For women who are not overweight, moderate exercise may be beneficial for hot flashes; more vigorous exercise may actually exacerbate them.

STRESS MANAGEMENT

The menopausal years can be a vulnerable time for many women. However, studies of women in midlife suggest that depression, as defined by the current Diagnostic and Statistical Manual of Mental Disorders (DSM-IV), is no more common in menopause than any other time of life (Freeman et al. 2004;

Schmidt et al. 2004). Most studies indicate that the perimenopause transition is associated with "subdiagnostic" depressive symptoms, meaning that women experience mood changes but fail to meet the DSM-IV criteria for the diagnosis of depression (Avis et al. 1994; Hunter 1990; Kaufert et al. 1992; Matthews et al. 1990). With this in mind, practitioners can support women with appropriate strategies for managing stress such as meditation, yoga, breathing exercises, going for walks, and even taking long baths.

DIETARY SUPPLEMENTS

There are a number of nutritional supplements that may be beneficial during the menopausal transition. Most women should probably take a good multivitamin that provides 70%–100% of the recommended daily intake of vitamins and minerals. The following dietary supplements are also sometimes used.

Bioflavonoids

Bioflavonoids, such as rutin, hesperidin, and quercetin, are known for their antioxidant and antiinflammatory properties and their ability to strengthen capillaries. Some older and less than optimal studies show that bioflavonoids, taken in combination with vitamin C, helps relieve menopausal hot flashes (Smith 1964). Ninety-four women with hot flashes were given a combination of 900 mg hesperidin, 300 mg hesperidin methylchalcone, and 1200 mg of vitamin C every day for 4 weeks. Hot flashes were relieved in 53% of women and reduced in an additional 34% by the end of one month.

Gamma-Oryzanol

Gamma-oryzanol was shown to have a therapeutic effect in relieving menopausal hot flashes in the early 1960s (Murase and Iishima 1963), with at least one additional study confirming that finding (Ishihara 1984). The dose used in the study was 300 mg/day.

BOTANICALS

Herbalists commonly use combinations of herbs to treat menopause. There has been limited research in this area and what follows are primarily studies of individual herbs. However, many of the OTC products that women use are in fact combinations.

Black Cohosh (Actaea racemosa, Cimicifuga racemosa)

Since the early 1980s, black cohosh has emerged as the most studied of the herbal alternatives to HRT for menopause symptoms. Numerous randomized clinical trials have studied black cohosh extract with encouraging, but mixed results (Bai et al. 2007; Borelli and Ernst 2002; Frei-Kleiner et al. 2005; Huntley and Ernst 2003; Jacobson et al. 2001; Liske et al. 2002; Newton et al. 2006; Osmers et al. 2005; Pockaj et al. 2006; Stolze 1985; Wuttke et al. 2003, 2006). In a study using the combination of black cohosh and St. John's wort (*Hypericum perforatum*), a popular treatment in Germany, the mean Menopause Rating Scale (MRS) score decreased 50% in the treatment group compared to 19.6% in the placebo group. The Hamilton Depression Rating Scale score decreased 41.8% in the treatment group and 12.7% in the placebo group. In both measures, the St. John's wort + black cohosh group was significantly superior to the placebo group (Uebelhack et al. 2006).

The average recommended dose of black cohosh extract is 40–80 mg/day. Clinical studies performed prior to 1996 used doses of 40–160 mg of standardized extract. There have been a small number of published case reports suggesting a rare, but possible, relationship between black cohosh consumption and liver damage. The United States Pharmacopeia Dietary Supplements Expert Information Council has published a thorough review of adverse events; they recommend that women with liver disease discontinue the use of black cohosh, as should any woman who develops nausea, vomiting, dark urine, or jaundice (Mahady et al. 2008).

Chasteberry (Vitex agnus castus)

One of the most common changes to occur in the menopause transition is irregular bleeding. Some women will experience significant bleeding problems

> Despite some negative studies, the collective research on black cohosh and my own clinical experience lead me to conclude that it is effective for hot flashes, mood swings, sleep disorders, and body aches.

because of menses that are either too frequent or too heavy. This set of symptoms is an indication for chaste tree berry. Chaste tree increases secretion of LH, an effect that favors progesterone (Haller 1961; Loch 1989). This shifts the ratio of estrogen to progesterone and creates a "progesterone-like" effect. In perimenopausal women, this is useful for managing dysfunctional uterine bleeding (DUB) associated with episodic anovulatory cycles. The dose is generally 500 mg/day taken continuously throughout the month. If using an extract (generally a strength of 12–16:1), the dose is generally 20–40 mg/day.

Dong Quai (Angelica sinensis)

A 12-week study using dong quai as a solo agent for the relief of menopausal symptoms such as hot flashes and sweats did not prove effective (Hirata et al. 1997). More research with dong quai is needed, and it should not be discounted just on the basis of this one study, especially since it was used as a solo herb and not, as is traditional, in combination with other herbal preparations.

> Dong quai may increase menstrual flow or bring on menstruation. In a perimenopausal woman who is having menorrhagia or who has not menstruated for several months, I recommend avoiding dong quai.

Ginseng (Panax ginseng)

Panax ginseng, also known as Korean or Chinese ginseng, is the most widely used of the ginseng species. A standardized extract of ginseng (200 mg/day) was studied in 384 postmenopausal women (Wiklund et al. 1999). While there was no improvement in hot flashes or night sweats, depression and well-being were significantly improved with ginseng. Another randomized controlled trial found that one month of Korean red ginseng increased energy, and decreased insomnia and depression in menopausal women (Tode et al. 1999).

Historically, ginseng has been used as a tonic. The German health authorities recognize its use as a "tonic for invigoration and fortification in times of fatigue and debility and for declining capacity for work and concentration." Ginseng can help in reducing mental or physical fatigue (D'Angelo et al. 1986; Hallstrom et al. 1982; Hikino 1991; Shibata et al. 1985), enhancing the ability to adapt to various physical and mental stressors by supporting the adrenal glands (Bombardelli et al. 1980). The dose is generally 100–300 mg ginseng extract standardized to 4%–6% ginsenosides. The use of ginseng in women with breast cancer is controversial and safety at this time is simply not known.

Kava (Piper methysticum)

Kava's properties have been most often associated with analgesic, sedative, anxiolytic, muscle relaxant, and anticonvulsant effects. Kava is not typically thought of as an herb for menopause. Anxiety, irritability, tension, nervousness, and sleep disruption are common symptoms for many menopausal women. Four randomized controlled trials have investigated the value of kava for menopausal symptoms (Cagnacci 2003; De Leo et al. 2000; Warnecke 1991; Warnecke et al. 1990). Two studies showed significant reduction in anxiety and menopausal symptoms, while another showed the greatest improvement with kava plus HRT. In the fourth, the study evaluated the effects of kava on anxiety, depression, and menopause symptoms in perimenopausal women for 3 months. Depression and anxiety were reduced in women receiving kava compared to the control group, but there was no improvement in hot flashes. The dose is typically 100–210 mg/ day of kava extract standardized to 60%–70% kavalactones. Women who have a liver disorder should avoid the use of kava, as should women who may be taking OTC or prescription medications that increase the risk of liver toxicity.

Maca (Lepidium peruvianum)

Results of a 2005 pilot study of a maca extract in 20 menopausal women (Meisner et al. 2005) paved the way for a larger clinical study of 168 postmenopausal women. Increased estradiol and lowered levels of luteinizing hormone, cortisol, and adrenocorticotropic hormone (ACTH) were noted. Reduced hot flashes, insomnia, depression; and improved memory, concentration, energy, and vaginal dryness were also found. Other promising effects were observed on lipids, blood pressure, body mass index, and bone density in early-postmenopausal women (Meisner et al. 2006). There are no other studies for review. The commonly recommended dose of maca extract is 2000 mg/day.

Red Clover (Trifolium praetense)

Six clinical trials have been conducted on semipurified red clover isoflavone extracts for vasomotor symptoms; three showed benefit and three did not. The first two published studies on red clover and vasomotor symptoms showed no statistically significant difference between the red clover standardized extract and the placebo (Baber et al. 1999; Knight et al. 1999). Two other studies showed positive results; one using 40 mg standardized extract of red clover produced a 75% reduction in hot flushes after 16 weeks in 30 women (Jeri and deRomana 1999), and a similar study, evaluating 40 mg of red clover standardized isoflavones found that red clover users had a 54% reduction in hot flushes versus 30% in the placebo group (Nachtigall et al. 1999). Two recent studies continue the contradictions. In 2002, 80 mg of isoflavones per day resulted in a significant reduction in hot flushes as compared to baseline (van de Weijer and Barentsen 2002). However, in 2003 the ICE study compared two different doses (82 and 57 mg) of red clover isoflavones with placebo for 12 weeks. The reductions in the mean daily hot flash count at 12 weeks were similar for all groups (Tice et al. 2003). The dose of red clover standardized extract is 40 mg total isoflavones taken one to two times per day.

St. John's Wort (Hypericum perforatum)

St. John's wort is the most thoroughly researched botanical antidepressant. (Please see the chapter on Depression for more information.) One 12-week open, controlled, drug monitoring study in women with menopausal symptoms found that 900 mg of St. John's wort standardized extract significantly improved psychological and psychosomatic symptoms and enhanced sexual well-being (Grube et al. 1999). As mentioned above, the combination of St. John's wort and black cohosh extract was superior to placebo for reducing scores in the general menopause rating and depression scales.

ADDITIONAL BOTANICALS

Numerous other herbs can be helpful for individual menopause symptoms. The German Commission E approved hops (*Humulus lupulus*) for anxiety, restlessness, and sleep disruptions. In one randomized, double-blind, placebo-controlled study, 67 menopausal women were given either a placebo, 100 mg, or 250 mg standardized hops extract for 12 weeks (Heyerick et al. 2006). At 6 weeks, the 100 and 250 mg doses were significantly superior to placebo, but not after 12 weeks. Even so, there was a more rapid decrease in menopause symptoms, especially hot flashes, for both doses of hops extract.

Valerian (*Valeriana officinalis*) has been used for centuries and is now popular for anxiety and insomnia. Three randomized clinical trials have shown improvement in sleep quality, although none of these studies were specific to menopausal women (Balderer and Borbely 1985; Leathwood and Chauffard 1985; Leathwood et al. 1982). Motherwort (*Leonurus cardiaca*) is another plant used historically in perimenopause and menopause. It can ease heart palpitations and act as a calming agent. The German Commission E has approved its use for nervous cardiac problems. The dose is generally 2 g/day of the herb.

HORMONE THERAPY

Choosing to use hormones, whether "bioidentical" or not, requires weighing the benefits and the risks. Hormonal therapies should be used in the lowest dose, for the shortest duration, and in the safest way possible. Each type of estrogen and progestogen, route of administration, timing of initiation, and duration of use have distinct benefits and adverse effects.

BIOIDENTICAL OR NATURAL HORMONES

One of the greatest areas of confusion in menopause management today is the subject of bioidentical, or natural hormones. The bioidentical hormones most commonly used in menopause include estradiol, estrone, estriol, progesterone, and to a lesser extent, testosterone and dehydroepiandrosterone (DHEA). Bioidentical hormones are made from either beta-sitosterol extracted from soybeans or from diosgenin extracted from Mexican Wild Yam (*Dioscorea villosa*). These compounds are then processed to create hormones that are biochemically identical to those the body produces.

Pharmaceutical estrogens can be bioidentical or not, synthetic, or derived from a natural substance (such as those found in the urine of pregnant mares). Nonbioidentical hormones include conjugated plant estrogens, conjugated equine estrogens (CEE), synthetic estrogens, synthetic progestogens, called progestins, and synthetic testosterone. It is the *chemical structure* of a hormone, not its *source,* that determines if a hormone is bioidentical or not.

Bioidentical estrogens require a prescription and are available from regular pharmacies or as nonpatented forms prepared by compounding pharmacies. Advantages of conventional pharmaceutical HRT include years of scientific study and the assurance of standardization. Insurance coverage generally pays for pharmaceutical hormone prescriptions but does not always pay for compounded hormones. Pharmaceutical preparations are limited in dosage forms and combinations; they also contain additives, binders, adhesives, and/or preservatives. Occasionally these substances can cause side effects including skin reactions, headaches, and digestive problems.

A popular practice for prescribing compounded natural estrogens is to combine estriol with small doses of estradiol and estrone. Triple estrogen, "Tri-Est," is typically prescribed in a formula composed of 80% estriol, 10% estradiol, and 10% estrone. Bi-est drops the estrone and is prescribed 80% estriol, 20% estradiol.

The advantages for using compounded forms include customized dosing regimens and a greater array of delivery options. Capsules, sublingual lozenges or pellets, creams, gels, vaginal creams/gels or tablets, nasal sprays, and even pellets that are implanted under the skin are available. Any combination of estradiol, estriol and estrone, progesterone, testosterone, and DHEA can be formulated in a compounded hormone prescription (Table 23.1).

Ideal prescribing Route

Estradiol has the least side effect on lipids and renin when delivered transdermally as it avoids the first pass effect on the liver. This also permits much lower doses to be used with equal efficacy. Micronized progesterone is available in both oral and vaginal forms. When symptoms are primarily uro-genital, vaginal forms of estrogen (CEE, Estradiol, and Estriol) can be used with minimal systemic absorption.

Table 23.1. Examples of Commercially Available Bioidentical Hormone Replacement Therapy

Generic Name	Brand Names
17 Beta estradiol (E2) Delivered as: Tablet Transdermal Vaginal cream	Estrace Climara, Vivelle Estrace
Progesterone	Prometrium Crinone gel

I am not suggesting that bioidentical hormones are innately good and other hormones are innately bad. There currently is no scientific evidence that bioidentical estradiol is safer than the non bioidentical estrogen.

Progesterone

For women with a uterus, a progestogen must be added to any estrogen preparation to prevent endometrial hyperplasia and uterine cancer. *Progesterone* is a natural hormone made by the ovaries and its main function is to support pregnancy. *Progestin* is the term applied to the synthetic derivatives, which differ in biochemical structure from progesterone. Progestins used in conventional HRT and birth control pills are what often account for the side effects that women experience such as irritability, depression, bloating, and mood swings. Progestins tend to cause water retention, can effect brain chemistry, and alter other steroid pathways. *Progestogen* is the term applied to any substance possessing progesterone qualities. It can refer to progesterone or progestin.

The advantages of bioidentical progesterone over progestins are better validated than they are for estrogens. Bioidentical progesterone minimizes the side effects associated with progestogens and has a more favorable effect on lipid profiles (The Writing Group for the PEPI Trial 1996), and cardiovascular function (Hermsmeyer et al. 2008). In some women, insomnia, fatigue, and mood swings may be more responsive to progesterone than estrogen.

Progesterone is available with a prescription as oral capsules, sublingual drops, sublingual pellets, lozenges, transvaginal or rectal suppositories, and by injection. Progesterone is also available OTC as a cream. Progesterone is added to a compounded biestrogen or triestrogen formulas at a minimum of 100 mg/day to protect the uterus (Table 23.2).

Table 23.2. Recommended Dose Ratios for Tri-estrogen and Bi-estrogen Formulations with Progesterone

Tri-estrogen formulation considered comparable to: 0.625 mg Premarin/2.5 mg Provera = Estriol 1 mg/estradiol 0.125 mg/estrone 0.125 mg/Prog 50 mg. 1 cap twice daily
Bi-estrogen formulation is considered comparable to: = 0.625 mg Premarin/2.5 mg Provera = Estriol 1 mg/estradiol 0.250 mg/Prog 50 mg. 1 cap twice daily
Vaginal estriol: Estriol cream 1 mg/g—insert 1 g nightly for 2 weeks then a maintenance of twice weekly

Testosterone

The majority of women treated with estrogen replacement have resolution of their menopausal symptoms. For those who do not, and especially for those women complaining of a loss of libido, estrogen with testosterone may be beneficial.

One study of early postmenopausal women (both natural and surgical) who were switched from estrogen alone to estrogen/testosterone therapy found overall symptom relief was superior to estrogen-only therapy. Sexual drive and satisfaction both increased (Dobay et al. 1996). A double-blind study of women dissatisfied with their HRT regimen showed that sexual desire, satisfaction, and frequency of sexual activity were increased when they used the estrogen/testosterone combination (Sarrel et al. 1998). Other studies have shown that the combination of 1.25 mg of esterified estrogen and 2.5 mg of methyltestosterone given daily for 2 years after surgical menopause significantly reduced the intensity of hot flashes and vaginal dryness in 81% and 73% of women, respectively (Watts et al. 1995). A 2008 RCT of 814 women with hypoactive sexual desire revealed that a 300 µg testosterone patch improved the frequency of satisfying sexual episodes and decreased distress in postmenopausal women (Davis et al. 2008). In this study, the women were not treated with estrogen or progesterone. Three excess cases of breast cancer were detected but not statistically significant in the study.

Formulations of CEE and methyltestosterone combine either 0.625 or 1.25 mg of CEE with 5 mg of methyltestosterone. Other preparations come as either 1.25 or 0.625 esterified estrogens, combined with 2.5 or 1.25 mg of methyltestosterone, respectively. At present, bioidentical testosterone can only be obtained from a compounding pharmacy. Two or three milligrams of bioidentical testosterone is generally formulated alone or together with the biestrogen or triestrogen formulation. Testosterone cream applied to the genital region can be used as an alternate delivery method. Common prescriptions are anywhere from 1 to 10 mg/g of cream. The cream is applied to the external genitalia right before sexual activity to enhance sensation to touch and orgasm. This should not exceed twice per week to avert local testosterone side effects, such as clitoral enlargement.

The North American Menopause Society (NAMS) concluded, "Postmenopausal women with decreased sexual desire who have no cause other than being postmenopausal, may be candidates for testosterone treatment." Other causes of low libido should be ruled out and laboratory testing of testosterone levels should be used to monitor for supraphysiologic levels before and during therapy. Testosterone therapy is contraindicated in women with breast or uterine cancer and in women with cardiovascular or liver disease. Testosterone should be given at the lowest dose for the shortest time that meets treatment objectives (North American Menopause Society, 2005).

> Naturopathic physicians often use estriol to treat menopausal symptoms as it is thought to have a better safety profile than estradiol and estrone. Estriol, is about one fourth as potent as estradiol (Head 1998). Estriol can be taken orally in capsules or tablets, and intravaginally as a cream. Vaginal estriol creams and suppositories have been shown to restore normal vaginal cytology (Hustin and Van der Eynde 1977), and decrease the incidence of bladder infections (Raz et al. 1993). These creams most likely work by restoring the vaginal flora, improving vaginal and bladder health, and increasing lubrication, elasticity, and thickness of vaginal cells. A common prescription is 1 mg of estriol per gram of cream inserted vaginally daily for 2 weeks and then twice a week for maintenance.

Additional Medications

Nonhormonal options for hot flashes include clonidine, usually 0.1 to 0.2 mg/day at bedtime. The neuroleptic, neurontin is administered 300 mg three times a day. Venlafaxine and paroxetine have shown a reduction in hot flashes in studies using 37.5–75 mg and 10–20 mg/day, respectively. However, selective serotonin reuptake inhibitor and selective norepinephrine reuptake inhibitor (SSRIs and SNRIs) have been occasionally shown to cause vasomotor symptoms in men and women. Bellergal, an ergot and belladonna combination, was used for many years for vasomotor symptoms, but is now only available from compounding pharmacies. There are no studies and empirical reports show mixed results.

Summary

Menopause is a normal and natural part of aging and each woman experiences it in her own way. Using natural therapies, hormone therapy, other pharmaceuticals, or some combination of each, is a personal decision for women. Menopause, aging, and our concerns about long-term health problems evolve over time. Balance is necessary and overmedicalization of menopause is inappropriate. The integrative provider can remind women that menopause can be a time of positive, life-changing insights, empowerment, and personal growth.

REFERENCES

Avis N, Brambilla D, McKinlay S, et al. A longitudinal analysis of the association between menopause and depression: results from the Massachusetts Women's Health Study. *Ann Epidemiol.* 1994;4:214–220.

Baber RJ, Templeman C, Morton T, et al. Randomized placebo-controlled trial of an isoflavone supplement and menopausal symptoms in women. *Climacteric.* 1999;2:85–92.

Bai W, Henneicke-von Zepelin H, Wang S, et al. Efficacy and tolerability of a medicinal product containing an isopropanolic black cohosh extract in Chinese women with menopausal symptoms: A randomized, double blind, parallel-controlled study versus tibolone. *Maturitas.* 2007;58:31–41

Balderer G, Borbely A. Effect of valerian on human sleep. *Psychopharmacology (Berl).* 1985;87:406.

Bombardelli E, Cirstoni A, Lietti A. The effect of acute and chronic (*Panax ginseng saponins*) treatment on adrenal function; biochemical and pharmacological. Proceedings 3rd International Ginseng Symposium 1980; Korean Ginseng Research Institute: 9–16.

Borrelli F, Ernst E. Cimicifuga racemosa: a systematic review of its clinical efficacy. *Eur J Clin Pharmacol.* 2002;58:235–241.

Cagnacci A, Arangino S, Rensi A, et al. Kava-Kava administration reduces anxiety in perimenopausal women. *Maturitas.* 2003;44:103–109.

Consensus Opinion. The role of isoflavones in menopausal health: consensus opinion of the North American Menopause Society. *Menopause.* 2000;7:215–229.

D'Angelo L, Grimaldi R, Caravaggi M, et al. A double-blind, placebo-controlled clinical study on the effect of a standardized ginseng extract on psychomotor performance in healthy volunteers. *J Ethnopharmacol.* 1986;16:15–22.

Davis SR, Moreau M, Kroll R, et al. APHRODITE Study Team Testosterone for Low Libido in Postmenopausal Women Not Taking Estrogen. *New Engl J Med.* 2008;359(19) 2005–2017.

De Leo V, Marca A, Lanzetta D, et al. Valutazione dell-associazione di estratto do Kava-Kava e terpie ormoale sostitutiva nel tratta mento d'ansia in postmenpausa. *Minerva Ginecol.* 2000;52:263–267.

Dobay B, Balos R, Willard N. *Improved menopausal symptom relief with estrogen-androgen therapy.* Presented at the Annual Conference of the North American Menopause Society, Chicago, IL, September 1996.

Fitzpatrick L, Santen R. Hot flashes: the old and the new, what is really true? *Mayo Clinic Proc.* 2002;77:1155–1158.

Freeman E, Sammel M, Liu L, et al. Hormones and menopausal status as predictors of depression in women in transition to menopause. *Arch Gen Psych.* 2004;61:62–70.

Frei-Kleiner S, Schaffner W, Rahlfs V, et al. *Cimicifuga racemosa* dried ethanolic extract in menopausal disorders: a double-blind placebo-controlled clinical trial. *Maturitas.* 2005;16;51(4):397–404.

Grube B, Walper A, Whatley D. St. John's wort extract: efficacy for menopasual symptoms of psychological origin. *Adv Ther.* 1999;16:177.

Haller J. The influence of plant extracts in the hormonal exchange between hypophysis and ovary. An experimental endocrinological animal study. *A Geburtsh Gynakol.* 1961;156:274–302.

Hallstrom C, Fulder S, Carruthers M. Effect of ginseng on the performance of nurses on night duty. *Comp Med East West.* 1982;6:277–282.

Head, K. Estriol: Safety and Efficacy. *Alt Med Rev.* 1998;3(2):101–113.

Hermsmeyer K, Thompson T, Pohost G, Kaski J. Cardiovascular effects of medroxyprogesterone acetate and progesterone: a case of mistake identity? *Nat Clin Pract Cardiovas Med.* 2008;5(7):387–395.

Heyerick A, Vervarcke S, Depypere H, et al. A first prospective, randomized, double-blind, placebo-controlled study on the use of a standardized hop extract to alleviate menopausal discomforts. *Maturitas.* 2006;54:164–175.

Hikino H. Traditional remedies and modern assessment: The case of ginseng. In: Wijeskera R, ed. *The Medicinal Plant Industry.* Boca Raton, FL: CRC Press; 1991:149–166.

Hirata J, Swiersz LM, Zell B, et al. "Does dong quai have estrogenic effects in postmenopausal women? A double-blind, placebo-controlled trial." *Fertil Steril.* 1997;68 (6):981–986.

Hunter M. Psychological and somatic experience of the menopause: a prospective study. *Psychosom Med.* 1990;52:357–367.

Huntley A, Ernst E. A systematic review of herbal medicinal products for the treatment of menopausal symptoms. Menopause. 2003;10:465–476.

Huntley A, Ernst E. Soy for the treatment of perimenopausal symptoms—a systematic review. *Maturitas.* 2004;47:1–9.

Hustin J, Van den Eynde J. Cytological evaluation of the effect of various estrogens given in postmenopause. *Acta Cytol.* 1977;21:225–228.

Ishihara M. Effect of gamma-oryzanol on serum lipid peroxide levels and climacteric disturbances. *Asia Oceania J Obstet Gynecol.* 1984;10:317.

Jacobson J, Troxel A, Evans J, et al. Randomized trial of black cohosh for the treatment of hot flushes among women with a history of breast cancer. *J Clin Oncol.* 2001;19:2739–2745.

Jeri A, deRomana C. The effect of isoflavone phytoestrogens in relieving hot flushes in Peruvian post-menopausal women. In Proceedings of the 9th International Menopause Society World Congress on Menopause. Yokohama, Japan: 1999.

Kaufert P, Gilbert P, Tate R. The Manitoba Project: a re-examination of the link between menopause and depressive. *Maturitas.* 1992;14:143–155.

Kemmler W, Engelke K, Weineck J, et al. The Erlangen fitness osteoporosis prevention study: a controlled exercise trial in early postmenopausal women with low bone density-first year results. *Arch Phys Med Rehabil.* 2003; 84:673–682.

Knight D, Howes J, Eden J. The effect of Promensil, an isoflavone extract, on menopausal symptoms. *Climacteric.* 1999;2:79–84.

Krebs E, Ensrud K, MacDonald R, Wilt T. Phytoestrogens for treatment of menopausal symptoms: a systematic review. *Obstet Gynecol* 2004;104:824–836.

Leathwood P, Chauffard F, Heck E, Munoz-Box R. Aqueous extract of valerian root (*Valeriana officinalis* L.) improves sleep quality in man. *Pharmacol Biochem Behav.* 1982;17:65.

Leathwood P, Chauffard F. Aqueous extract of valerian reduces latency to fall asleep in man. *Planta Med.* 1985;144.

Liske E, Hanggi W, Henneicke-von Zepelin H, et al. Physiological investigation of a unique extract of black cohosh: a 6 month clinical study demonstrates no systemic estrogenic effect. *J Womens Health Gend Based Med.* 2002;11:163–174.

Loch E. Diagnosis and therapy of hormonal bleeding disturbances. *TW Gynakol.* 1989;2:379–385.

Mahady GB, Low Dog T, Sarma D, et al. Review of case reports concerning hepatotoxicity and black cohosh (*Cimicifuga racemosa*). *Menopause.* 2008;15(4 Pt 1):628–638.

Manson J, Greenland P, LaCroix AZ, et al. Walking compared with vigorous exercise for the prevention of cardiovascular events in women. *N Engl J Med.* 2002; 347:716–725.

Matthews K, Wing R, Kuller L, et al. Influenes of natural menopause on psychological characteristics and symptoms of middle-aged healthy women. *J Consult Clin Psychol.* 1990;5:345–351

McTiernan A, et al. Recreational physical activity and the risk of breast cancer in postmenopausal women: The Women's Health Initiative Cohort Study. *JAMA.* 2003;290:1331–1336.

Meissner H, et al. Hormone-Balancing effect of pre-gelatinized organic Maca (*Lepidium peruvianum* Chacon): (III) Clinical responses of early-postmenopausal women to Maca in double blind, randomized, placebo-controlled, crossover configuration, outpatient study. *Int J Biomed Sci.* 2006;2(4):375–394.

Meissner H., Kapczynski W., Mscisz A, et al. Use of a gelatinised maca (*Lepidium peruvianum*) in early-postmenopausal women—a pilot study. *Int J Biomed Sci.* 2005;I(1):33–45.

Murase Y, Iishima H. Clinical studies of oral administration of gamma-oryzanol on climacteric complaints and its syndrome. *Obstet Gynecol Prac.* 1963;12:147–149.

Nachtigall L, La Grega L, Lee W, Fenichel R. *The effects of isoflavones derived from red clover on vasomotor symptoms and endometrial thickness.* In: Proceedings of the 9th International Menopause Society World Congress on the Menopause. Yokohama, Japan: 1999.

Newton K, Reed S, LaCroix A, Grothaus L, Ehrlich K, Guiltinan J. Treatment of vasomotor symptoms of menopause with black cohosh, multibotanicals, soy, hormone therapy, or placebo: a randomized trial. *Ann Intern Med.* 2006;145(12):869–879.

North American Menopause Society. The role of testosterone therapy in postmenopausal women: position statement of the North American Menopause Society. *Menopause*. 2005;12(5):497–511.

Osmers R, Friede M, Liske E, et al. Efficacy and safety of isopropanolic black cohosh extract for climacteric symptoms. *Obstet Gynecol*. 2005;105:1074–1083.

Pockaj B, Gallagher JG, Loprinzi CL, et al. Phase III double-blind, randomized, placebo-controlled crossover trial of black cohosh in the management of hot flashes: NCCTG Trial NO1CC1. *J Clin Oncol*. 2006;24:2836–2841.

Pruthi SL, Thompson PJ, Novotny DL, et al. Pilot evaluation of flaxseed for the management of hot flashes. *J Soc Integ Oncol*. 2007;5(3):106–112.

Raz et al. A controlled trial of intravaginal estriol in postmenopausal women with urinary tract infections. *N Engl J Med*. 1993;329:753–756.

Sarrel P, Dobay B, Wiita B. Sexual behavior and neuroendocrine responses to estrogen and estrogen-androgen in postmenopausal women dissatisfied with estrogen-only therapy. *J Reprod Med*. 1998;43(10):847–856.

Schmidt P, Haw N, Rubinow D. A longitudinal evaluation of the relationship between reproductive status and mood in perimenopausal women. *Am J Psychiatry*. 2004;161:2238–2244.

Shibata S, Tanaka O, Shoji J, Saito H. Chemistry and pharmacology of Panax. *Econ Med Plant Res*. 1985;1:217–284.

Smith C. Non-hormonal control of vaso-motor flushing in menopausal patients. *Chic Med*. 1964;67:193–195.

Stolze H. An alternative to treat menopausal symptoms with a phytotherapeutic agent. *Med Welt*. 1985;36:871–874.

The Writing Group for the PEPI Trial. Effects of hormone replacement therapy on endometrial histology in postmenopausal women. The Postmenopausal Estrogen/Progestin Interventions (PEPI) Trial. *JAMA*. 1996;275(5):370–375.

Thompson L, Robb P, Serraino M, Cheung F. Mammalian lignan production from various foods. *Nutr and Canc*. 1991;16(1):43–52.

Tice J, Ettinger B, Ensrud K, et al. Ph-ytoestrogen supplements for the treatment of hot flashes: the isoflavone clover extract (ICE) study. *JAMA*. 2003;290:207–214.

Tode T, Kikuchi Y, Hirata J, et al. Effect of Korean red ginseng on psychological functions in patients with severe climacteric syndromes. *Int J Gynaecol Obstet*. 1999;67:169.

Uebelhack R, Blohmer JU, Graubaum HJ, et al. Black cohosh and St. John's wort for climacteric complaints. *Obstet Gynecol*. 2006;107:247–255.

van de Weijer P, Barentsen R. Isoflavones from red clover Promensil significantly reduce menopausal hot flush symptoms compared with placebo. *Maturitas*. 2002;42:187–193.

Warnecke G. Psychomatic dysfunction in the female climacteric. Clinical effectiveness and tolerance of kava extract WS 1490 (in German). *Fortschr Med*. 1991;109:119–122.

Warnecke G. Pfaender H, Gerster G, Gracza E. Wirksamkeit von Kawa-Kawa-Extrakt beim klimakterischen Syndrom. *Zeitschrift Phytotherapie*. 1990;11:81–86.

Watts N, Notelovitz M, Timmons M, et al. Comparison of oral estrogens and estrogens plus androgen on bone mineral density, menopausal symptoms, andlipid-lipoprotein profiles in surgical menopause. *Obstet Gynecol*. 1995;85:529–537.

Wiklund I, Mattsson L, Lindgren R, Limoni C. Effects of a standardized ginseng on the quality of life and physiological parameters in symptomatic postmenopasual women: a double-blind, placebo-controlled trial. *Int J Clin Pharm Res.* 1999;XIX:89–99.

Wuttke W, Gorkow C, Seidlova-Wuttke D. Effects of black cohosh on bone turnover, vaginal mucosa, and various blood parameters in postmenopausal women: a double-blind, placebo-contrlled, and conjugated estrogens-controlled study. *Menopause.* 2006;13(2):185–196.

Wuttke W, Seidlova-Wuttke D, Gorkow C. The Cimicifuga preparation BNO 1055 vs. conjugated estrogens in a double-blind placebo-controlled study: effects on menopause symptoms and bone markers. *Maturitas.* 2003;44:S67–77.

24

Sexuality

LANA L. HOLSTEIN

CASE STUDY

"My sex life is not satisfying, it's not the way I want it."—Cindy W., in for her yearly examination, was complaining generally about her sexual intimacy. She was 45, a year post TAH/BSO, had two teenagers stirring up her two-career household, and an increasingly responsible and exhausting position at work. She spoke of plummeting desire and vaginal soreness after sex although she could still be orgasmic once "they got going." She wanted that deep, exhilarating love-making back, and understandably rejected merely servicing her husband's libido. Now it is up to you to figure out Cindy's problem.

The confusion for most practitioners who seek to help patients with sexuality complaints comes from the lack of a template to sort out the issues. Is there a hormonal lack, a childhood trauma, an affair, unrelenting boredom, or a spiritual crisis? What are the roots of the dysfunction and how can the energy and vitality of sexual exchange be rekindled? The development of the Seven Dimensions of Sexuality (Holstein 2001) came from confronting this need for a coherent approach in my own practice.

All dimensions have their own essential energetic quality and are integral to a complete sexual life although each partner in the sexual dyad contributes unique dimensional strengths. In addition, each dimension has positive and negative qualities and, perhaps most commonly, a stagnant aspect where individuals and couples generate little energy and are often in the sexual doldrums (Holstein and Taylor 2004).

The Dimensions

- Biologic, sensual, desire, comprising the physical aspects
- Heart and intimacy, expressing the emotional aspects
- Esthetic and ecstatic, representing the soul qualities

THE BIOLOGIC DIMENSION

Most practitioners are familiar with this dimension, the one elucidated initially by Masters and Johnson (1966). The positive aspects of sexual biology start with the basics of good physical function and knowing what's what anatomically and physiologically, then progress to an inner experience of sexual confidence as a lover, and finally mature into the deepest level of understanding that sex is how the species perpetuates itself. Sex always contains the awe-inspiring potential for making babies, maybe even our own child.

The negative energy is physical dysfunction, whether due to hormonal decline, infertility issues, medications, surgeries, or aging. There is not much mystery about the negative pole of the biologic dimension. The static zone in this dimension is ignorance, inattention, and silence. Something is wrong but corrective action is avoided.

Health – Ignorance – Dysfunction

A myth about the biological dimension is that sex necessarily disappears with advancing age. This is probably the most common and depressing misconception people have about sex. Whether couples have great sex, adequate sex, or no sex at all does not have a lot to do with their age. There are celibate couples in their twenties and ecstatic lovers in their seventies. So while it is perfectly true that bodies change over time, those changes do not determine the quality or frequency of sexual connections.

Do aging hormonal levels affect sexuality? Yes. Not enough estrogen in women causes problems with lubrication and comfort (Basson et al. 2004). Declining testosterone levels can also cause problems, for women as well as men. While we know testosterone is crucial to libido (an aspect of the desire dimension), inadequate levels of testosterone in postoophorectomy women can in addition directly affect physical arousal and orgasmic potential (Braunstein et al. 2005; Shifren et al. 2000; Simon et al. 2005). In contrast, recent studies have not supported wholesale use of testosterone in women with functioning ovaries since placebo effects are often equal to treatment (Davis et al. 2008).

Oral contraceptives and oral estrogens do increase sex hormone–binding globulin (SHBG), which preferentially binds testosterone, causing decreased desire and responsiveness in some patients (Nachtigall et al. 2008). Other medications, most notably the antidepressants, have a 30%–50% inhibitory effect on arousal and orgasm no matter what the age of their users (Balon 2006). The integrative medicine practitioner will address these biologic concerns of course, but they are often just the portal into much more complex sexual issues.

> Measuring Cindy's morning total and free testosterone and examining her for vaginal atrophy will be important in determining if hormonal supplementation is indicated. She does not want to use systemic estrogen but has indicated that she would consider a vaginal product if the OTC lubricants do not ease her discomfort.

THE SENSUAL DIMENSION

The sensual dimension is all about pleasure, which after all is our usual motivation for having sex. Masters and Johnson developed the Sensate Focus activity of nondemand sensual touching specifically for couples who had lost this dimension.

One reason that the pleasure sex gives us is so intense is that it involves all five of the traditional senses—sight, hearing, smell, taste, and touch—plus the sixth sense, the kinesthetic. However, most of us damp down our senses. It is easy to stray out of our sensory bodies and into our left brains. We tend to emphasize abstract functions over the more intuitive, immediate concerns of the right brain, so we end up automatically preferring language to image, debate to feeling, and analysis to intuition.

Pleasure means being awake sensually. This requires a "pleasure alert" multiple times a day. Stopping to enjoy the deep color of that flower, smell your lover's hair, and paste your bodies together in a mega-hug. Pleasure also includes conscious appreciation of physical sensations both outside and inside the bedroom. It is one thing to give the kiss, listen to the wind in the trees, or smell the salt air, but when we specifically value our sensual involvement with the world, and most especially with our lover, we begin to automatically seek opportunities to increase sensuality. And, at the deepest level of sensuality, we merge with the experience itself. Any sensual experience can be entered into in this way, so that we feel no difference between our selves and our perceptions. All it requires is letting go fully into our wonderful, sensitized, sensual bodies, and becoming pleasure itself.

The negative pole is, as you might expect, pain, either physical or emotional. Pain can ruin sex. It may be simple, temporary, or avoidable—after childbirth, sex is the last thing you want, or there is a urinary infection, or that hip arthritis means certain positions hurt. But pain can also be emotional.

For people who have been sexually traumatized, the most loving touch can trigger memories of rape or forced sex or something else frighteningly associated with sex. A woman who has had a bad experience may love and want her partner, but if he happens to touch her neck in just the way her attacker did long ago, she may flash back to fear and humiliation and pain. The good news is that these wounds can be healed. Psychological help is often necessary, but healing can also occur through sensual awakening with a completely trustworthy partner.

What's the stagnant no man's land? Numbness. This may also be the result of frightening sexual encounters—it is just easier to shut down rather that confront fear—but often the cause is more ordinary: we are just busy elsewhere in our minds.

Pleasure – Numbness – Pain

The way out of numbness is simply to start attending to the senses. They are the channels of physical awareness and they bring the sensual dimension to fruition. It is easy to give patients a "sense of the week" prescription: emphasize a new sense every week with her partner both in and out of bed, and this dimension will blossom.

> Cindy has never suffered from sexual trauma but she is constantly preoccupied with work and needs to get back into her body. She loves the idea of emphasizing a "sense of the week" and will begin with touch and include massage with new oils and lotions during sex.

THE DESIRE DIMENSION

The next dimension, the last of the three physical dimensions, is desire. This dimension is what we may think of as sex itself; desire is the crackling charge created when masculine and feminine energies come close. Helen Kaplan added this quality to the Masters and Johnson paradigm (Kaplan 1974). And Rosemary Basson found that women feel desire after they experience love, trust, and closeness in their relationship (Basson 2005, 2006). In fact, functional magnetic resonance imaging (MRI) studies have shown that unless the brain center for fear and vigilance, the amygdala, is suppressed, orgasm does not occur in women (Holstege 2006).

The positive aspect of this dimension is attraction—outwardly presenting an engaging, "I'm vital and sexual" persona to the world. This attraction is basic, fundamental—it is the powerful energy inherent in the mating drive and the current of sexuality flowing between lovers that energize daily life. It is the masculine and feminine, the yin and yang, joining up to create a dynamic fusion.

Mutual desire is the nuclear fuel of coupleship. Without that essential fuel, the most caring, committed, loving couple in the world is not going to have great sex, or much sex, or maybe any sex at all.

Desire does have many everyday enemies. Negative energy in this dimension shows up as avoidance, the flip-side of personal power that says "no" to sex and mating. For women, this negative energy is usually generated by one of the "three F's": fatigue, fury, or fear with its activation of the amygdala. These problems result in many women accommodating their man by "providing" sex rather than making love. The woman is participating in the sex act, but is not really there. Sex happens, but energy is not flowing in this dimension: one partner may be generating it, but the other isn't receptive, and the encounter ends up feeling dead for both.

Erotic Power – Indifference – Avoidance

And then there is the ultimate dead zone of the desire dimension, the celibate relationship. The sexless (or nearly sexless) state develops as couples become increasingly awkward and distanced by the daily wear and tear of living, "no time," deep-seated worries, or simmering anger. They avoid confronting the three F's by sidestepping fury, fear, and fatigue and withdrawing their sexual energy. They effectively protect themselves from further humiliation and disappointment by denying desire. The typical process goes like this: one partner refuses to respond to the advances of the other, and the other, tired of the humiliation of being rejected, gradually gives up. The situation deteriorates into a profound and chronic power struggle in which the partner who wants sex *least* is the one with control in the bedroom, and once-loving partners silently vie for the coveted title of "least interested." When the sexual charge of the desire dimension is diverted into power games like this, its creative potential energy is squelched. And the longer sexual energy is untapped, the greater the inertia to be overcome in order for things to start up again.

R-energizing desire means recognizing and deconstructing old beliefs about sex that block its natural flow. If the beliefs that sap desire go very deep, people with trouble in this dimension may want to talk to a skillful counselor. But for many couples, seeing the nature of the problem clearly is half the battle. The most desire-sapping belief of all is that lust always grows cold. It does not once a couple consciously reunites with the life-affirming, erotic life force.

> Cindy has appropriately rejected "servicing" her husband but she needs to energize her desire by receiving and giving teasing touches, looks, and words as well as creating private, erotic time for the two of them at least once a week. She is actually excited by this assignment and knows her husband will enjoy it immensely.

THE HEART DIMENSION

Rosemary Basson has documented that for women the heart and intimacy dimensions are crucial to the willingness to engage sexually (Basson 2006); so what does the emotional heart dimension look like? At the positive pole are the exquisite experiences of falling in love and welcoming commitment. Tokens and symbols—valentines, flowers, and little gifts—are the natural currency of the heart, because love truly is about joyful giving and receiving. Of course, the giddiness of new love is bound to fade, but here is where that unbounded give and take can expand throughout life if we give it the sustenance it needs. As with the other dimensions of sex, when *attention* is paid to the heart dimension, it becomes stronger and deeper.

The deepest level of heart connection manifests sexually when the beauty of complete, emotional dedication is experienced physically. As so many couples solidly acknowledge, this is the foundation of commitment, the place where their physical joining of bodies is infused with potent heart energy. This is *making love* rather than having sex.

The negative pole of the heart dimension is abandonment. Every one of us has felt abandoned and unloved at some time or other. This, too, is embedded in language—and in every classic country-western song: broken-hearted, disheartened, living in heartbreak hotel. If old scars and new hurts are allowed to pull the heart closed, the open heart that easy love requires is lost.

Commitment – Stinginess – Abandonment

The trap here, the place where the positive energy of love and commitment is neutralized by the negative energy of abandonment fears, is stinginess of heart. The stingy heart devotes all its energy not to giving and receiving love but to building walls and guarding gates, and one sure sign of it is counting and keeping score of all the emotional injuries. This kind of stagnant, dank thinking—which can quickly become a habit—destroys the act of making love. Conversely, an open heart gives and forgives, sympathizes and admires and enjoys, not because of a desire to be declared saintly, but because we want to be happy and secure in our love. Only by giving will we receive. If we want to live, now and forever, in that warm, safe, comfortable space that two open-hearted people can create between them, there is no other way but to be vigilant to our stinginess and to open the heart.

> Cindy admitted to having a stingy heart toward her husband because of the disagreements about disciplining their teenagers. She is open to leaving that issue at the bedroom door so that they can get back to "making love" again.

THE INTIMACY DIMENSION

The positive pole of the other emotional dimension—intimacy—is trust. At first glance, distinguishing intimacy from the heart dimension, trust from commitment, may seem odd. How is there love without intimacy? How can we be intimate without love? Easily, and we do it all the time. We may love our parents or grandparents dearly without knowing very much about what goes on deep inside them. We can trust and confide in a therapist, a financial advisor, or a colleague without investing any emotion in the connection. Love and intimacy are different emotions.

We tend to confuse them, in part, because these two dimensions must fuse if an important relationship is to be joyful and free and strong. When we trust as well as love, the emotional core of the relationship is solid. Without trust—when lovers have stopped talking to one another, or have wandered off into lying and cheating—love is on shaky ground, and the quality of our sexual connection erodes. Trust is fundamental to great sexual connection because we make ourselves exquisitely vulnerable when we make love. Consequently, we can only really let go with someone we know is not lying to us.

In many relationships, the partners start out telling each other everything, but have clammed up because they fear that the truth will be disregarded or lead to an argument. Or they may become so overwhelmed by the demands of daily life that they have gradually stopped talking about anything other than what needs to get done.

It is easy to imagine the flip side of unrestricted truth, self-revelation, and deep understanding—betrayal. For some couples, an affair has ripped the fabric of trust in a terribly painful way. One partner feels betrayed and bewildered and unable to believe anything the other says; the other feels permanently guilty and defensive and beaten up. It is important, though, to look deeper than "who wronged whom." Often an affair is as much the product of silence as the source of it: most people who stray are, at some level, looking for intimacy their marriage does not provide: more than sex, they want *to be known*. Affairs are never okay, of course, but often they do break through the hard, dry surface of relationships that are quietly dying from lack of communication. For couples whose love is still there, the shock of betrayal may be an opportunity for renewal. However, betrayal causes such deep wounds that couples who want to heal must seek help from an objective, compassionate third party. The feelings that an affair brings to the surface are too intense to work though independently. Whether a couple wants to rebuild or call it quits after the revelation of an affair, *both* partners need counseling.

If the positive pole of the intimacy dimension is trust, and the negative end is betrayal, then the static zone is withholding. Some couples maintain a civil façade while giving nothing away. This type of withholding is an insidious relationship-wrecker. This is how two people, who once felt that they knew one another, completely transform themselves into unhappily married strangers.

Trust – Withholding – Betrayal

Sharing the most inspiring truths, our hopes, dreams, and visions for the most passionate life possible is what we need to make time for our ultimate, profound potential, because this is what we find erotic in one another; this is the turn-on, this is vitality and purpose. We want to make love to this potent person, to the genuine being, and we deepen our knowledge with the sexual exchange—discovering ever more of their unveiled self through pillow talk and love whispers.

Cindy considers her relationship truthful and trusting. There have never been sexual betrayals although she relates that her father's affairs have made her perpetually cautious about trusting men. She acknowledges she could reach out more to her own man.

THE ESTHETIC DIMENSION

Poets and novelists have long described the deeper aspects of sexuality although clinicians have rarely addressed them in their patients. Great sex requires that the first five dimensions are energized, but really spectacular, multidimensional lovemaking involves body, heart, *and* soul.

The esthetic, soul dimension is all about beauty, and, at its deepest level, the positive pole is awe in the presence of radiance. When we are attentive to beauty we might call our lover's attention to a crystalline blue sky while walking out the door; we may devote loving effort to making the bedroom beautiful. Or we might share an evening at the ballet: such human grace and powerful movement is beautiful—and erotic. Being aware of beauty is a turn-on because it heightens our connection to our world and ultimately to our lover.

We also need to include our self and our partner in the experience of beauty. The skill here is awakening the radiance and beauty in our beloved. An even bigger challenge is to claim one's own beauty. Being looked at during sex, even by our trusted lover, can be quite intimidating, but allowing our partner to bask in the radiance of our sexual arousal is an enormous gift.

Finally, the most potent positive feature of the esthetic is the transformation that takes place when meaning cleaves to gratitude—when your soul thanks this beautiful being for making love to you. At the same time, of course, we are probably aware that our beloved is filled with gratitude for our existence. At this point, both have entered rarified space where the esthetic becomes powerfully sexual.

The negative pole of the esthetic is shame. Shame is the dark side of seeing and being seen, and it is an unending source of human unhappiness. It begins to develop as soon as we realize that we are observed, judged, and found wanting.

Everyone is susceptible to shame, but cultural and religious attitudes about sex, the body and desire usually have greater impact on women than men. Our culture is crazily fixated on the image of a certain type of young woman, an obsession that gives another twist to women's anxieties. "My looks aren't perfect and I'm getting older every day." That's obviously unattractive and certainly not sexually appealing. "Must hide everything!" Among the most precious gifts deadened by shame are radiance and freedom of sexual expression. The typical man, in my experience, does not look at the woman he loves with the eye of a judge at a beauty contest although she may be convinced that he does. He yearns for the depth of a full sexual encounter with the person he loves.

The burnt-out zone of the esthetic dimension is blindness. Blindness can develop from a number of sources. Usually, it stems from the habit of inattention to beauty; there is so much to *do* each day. We have the lists, the family obligations, and even the usual sex. You know the kind: same bed, same person, same positions, and definitely the same uninspiring experience. We forget to really look at our partner when we kiss them, we underestimate the power we have to awaken their glow, we ignore chances to amp up the smile, and then we wonder why we are bored.

Radiance – Blindness – Shame

The way to a radiant sensual connection lies through the doorway of self-acceptance of our grace and beauty as part of the human race. When we accept ourselves and our lover in all our imperfection *and* in all our essential beauty, we create a secret garden for two, a place where shame falls away and beauty reigns. This is the place where ecstatic sex happens.

> Cindy has had a lot of doubts about her sexiness after the complete hysterectomy. She is glad not to have the monthly hemorrhaging but she somehow feels less of a woman and has not really discussed that with her mate. She also admits to boredom and an apathetic approach to their lovemaking and is confident she can change that by putting more of her own energy into their connections.

THE ECSTATIC DIMENSION

Ecstatic, transcendent, gone-to-heaven sex is the realm of the final dimension. Here we venture beyond the merely human and connect with universal divine energy. This is not as rare or as impossible as it sounds. Ecstatic sexual experiences can be created: repeatedly, reliably, and as part of an otherwise prosaic, everyday life.

Once an open exchange of energy has been established in the first six dimensions, just two things are needed to make sexual connection sacred and transformative. One is the simple belief that such a connection is possible and worth creating. The second is an advanced technology of sex. Fortunately, this technology has existed for at least 3000 years. The discipline known as Tantra developed in classical India as one of the eight traditional yogic paths to enlightenment. All the practices of yoga, which literally means "union," promote the spiritual evolution and integration of the individual; Tantra is the branch of yoga that includes sexual ritual, considered sacred physical practice, and its aim is to unite and balance the energies of male and female through perfected sex

(Anand 2006). In Tantra, the woman is the eternal source of life energy, and her partner appreciates her as such.

Tantra is not about feats of sexual prowess, but rather about the generation and release of sacred energy for the good of the universe. In the fullness of transcendent sex, the divine is awakened within our lover, radiance is sensed within us, and partners gratefully exchange energies. Sexual connection becomes profoundly healing as couples bathe in the stream of loving energy that flows through the world.

Letting go of boundaries, being willing to merge, and turning a deaf ear to the warnings of the ego, which wants to maintain separateness above all, are all tasks to be accomplished before entering the sweet space of ecstatic sex. We may know, believe, and even cry out for this sexual bliss, but unless we are ready to surrender the egoic safety of being two, we will not enjoy the exhilarating expansion of becoming one.

So the positive pole of the ecstatic dimension is the sacred. The negative pole is the profane: the belief that sex is, at best, worldly rather than heavenly, and at worst, the work of the devil. The Puritanical tradition in our culture is that sex is shameful, sinful, a temptation that leads us astray from the good and righteous life. While few people today subscribe to such a negative view of sexuality, it remains a heavy undercurrent, coexisting uneasily and ambiguously with the overtly sexual imagery that saturates popular culture. Sadly, neither of these currents evokes the sacred feeling so crucial to energizing this dimension.

Sacred – Cynicism – Profane

In fact, most of us are stuck in the middle space, between heaven and hell, if you will, in a purgatory where disbelief in the sacred power of sex allows no sexual energy to flow; where the conflict between sacred and profane, soul and ego, chokes off this energy. We need to discard these limiting beliefs and embrace a higher view of sexuality if we are to tap into the vast power of the ecstatic dimension. This may sound like an overwhelmingly difficult or implausible task. Yet I have found that it is easily within reach of most of the ordinary couples I have taught: It is easy because the soul yearns for it. Ultimately, there is no limit to the flow of energy that is possible in the ecstatic dimension of sex.

Cindy has a visceral memory of this type of experience and is eager to explore this again with her husband. When taught tantric soul gazing—holding hands and breathing together while looking into each other's eyes—she is ready to initiate this at home and believes it will be welcomed by her partner. In fact she is delighted with your discussion of sex with her and feels enthused once again about establishing an emotionally satisfying, body and soul sexual connection.

Use of the Dimensions in Practice

Allowing a patient to unravel their sexual concerns is best accomplished in a consultation with an integrative practitioner who is listening with the framework of the seven dimensions in mind. Quickly it will be established which dimensions are in the negative or static zone and which are positive. Approaching each of the dimensions with specific suggestions allows for a stepwise approach to reenergizing the sexual connection.

The scenarios your patients will present are infinite and inevitably fascinating and the rewards for helping a couple establish a multidimensional love life are enormous.

REFERENCES

Anand M. *The Art of Sexual Ecstasy*. Los Angeles: Tarcher; 2006.

Balon R. SSRI-associated sexual dysfunction. *Am J Psychiatry*. 2006;163(9):1504–1509.

Basson R, Althof S, Davis S, et al. Summary of the recommendations on sexual dysfunctions in women. *J Sex Med*. 2004;1(1):24–34.

Basson R. Sexual desire and arousal disorders in women. *N Engl J Med*. 2006;354(14):1497–1506.

Basson R. Women's sexual dysfunction: revised and expanded definitions. *CMAJ*. 2005;172(10):1327–1333.

Braunstein GD, Sundwall DA, Katz M, et al. Safety and efficacy of a testosterone patch for the treatment of hypoactive sexual desire disorder in surgically menopausal woman: a randomized placebo-controlled trial. *Arch Intern Med*. 2005;165(14):1582–1589.

Davis S, Papalia M, Norman RJ, et al. Safety and efficacy of a testosterone metered-dose transdermal spray for treating decreased sexual satisfaction in premenopausal women: a randomized trial. *Ann Intern Med*. 2008;148:569–577.

Holstege G. Regional cerebral blook flow changes associated with clitorally induced orgasm in healthy women. *Eur J Neurosci*. 2006;24:3305–3316.

Holstein LL. *How to Have Magnificent Sex: The 7 Dimensions of a Vital Sexual Connection*. New York: Harmony Books; 2001.

Holstein LL, Taylor DJ. *Your Long Erotic Weekend: Four Days of Passion for a Lifetime of Magnificent Sex*. Gloucester, MA: Fair Winds Press; 2004.

Masters WH, Johnson VE. *Human Sexual Response.* Boston: Little, Brown & Co; 1966.

Nachtigall LE, Raju U, Bannerjee S, et al. Serum estradiol-binding profiles in post-menopausal women undergoing three common estrogen replacement therapies Associations with sex hormone-binding globulin, estradiol and estrone levels. *Menopause.* 2000;7:243–250.

Kaplan HS, ed. *The New Sex Therapy.* New York: Brunner/Mazel; 1974.

Shifren JL, Braunstein GD, Simon JA, et al. Transdermal testosterone treatment in women with impaired sexual function after oophorectomy. *N Engl J Med.* 2000:343(10):682–688.

Simon J, Braunstein GD, Nachtigall L, et al. Testosterone patch increases sexual activity and desire in surgically menopausal women with hypoactive sexual desire disorder. *J Clin Endocrinol Metab.* 2005;90(9):5226–5233.

PART IV

Common Illnesses in Women

25

Urinary Tract Infections

PRISCILLA ABERCROMBIE

CASE STUDY

Rosemary is a 27-year-old college student who suffers from frequent bladder infections. She is worried about taking so many antibiotics. It seems like every time she goes home on vacation from school and has sex with her boyfriend she gets another infection. She is wondering what she can do to prevent these infections. Can she prevent bladder infections without taking antibiotics?

Introduction

More than 50% of all women will develop a urinary tract infection (UTI) in their lifetime (Fihn 2003). Eighty to ninety percent of UTIs are caused by *Escherichia coli* (Fihn 2003). Twenty five percent of women will have a recurrence of their UTI in their lifetime (Franco 2005).

Definitions

Acute lower UTI also called acute bacterial cystitis is characterized by urinary frequency, dysuria, and urgency. A combination of these symptoms without vaginal symptoms increases the diagnostic probability of UTI to more than 90% (Fihn 2003).Other symptoms may include suprapubic pressure and gross hematuria.

Recurrent UTI is most commonly caused by reinfection with the same or different organism and occurs after resolution of a previously treated infection (Franco 2005).

Interstitial cystitis (IC) is characterized by urinary frequency, urgency, and pelvic pain and is frequently misdiagnosed as recurrent UTI (Dell 2007). IC can be differentiated from recurrent UTI by the absence of pyuria or bacteria on urine culture. Standardized symptom surveys such as the Pelvic Pain and Urgency/Frequency (PUF) questionnaire have been used to identify women with IC but the reliability of this tool has been questioned (Brewer et al. 2007). IC remains a diagnosis made by exclusion.

Women who present with fever, chills, and flank pain are more likely to have a complicated upper UTI or pyelonephritis, requiring more aggressive treatment and vigilant follow-up. The focus of this chapter will be on the management of uncomplicated lower UTI.

CLINICAL TIP

In young women under age 23, infection with the sexually transmitted infections *Neisseria gonorrhoeae* or *Chlamydia trachomatis* urethritis should be ruled out. All women with vaginal symptoms including burning with urination on the external genitalia should be evaluated for vaginitis.

Risk Factors for UTI

See Table 25.1 comparing acute UTI, UTI in postmenopausal women, and recurrent UTI. The most common risk factor for acute and recurrent UTI in women of all ages is sexual intercourse.

LABORATORY TESTING

Those with classic UTI symptoms should be treated empirically. A telephone consultation is an acceptable method of identifying and treating women with a UTI (Schauberger et al. 2007). Women with a history of recent UTI, recurrent UTI, or symptoms of vaginitis or cervicitis should be seen for an evaluation.

A urine analysis by dipstick is sufficient for diagnosis in most cases. Either nitrite positive or leukocyte esterase and blood on dipstick are sufficient for diagnosis (70% sensitivity and 70% specificity) (Little et al. 2006). All women with a positive dipstick with clinical symptoms should be treated. Patients with

Table 25.1. Risk Factors for UTI

Risk Factors	Acute UTI (Fihn 2003)	UTI Postmenopause (Hu et al. 2004)	Recurrent UTI (Franco 2005)
Previous UTI	X	X	X
Sexual intercourse	X	X	X
Use of spermicide	X		X
Diabetes		X	
Incontinence		X	
Antimicrobials			X
Contraception			X
Genetics			X
Distance from urethra to anus			X

a negative urine dipstick, upper urinary tract symptoms, or with recurrent UTI should have a urine culture.

MANAGEMENT STRATEGIES

Although evidence-based guidelines for the treatment of UTI are available from many organizations such as The Infectious Disease Society of America and the American College of Obstetricians and Gynecologists, many clinicians continue to conduct unnecessary tests and treat with inappropriate antimicrobials. One study conducted by the Mayo Clinic (Grover et al. 2007) found that only 30% of patients with UTI seen in a family residency clinic setting were managed

Clinical Management Guidelines

ACOG Practice Bulletin: Treatment of Urinary Tract Infections (American College of Obstetricians and Gynecologists 2008)
   Diagnosis and Management of Uncomplicated Urinary Tract Infections, American Family Physician 2005 (Mehnert-Kay 2005)
   Guidelines for Antimicrobial Treatment of Uncomplicated Acute Bacterial Cystitis and Acute Pyelonephritis in Women, Infectious Disease Society of America, 1999 (Warren et al. 1999)

within clinical guidelines. Less than 25% of patients received empiric treatment, urine cultures were done despite positive dipsticks, and although SMX-TMP is effective in most cases, it was prescribed less often than expected.

ANTIMICROBIALS

Three-day antimicrobial therapy is now the standard treatment regimen for acute UTI and is effective in over 90% of cases (American College of Obstetricians and Gynecologists 2008). Trimethoprim–sulfamethoxazole remains the treatment of choice for women with acute UTI (Warren et al. 1999). In community settings where there is a greater than 15%–20% resistance to trimethoprim–sulfamethoxazole, other antimicrobials should be prescribed (American College of Obstetricians and Gynecologists 2008). Recurrences can be treated with a 3-day or 7-day antimicrobial regimen. Women should be evaluated and counseled for risk factors for recurrence such as sexual intercourse and the use of spermicides. Women with more than two UTIs in a year should be referred to an urologist or urogynecologist to rule out structural abnormalities. Prophylaxis with an antimicrobial such as nitrofurantoin once daily has been shown to reduce the risk of recurrence by 95% (Franco 2005). A Cochrane analysis found that daily prophylaxis for 6–12 months successfully reduced recurrent UTIs compared to placebo (Albert et al. 2004). Of note, there were no differences between the groups when the antimicrobials were discontinued and there was an increase in side effects among the antimicrobial group. For women with recurrent UTI associated with sexual intercourse, a single dose of an antimicrobial after intercourse for prophylaxis has been found to be effective (Melekos et al. 1997). Health behaviors such as postcoital voiding, wiping pattern, and the wearing of pantyhose do not appear to reduce the recurrence of UTIs (Fihn 2003). See Table 25.2 for a Quick Guide to Antimicrobial Treatment of UTIs.

CLINICAL TIP

Of particular note, the use of certain antimicrobials may adversely affect normal genital flora such as lactobacilli increasing colonization of uropathogens (Franco 2005). Trimethoprim and nitrofurantoin are thought to have less effect on normal genital flora than amoxicillin and beta-lactam antibiotics. Similarly, spermicides have been found to alter the vaginal microflora increasing the risk of UTI (Gupta et al. 2000).

Table 25.2. Quick Guide: Treatment of Uncomplicated UTIs

	Drug	*Dose*
Acute UTI	Trimethoprim–sulfamethoxazole	One twice a day for 3 days, category C for pregnancy and breastfeeding
	Trimethoprim	100 mg, twice daily for 3 days
	Ciprofloxacin	250 mg twice daily for 3 days, do not use in pregnancy or breastfeeding
	Nitrofurantoin	100 mg twice daily for 7 days, Category B for pregnancy and breastfeeding
Recurrent UTI	Ciprofloxacin	250 mg twice daily for 3 or 7 days
	Nitrofurantoin	100 mg twice daily for 7 days,
Prophylaxis	Nitrofurantoin	100 mg once daily for 6–12 months
	Nitrofurantoin	100 mg once daily after intercourse

Refer to ACOG Guidelines.

*See current guidelines for a more comprehensive list of antimicrobials.

ESTROGEN IN POSTMENOPAUSAL WOMEN

A recent Cochrane review (Perrotta et al. 2008) found that the use of oral estrogen did not reduce the risk of recurrent UTI in the four RCTs reviewed. On the other hand, in two small RCTs, vaginal estrogen did successfully reduce the number of UTIs in postmenopausal women with recurrent UTIs. Vaginal estrogen improves tissue integrity and promotes the growth of healthy microflora. This may explain its role in the prevention of UTI in the postmenopausal woman.

LACTOBACILLI

Lactobacilli are probiotics that are thought to play a role in the prevention of UTIs. A variety of strains of lactobacilli, particularly hydrogen-producing lactobacilli, prevent the growth of uropathogens and promote the restoration of normal genitourinary microflora. A decrease in hydrogen peroxide–producing lactobacilli is thought to increase risk of recurrent UTI by facilitating colonization of *E. coli* (Gupta et al. 1998). Only two strains of lactobacilli, *L. rhamnosus* GR-1 and *L. reuteri* B-54 and RC-14, have been found to be effective in the treatment of UTIs (Reid and Bruce 2006). Numerous issues plague clinical research on the use of probiotics for genitourinary health: small sample size, lack of quantitative evidence of colonization of lactobacilli, issues regarding product stability and quality, lack of knowledge regarding the role of specific lactobacilli strains in the genitourinary ecosystem, and the need for validated dosing strategies (Barrons and Tassone 2008).

Barrons and Tassone (2008) reviewed four randomized clinical trials conducted with various strains of lactobacilli to prevent the recurrence of UTIs. Only one study showed a significant reduction in the episodes of recurrent UTIs (Bruce and Reid, 1988). In this study, participants used vaginal suppositories containing either *L. rhamnosus* GR-1 and *L. fermentum* B-54 (>1.0 × 10^9 CFU per suppository) or Lactobacillus growth factor (LGF) once a week for 12 months. LGF is thought to stimulate the growth of indigenous lactobacilli. Although there was no significant difference between the groups in UTI recurrence, both groups experienced a 73% reduction ($P = 0.001$) in the rates of UTI compared to the previous year.

Clinical Pearl

Currently, there is one over-the-counter product containing *L. rhamnosus* GR-1 and *L. reuteri* RC-14 available in the United States. One capsule taken orally contains 5 billion CFU Fem-Dophilus Jarrow.

UVA URSI (*ARCTOSTAPHYLOS UVA URSI*)

Uva ursi or bearberry leaf has a long history of traditional use for inflammatory conditions of the urinary tract. The main constituent of dried uva ursi leaf is the glycoside arbutin. The antimicrobial effect of the herb is associated with the glycone hydroquinone that is released from the arbutin. The hydroquinone acts as an antiseptic and antimicrobial in the bladder. It was originally thought that the urine must be alkaline for the hydroquinone glucuronide to decompose sufficiently to release the hydroquinone and have its antimicrobial effect (Yarnell 2002). A recent study showed that alkalinization of the urine was not a requirement for hydroquinone to maintain its antimicrobial effects (Siegers et al. 2003). According to the German E Commission, uva ursi has effects in vitro against common uropathogens such as *E. coli*, *Proteus vulgaris*, *Ureaplasma urealyticum*, and *Staphylococcus aureus* (Blumenthal and Bundesinstitut für Arzneimittel und Medizinprodukte. Commission E 2000).

Although uva ursi is traditionally used as a treatment for mild acute UTI, one double-blinded placebo controlled trial demonstrated that the botanical could be successfully used as a preventive therapy (Larsson et al. 1993). Fifty seven women with recurrent cystitis were randomized to either receive standardized uva ursi extract combined with dandelion or placebo for 1 month. In the following year, there were no UTIs in the treatment group and 23% in the placebo group.

The German E Commission has approved uva ursi for the treatment, not prevention, of UTI. No clinical trials have been conducted to support its effectiveness for treating UTI. The recommended dose is that which provides 400–800 mg/day arbutin, divided into two to three doses. This is equivalent to 1.5–2.5 g in infusion or cold aqueous extract or 2–4 mL of a tincture (1:5) 3 times/ day. Most authorities recommend using uva ursi for no longer than 1–2 weeks at a time and no more than 5 times a year due to the potential toxic effects of hydroquinone. One case of Bull's eye maculopathy secondary to prolonged use of uva ursi was reported in the literature (Wang and Del Priore 2004). Uva ursi is a known melanin inhibitor and has been used to treat hyperpigmentation of the skin (Arndt and Fitzpatrick 1965; Fitzpatrick et al. 1966). It should not be used during pregnancy or breastfeeding.

CRANBERRY (*VACCINIUM MACROCARPON*)

Cranberry is used widely for the prevention of UTI but should not be used for the treatment of UTI. It was originally thought that it worked by acidifying the urine but subsequent studies have shown that the active ingredient proantho-cyanadin inhibits the adherence of bacteria to the uroepithelial cells lining the urinary tract (Sobota 1984; Zafriri et al. 1989). Studies show efficacy of cran-berry against uropathogens such as *E. coli* (Sobota 1984). Blueberry (*Vaccinium augustifolium*), cranberry's close cousin, has similar active ingredients and anti-adhesion properties (Ofek et al. 1996) although it has been studied less.

In a recent Cochrane review (Jepson and Craig, 2008), seven studies with cranberry juice and four with cranberry tablets (one with both juice and tablets) showed that cranberry significantly reduced symptomatic UTI over a 12-month period (RR 0.65, 95% CI 0.46–0.90) compared to a control or placebo. Cranberry was less effective in the elderly and those catheterized. Dosages, concentrations, and the length of the intervention were variable across studies. The high drop-out rates may be attributed to the participants' inability to drink large quantities of cranberry juice over long periods of time. Cranberry tablets appeared to be better tolerated and less expensive.

Cranberry is available as a sweetened and unsweetened juice and as a concentrated juice extract tablet with or without other active ingredients. One well-designed study used Ocean Spray cranberry cocktail 300 mL/day (10 oz). Recommended juice dosages vary from 250 to 500 mL/day. Capsules of concentrated juice extract in 300–500 mg can be given 2–3 times/day. Cranberry is safe to use during pregnancy and lactation.

Clinical Pearl

For my patients at risk for recurrent UTI, I recommend the use of 500 mg of cranberry extract in tablet form 1–3 times/day. The tablets are more convenient, do not contain sugar, and are better tolerated than unsweetened cranberry juice. Supplements containing both cranberry and D-mannose are also available over-the-counter.

OTHER BOTANICALS

There are a few other botanicals that should be mentioned because of their long-standing traditional use. The leaves and oil of buchu (*Agathosma betulina*), a South African plant, have been used as a diurectic and to treat bladder infections (Simpson 1998). Unfortunately, one study found buchu had very little antimicrobial activity against *E. coli* when tested in vitro (Lis-Balchin et al. 2001). Corn silk (stigma of *Zea mays*) has been found to have diuretic effects (Maksimovic et al. 2004; Masteikova et al. 2007; Velazquez et al. 2005) and its other active constituents may be helpful in the treatment of UTI. The saponins are thought to decrease inflammation and the allantoin is thought to soothe the irritated lining of the bladder. Finally, *Echinacea purpurea* has been approved by the German E Commission for treatment of chronic infections of the lower urinary tract (Blumenthal and Bundesinstitut für Arzneimittel und Medizinprodukte. Commission E 2000) though a search of Pubmed found no studies investigating its use for the urinary tract.

D-MANNOSE

D-Mannose is a sugar found in fruit such as peaches, oranges, cranberries, and blueberries. It is also present in the epithelial cells that line the urinary tract. Unlike most sugars, it is not broken down in the bloodstream but instead it is excreted in the urine. In the urinary tract, D-mannose coats *E. coli*, essentially inactivating the bacteria, rendering it unable to stick to the uroepithelial cells (Toyota et al. 1989). D-Mannose has been shown to decrease bacturia due to *E. coli* in rats (Michaels et al. 1983). Numerous in vitro studies document the useful role D-mannose plays in the urinary tract but clinical trials are lacking.

Summary

Antimicrobials remain the standard choice for the treatment of acute UTI because of the strong evidence for its effectiveness. Uva ursi is an alternative treatment though there is little clinical research to support its use. While the strongest evidence exists for the use of antimicrobials for the prevention of recurrent UTI, there is good evidence for the use of cranberry also. It offers additional health because of its antioxidant properties and does not contribute to antimicrobial resistance. Vaginal estrogen may play a role in the prevention of UTI in postmenopausal women. Probiotics and D-mannose have not been adequately studied but pose few safety concerns and are well tolerated.

Let us revisit Rosemary, our college student with recurrent UTI related to sexual intercourse. What treatment options does she have? She could take a single dose of an antibiotic after each episode of intercourse; there is good evidence to support this. But Rosemary has expressed concern about using antibiotics. It seems to me we could offer her three choices for the long-term prevention of UTI: cranberry, D-mannose, or probiotics. Since Rosemary is a college student, she will want to consider which of her options is most likely to fit into her lifestyle and is the most affordable.

REFERENCES

Albert X, Huertas I, Pereiro II., Sanfelix J, Gosalbes V, Perrota C. Antibiotics for preventing recurrent urinary tract infection in non-pregnant women. *Cochrane Database Syst Rev.* 2004;(3):CD001209.

American College of Obstetricians and Gynecologists. ACOG practice bulletin no. 91: Treatment of urinary tract infections in nonpregnant women. *Obstetr Gynecol.* 2008;111(3):785–794.

Arndt KA, Fitzpatrick TB. Topical use of hydroquinone as a depigmenting agent. *JAMA.*1965;194(9):965–967.

Barrons R, Tassone D. Use of lactobacillus probiotics for bacterial genitourinary infections in women: a review. *Clin Ther.* 2008;30(3):453–468.

Blumenthal M, Bundesinstitut für Arzneimittel und Medizinprodukte. Commission E. *Herbal Medicine: Expanded Commission E Monographs.* 1st ed. Newton, MA: Integrative Medicine Communications; 2000.

Brewer ME, White WM, Klein FA, Klein L M, Waters WB. Validity of pelvic pain, urgency, and frequency questionnaire in patients with interstitial cystitis/painful bladder syndrome. *Urology.* 2007;70(4):646–649.

Bruce AW, Reid G. Intravaginal instillation of lactobacilli for prevention of recurrent urinary tract infections. *Can J Microbiol.* 1988;34(3):339–343.

Dell JR. Interstitial cystitis/painful bladder syndrome: appropriate diagnosis and management. *J Women Health.* 2007;16(8):1181–1187.

Fihn SD. Clinical practice. acute uncomplicated urinary tract infection in women. *N Engl J Med.* 2003;349(3):259–266.

Fitzpatrick TB, Arndt KA, el-Mofty AM, Pathak MA. Hydroquinone and psoralens in the therapy of hypermelanosis and vitiligo. *Arch Dermatol.* 1966;93(5):589–600.

Franco AV. Recurrent urinary tract infections. *Best Pract Res Clin Obstetr Gynaecol.* 2005;19(6):861–873.

Grover ML, Bracamonte JD, Kanodia AK, et al. Assessing adherence to evidence-based guidelines for the diagnosis and management of uncomplicated urinary tract infection. *Mayo Clin Proc.* 2007;82(2):181–185.

Gupta K, Hillier SL, Hooton TM, Roberts PL, Stamm WE. Effects of contraceptive method on the vaginal microbial flora: a prospective evaluation. *J Infect Dis.* 2000;181(2):595–601.

Gupta K, Stapleton AE, Hooton TM, Roberts PL, Fennell CL, Stamm WE. Inverse association of H₂O₂-producing lactobacilli and vaginal *Escherichia coli* colonization in women with recurrent urinary tract infections. *J Infect Dis.* 1998;178(2);446–450.

Hu KK, Boyko EJ, Scholes D, et al. Risk factors for urinary tract infections in postmenopausal women. *Arch Intern Med.* 2004;164(9):989–993.

Jepson RG, Craig JC. Cranberries for preventing urinary tract infections. *Cochrane Database Syst Rev.* 2008;(1):CD001321.

Larsson B, Jonasson A, Fianu S. Prophylactic effect of uva-E in women with recurrent cystitis: a preliminary report. *Curr Ther Res.* 1993;53(4):441–443.

Lis-Balchin M, Hart S, Simpson E. Buchu (*Agathosma betulina* and *A. crenulata, rutaceae*) essential oils: Their pharmacological action on guinea-pig ileum and antimicrobial activity on microorganisms. *J Phar Pharmacol.* 2001;53(4):579–582.

Little P, Turner S, Rumsby K, et al. Developing clinical rules to predict urinary tract infection in primary care settings: sensitivity and specificity of near patient tests (dipsticks) and clinical scores. *Br J Gen Practice; J R Coll Gen Practition.* 2006;56(529):606–612.

Maksimovic Z, Dobric S, Kovacevic N, Milovanovic Z. Diuretic activity of maydis stigma extract in rats. *Die Pharmazie.* 2004;59(12):967–971.

Masteikova R, Klimas R, Samura BB, et al. An orientational examination of the effects of extracts from mixtures of herbal drugs on selected renal functions. [Orientacni sledovani vlivu vyluhu ze smesi rostlinnych drog na vybrane funkce ledvin] *Ceska a Slovenska Farmacie: Casopis Ceske Farmaceuticke Spolecnosti a Slovenske Farmaceuticke Spolecnosti.* 2007;56(2):85–89.

Mehnert-Kay SA. Diagnosis and management of uncomplicated urinary tract infections. *Am Fam Phys.* 2005;72(3):451–456.

Melekos MD, Asbach HW, Gerharz E, Zarakovitis IE, Weingaertner K, Naber KG Post-intercourse versus daily ciprofloxacin prophylaxis for recurrent urinary tract infections in premenopausal women. *J Urol.* 1997;157(3):935–939.

Michaels EK, Chmiel JS, Plotkin BJ, Schaeffer AJ. Effect of D-mannose and D-glucose on *Escherichia coli* bacteriuria in rats. *Urolog Res.* 1983;11(2):97–102.

Ofek I, Goldhar J, Sharon N. Anti-*Escherichia coli* adhesin activity of cranberry and blueberry juices. *Adv Exp Med Biol.* 1996;408:179–183.

Perrotta C, Aznar M, Mejia R, Albert X, Ng C. Oestrogens for preventing recurrent urinary tract infection in postmenopausal women. *Cochrane Database Syst Rev.* 2008;(2):CD005131.

Reid G, Bruce AW. Probiotics to prevent urinary tract infections: The rationale and evidence. *World J Urol.* 2006;24(1):28–32.

Schauberger CW, Merkitch KW, Prell AM. Acute cystitis in women: experience with a telephone-based algorithm. *WMJ Off Pub State Med Soc Wisconsin.* 2007;106(6):326–329.

Siegers C, Bodinet C, Ali SS, Siegers CP. Bacterial deconjugation of arbutin by *Escherichia coli*. *Phytomed Int J Phytother Phytopharmacol.* 2003;10(Suppl 4);58–60.

Simpson D. Buchu—South Africa's amazing herbal remedy. *Scot Med J.* 1998; 43(6):189–191.

Sobota AE. Inhibition of bacterial adherence by cranberry juice: potential use for the treatment of urinary tract infections. *J Urol.* 1984;131(5):1013–1016.

Toyota S, Fukushi Y, Katoh S, Orikasa S, Suzuki Y. Anti-bacterial defense mechanism of the urinary bladder. role of mannose in urine. *Nippon Hinyokika Gakkai Zasshi. Jpn J Urol.* 1989;80(12):1816–1823.

Velazquez DV, Xavier HS, Batista JE, de Castro-Chaves C. Zea mays L. extracts modify glomerular function and potassium urinary excretion in conscious rats. *Phytomed Int J Phytother Phytopharmacol.* 2005;12(5):363–369.

Wang L, Del Priore LV. Bull's-eye maculopathy secondary to herbal toxicity from uva ursi. *Am J Ophthalmol.* 2004;137(6):1135–1137.

Warren JW, Abrutyn E, Hebel JR, Johnson JR, Schaeffer AJ, Stramm WE. Guidelines for antimicrobial treatment of uncomplicated acute bacterial cystitis and acute pyelonephritis in women. *Clin Infect Dis.* 1999;2:745–758.

Yarnell E. Botanical medicines for the urinary tract. *World J Urol.* 2002;20(5):285–293.

Zafriri D, Ofek I, Adar R, Pocino M, Sharon N. Inhibitory activity of cranberry juice on adherence of type 1 and type P fimbriated *Escherichia coli* to eucaryotic cells. *Antimicrob Agent Chemother.* 1989;33(1):92–98.

26

Irritable Bowel Syndrome

CYNTHIA A. ROBERTSON

CASE STUDY

Lori presented herself at my office with symptoms of irritable bowel syndrome with alternating diarrhea and constipation in 1993. She was treated with bulking agents, antispasmodic medications, and eventually a low dose tricyclic antidepressant over the course of several years. Although initially she seemed to respond to these therapies, her symptoms would return within a month or two. After some time, Lori cancelled her follow-up appointment and stopped coming to the office.

After 9 months, Lori returned to my office reporting that her symptoms had been well controlled during that period. She explained that she did appreciate all that we had tried, but that she had found something different that was working very well for her. In fact, she was actually in the office because she needed a prescription for her insurance company for the acupuncture that had controlled her symptoms.

That day, Lori opened my eyes to the potential benefits of complementary and alternative therapies, and I began my journey into integrative medicine. In this chapter, I hope to share with you some ideas and potential solutions that will be of help in your treatment of women with irritable bowel syndrome.

Introduction

Gastrointestinal complaints rank among the most frequent reasons for primary care visits in the United States. Direct costs are in excess of $85 billion annually (Sandler et al. 2002), with an additional indirect cost of $20 billion due to days off work (Mullin 2008). This chapter will discuss the most common digestive disorder that affects women in the United States: irritable bowel syndrome. On a worldwide basis, the prevalence of IBS is between 10% and 15%. It occurs twice as often in women than men (Mayer 2008); women are also more likely to seek medical care (Whitehead et al. 2002).

The etiology of IBS is multifactorial and not fully understood. Alterations in visceral perception, brain pain modulation, motor function, and neuroendocrine function are present. Immune activation and changes in intestinal flora may contribute to symptoms (Mayer 2008).

As defined by the Rome III criteria, IBS is divided into diarrhea predominant (IBS-D); constipation predominant (IBS-C); a combination of the two as a mixed classification (IBS-M); and unspecified (IBS-U) (Table 26.1). Among women, IBS-C occurs most frequently. The reader is directed to other sources for a more detailed description of the warning signs, differential diagnosis, and appropriate workup.

In as many as 30% of cases, IBS develops following a gastrointestinal infection. These individuals have evidence of ongoing inflammation for years with increased numbers of enterochromaffin cells and inflammatory cells in the intestinal mucosa (Spiller 2007).

Women are more likely to experience associated extraintestinal conditions including temporomandibular joint disorder, chronic fatigue syndrome, chronic pelvic pain, and fibromyalgia. Among women with IBS seen in gynecology

Table 26.1. Rome III Criteria Irritable Bowel Syndrome

Symptoms of recurrent abdominal pain or discomfort and a marked change in bowel habit for at least 6 months, with symptoms experienced on at least 3 days of at least 3 months. Two or more of the following must apply:

1. Pain is relieved by a bowel movement.
2. Onset of pain is related to a change in frequency of stool.
3. Onset of pain is related to a change in the appearance of stool.

practices, dysmenorrhea, dyspareunia, and urinary frequency, and also urgency are prevalent (Whitehead et al. 2002).

Abuse

In studies of women with functional bowel disease, including IBS, 30%–40% have a history of physical or sexual abuse (Drossman et al. 1990; Talley et al. 1998). In the evaluation of women with gastrointestinal illness it is important to be aware of the possibility of a prior history of abuse. For women who have experienced abuse, psychological counseling plays an important role in the treatment of IBS.

Conventional Therapies

One of the challenges of evaluating therapies for irritable bowel syndrome is the high placebo response rate; rates of approximately 40% have been found (Dorn et al. 2007). Historically, conventional treatments for irritable bowel have included bulking agents, antispasmodic and antidepressant medications. A Cochrane review only found evidence to support the use of antispasmodic medications for abdominal pain and overall well-being (Quartero et al. 2005). The review further concluded that despite numerous studies there was no clear evidence for antidepressants or bulking agents in IBS. Bulking agents, however- have been found to improve constipation (Schoenfeld 2005). For patients with diarrhea-predominate IBS-D, over-the-counter agents, including low dose loperamide, can reduce urgency and soiling.

Lubiprostone, a selective chloride channel activator, has demonstrated efficacy in chronic constipation (Rivkin et al. 2006). It is beneficial as well in the treatment of IBS-C (Johanson et al. 2008) for which it has received FDA approval (FDA 2008). [Pregnancy Category C; not recommended during breast-feeding.] The selective serotonergic agonist, tegaserod and antagonist, alosetron, were found beneficial in studies of women with IBS-C and IBS-D respectively. However, both were withdrawn by the FDA due to serious adverse effects (Mayer 2008).

Diet

Most women with IBS are aware of a relationship between their diet and symptoms. Malabsorption of the sugars lactose, fructose, and sorbitol produces gas, bloating, abdominal pain, and diarrhea. Lactase deficiency is common and affects approximately 70% of the world's population (Lomer et al. 2008). While some women may have sugar intolerances alone, others have coexisting IBS. Breath testing can be performed to identify specific problems, and empiric trials are useful as they are often diagnostic and therapeutic.

Although women may be certain of specific food culprits, it is not uncommon for inconsistency to exist, and this factor adds further confusion to this frustrating disorder. Diet, activity, stressor, and symptom logs will help elucidate foods and circumstances that precipitate attacks.

A review of studies of sugar intolerance in patients with IBS found four uncontrolled studies all of which demonstrated an improvement in IBS symptoms with elimination of the offending sugar (Spanier et al. 2003). In addition, a small (n = 25) double-blind placebo-controlled study found a significant correlation of resumption of IBS symptoms with the addition of fructose or fructans, compared to adding glucose alone, $p \leq 0.002$ (Shepherd et al. 2008). Addressing issues of potential lactose, fructose, and sorbitol intolerance will provide benefit to some women with IBS.

The removal of specific offending foods has been used in the treatment of IBS. Elimination diets have been performed both empirically and based on IgG and IgE food antibodies. Empiric elimination diets with subsequent reintroduction of foods can be helpful, but they are time-consuming with varying patient compliance.

Elimination diets based on IgG and IgE food antibodies have shown benefit in IBS (Atkinson et al. 2004; Drisko et al. 2006; Zar et al. 2005). In one small pilot study (n = 20), elimination and rotation diets that were based on IgG and IgE food and mold panels demonstrated an improvement in abdominal pain, stool frequency, and quality of life scores (Drisko et al. 2006). In another three-month study, 150 patients were given either a sham elimination diet or an elimination diet based on IgG food antibodies. Those patients who were compliant with the antibody-directed diet demonstrated a statistically significant improvement in symptoms and global rating (Atkinson et al. 2004). Reintroduction of the targeted foods led to increased symptoms in both groups but more so in the antibody-directed diet. Critics have questioned how well controlled the sham diet was.

Gut Flora

Changes in intestinal flora, including small bowel overgrowth, have been found in some patients with IBS (Mullin et al. 2008). Symptom reduction has been demonstrated following treatment with luminal acting antibiotics (Pimentel et al. 2000). However, several subsequent studies failed to reveal a difference in IBS patients with and without small intestinal bacterial overgrowth (Grover et al. 2008; Posserud et al. 2007).

Modification of intestinal flora with probiotics reduces symptoms of IBS. Individual strains of Lactobacillus and Bifidobacteria have been tested (Nobaek et al. 2000; Whorwell et al. 2006) as well as multi-species products (Kajander et al. 2005, 2008; Kim et al. 2003; O'Mahony et al. 2005). *Bifidobacterium infantis* 3564 demonstrated an improvement in abdominal pain and in a composite score of abdominal pain/discomfort, bloating/distension, and bowel movement satisfaction in women (Whorwell et al. 2006) (Table 26.2). It has been proposed that probiotics work not only by impacting the bacterial milieu, but also via changes in motility and immune function (Camilleri 2006).

Table 26.2. Studies of Probiotics in Irritable Bowel Syndrome

Author	Species Studied	Duration n=	Significant Findings
Kim et al. (2003)	Mixture of: *Lactobacillus casei, L. plantarum, L. acidophilus L. delbrueckii* ssp. *bulgaricus Bifidobacterium longum, B. breve, B. infantis and Streptococcus salivarius* ssp. *thermophilus*	8 weeks $n = 25$	Decreased abdominal Bloating, $p < 0.05$
Kajander et al. (2005)	Mixture of: *Lactobacillus rhamnosus* GG, *L. rhamnosus* LC705, *Bifidobacterium breve* Bb99, *Propionibacterium freudenreichii* ssp. Shermanii JS	6 months $n = 103$	Reduced total IBS symptom score, $p < 0.02$.
O'Mahoney et al. (2005)	1. *Lactobacillus salivarius* UCC4331 2. *Bifidobacterium infantis* 35624 (Each compared to the other, and control)	8 weeks $n = 75$	1. Improved Quality of life-dysphoria score, $p < 0.1$ No other significant improvement after 8 weeks 2. Lower composite IBS score, $p < 0.05$ Lowered bowel difficulty compared to *L. salivarius*, $p < 0.05$ Improved quality of life-health worry score, $p < 0.05$

(continued)

Author	Species Studied	Duration n=	Significant Findings
Whorwell et al. (2006)	*Bifidobacterium infantis* 35624	4 weeks n = 362	Decreased abdominal pain, $p < 0.02$ Improved composite score, (pain-discomfort, bloating-distension, bowel movement satisfaction), $p < 0.02$
Kajander et al. 2008	Mixture of: *Lactobacillus rhamnosus* GG *L. rhamnosus* Lc705 *Propionibacterium freudenreichii* ssp. Shermanii JS *Bifidobacterium animalis* ssp. Lactis Bb12	5 months n = 86	Composite IBS score decreased, $p < 0.01$

A meta-analysis of probiotics found evidence of improvement in global IBS symptoms and a reduction in abdominal pain (McFarland and Dublin 2006). There is, however, no current consensus as to the preferred probiotics or whether to use individual or multiple species.

Taking into consideration the wide range of individual variation, I generally recommend a probiotic with multiple species for women with IBS.

Exercise

Exercise has demonstrated benefit in a variety of gastrointestinal diseases (Bi and Trandafilopoulos 2003; Peters et al. 2001). Epidemiological studies have shown that exercise is a protective factor for gastrointestinal symptoms in obese patients (Levy et al. 2005). In one small study ($n = 8$), mild physical activity was associated with improved intestinal gas clearance (Villoria et al. 2006).

There are limited studies of exercise in women with IBS. One trial evaluating a class that taught health-promoting behaviors, which included exercise instruction, found a significant reduction in IBS pain after one month, $p < 0.05$ (Colwell et al. 1998). In a small trial of yoga in adolescents with IBS ($n = 25$), a significant improvement in gastrointestinal symptoms, lower levels of functional disability, and lower anxiety after 4 weeks were demonstrated (Kuttner et al. 2006). A recent study of exercise in patients with IBS found no differences in overall quality of life; however, those with IBS-C did show significant symptom improvement (Daley et al. 2008).

Sleep

Nearly one-quarter of patients with IBS have sleep disturbance (Jarett et al. 2000). Women with both IBS and depressive symptoms have greater sleep complaints and take longer to enter initial rapid-eye movement period than healthy controls (Robert et al. 2004). The optimization of sleep with instructions in good sleep hygiene and the use of relaxation techniques are a reasonable part of the treatment plan.

Traditional Chinese Medicine

With highly individualized treatments designed to address all of the health issues of an individual, traditional Chinese medicine (TCM) seems ideally suited to the treatment of irritable bowel syndrome. However, the individual nature of TCM therapies makes evaluation using double-blind placebo-controlled studies difficult.

The data on the use of acupuncture for IBS is mixed. Challenges exist in studying identical acupuncture treatments with well-matched IBS patients and an appropriate placebo. Trials using sham acupuncture are complicated by the potential activation of other meridians that may indirectly impact the gut or modulate pain (Lim et al. 2006). A Cochrane review concluded that there is insufficient evidence to support the use of acupuncture for IBS and advised further study (Lim et al. 2006).

The research on Chinese herbal therapies present similar challenges. Chinese medicines are generally mixtures of as many as 20 different herbs, and concerns exist regarding potential adulteration of imported herbs with toxic substances (Liu et al. 2006). In 1998, a controlled trial of a single formula as well as a separate arm with individualized formulas showed a significant improvement in symptoms over a 14-week treatment period. The patients who received individualized treatments showed continued benefit for 3 months following the conclusion of treatment (Bensoussan et al. 1998).

TCM typically addresses multiple health concerns of a woman with several therapies rather than the one problem–one treatment approach used in Western medicine. Although trials of these more comprehensive treatment programs are not available, it has been my experience that many women with IBS do well with TCM therapies.

AYURVEDIC MEDICINE

In Ayurvedic medicine, IBS is described as an imbalance in a woman's dosha. Treatment typically incorporate changes in diet, meditation, stress management, and herbs. In a double-blind randomized trial *Aegle marmelos* plus *Bacopa monnieri* was compared with placebo or standard therapy. The standard therapy consisted of Chlordiazepoxide with an antispasmodic (clidinium bromide), and psyllium. The Ayurvedic preparation demonstrated improvement at 6 weeks of 64.9%, versus placebo at 32.7%. However, the standard therapy response rate was highest at 78.3% (Yadav et al. 1989). Triphala is an ayurvedic formulation containing *Emblica officinalis, Terminalia belerica, Terminalia chebula*, which has long been used as a stool softener and bowel regulator (Low Dog T. personal communication, September 28, 2008). Triphala is often advised for regular daily use (Weil 2004).

Botanicals

Perhaps the most widely studied Western botanical for IBS is peppermint oil (*Mentha piperita*). Peppermint oil is a smooth muscle relaxant that acts directly on the gastrointestinal tract. The menthol component of peppermint oil interferes with the movement of calcium across the cell membrane and leads to smooth muscle relaxation (Capello et al. 2007). Multiple clinical trials have studied peppermint for the treatment of IBS. In a review of 16 trials, peppermint was found to demonstrate a statistically significant benefit in 8 of the studies, whereas in 3 of the other trials peppermint and anticholinergic medications showed comparable benefits (Grigoleit and Grigoleit 2005). A subsequent double-blind placebo-controlled trial of peppermint oil demonstrated significant improvement in IBS symptoms after 4 weeks of treatment (Capello et al. 2007).

Because peppermint oil is rapidly destroyed by gastric acid, it must be enteric-coated to reach the intestines. Optimum results are achieved when taken three times a day after meals. Some women develop anal-burning with larger doses (Jellin et al. 2006), which may resolve with dose reduction.

> The antispasmodic property of peppermint oil has also been used to quiet the spasmodic colon during barium and endoscopic exams and is applied directly to the colon lumen.

In 2006, a Cochrane review evaluated 75 randomized trials of herbal medicines for the treatment of IBS (Liu et al. 2006). The quality of the majority of trials was considered poor with only three double-blind, placebo-controlled trials that are considered of high methodological quality. These three trials include the aforementioned 1998 Chinese Medicine trial by Bensoussan et al. and two herbal formulas; STW 5, (a combination of 9 herbs), and a Tibetan formula, Padma Lax (Table 26.3).

STW 5 was evaluated in a multicenter randomized trial in Germany; a significant improvement was found in total abdominal pain ($p < 0.001$), and irritable bowel symptom score ($p < 0.001$) after 4 weeks (Madisch et al. 2004). Further, in a double-blind placebo-controlled randomized study for IBS-C, Padma Lax demonstrated significant improvement after 3 months in constipation, abdominal pain severity, incomplete evacuation, distension, gas, and daily activities (Sallon et al. 2002). Some concerns have been raised regarding the safety of the celandine component of the formula (Low Dog T. personal communication, September 28, 2008). The Cochrane review concluded that while these herbal medicines may improve symptoms, additional well-designed studies are needed (Liu et al. 2006).

Western and Chinese herbalists generally include digestive bitters such as dandelion and gentian in formulas for IBS. Bitters act as a GI tonic; they increase gastric secretions, provide exocrine pancreatic support, and act as mild laxatives (Abascal and Yarnell 2005; Low Dog T. personal communication, September 28, 2008).

Table 26.3. STW 5 Formula

- German Chamomile flower (*Matricaria recutita*)
- Clown's Mustard plant (*Iberis amara*)
- Angelica root and rhizome (*Angelica archangeica*)
- Caraway fruit (*Carum carvi*)
- Milk Thistle fruit (*Silybum marianum*)
- Lemon Balm leaf (*Melissa officinalis*)
- Celandine aerial part (*Chelidonium majus*)
- Licorice root (*Glycyrrhiza glabra*)
- Peppermint leaf (*Mentha* × *peperita*)

Source: Adapted from Jellin JM, Gregory PJ, Batz, Hitchens K, et al. *Pharmacist's Letter/Prescriber's Letter Natural Medicines Comprehensive Database*. 8th ed. Stockton, CA: Therapeutic Research Faculty; 2006:1776.

Mind–Body Medicine

The importance of listening to women with IBS and developing a compassionate therapeutic relationship cannot be overemphasized. In the past, women were often told that IBS was all in their head. Acknowledgment of women's symptoms and the actual pathophysiological changes that occur with IBS has been found to foster a healing relationship (Mayer 2008).

> In working with women with IBS, I have found that taking the additional time to listen, answer questions, and thoroughly explain treatments results in better outcomes in shorter time frames. Many women comment that working with a practitioner who listens and explains things has been therapeutic in and of itself.

Hypnosis and cognitive behavioral therapy (CBT) are the most widely studied mind–body therapies in the treatment of IBS. Reviews have found hypnotherapy to produce sustained benefits that can last for years (Naliboff et al. 2007; Whitehead 2006; Whorwell 2008). Overall response rates from 70% to 87% have been demonstrated, with an improvement of 50% in digestive symptoms and quality of life (Whitehead 2006). In addition to clinician directed hypnosis, self-directed hypnosis tapes have shown benefit in typical and refractory IBS (Forbes et al. 2000; Palsson et al. 2006). Hypnotherapy is best utilized as part of an integrated approach to IBS (Whorwell 2006).

A meta-analysis of 17 cognitive and behavioral treatments found those patients receiving CBT had a 50% reduction in symptoms (Lackner et al. 2004; Mayer 2008). In women with moderate to severe IBS, CBT demonstrated a significant benefit compared to education (Drossman et al. 2003). Two European studies showed that a combination of an antispasmodic and CBT was significantly more effective than an antispasmodic alone (Kennedy et al. 2006), and this treatment combination was cost-effective as well (McCrone et al. 2008).

Manual Medicine

Osteopathy is often used for treatment of abdominal complaints. In one small study ($n = 20$), osteopathy was found to have a significant impact on overall symptoms and improved quality of life (Hundscheid et al. 2007). Further studies will help to define the role osteopathy in IBS.

Summary

Irritable bowel syndrome is common among women. Among the types, constipation predominant (IBS-C) occurs most frequently. In contrast to conditions like hypertension, conventional medications have limited efficacy in IBS. Taking the time to listen to women, becoming cognizant of significant personal issues including abuse, and creating a strong supportive partnership is essential in the treatment of IBS. Efforts to create a treatment plan that addresses the mind, body, and spirit using multiple modalities will offer additional opportunities for healing.

Acknowledgment

Special thanks to Sarah E. Hoefker for assistance in the preparation of the tables and references.

REFERENCES

Abscal K, Yarnell E. Combing herbs in a formula for irritable bowel syndrome. *Alter Complement Ther.* 2005;11(1):17–23.

Atkinson W, Sheldon TA, Shaath N, Whorwell PJ. Food elimination based on IgG antibodies in irritable bowel syndrome: a randomised controlled trial. *Gut.* 2004;53:1459–1464.

Barucha AE. Mayo Clinic Gastroenterology and hepatology board review. In: Hauser SC, ed. Mayo Clinic Scientific Press; 2006;233–244.

Bensoussan A, Talley NJ, Hing M, et al. Treatment of irritable bowel syndrome with Chinese herbal medicine: a randomized controlled trial. *JAMA.* 1998;280: 1585–1589.

Bi L, Triadafilopoulos G. Exercise and gastrointestinal function and disease: an evidence-based review of risks and benefits. *Clin Gastroenterol Hepatol.* 2003;1(5):345–355.

Blumenthal M, Busse W, Goldberg A, et al. eds. *The Complete German Commission Monographs: Therapeutic Guide to Herbal Medicines.* Boston: Integrative Medicine Communications; 1998.

Bouchoucha M, Devroede G, Dorval E, Faye A, Arhan P, Arsac M, Different segmental transit times in patients with irritable bowel syndrome and "normal" colonic transit time: is there a correlation with symptoms? *Tech Coloproctol.* 2006;10(4):287–296.

Capello G, Spezzaferro M, Grossi L, Manzoli L, Marzio L. Peppermint oil (Mintoil) in the treatment of irritable bowel syndrome: a prospective double-blind placebo-controlled randomized trial. *Dig Liver Dis.* 2007;39(6):530–536.

Camilleri M. Probiotics and irritable bowel syndrome: rationale, putative mechanisms, and evidence of clinical efficacy. *J Clin Gastroenterol.* 2006;40:264–269.

Cappello G, Spezzaferro M, Grossi L, Manzoli L, Marzio L. Peppermint oil (Mintoil) in the treatment of irritable bowel syndrome: a prospective double-blind placebo-controlled randomized trial. *Dig Liver Dis.* 2007;39(6):530–S536.

Colwell LJ, Prather CM, Phillips SF, Zinsmeister AR. Effects of an irritable bowel syndrome educational class on health-promoting behaviors and symptoms. *Am J Gastroenterol.* 1998;93(6):901–905.

Daley AJ, Grimmett C, Roberts L, et al. The effects of exercise upon symptoms and quality of life in patients diagnosed with irritable bowel syndrome: a randomised controlled trial. *Int J Sports Med.* 2008. 2008;29(9):778–782.

Dorn SD, Kaptchuk TJ, Park JB, et al. A meta-analysis of the placebo response in complementary and alternative medicine trials of irritable bowel syndrome. *Neurogastroenterol Motil.* 2007;19(8):630–637.

Drisko J, Bischoff B, Hall M, McCallum R. Treating irritable bowel syndrome with a food elimination diet followed by food challenge and probiotics. *J Am Coll Nutr.* 2006;25:514–522.

Drossman DA, Leserman J, Nachman G, et al. Sexual and physical abuse in women with functional or organic gastrointestinal disorders. *Ann Intern Med.* 1990;113(11):828–833.

Drossman DA, Toner BB, Whitehead WE, et al. Cognitive-behavioral therapy versus education and desipramine versus placebo for moderate to severe functional bowel disorders. *Gastroenterology.* 2003;125(1):19–31.

Food and Drug Administration. FDA approves Amitiza, (lubiprostone), for IBS-C. *FDA News.* April 30, 2008.

Forbes A, MacAuley S, Chiotakakou-Faliakou E. Hypnotherapy and therapeutic audio-tape: effective in previously unsuccessfully treated irritable bowel syndrome? *Int J Colorectal Dis.* 2000;15(5–6):328–334.

Grigoleit HG, Grigoleit P. Peppermint oil in irritable bowel syndrome. *Phytomedicine.* 2005;12(8):601–606.

Grover M, Kanazawa M, Palsson OS, et al. Small intestinal bacterial overgrowth in irritable bowel syndrome: association with colon motility, bowel symptoms, and psychological distress. *Neurogastroenterol Motil.* 2008.

Hundscheid H, Pepels M, Engels L, Loffeld R. Treatment of irritable bowel syndrome with osteopathy: results of a randomized controlled pilot study. *J Gastroenterol Hepatol.* 2007;22(9):1394–1398.

Jarrett ME, Burr RL, Cain KC, Rothermel JD, Landis CA, Heitkemper MM. Autonomic nervous system function during sleep among women with irritable bowel syndrome. *Dig Dis Sci.* 2008;53(3):694–703.

Jellin JM, Gregory PJ, Batz, Hitchens K, et al. *Pharmacist's Letter/Prescriber's Letter Natural Medicines Comprehensive Database.* 8th ed. Stockton, CA: Therapeutic Research Faculty; 2006:982–985.

Johanson JF, Drossman DA, Panas R, Wahle A, Ueno R. Clinical trial: phase 2 study of lubiprostone for irritable bowel syndrome with constipation. *Aliment Pharmacol Ther.* 2008;27(8):685–696.

Kajander K, Myllyluoma E, Rajilic-Stojanovic§ M, et al. Clinical trial: multispecies probiotic supplementation alleviates the symptoms of irritable bowel syndrome and stabilizes intestinal microbiota. *Aliment Pharmacol Ther.* 2008;27:48–57.

Kennedy TM, Chalder T, McCrone P, et al. Cognitive behavioural therapy in addition to antispasmodic therapy for irritable bowel syndrome in primary care: randomised controlled trial. *Health Technol Assess.* 2006;10(19):1–2.

Kim HJ, Camilleri M, McKinzie S, et al. A randomized controlled trial of a probiotic, VSL#3, on gut transit and symptoms in diarrhoea-predominant irritable bowel syndrome. *Aliment Pharmacol Ther.* 2003;17(7):895–904.

Kuttner L, Chambers CT, Hardial J, Israel DM, Jacobson K, Evans K. A randomized trial of yoga for adolescents with irritable bowel syndrome. *Pain Res Manag.* 2006;11(4):217–223.

Lackner JM, Mesmer C, Morley S, Dowzer C, Hamilton S. Psychological treatments for irritable bowel syndrome: a systematic review and meta-analysis. *J Consult Clin Psychol.* 2004;72(6):1100–1113.

Levy RL, Linde JA, Feld KA, Crowell MD, Jeffery RW. The association of gastrointestinal symptoms with weight, diet and exercise in weight-loss program participants. *Clin Gastroenterol Hepatol.* 2005;3(10):992–996.

Lim B, Manheimer E, Lao L, et al. Acupuncture for treatment of irritable bowel syndrome. *Cochrane Database Syst Rev.* 2006;(4):CD005111.

Liu JP, Yang M, Liu YX, Wei ML, Grimsgaard S. Herbal medicines for treatment of irritable bowel syndrome. *Cochrane Database Syst Rev.* 2006;(1):D004116.

Lomer MC, Parkes GC, Sanderson JD. Review article: lactose intolerance in clinical practice—myths and realities. *Aliment Pharmacol Ther.* 2008;27(2):93–103.

Madisch A, Holtmann G, Plein K, Hotz J. Treatment of irritable bowel syndrome with herbal preparations: results of a double-blind, randomized, placebo-controlled, multi-centre trial. *Aliment Pharmacol Ther.* 2004;19(3):271–279.

Mayer E. Irritable bowel syndrome. *N Engl J Med.* 2008;358(16):1692–1699.

McFarland LV; Dublin S. Meta-analysis of probiotics for the treatment of irritable bowel syndrome. *World J Gastroenterol.* 2008;14(17):2650–2661.

McCrone P, Knapp M, Kennedy T, Seed P, Jones R, Darnley S, Chalder T. Cost-effectiveness of cognitive behaviour therapy in addition to mebeverine for irritable bowel syndrome. *Eur J Gastroenterol Hepatol.* 2008;20(4):225–263.

Mullin GE, Pickett-Blakey O, Clarke JO. Integrative medicine in gastrointestinal disease: evaluating the evidence. *Expert Rev Gastroenterol Hepatol.* 2008;2(2): 261–280.

Naliboff BD, Fresé MP, Rapgay L. Mind/body psychological treatments for irritable bowel syndrome. *Evid Based Complement Alternat Med.* 2008;5(1):41–50.

Nobaek S, Johansson ML, Molin G, Ahrné S, Jeppsson B. Alteration of intestinal microflora is associated with reduction in abdominal bloating and pain in patients with irritable bowel syndrome. *Am J Gastroenterol.* 2000;95(5):1231–1238.

O'Mahony L, McCarthy J, Kelly P, et al. Lactobacillus and Bifidobacterium in irritable bowel syndrome: symptom responses and relationship to cytokine profiles. *Gastroenterology.* 2005;128(3):541–551.

Palsson OS, Turner MJ, Whitehead WE. Hypnosis home treatment for irritable bowel syndrome: a pilot study. *Int J Clin Exp Hypn.* 2006;54(1):85–99.

Peters HP, De Vries WR, Vanberge-Henegouwen GP, Akkermans LM. Potential benefits and hazards of physical activity and exercise on the gastrointestinal tract. *Gut.* 2001;48(3):435–439.

Pimentel M, Chow EJ, Lin HC. Eradication of small intestinal bacterial overgrowth reduces symptoms of irritable bowel syndrome. *Am J Gastroenterol.* 2000;95(12):3503–3506.

Posserud I, Stotzer PO, Björnsson ES, Abrahamsson H, Simrén M. Small intestinal bacterial overgrowth in patients with irritable bowel syndrome. *Gut.* 2007;56(6):802–808.

Quartero AO, Meineche-Schmidt V, Muris J, Rubin G, de Wit N. Bulking agents, antispasmodic and antidepressant medication for the treatment of irritable bowel syndrome. *Cochrane Database Syst Rev.* 2005;(2):CD003460.

Rivkin A, Chagan L. Lubiprostone: chloride channel activator for chronic constipation. *Clin Ther.* 2006;28(12):2008–2021.

Robert JJ, Elsenbruch S, Orr WC. Sleep-related autonomic disturbances in symptom subgroups of women with irritable bowel syndrome. *Dig Dis Sci.* 2006;51(12): 2121–2127.

Robert JJ, Orr WC, Elsenbruch S. Modulation of sleep quality and autonomic functioning by symptoms of depression in women with irritable bowel syndrome. *Dig Dis Sci.* 2004;49(7–8):1250–1258.

Sadik R, Abrahamsson H, Stotzer PO. Gender differences in gut transit shown with a newly developed radiological procedure. *Scand J Gastroenterol.* 2003;38(1):36–42.

Sallon S, Ben-Arye E, Davidson R, Shapiro H, Ginsberg G, Ligumsky M. A novel treatment for constipation-predominant irritable bowel syndrome using Padma Lax, a Tibetan herbal formula. *Digestion.* 2003;65(3):161–167.

Sandler RS, Everhart JE, Donowitz M, et al. The burden of selected digestive diseases in the United States. *Gastroenterology.* 2002;122(5):1500–1511.

Schoenfeld P. Efficacy of current drug therapies in irritable bowel syndrome: what works and does not work. *Gastroenterol Clin North Am.* 2005;34(2):319–335.

Shepherd SJ, Parker FC, Muir JG, Gibson PR. Dietary triggers of abdominal symptoms in patients with irritable bowel syndrome: randomized placebo-controlled evidence. *Clin Gastroenterol Hepatol.* 2008;6(7):765–771.

Spanier JA, Howden CW, Jones MP. A systematic review of alternative therapies in the irritable bowel syndrome. *Arch Intern Med.* 2003;163:265–274.

Spiller RC. Role of infection in irritable bowel syndrome. *J Gastroenterol.* 2007;42 (Suppl 17):41–47.

Stewart WF, Liberman JN, Sandler RS, et al. Epidemiology of constipation (EPOC) study in the United States: relation of clinical subtypes to sociodemographic features. *Am J Gastroenterol.* 1999;94(12):3530–3540.

Talley NJ, Boyce PM, Jones M. Is the association between irritable bowel syndrome and abuse explained by neuroticism? A population based study. *Gut.* 1998;42(1): 47–53.

Thompson FE, Midthune D, Subar AF, McNeel T, Berrigan D, Kipnis V. Dietary intake estimates in the National Health Interview Survey, 2000: methodology, results, and interpretation. *J Am Diet Assoc.* 2005;105(3):352–363.

Villoria A, Serra J, Azpiroz F, Malagelada JR. Physical activity and intestinal gas clearance in patients with bloating. *Am J Gastroenterol.* 2006;101(11):2552–2557.

Weil A. *Natural Health, Natural Medicine: The Complete Guide to Wellness and Self-Care for Optimum Health.* rev. ed. Boston: Houghton Mifflin; 2004:313.

Whitehead WE, Palsson O, Jones KR. Systematic review of the comorbidity of irritable bowel syndrome with other disorders: what are the causes and implications? *Gastroenterology.* 2002;122(4):1140–1156.

Whitehead WE. Hypnosis for irritable bowel syndrome: the empirical evidence of therapeutic effects. *Int J Clin Exp Hypn.* 2006;54(1):7–20.

Whorwell PJ. Effective management of irritable bowel syndrome—the Manchester Model. *Int J Clin Exp Hypn.* 2006;54:21–26.

Whorwell PJ. Hypnotherapy for irritable bowel syndrome: the response of colonic and noncolonic symptoms. *J Psychosom Res.* 2008;64:621–623.

Whorwell P, Altringer L, Morel J, et al. Efficacy of an encapsulated probiotic *Bifidobacterim infantis* 35624 in women with irritable bowel syndrome. *Am J Gastroenterol.* 2006;101(7):1581–1590.

Yadav SK, Jain AK, Tripathi SN, Gupta JP. Irritable bowel syndrome: therapeutic evaluation of indigenous drugs. *Indian J Med Res.* 1989;90:496–503.

Zar S, Mincher L, Benson MJ, Kumar D. Food-specific IgG4 antibody-guided exclusion diet improves symptoms and rectal compliance in irritable bowel syndrome. *Scand J Gastroenterol.* 2005;40(7):800–807.

27

Headaches

KELLY McCANN

CASE STUDY

As Justine entered her 40s and perimenopause, she developed debilitating menstrual migraines. She tried conventional pharmaceutical therapies, but preferred a more holistic approach in keeping with her yogic lifestyle. So we suggested an elimination diet whose effects were also assessed. She discovered that avoiding alcohol and cheese reduced her frequency of migraines. Lifestyle considerations were also factored in her migraine frequency, and when she got 9 hours of sleep, reduced her stress, and maintained her dedicated yoga practice, her symptoms occurred less often and resolved faster. Lastly, when she added riboflavin, magnesium, and the botanical feverfew to her daily regimen, together with acupuncture treatments around the time of her menses, Justine's menstrual migraines were greatly improved. Now at 52, her menstrual cycles have stopped and subsequently her migraines have virtually disappeared. However, she continues to practice the diet and lifestyle changes that she learned, as she moves gracefully into this new phase in her life.

Introduction

Patients experience headaches more than any other type of pain. In all, 45 million Americans suffer from chronic headaches and 7 in 10 people will have at least one headache a year. The majority of headaches are considered benign in that they are symptomatically treatable and non-disabling. Roughly 90% of headaches fall into three categories: migraine, tension-type, and cluster headaches (Table 27.1).

Table 27.1. Characteristics of Common Headache Syndromes

Symptom	Migraine Headache	Tension Headache	Cluster Headache
Location	Unilateral in 60%–70%; global in 30%	Bilateral	Always unilateral, usually begins around the eye or temple
Characteristics	Gradual in onset; crescendo pattern; dull, deep and steady when mild to moderate; throbbing and pulsating when moderate to severe in intensity; aggravated by routine physical activity	Pressure or tightness which waxes and wanes	Pain begins quickly, reaches peak in minutes; pain is deep, continuous, excruciating, and explosive in quality
Patient appearance	Patient prefers resting in a dark, quiet room	Patient may remain active	Patient remains active
Duration	4 to 72 hours	Variable	30 minutes to 3 hours
Associated symptoms	Nausea, vomiting, photophobia, phonophobia; may have aura which is usually visual but may involve other senses	None	Ipsilateral lacrimation and eye redness; nasal congestion, rhinorrhea, pallor, sweating, and Horner's syndrome; focal neurologic symptoms are rare

Aura is defined as a recurrent disorder manifesting in attacks of reversible neurological symptoms that develop gradually over 5–20 minutes and last for less than 60 minutes.

Tension headaches are the most common type of headache, 1-year prevalence rates are approximately 60%. Tension-type headaches (TTH) are more common in women, in a ratio of 1.5:1 (Rasmussen 1994). Migraine headaches are less prevalent but are often more distressing for the patient. The overall prevalence of migraine is estimated to be 12%–16% in North America; however, rates for women are significantly higher than those for men (18% vs. 6%) (Lipton et al. 2001). Migraineurs often experience TTH as well. Prevalence for cluster headaches in the general population is low, around 0.1%, making it an infrequent diagnosis. Overall, 85% of cluster headache sufferers are men (Bahra et al. 2002). The remaining 10% of headache diagnostic possibilities include the following:

> systemic disease, infections, autoimmune conditions such as temporal arthritis
>
> neurologic disorders including post traumatic headaches and intracranial lesions
>
> sinus conditions, TMJ dysfunction, refractive errors, and medication overuse syndromes.

A thorough history is essential for establishing the proper diagnosis and determining further evaluation and treatment plans. Questions should screen for space- occupying mass, metabolic disturbance, or systemic problems. In benign headaches, the physical/neurological exam will usually be normal. Barring an abnormal neurological exam, a sudden onset of symptoms, or atypical features, imaging is unnecessary. Once an accurate diagnosis is reached, appropriate therapies can be instituted. Therapies can be divided into two main categories: preventive and abortive. This chapter will explore integrative therapies for migraine and TTH.

Migraines

Approximately 28 million people in the United States suffer from migraines. Nearly 40% are not given the diagnosis of migraine and most don't receive appropriate treatment (Lipton et al. 1998). Nearly 6 out of 10 migraineurs use over-the-counter medications to manage their headaches. An average of 80% migraineurs say their headaches are severe or extremely severe (Lipton et al. 2001) and 51% of migraine sufferers report 50% or more reduction in productivity (Hu et al. 1999). Women account for over 75% of the over 3 million days/month that migraineurs spend bedridden (Stang and Osterhaus 1993). They report more frequent and severe pain (Celentano et al. 1990), longer duration of migraine (Stewart et al. 1994), and more depression than men do (Phillips and Jahanshahi 1985).

MIGRAINE TRIGGERS

A migraine trigger is any factor that on exposure or withdrawal leads to the development of an acute migraine (Table 27.2). Mechanisms, exposure time, and frequency all vary. General lifestyle recommendations for migraine patients include limiting caffeine, maintaining regular sleep, eating regular meals, and minimizing stress with regular exercise and relaxation. Dietary triggers impact 30% of migraineurs. A headache diary can help elucidate triggers. It may take 24–48 hours to develop symptoms following a trigger and triggers may be additive (Martin and Behbehani 2001).

Table 27.2. Systematic History for Headache Evaluation

Frequency, intensity, duration of attack
Recent change in the pattern, frequency or severity of headaches
Worsening of headache despite appropriate therapy
Presence or absence of aura and prodrome
Age at onset (concern for development after age 40)
Number of headache days per month
Time and mode of onset (concern for development with cough, exertion or sexual activity)
Quality, site and radiation of pain
Associated symptoms and abnormalities
Family history of migraine
Precipitating and relieving factors
Effect of activity on pain and pain on activity
Relationship with food/alcohol
Relationship with pain medications
Response to any previous treatment
Any recent change in vision
Any recent changes in sleep, exercise, weight, or diet

(continued)

State of general health

Associated psychological conditions, i.e., depression

Change in work or lifestyle (evaluating disability)

Change in method of birth control (women)

Environmental factors

Effects of menstrual cycle and exogenous hormones (women)

ESTROGEN-ASSOCIATED MIGRAINE

The menstrual migraine, also called catamenial migraine, occurs exclusively in close temporal relationship to menses, typically two days before to three days after the onset of menstrual bleeding. Women may experience migraines at other times of the cycle; however, menstrual migraines may be more severe, may last longer and may be less responsive to treatment (MacGregor et al. 2004).

Migraine occurs in 2.5%–4% of girls, prior to puberty; the prevalence is slightly higher among boys. After menarche, migraine becomes more prevalent in females reaching peak prevalence by age 40. After menopause, the prevalence falls, at least partly as a result of hormonal stability (Waters and O'Connor 1971).

Menstrual migraines (MM) resemble other migraines, though MM are typically without aura even in women who have migraine with aura at other times (Johannes et al. 1995). Estrogen associated migraines tend to occur in settings of estrogen decline, either natural declines such as during the luteal phase of menstrual cycle and menopause or during withdrawal from hormonal products. Women with MM appear to have a pathologic response to normal declines in estrogen concentrations (Brandes 2006). In women, serotonergic tone is positively correlated with estrogen levels; as estrogen levels fall, serotonin concentrations fall due to a decline in production and increase in elimination.

Most women (48%–79%) report improvement in their migraines during pregnancy. Fewer than 5% describe worsening and the rest remain unaffected. Pregnancy outcome does not appear to be affected by migraine (Sances et al. 2003). Recurrence of migraine is lower in women who breastfeed.

Conventional Treatment

After lifestyle recommendations, conventional treatment relies on pharmaceutical agents for abortive and preventive therapy (Table 27.3). Prophylactic measures are indicated for women with more than two severe attacks in a month, women who use abortive therapies more than 2 times a week, and women for whom acute medications are ineffective or contraindicated (Silberstein 2000). Medications may be effective for managing symptoms, but they are often expensive and fail to address the underlying causes of headaches. A high proportion of headache patients use and report benefit from behavioral modifications and non-pharmacologic interventions. In one small study, the most useful integrative therapies in alleviating head pain were acupuncture, exercise, chiropractic manipulation, relaxation therapy, massage, biofeedback, and herbs (von Peter et al. 2002).

Table 27.3. Headache Triggers

Behavioral factors

   Irregular meal patterns

   Schedule changes

   Travel (across time zones)

   Irregular physical activity

Environmental factors

   Weather changes

   Altitude changes

   Loud noises

   Strong odors

   Bright or glaring lights

   Cigarette smoke

Dietary factors

   Chocolate

   Aged cheeses

   Caffeinated beverages

   Nuts

   Alcoholic beverages

   Ice cream

Emotional factors

   Crisis

   Times of intense activity

(continued)

Excitement

Fear

Anxiety

Anger

Stress let down

Change or loss (death, separation, divorce, job change)

Food and chemical additive factors

Monosodium glutamate

Aspartame (Nutrasweet)

Tyramine

Nitrites and Nitrates

Sleep disturbances

Irregular sleep patterns

Too much or too little sleep

Hormonal factors

Menstruation

Oral Contraceptives

Estrogen replacement

Source: From Martin and Behbehani (2001).

Nutrition

Avoidance of particular foods and food additives may significantly reduce migraines in some people. The most frequent triggers are caffeine, chocolate, alcoholic beverages, monosodium glutamate (MSG), processed meats, dairy products including cheese, yogurt, sour cream and buttermilk, nuts and nut butters, citrus fruits, onions, some beans, and artificial sweeteners such as aspartame and saccharin. Elimination diets have been shown to be valuable in managing migraine. When 88 children were put on an oligoantigenic diet, 93% improved (Egger et al. 1983). An oligoantigenic, or hypoallergenic, diet consists of foods that are thought to be well-tolerated and avoids foods known to cause symptoms such as wheat, dairy, soy, corn, nuts, citrus, plus additives and preservatives. Foods are then re-introduced and symptoms monitored. For women who do not appear to have specific food triggers, a general anti-inflammatory diet is recommended, as some data suggest migraine is an inflammatory process (Waeber and Moskowitz 2005). Hypoglycemia, fasting, and dehydration may also increase migraine frequency.

Dietary Supplements

Impaired mitochondrial energy metabolism may play a role in migraine pathogenesis (Lodi et al. 1997; Montagna et al. 1994). This is the proposed mechanism by which magnesium, riboflavin, and coenzyme Q10 are thought to work. The following is a brief review of each.

MAGNESIUM

Magnesium plays an important role in mitochondrial energy production, cell communication, muscle relaxation, and neurotransmitter production and regulation. Low serum, intracellular, cerebrospinal and salivary magnesium levels have been demonstrated in migraine and headache patients. Magnesium deficiency can lead to physiological changes including cerebrovascular spasm and release of pain mediators (Mauskop and Altura 1998; Welch and Ramada 1995). Some research suggests that magnesium depletion is inversely correlated with migraine severity (Lodi et al. 2001). Mechanisms might include magnesium dependent alterations in circadian regulation (Durlach et al. 2002), reduction in neuron excitability (Boska et al. 2002), or in the case of menstrual migraine, estrogen may exert effects on intracellular magnesium levels of cerebral vascular smooth muscle cells (Li et al. 2001).

Oral magnesium has been found effective for migraine prophylaxis (Wang et al. 2004). In one study, 600 mg of trimagnesium dicitrate daily for 12 weeks reduced migraine frequency by 41.6% compared to 15.8% in the control group. Adverse effects were diarrhea and gastric irritation (Peikert et al. 1996). In another study, a daily administration of 360 mg of pyrrolidine carboxlic acid magnesium resulted in greater pain relief for women with menstrual migraine (Facchinetti et al. 1991).

Intravenous magnesium sulfate in the setting of acute migraine has also been studied. A small study of 30 patients found that every subject in the treatment group responded to 1 g of magnesium sulfate with pain elimination in 86.6% and reduction in the remaining two patients; there was also 100% elimination of accompanying symptoms of nausea and vomiting, whereas the placebo response rate was 7% with no subjects pain free (Demirkaya et al. 2001).

The treatment was well-tolerated, with rare side effects including a brief flushed feeling (Mauskop et al. 1996). It may be that IV magnesium for acute treatment of migraines may be more effective in patients with aura (Bigal et al. 2002). Magnesium is safe for use in pregnancy and lactation.

Rich sources of magnesium include nuts (almonds and cashews), red meat, legumes, green leafy vegetables, whole grains, and seafood. Despite these abundant sources, up to 75% of the US population may have inadequate dietary intake (Altura et al. 1994). Magnesium levels are also depleted by stress, hormonal imbalances of estrogen, progesterone, thyroid, and parathyroid hormones

RIBOFLAVIN

Riboflavin (vitamin B2) is a precursor required for the electron transport chain. A randomized controlled trial(RCT) of 55 patients taking 400 mg of riboflavin for migraine prophylaxis revealed a reduction in headache frequency and duration in greater than 50% of the subjects, but the effects appeared to be maximal only after 3 months of treatment. Side effects were mild and included diarrhea, polyuria, and abdominal cramps (Schoenen et al. 1998). Riboflavin appears to act via a different mechanism than do beta-blockers and combining treatments might enhance efficacy (Sandor et al. 2000). Riboflavin is a reasonable, safe, and inexpensive choice for migraine prophylaxis. It is not known if it is safe for pregnant and lactating women at this dose.

COENZYME Q10

Co Q10 may also play a role in mitochondrial dysfunction and energy production (Littarru and Tiano 2005). An open label trial of 32 migraineurs taking 150 mg of Co Q10 daily revealed that 61% of the patients had a 50% reduction in the number of days with migraine headache (Rozen et al. 2002). A subsequent placebo-controlled trial of 42 patients utilizing 100 mg three times per day (TID) resulted in a reduction in attack frequency of 47.6% compared to 14.4% in controls at 3 months. Adverse events were similar in active and placebo arms. Safety in pregnancy and lactation has not been determined.

FISH OIL

Omega-3 fatty acids, eicosapentaenoic acid (EPA), and docosahexaenoic acid (DHA), found in fish oil have effects including anti-inflammatory, vasorelaxation, and inhibition of 5-hydroxytryptophan release from platelets

(Simopoulos 2002; McCarthy 1996). A RCT of 27 adolescents comparing an omega-3 fatty acid versus olive oil placebo demonstrated significant reduction in frequency (87% vs. 78%), duration (74% vs. 70%), and severity (83% vs. 65%) with both oils, suggesting that further studies are warranted (Harel et al. 2002). A 16-week RCT of 196 subjects using a dose of 6 g/day failed to show any statistically significant difference between omega-3s and placebos, though a very strong placebo effect was observed (Pradalier et al. 2001). Doses range from 2 to 6 g/day. Side effects include mild gastrointestinal distress. Fish oil at these doses is likely to be safe in pregnancy and lactation.

5-HTP

5-Hydroxytryptophan (5-HTP) is a precursor to serotonin (5-HT), a neurotransmitter that may play a role in the pathophysiology of migraines. It is suspected that migraneurs suffer a low serotonin state that leads to a decrease in pain threshold (Sicuteri 1976). For example, sumatriptan (Imitrex), a selective agonist for serotonin, binds the 5-HT_{1D} receptor to mimic the effect of serotonin and relieve migraines. One hundred twenty four migraine patients underwent a 6 month comparative study between 5-HTP (600 mg/day) and methysergide (3 mg/day), a known preventive agent. Seventy-five percent of the methysergide group and 71% of the 5-HTP patients showed significant improvement in frequency, intensity, and duration of attacks (Titus et al. 1986). Other studies have had mixed outcomes (Maissen and Ludin 1991; Bono et al. 1982). For TTH, 400 mg of 5-HTP daily was slightly more effective than placebo but not to statistical significance; the 8 week study duration may have been too short (Riberio 2000; De Benedittis and Massei 1985). The effective dose appears to range from 100 mg TID to 600 mg/day in divided doses, though it may be possible to reduce the dose once it begins to work. No significant adverse effects have been reported in clinical trials; side effects include mild digestive distress and allergies. Safety in pregnant or lactating women has not been determined. 5-HTP should not be combined with medications that raise serotonin levels such as SSRIs, MAOIs or Tramadol for concern of serotonin syndrome.

THIOCTIC ACID (ALPHA-LIPOIC ACID)

For addressing the mitochondrial dysfunction hypothesis, researchers have studied thioctic acid for migraine prophylaxis. Fifty-four migraineurs were given 600 mg of thioctic acid versus placebo for 3 months. There was reduction in the frequency, headache days, and severity. While additional studies need to be performed, it may be a reasonable choice for people with diabetes (Magis et al. 2007). Safety and efficacy in pregnancy and breastfeeding is lacking.

MELATONIN

Environmental factors such as irregular sleep patterns are known triggers for migraines. Preliminary research reveals that migraineurs, especially women, have altered levels in melatonin overall and during migraine attacks (Gagnier 2001). Small studies suggest that melatonin administration may improve headaches, particularly in patients with delayed sleep phase syndrome (Claustrat et al. 1997; Nagtegaal et al. 1998). Women with sleep disturbance and migraines may derive benefit from melatonin. Recommended dose is 0.3–1 mg at bedtime. Melatonin administration , particularly those higher than the physiologic dose of 0.3 mg, should be avoided in pregnant women, due to possible hormonal effects. In animal studies, melatonin is detected in breast milk and should be avoided while breastfeeding.

Sleep disturbance and anxiety often co-exist with migraines and headaches. Patients appear to be in a state of hyperarousal or sympathetic overdrive. From a Traditional Chinese Medicine perspective, these conditions reflect a singular, cascading imbalance. Illuminating the etiological relationship of conditions, we as providers empower our patients to see themselves as an integral whole. They begin to learn that what they do, how they do it, and what they think and believe all can impact their health in positive or not-so-positive ways.

Botanicals

PETASITES (PETASITES HYBRIDUS)

Commonly known as butterbur, this perennial herb has been used medicinally for more than 2,000 years. Active constituents appear to have anti-inflammatory, vasodilatory and smooth muscle relaxant activity, which may account for its efficacy in migraine prophylaxis. Most trials used the patented, standardized extract of butterbur root, Petadolex (Weber and Weber GmbH & Co, Germany), which provides 7.5 mg of petasin and isopetasin per 50 mg tablet. A 4 month RCT of 245 patients revealed that migraine frequency was reduced 48% in the 75 mg BID dose versus 26% for placebo (Agosti et al. 2006).

One hundred and eight children and adolescents aged 6 to 17 years were given 50 to 150 mg of Petadolex extract for 4 months in an open prospective study. Seventy seven percent reported migraine frequency reduction and 91% of patients felt substantially or partially improved. Side effects included eructation (burping) with no serious adverse events (Pothmann and Danesch 2005). It is unclear if butterbur is safe during pregnancy and lactation. The plant naturally contains pyrrolizidine alkaloids (PA), which can be hepatotoxic, thus patients should only use those products that are standardized to be PA free.

FEVERFEW (*TANACETUM PARTHENIUM*)

The leaf of feverfew, a member of the *Asteraceae* family, has been studied in the prophylaxis of migraine headache. It is generally thought that the active ingredient is parthenolide, though this has been recently challenged (Awang 1998). Early, small RCTs of the dried whole leaves appeared to show benefit (Murphy et al. 1988; Johnson et al. 1985), whereas an ethanolic extract did not (De Weerdt et al. 1996). A Cochrane review of 5 trials and 343 patients found insufficient evidence to recommend feverfew over placebo for preventing migraine (Pittler et al. 2004).

More recently, a CO_2 extract of feverfew (MIG-99, manufactured by Schaper & Brummer GmbH & Co. KG in Germany) was investigated in 170 migraine patients for 16 weeks at a dose of 6.25 mg three times daily. Migraine frequency decreased by 1.9 attacks per month in the treatment group compared to 1.3 headaches in the placebo group. Adverse reactions were comparable (Diener et al. 2005). A combination of riboflavin, magnesium and feverfew for migraine prophylaxis failed to show benefit over a placebo of low dose riboflavin (Maizels et al. 2004), whereas an open label study combination of feverfew with white willow (*Salix alba*) looked promising (Shrivastava et al. 2006).

Adverse events include sore mouth, oral ulcers, and GI disturbance. Mouth sores appear to be primarily associated with chewing the fresh leaf, though there is some suggestion that ulceration is a systemic effect (Johnson et al. 1985). Feverfew should not be used in pregnant women due to possible inhibition of platelets and history of use as an abortifacient (Evans and Taylor 2006).

Mind–Body Medicine

When researchers assessed the power of the mind to affect the body, they found that these modalities are valuable for most women and that they are especially useful in situations when medication may be contraindicated, such as pregnancy and lactation. Behavioral treatments for migraine headache, including biofeed-back, relaxation, cognitive-behavioral therapy and hypnosis/guided imagery, have demonstrated efficacy and enduring effects (Andrasik 2007).

BIOFEEDBACK

Biofeedback involves the use of monitoring equipment that amplifies, or "feeds back" to patients, physiological processes of which they are not normally aware. A meta-analysis of 55 studies found that biofeedback (BFB) was more effective than controls, for the treatment of migraine, with strongest improvements in frequency of attacks and self-efficacy (Nestoriuc and Martin 2007). According to the US Headache Consortium guidelines, thermal biofeedback showed an average of 37% improvement and electroencephalogram (EEG) biofeedback therapy revealed an averaged improvement in migraines of 40%. When compared to drug treatments (propanolol or ergotamine), behavioral treatments were as efficacious as drug treatments (Campbell et al. 2008). Biofeedback was more effective than relaxation training in reducing frequency, muscle tension, anxiety, depression, and medication usage, but the combination of the two was the most effective (Nestoriuc et al. 2008).

RELAXATION TRAINING

Relaxation training includes progressive muscle relaxation, autogenic training (using self-instructions of warmth and heaviness to promote deep relaxation and reduced sympathetic arousal), and meditation (Holroyd and Mauskop 2003). A meta-analysis of 10 trials yielded an average improvement of 32%–41% (Campbell et al. 2008).

COGNITIVE BEHAVIORAL THERAPY

Cognitive behavioral therapy (CBT) alerts patients to the fact that their thoughts and beliefs contribute to stress and maladaptive patterns. Patients are then taught effective coping strategies and self counseling skills that enable them to think and act differently (Holroyd and Mauskop 2003). Seven trials revealed a 49% improvement in headache activity (Campbell et al. 2008). The American Academy of Neurology acknowledges that cognitive and behavioral treatments have strong level of evidence to support their use as adjunctive therapies (Silberstein 2000).

HYPNOSIS/GUIDED IMAGERY

Multiple studies support Hypnosis as an effective modality for the prevention of headache and migraines (Hammond 2007). Most studies included self-hypnosis instruction or use of self hypnosis recordings, resulting in significant reductions in frequency, duration, and intensity of headaches compared to wait list controls (Melis 1991, Kohen 2007). In one trial, six sessions of hypnotherapy were compared to prochlorperazine (10 mg/day for first month, then 20 mg/day for 11 months). Patients in the hypnotherapy group had a statistically significant reduction in headache frequency (Anderson et al. 1975). Hypnotizability appeared to play a part in therapeutic effectiveness, though this is still under debate (Hammond 2007).

Manual Therapies

PHYSICAL THERAPY

Although not effective by itself in the treatment of migraine, physical therapy is a useful adjunct to biofeedback and relaxation training in the setting of muscle tension and limited head and neck mobility (Marcus et al. 1998).

SPINAL MANIPULATION

Manipulative therapies as practiced by chiropractors and osteopathic physicians have been shown to be as effective for the prophylaxis of migraine as amitriptyline (Bronfort et al. 2004). An RCT of migraine prophylaxis with 88 patients receiving 8 weeks of manipulation therapy, twice weekly, revealed a non-significant trend favoring spinal manipulative therapy (Parker et al. 1990). Although there are reports in the literature of complications from manipulation (Mauskop 2001), reviews suggest a very low risk of side effects.

EXERCISE/PHYSICAL ACTIVITY

Engaging in regular vigorous exercise is fundamental to any integrative medicine prescription. The physical and psychological benefits of regular exercise are well known. Fortunately, the benefits of consistent exercise extend to management of headaches, although the mechanism is unclear. Stress reduction, endogenous endorphin release, lowering sympathetic tone, lowering of nitric oxide levels, and muscular relaxation may all play a role (Kay et al. 2005; Narin et al. 2003; Yerdelen et al. 2008). Two studies with control groups showed that regular aerobic exercise reduced pain severity, trends towards decreased frequency, intensity, and duration of migraine headache (Lockett and Campbell 1992; Narin et al. 2003).

YOGA

Both a physical practice and a meditation practice, yoga programs have been shown to be helpful for headache relief in several studies. In a recent study, yoga therapy was contrasted with self-care for 72 randomized migraneurs. Intensity, frequency, pain, medication use, and anxiety and depression scores were statistically lower in the yoga group (John et al. 2007).

Bioenergetic Therapies

ACUPUNCTURE

Acupuncture and Traditional Chinese Medicine (TCM) view migraine and tension headaches as imbalances of energies. The disturbances vary between women, and subsequently the treatment may also vary (Coeytaux et al. 2006). Several systematic reviews support the use of acupuncture for prophylactic treatment of recurrent headaches. However, the quality and amount of the evidence is not fully convincing (Melchart et al. 1999, 2000; Manias et al. 2000). More recent RCTs comparing sham and acupuncture for migraine (Alecrim-Andrade et al. 2006, 2008; Diener et al. 2006; Linde et al. 2005) have found both sham and verum acupuncture are more effective than no treatment. Acupuncture compared well with metoprolol for prophylaxis, though there was a high drop-out rate in the metoprolol group, confounding results (Streng et al. 2006). Scalp acupuncture may be effective though rigorous evidence is lacking (Wenzhong 2002).

In a trial of 179 migraineurs with acute attacks, acupuncture (35%) and sumatriptan (36%) were both more effective than placebo (18%). If an attack could not be prevented, sumatriptan was more effective than acupuncture in relieving the headache (Melchart et al. 2003).

Rare risks include infection, pneumothorax, and localized bleeding (Audette and Blinder 2003). Some practitioners may avoid needling in pregnancy, though risks for complications are low in the hands of qualified practitioners and may outweigh the risks of medications.

ELECTRICAL NERVE STIMULATION

Percutaneous electrical nerve stimulation (PENS), a technique that adds electrical stimulation to acupuncture needles, was helpful in one small study (Ahmed et al. 2000), but transcutanous electrical nerve stimulation (TENS) was not (Sheftell et al. 1989; Solomon and Guglielmo 1985). Use of pulsing electromagnetic fields (PEMFs) for migraine appeared to be potentially effective in a study of 42 migraineurs; however, the therapy was prohibitively time intensive (Sherman et al. 1999).

REFLEXOLOGY

An exploratory study of 220 patients suggested reflexology may be an effective treatment for chronic headaches (Launso et al. 1999).

THERAPEUTIC TOUCH

A modern version of "laying on of hands," therapeutic touch helps balance the body's energy fields. Evaluating therapeutic touch and placebo simulation in a randomized study of 60 patients with tension headaches revealed that the treatment group had statistically significant reduction in their pain scores, although the effect only lasted up to 4 hours after the intervention (Keller and Bzdek 1986). Craniosacral therapy, derived from osteopathic manipulation, is a gentle hands-on healing modality that may have beneficial effects for migraine and headache (Upledger 1995).

Homeopathy

A number of randomized trials have failed to demonstrate the effectiveness of homeopathy in the treatment of headache and migraine (Termine et al. 2004; Whitmarsh et al. 1997). A rigorous study of 98 chronic headache and migraine patients having randomized to individualized homeopathic remedies or placebo for 12 weeks failed to show benefits greater than due to placebo. At the completion of the 12 weeks, patients were offered free treatment for a year and 18 of the 98 accepted the offer. At the one year mark, all participants (87 respondents) were sent

6 week headache diaries and follow-up questionnaires. About 30% of the patients receiving free treatment for the year had improvement. Any improvements seen in the first 12 weeks tended to be stable at a year (Walach et al. 1997, 2000).

BOTULINUM TOXIN

An evidence-based review of the literature revealed that botulinum toxin is probably ineffective for episodic migraine and TTH (Naumann et al. 2008).

HYPERBARIC OXYGEN

One small trial examined hyperbaric oxygen at two atmospheres of pressure versus normobaric oxygen for the treatment of acute migraine. After 40 minutes of treatment, the results were statistically significant in favor of hyperbaric oxygen (Myers and Myers 1995).

Tension-type Headaches

Phyllis suffered with TTH for years. She had developed them when she was commuting 2 hours a day to a job she despised. Sometimes the headache episodes would come on just prior to a vacation. Over time they began to take on a life of their own, lasting daily for up to ten weeks in a row. Conventional medications took the edge off, but nothing seemed to resolve them. Eventually psychotherapy coupled with healthy lifestyle choices and acupuncture helped her decide to leave her job and return to school.

Tension- Type Headache Classification and Epidemiology

TTH are common and relatively non-specific, symptoms often described as mild to moderate intensity, with non-throbbing headache. They are the least studied headaches despite having the highest socioeconomic burden. TTH are classified as infrequent episodic, occurring less than once monthly; frequent episodic, occurring between 1 and 14 days per month and chronic TTH, occurring more than 15 days a month. The overall one year prevalence appears to be 86% in one study (Russell et al. 2006), though by classification episodic and chronic prevalences were 38.3% and 2.2% respectively (Schwartz et al. 1998).

Women have a higher prevalence of TTH than men. Lifetime prevalence for episodic TTH was 88% for women and 69% for men (Rasmussen et al. 1991).

Integrative Therapies for Tension-type Headaches

The primary conventional treatments for TTH are non-steroidal anti-inflammatory drugs (NSAIDs) and acetaminophen. Analgesics containing caffeine may be more effective but have more side effects. The use of butalbital and codeine or other opiates is not recommended due to the propensity of overuse, which can transform episodic to chronic headaches. Triptans may be helpful for migraineurs with TTH. Prophylactic therapies are indicated for chronic TTH and most frequent episodic TTH patients. Pharmaceutical preventive strategies for TTH include tricyclic antidepressants, especially amitriptyline, serotonin-norephiphrine reuptake inhibitors, but not SSRIs. There is limited evidence for anticonvulsants, gabapentin, and topiramate.

Many of the lifestyle recommendations for prevention of migraines extend to TTH. Although there is less evidence to suggest that specific foods trigger TTH, an anti-inflammatory diet is recommended. In addition stress, hunger, dehydration, and sleep deprivation tend to precipitate headaches and should be managed accordingly (Spierings et al. 2001).

Mind–Body Medicine

A meta-analysis of 78 trials and 2866 patients on behavioral treatment for TTH showed 37%–50% reduction in symptoms compared with 2%–9% in control patients. Therapies included relaxation training, EMG biofeedback alone and combined with relaxation training, cognitive behavioral therapy, and stress management training. Findings suggested that patient characteristics may affect treatment outcome more than type of treatment (Bogaards and ter Kuile 1994). Another meta-analysis found at least 50% improvement in headache reduction using psychologically based modalities (Trautmann et al. 2006). Behavioral strategies present a viable option for women who are pregnant, planning pregnancy, or breast-feeding.

HYPNOSIS

In an experiment 26 unsuccessfully treated chronic TTH patients, randomized in a single-blinded study, underwent 4 weeks of hypnosis sessions with home practice tapes. The hypnosis group experienced significant reductions in headache days, hours, and intensity. The subjects reported an increase in sense of control, altered pain perception, and reduced tensions (Melis et al. 1991).

An RCT of 230 patients with chronic TTH were assigned to one of four arms, tricyclic anti-depressant medication placebo stress management therapy or both therapies combined. Both the medication and therapy groups showed significant improvement in headache activity and decline in medication use than placebo. Although the medication group responded more rapidly, the combination provided more than 50% reduction in 64% of the participants which was almost double than respondents for either monotherapy group (Holroyd et al. 2001).

Physical Therapy

Patients with chronic headaches may benefit from physical or manipulative therapies as part of their treatment strategy (Mills Roth 2003). One trial of 81 patients with TTH randomly assigned to a program of craniocervical endurance exercises with physical therapy (massage, postural techniques) or physical therapy alone, favored the combined program and the benefit was sustained and statistically significant at 6 months (van Ettekoven and Lucas 2006).

Spinal Manipulation Therapy

Manipulative therapies have been shown to be slightly less effective for the prophylaxis of TTH than amitriptyline but longer lasting (Bronfort et al. 2004). Unfortunately, no high quality studies exist with placebo and sham controls, though three studies in a systematic review report a benefit of spinal manipulation therapy (SMT) (Vernon et al. 1999). A Cochrane review determined SMT to be of limited usefulness (Bronfort et al. 2004).

Exercise/Yoga

A trial of six weeks of exercise therapy compared to SMT and no treatment found moderate evidence that exercise is superior to no treatment in reducing headache pain initially and 12 months following treatment. Exercise was similar to SMT in effect (Bronfort et al. 2004). A 4 month yoga-based intervention of 20 headache patients showed statistically significant reductions in frequency, duration, and intensity and decreased use of pain medications compared to controls (Latha and Kaliappan 1992). When treatments based on yoga were compared with antidepressants or anti-anxiety medications in 85 participants with chronic tension headaches, it was found that both groups improved, though the improvements were greater in the yoga group (Prabhakar 1991).

Acupuncture

It was found in a trial of 270 patients with chronic TTH that true acupuncture was statistically superior to no treatment but equivalent to sham acupuncture. The remainder of the trials was of average to low quality, with small sample sizes and mixed results, though there were some favorable tendencies towards acupuncture (Melchart et al. 2005). For TTH, conventional and laser acupuncture may also have benefits (Ebneshahidi et al. 2005; Endres et al. 2007). Although acupuncture for prevention of TTH is of unproven benefit, it is a relatively safe modality and may be used in those patients who decline other modalities or pharmaceuticals.

Aromatherapy

Oleum menthae piperitae, or peppermint oil solution, when applied to the forehead was comparable to 1000 mg of acetaminophen in alleviating TTH in 41 patients in a placebo-controlled, cross-over, randomized study (Gobel et al. 1996). An earlier study of peppermint and eucalyptus oils increased cognitive function and relaxed muscles in 32 healthy subjects but had little influence on pain sensitivity (Gobel et al. 1994).

Summary

Women are frequent sufferers of migraines and TTH. Health care practitioners need to inquire and then partner with their patients to assist them in making healthy lifestyle modifications, identifying and avoiding triggers and determining appropriate treatment modalities. A multimodal approach incorporating nutrition, supplements, mind–body medicine, manual therapies, and potentially other bioenergetic modalities is warranted for an integrative approach to the prevention and treatment of migraine and TTH.

REFERENCES

Agosti R, Duke RK, Chrubasik JE, Chrubasik S. Effectiveness of *Petasites hybridus* preparations in the prophylaxis of migraine: a systemic review. *Phytomedicine.* 2006;13(9–10):743–746.

Ahmed HE, White PF, Craig WF, et al. Use of percutaneous electrical nerve stimulation in the short-term management of headache. *Headache*. 2000;40:311–315.

Alecrim-Andrade J, Maciel-Junior JA, Cladellas XC, Correa-Filho HR, Machado HC. Acupuncture in migraine prophylaxis. *Cephalalgia*. 2006;26(5):520–529.

Alecrim-Andrade J, Maciel-Junior JA, Carne X, Severino-Vasconcelos GM, Correa-Filho HR. Acupuncture in migraine prevention. *Clin J Pain*. 2008;24(2):98–105.

Altura BM, Brodsky MA, Elin RJ, et al. Magnesium: growing in clinical importance. *Patient Care*. 1994;10:130–150.

Anderson JA, Basker MA, Dalton R. Migraine and hypnotherapy. *Int J Clinc Exp Hypn*. 1975;23(1):48–58.

Andrasik, F. What does the evidence show? Efficacy of behavioural treatments for recurrent headache in adults. *Neurol Sci*. 2007;28(Suppl 2):S70–S77.

Audette JF, Blinder RA. Acupuncture in the management of myofascial pain and head-ache. *Curr Pain Headache Rep*. 2003;7:395–401.

Awang, D. Prescribing therapeutic feverfew (*Tanacetum parthenium*). *Integr Med*. 1998;1(1):11–13.

Bahra, A, May, A, Goadsby, PJ. Cluster headache: a prospective clinical study with diag-nostic implications. *Neurology*. 2002;42:256.

Bigal ME, Bordini CA, Tepper SJ, Specilai JG. Intravenous magnesium sulfate in the acute treatment of migraine without aura and migraine with aura. A randomized, double-blind, placebo-controlled study. *Cephalalgia*. 2002;22(5):345–353.

Bigal ME, Liberman JN, Lipton RB. Obesity and migraine: a population study. *Neurology*. 2006;66:545–550.

Billie BS. Migraine in school children. *Acta Paediatr*. 1962;51(Supp 136):1.

Bogaards MC, ter Kuile MM. Treatment of recurrent tension headache: a meta-analytic review. *Clin J Pain*. 1994;10(3):174–190.

Bono G, Criscuoli M, Martignoni E, et al. Serotonin precursors in migraine prophy-laxis. *Adv Neurol*. 1982;33:357–363.

Boska MD, Welch KM, Barker PB, et al. Contrasts in cortical magnesium, phospholipid, and energy metabolism between migraine syndromes. *Neurology*. 2002;58:1227–1233.

Brandes, JL. The influence of estrogen on migraine: a systematic review. *JAMA*. 2006;295:1824.

Bronfort G, Nilsson N, Haas M, et al. Non-invasive physical treatments for chronic/ recurrent headache. *Cochrane Database Syst Rev*. 2004; CD001878.

Campbell JK, Penzien D, Wall EM for the U.S. Headache Consortium. Evidence-based guidelines for migraine headache: behavioral and physical treatments. Available at http:www.aan.com/professionals/practice/pdfs/gl0089.pdf. Accessed May 2008.

Celentano DD, Linet MS, Stewart WF. Gender differences in the experience of head-ache. *Soc Sci Med*. 1990;30:1289–1295.

Claustrat B, Brun J, Geoffriau M, et al. Nocturnal plasma melatonin kinetics pro-file and melatonin kinetics during infusion in status migrainosus. *Cephalalgia*. 1997;17:511–517.

Coeytaux RR, Chen W, Lindemuth CE, Tan Y, Reilly AC. Variability in the diagnosis and point selection for persons with frequent headache by traditional Chinese medi-cine acupuncturists. *J Alternat Complement Med*. 2006;12(9): 863–872.

Demirkaya S, Vural O, Dora B, Topcuoglu MA. Efficacy of intravenous magnesium sulfate in the treatment of acute migraine attacks. *Headache*. 2001;41(2):171–177.

De Benedittis G, Massei R. Serotonin precursors in chronic primary headache. A double-blind cross-over study with L-5-hydroxytrytophan vs. placebo. *J Neurosurg Sci*. 1985;29(3):239–248.

De Weerdt CJ, Bootsma HPR, Hendricks H. Herbal medicines in migraine prevention: randomized double-blind placebo-controlled crossover trial of feverfew preparation. *Phytomedicine*. 1996;3:225–230.

Diener HC, Pfaffenrath V, Schnitker J, Fried M, Henneicke-von Zepelin HH. Efficacy and safety of 6.25 mg of tid feverfew CO2-extract (MIG-99) in migraine prevention—a randomized, double-blind, multicentre placebo-controlled study. *Cephalalgia*. 2005;25(11):1031–1041.

Diener HC, Kronfeld K, Boewing G, et al. Efficacy of acupuncture for the prophylaxis of migraine: a multi-centre randomized controlled clinical trial. *Lancet Neurol*. 2006;5(4):310–316.

Durlach J, Pages N, Bac P, Bara M, Guiet-Bara A. Biorhythms and possible central regulation of magnesium status, phototherapy, darkness therapy and chronopathological forms of magnesium depletion. *Magnes Res*. 2002;15(1–2):49–66.

Ebneshahidi NS, Heshmatipour M, Moghaddami A, Eghtesadi-Araghi P. The effects of laser acupuncture of chronic tension headache—a randomized controlled trial. *Acupuncture Med*. 2005;23(1):13–18.

Egger J, Cater CM, Wilson J, Turner MW, Soothill JF. Is migraine food allergy? A double-blind controlled trial of oligoantigenic diet treatment. *Lancet*. 1983;2(8355):865–869.

Endres HG, Bowing G, Diener HC, et al. Acupuncture for tension-type headache: a multicentre, sham-controlled, patients and observer blinded, randomized trial. *J Headache Pain*. 2007;8(5):306–314.

Evans RW, Taylor FR. Natural or alternative medications for migraine prevention. *Headache*. 2006;46:1012–1018.

Facchinetti F, Sances G, Borella P, et al. Magnesium prophylaxis of menstrual migraine: effects on intracellular magnesium. *Headache*. 1991;31:298–301.

Gagnier JJ. The therapeutic potential of melatonin in migraines and other headache types. *Altern Med Rev*. 2001;6(4):383–389.

Gobel H, Schmidt G, Soyka D. Effects of peppermint and eucalyptus oil preparations on the neurophysiological and experimental algesimetric headache parameters. *Cephalalgia*. 1994;14:228–234.

Gobel H, Fresenius J, Heinze A, et al. Effectiveness of Oleum menthae piperitae and paracetamol in therapy of headache of the tension type. *Nervenarzt*. 1996;67:672–681.

Grant, EC. Food allergies and migraines. *Lancet*. 1979;5:1(8123):966–969.

Hammond DC. Review of the efficacy of hypnosis with headache and migraines. *Int J Clin Exp Hypn*. 2007;55(2):207–219.

Harel Z, Gascon G, Riggs S, Vaz R, Brown W, Exil G. Supplementation with omega-3 polyunsaturated fatty acids in the management of recurrent migraines in adolescents. *J Adolesc Health*. 2002;31(2):154–161.

Holroyd KA, O'Donnell FJ, Stensland M, Lipchik GL, Cordingley GE, Calrson BW. Management of chronic tension type headache with tricyclic antidepressant medication, stress management therapy and their combination: a randomized controlled trial. *JAMA*. 2001;285(17):2208–2215.

Holroyd KA, Mauskop A. Complementary and alternative treatments. *Neurology*. 2003;60(7):1–9.

Hu HX, Markson LE, Lipton RB, Stewart WF, Berger MC. Burden of migraine in the United States. *Arch Intern Med*. 1999;159:813–818.

Johannes CB, Linet MS, Stewart WF, et al. Relationship of headache to phase of the menstrual cycle among young women: a daily diary study. *Neurology*. 1995;45:1076.

John PJ, Sharms N, Sharma CM, Kankane A. Effectiveness of yoga therapy in the treatment of migraine without aura: a randomized controlled trial. *Headache*. 2007;47(5):654–661.

Johnson ES, Kadam NP, Hylands DM, Hylands PJ. Efficacy of feverfew as prophylactic treatment of migraine. *Br Med J (Clin Res Ed)*. 1985;291(6495):569–573.

Kay TM, Gross A, Goldsmith C, et al. Exercises for mechanical neck disorders. *Cochrane Database Syst Rev*. 2005;(3):CD004250.

Keller E, Bzdek VM. Effects of therapeutic touch on tension headache pain. *Nurs Res*. 1986;35(2):101–105.

Kohen DP, Zajac R. Self-hypnosis training for headaches in children and adolescents. *J Pediatrics*. 2007;150:635–639.

Latha S, Kaliappan KV. Efficacy of yoga therapy in the management of headaches. *J Ind Psychol*. 1992;10(1–2):41–47.

Launso L, Brendstrup E, Arnber S. An exploratory study of reflexological treatment for headache. *Altern Ther Health Med*. 1999;5(3):57–65.

Li W, Zheng T, Altura BM, Altura BT. Sex steroid hormones exert biphasic effects on cyctolic magnesium ions in cerebral vascular smooth muscle cells: possible relationships to migraine frequency in premenstrual and stroke incidence. *Brain Res Bull*. 2001;54(1):83–89.

Linde K, Streng A, Jurgens S, et al. Acupuncture for patients with migraine—a randomized controlled trial. *JAMA*. 2005;293(17):2118–2125.

Lipton, RB, Stewart, WF, Simon, D. Medical consultation for migraine: results from the American Migraine Study. *Headache*. 1998;38(2):87–96.

Lipton RB, Stewart WF, Diamond S, et al. Prevalence and burden of migraine in the United States: data from the American Migraine Study II. *Headache*. 2001;41:646.

Littarru GP, Tiano L. Clinical aspects of coenzyme Q10: an update. *Curr Opin Clin Nutr Metab Care*. 2005;8(6):641–646.

Lockett DM, Campbell JF. The effects of aerobic exercise on migraine. *Headache*. 1992;32(1):50–54.

Lodi R, Montagna P, Soriani S, et al. Deficit of brain and skeletal muscle bioenergetics and low brain magnesium in juvenile migraine: an in vivo 31P magnetic resonance spectroscopy interictal study. *Pediatr Res*. 1997;42(6):866–871.

Lodi R, Iotti S, Cortelli P, et al. Deficient energy metabolism is associated with low free magnesium in brains of patients with migraine and cluster headache. *Brain Res Bull*. 2001;54(4):437–441.

Macgregor A, Hacksaw, A. Prevalence of migraine on each day of the natural menstrual cycle. *Neurology*. 2004;63:351.

Magis D, Ambrosini A, Sandor P, Jacquy J, Laloux P, Schoenen J. A randomized double-blind placebo-controlled trial of thioctic acid in migraine prophylaxis. *Headache.* 2007;47(1):52–57.

Maizels M, Blumenfeld A, Burchette R. A combination of riboflavin, magnesium and feverfew for migraine prophylaxis: a randomized trial. *Headache.* 2004;44(9):885–890.

Maissen, CP, Ludin HP. Comparison of the effect of 5-hydroxytryptophan and propanolol in the interval treatment of migraine (In German). *Schweiz Med Wochenschr.* 1991;121(43):1585–1590.

Manias P, Tagaris G, Karageorgiou K. Acupuncture in Headache: a critical review. *Clin J Pain.* 2000;16(4):334–339.

Marcus DA, Scharff L, Mercer S, Turk DC. Nonpharmacologica treatment for migraine: incremental utility of physical therapy with relaxation and thermal biofeedback. *Cephalagia.* 1998;18:266–272.

Martin, VT, Behbehani, MM. Toward a rational understanding of migraine trigger factors. *Med Clin N Am.* 2001;85(4):911–941.

Mauskop A, Altura BT, Cracco RQ, Altura BM. Intravenous magnesium sulfate rapidly alleviates headache of various types. *Headache.* 1996;36:154–160.

Mauskop A, Altura BM. Role of magnesium in the pathogenesis and treatment of migraines. *Clin Neurosci.* 1998;5(1):24–27.

Mauskop A. Alternative therapies in headache: is there a role? *Med Clin North Am.* 2001;85:1077–1084.

Melchart D, Linde K, Fischer P, White A, Allais G, Vickers A, Berman B. Acupuncture for recurrent headache: a systematic review of randomized controlled trials. *Cephalalgia.* 1999;19(9):779–786.

Melchart D, Thormaehlen J, Hager S, Liao J, Linde K, Weidenhammer W. Acupuncture versus placebo versus sumatriptan for early treatment of migraine attacks: a randomized controlled trial. *J Internal Med.* 2003;253(2):181–188.

Melchart D, Streng A, Hoppe A, et al. Acupuncture in patients with tension-type headache: a randomized controlled trial. *BMJ.* 2005;331(7513):376–382.

Melis PM, Rooimans W, Spiering EL, Hoogduin CA. Treatment of chronic tension-type headache with hypnotherapy: a single-blind, time-controlled study. *Headache.* 1991;31:686–689.

Mills Roth, J. Physical therapy in the treatment of chronic headache. *Curr Pain Headache Rep.* 2003;7:482.

Montagna P, Cortelli P, Monari L, et al. 31P-magnetic resonance spectroscopy in migraine without aura. *Neurology.* 1994;44(4):666–669.

Murphy JJ, Heptinstall S, Mitchell JR. Randomised double-blind, placebo controlled trial of feverfew in migraine prevention. *Lancet.* 1988;2(8604):189–192.

Myers DE, Myers RA. A preliminary report on hyperbaric oxygen in the relief of migraine headache. *Headache.* 1995;35(4):197–199.

Nagtegaal JE, Smits MG, Swart AC, et al. Melatonin-responsive headache in delayed sleep phase syndrome: preliminary observations. *Headache.* 1998;38:303–307.

Narin SO, Pinar L, Erbas D, Ozturk V, Idiman F. The effects of exercise and exercise-related changes in blood nitric oxygen level on migraine headache. *Clin Rehabil.* 2003;17(6):624–630.

Naumann M, So Y, Argoff CE, et al. Assessment: Botulinum neurotoxin in the treatment of autonomic disorders and pain (an evidence-based review): report of the therapeutics and technology assessment subcommittee of the American Academy of Neurology. *Neurology.* 2008;70(19):1707–1714.

Nestoriuc Y, Martin A. Efficacy of biofeedback for migraine: a meta-analysis. *Pain.* 2007;128(1–2):111–127.

Nestoriuc Y, Rief W, Martin A. Meta-analysis of biofeedback for tension-type headache: efficacy, specificity, and treatment of moderators. *J Consult Clin Psychol.* 2008;76(3):379–396.

Butterbur root extract and music therapy in the prevention of childhood migraine: an explorative study. *Eur J Pain.* 2008;12(3):301–313.

Parker GB, Pryor DS, Tupling H. Why does migraine improve during a clinical trial? Further results from a trial of cervical manipulation for migraine. *Aust N Z J Med.* 1980;10:192–198.

Peikert A, Wilimzig C, Kohne-Volland R. Prophylaxis of migraine with oral magnesium: results from a prospective, multi-center, placebo-controlled and double-blinded randomized study. *Cephalgia.* 1996;16(4):257–263.

Phillips HC, Jahanshahi, M. The effects of persistent pain: chronic headache sufferer. *Pain.* 1985;21:163–176.

Pittler MH, Vogler BK, Ernst E. Feverfew for preventing migraine. *Cochrane database Syst Rev.* 2004;(1):CD00286.

Pothmann R, Danesch U. Migraine prevention in children and adolescents: results of an open study with a special butterbur root extract. *Headache.* 2005;45(3):196–203.

Pradalier A, Bakouche P, Baudesson G, et al. Failure of omega-3 fatty acids in prevention of migraine: a double-blind study versus placebo. *Cephalalgia.* 2001;21(8):818–822.

Rasmussen BK, Jensen R, Schroll M, Olesen J. Epidemiology of headache in a general population: a prevalence study. *J Clin Epidemiol.* 1991;44:1147.

Rasmussen BK. Epidemiology of headache in Europe. In: Olesen J, ed. *Headache Classification and Epidemiology.* New York: Raven Press; 1994:231–237.

Ribeiro CA. L-5-Hydroxytryptophan in the prophylaxis of chronic tension-type headache: a double-blind, randomized, placebo-controlled study. *Headache.* 2000;40(6):451–456.

Rozen TD, Oshinsky ML, Gebeline CA, et al. Open label trial of Coenzyme Q10 as a migraine preventive. Cephalalgia 2002;22:137–141.

Russell MB, Levi N, Saltyte-Benth J, Fenger K. Tension-type headache in adolescents and adults: a population based study of 33,764 twins. *Eur J Epidemiol.* 2006;21:153.

Sances G, Granella F, Nappi RE, et al. Course of migraine during pregnancy and postpartum: a prospective study. *Cephalalgia.* 2003;23:197.

Sandor PS, Afra J, Ambrosini A, Schoenen J. Prophylactic treatment of migraine with beta-blockers and riboflavin: differential effects on the intensity dependence of auditory evoked cortical potentials. *Headache.* 2000;41(1):30–35.

Schoenen J, Jacquy J, Lenaerts, M. Effectiveness of high-dose riboflavin in migraine prophylaxis: a randomized controlled trial. *Neurology*. 1998;50(2);466–70.

Schwartz BS, Stewart WF, Simon D, Lipton RB. Epidemiology of tension-type headache. *JAMA*. 1998;279:381.

Sheftell F, Rapoport A, Kudrow L. Efficacy of cranial electrotherapy stimulation in the prophylactic treatment of migraine and chronic muscles contraction headaches. *Cephalalgia*. 1989;9(Supp10):379–380.

Sherman RA, Acosta NM, Robson L. Treatment of Migraine with pulsing electromagnetic fields: a double-blind, placebo-controlled study. *Headache*. 1999;39:567–575.

Shrivastava R, Pechadre JC, John GW. Tanacetum parthenium and Salix alba (Mig-RL) combination in migraine prophylaxis: a prospective, open-label study. *Clin Drug Investig*. 2006;26(5):287–296.

Sicuteri F. Hypothesis: migraine, a central biochemical dysnociception. *Headache*. 1976;16:145–149.

Silberstein, SD for the US headache Consortium. Practice parameter: evidence based guidelines for migraine headache. *Am Acad Neuro*. 2000;1–11.

Simopoulos AP. Omega-3 fatty acids in inflammation and autoimmune disease. *J Am Coll Nutr*. 2002;21(6):495–505.

Solomon S, Guglielmo KM. Treatment of headache by transcutaneous electrical stimulation. *Headache*. 1985;25(1):12–15.

Spierings EL, Ranke AH, Honkoop PC. Precipitating and aggravating factors of migraine versus tension-type headache. *Headache*. 2001;41(6):554–558.

Stang PE, Osterhaus JT. Impact of migraine in the United States: data from the National Health Interview Survey. *Headache*. 1993;33(1):29–33.

Stewart WF, Schecter A, Lipton RB. Migraine heterogeneity: disability, pain intensity, and attack frequency and duration. *Neurology*. 1994;44(S4):S24–39.

Streng A, Linde K, Hoppe A, et al. Effectiveness and tolerability of acupuncture compared with metoprolol in migraine prophylaxis. *Headache*. 2006;46(10):1492–1502.

Termine C, Ginevra OF, D'Arrigo S, Rossi M, Lanzi G. Alternative therapies in the treatment of headachesin childhood, adolescence and adulthood. *Funct Neurol*. 2005;20(1):9–14.

Titus F, Davalos A, Alom J, Codina A. 5-Hydroxytryptophan versus methysergide in the prophylaxis of migraine. *Eur Neurol*. 1986;25(5):327–329.

Trautmann E, Lackschewitz H, Kroner-Herwig B. Psychological treatment of recurrent headache in children and adolescents—a meta-analysis. *Cephalagia*. 2006;26(12):1411–1426.

Upledger JE. Craniosacral therapy. *Phys Ther*. 1995;75:328–330.

Van Ettekoven H, Lucas C. Efficacy of physiotherapy including craniocervical training programme for tension-type headache: a randomized clinical trial. *Cephalagia*. 2006;26:983.

Vernon H, McDermaid CS, Hagino C. Systematic review of randomized clinical trials of complmentary/alternative therapies in the treatment of tension-type and cervicogenic headache. *Complement Ther Med*. 1999;7(3):142–155.

Von Peter S, Ting W, Scrivani S, et al. Survey on the use of complementary and alternative medicine among patients with headache syndromes. *Cephalalgia*. 2002;22:395–400.

Waeber C, Moskowitz M. Migraine as an inflammatory disorder. *Neurology*. 2005;64(S2):S9–S15.

Walach H, Haeusler W, Lowes T, et al. Classical homeopathic treatment of chronic headaches. *Cephalagia*. 1997;17:119–126.

Walach H, Lowes T, Mussbach D, et al. The long term effects of homeopathic treatment of chronic headaches: one year follow-up. *Cephalalgia*. 2000;20:835–837.

Wang F, Van Den Eden SK, Ackerson LM, Salk SE, Reince RH, Elin RJ. Oral magnesium oxide prophylaxis of frequent migraine headache in children: a randomized, double-blinded, placebo-controlled trial. *Headache*. 2004;44(5):445–446.

Waters WE, O'Connor PJ. Epidemiology of headache and migraine in women. *J Neurol Neurosurg Psychiatry*. 1971;34:148.

Welch KM, Ramada NM. Mitochondria, magnesium and migraine. *J Neuro Sci*. 1995;134:9–14.

Wenzhong T. Clinical observation on scalp acupuncture treatment in 50 cases of headache. *J Trad Chin Med*. 2002;22(3):190–192.

Whitmarsh TE, Coleston-Shields DM, Steiner TJ. Double blind randomized placebo-controlled study of homeopathic prophylaxis of migraine. *Cephalalgia*. 1997;17:600–604.

Yerdelen D, Acil T, Goksel B, Karatas M. Heart rate recovery in migraine and tension-type headache. *Headache*. 2008;48(2):221–225.

28

Fibromyalgia–Chronic Fatigue

MELINDA RING

CASE STUDY

Janet is a successful professor of literature at a Midwestern university. In 2007, she presented to her primary care physician with overwhelming fatigue. Janet underwent a thorough battery of tests, with no clear cause identified for her symptoms. She was referred for an evaluation at the Northwestern Center for Integrative Medicine and Wellness. After an extensive history and physical exam, I felt her symptoms consistent with chronic fatigue syndrome and recommended a regimen of supplements and complementary therapies. As is not atypical, her symptoms evolved to include the widespread pain characteristic of fibromyalgia, leading to adjustments in her treatment. Janet's progress has been slow, but she was able to return to work and has improved compared with last year. Throughout this chapter, comments from the Northwestern team of practitioners who care for Janet will show the benefits of an integrative team approach achieved by uniting diverse philosophies of health and moving beyond the Western view of disease.

Introduction

ibromyalgia (FM) and Chronic fatigue syndrome (CFS) are conditions that confound the physician for many reasons. Patients present with a wide-range of symptoms, and no confirmatory diagnostic test is currently available. There is no unanimous agreement on the etiology and management, and patient responses to interventions are inconsistent. In general, medical trainees receive minimal education about FM/CFS. As a result, many doctors discredit the diagnoses as psychosomatic or psychiatric conditions (Chew-Graham et al. 2008).

Interestingly, these diseases are not new to this century but have been described in the literature as early as the relative diagnoses of "little fever" in 1750 and "rheumatism" in the sixteenth century (Inanici and Yunus 2004; Kim 1994). Today, however, we know more about the underlying pathophysiology and effective management than ever before, as the evidence base grows through research. Combining this knowledge with a patient-centered approach, the integrative medicine physician is uniquely situated to help relieve suffering and reduce disability across the full spectrum of FM/CFS symptoms.

My sister-in-law was diagnosed with CFS when I was still an internal medicine resident. Like many physicians, I had a poor understanding of her condition. She looked healthy; it was a challenge for my family to understand why she couldn't come to some gatherings because of her fatigue. Over the years, as I gained a better understanding of CFS I appreciated her bravery and the struggle of battling not just her disease, but also the misconceptions of everyone around her. I now appreciate fully that when she spends time playing with my two boisterous young boys she is making a sacrifice, as the following day she may be too exhausted to do more than the minimum necessary activities. This personal experience helped me become more supportive toward my own patients, such as Janet. For many CFS/FM patients, finding a physician willing to listen and acknowledge their condition provides significant relief and begins the healing process.

This chapter on FM/CFS offers an introduction to the symptoms, current hypotheses of the pathophysiology, and practical diagnostic algorithms, with special attention to issues specific to female patients. The remainder of the chapter explores the evidence for available treatment modalities, including conventional pharmacology and complementary therapies. Current research suggests that CFS and FM fall along a continuum of related disorders with common pathogenesis: 50%–70% of CFS and FM patients meet both diagnostic criteria (Aaron et al. 2000; Goldenberg et al. 1990). In this chapter the two diseases will be discussed as such, with distinctions noted when relevant.

Definition and Symptomatology

The CDC criteria for CFS and ACR criteria for FM are of utility primarily to researchers needing to identify a uniform patient population (Tables 28.1 and 28.2) (Fukuda et al. 1994; Wolfe et al. 1990). In practice, expanding beyond these definitions allows the physician to identify thousands of people with chronic fatigue and widespread pain, likely arising from similar immunologic and hormonal imbalances and appropriate for the same interventions (Harth and Nielson 2007). The hallmark symptoms common to both CFS/FM patients include the following: overwhelming fatigue which is exacerbated post-exertion, concentration issues (brain fog) and disequilibrium, unrefreshing sleep and sleep disturbances, flu-like feelings and myalgias, and headaches. The physical examination is usually unremarkable except for tender points. Patients often have co-existing conditions such as irritable bowel syndrome, interstitial cystitis, dyspareunia, allergies, chemical sensitivities and depression or anxiety.

Epidemiology

CFS and FM are much more common in women compared to men. The prevalence of FM is estimated at 2%–4% in the general U.S. population, with a breakdown of 3.4% of all women and only 0.5% of men (Wolfe et al. 1995). It is a challenge to ascertain the prevalence of CFS; one study of a primary care population estimates 8.5% of patients have debilitating fatigue lasting over 6 months, but as per the stricter CDC definition less than 15% of these patients would be diagnosed with CFS (Bates et al. 1993). Both conditions have a modal age distribution, with most cases diagnosed from age 20 to 50; onset in childhood and postmenopause occurs to a much lesser degree.

Pathophysiology

Research over the past decade has identified pathophysiologic abnormalities in multiple arenas including central nervous system pain processing, neuroendocrine and autonomic nervous system function, neurotransmitter levels, and

Table 28.1. CFS Fibromyalgia Chapter

A case of chronic fatigue syndrome is defined by the presence of:

1. Clinically evaluated, unexplained, persistent or relapsing fatigue that is of new or definite onset; is not the result of ongoing exertion; is not alleviated by rest; and results in substantial reduction in previous levels of occupational, educational, social, or personal activities

And

2. Four or more of the following symptoms that persist or recur during six or more consecutive months of illness and that do not predate the fatigue:

Self-reported impairment in short term memory or concentration

Sore throat

Tender cervical or axillary nodes

Muscle pain

Multijoint pain without redness or swelling

Headaches of a new pattern or severity

Unrefreshing sleep

Post-exertional malaise lasting 24 hours

Table 28.2. CFS Fibromyalgia

American College of Rheumatology Criteria for Fibromyalgia	Pope and Hudson Criteria for Fibromyalgia
Widespread pain ≥3-months duration	Widespread pain ≥3-months duration
Pain at ≥ 11 of 18 tender points	Pain at ≥11 of 18 tender points **or**
	≥4 of 6 of the following symptoms:
	Generalized fatigue
	Headaches
	Sleep disturbance
	Neuropsychiatric complaints
	Numbness or tingling sensations
	Irritable bowel symptoms

Source: Based on Wolfe et al. 1990 and Pope and Hudson 1996.

oxidative stress (Afari and Buchwald 2003; Bradley 2008). Current hypotheses suggest the manifestation of FM/CFS and related conditions are multifactorial, a complex interplay of environmental triggers, genetic susceptibility, and disordered biochemical functioning. Briefly, some of the documented risk factors and abnormalities that contribute to symptoms include the following:

- *Genetics:* Familial studies in both CFS and FM have identified a familial predisposition, with a greater than 8 odds ratio of FM occurrence in first-degree relatives (Arnold et al. 2004a). In FM the foremost genes include those that impact on neurotransmitter/monoamine levels such as serotonin and dopamine receptors and transporters (Cohen et al. 2002; Offenbaecher et al. 1999). In CFS 88 genes have differential expression compared to normal controls; those identified have links to hematological function, immunologic disease, cancer, cell death, immune response, and infection (Kerr et al. 2008b). One group identified seven genomically distinct subtypes, which may correlate with variable phenotypic expression (Kerr et al. 2008a).

- *Triggers:* A significant number of patients identify a triggering event prior to the onset of symptoms. Frequent offenders are physical trauma (motor vehicle accident), psychological stressors (grief, stressful life events), and infections (viral, gastroenteritis, Lyme disease). It is important for the treating physician to help patients understand that these events are considered triggers in someone with an underlying predisposition, rather than the ultimate etiology. Without this clarification, some patients seek costly and invasive testing to identify the perceived cause and pursue potentially harmful treatments.

- *Central Pain Augmentation:* Central sensitization causes hyperalgesia, allodynia, and referred pain, leading to chronic widespread pain. FM studies support the existence of triggers for sensitization: wind-up or temporal summation (pain augmentation at the dorsal horn neuron whereby repeated pain stimuli lead to augmented pain response), dysregulated descending inhibitory pathways, and upregulated facilitatory modulation (stimulated by behavioral and cognitive factors) (Meeus and Nijs 2007). Objective central abnormalities noted include hyperexcitability of the spinal cord, decreased perfusion of pain-related brain structures on functional MRI, and high CSF levels of substance P. Cognitive central sensitization can also derive from pain hypervigilance, maladaptive coping strategies, and catastrophizing often found on presentation.

- *Autonomic/Neuroendocrine Dysfunction:* A review of recent neuroendocrine studies reported that aberrations in the hypothalamic-pituitary-adrenal (HPA) axis and serotonin pathways have been identified in CFS, suggesting an altered stress response (Demitrack 1997). About one-third of patients exhibit low cortisol, as well as decreased DHEA-S and insulin-like growth factor.

- **Immune Dysfunction:** Multiple immune disturbances have been noted in CFS and FM patients. The impact of this dysregulation is unclear, with studies showing conflicting results in markers such as levels of circulating immunoglobulin and immune complexes, natural killer (NK) cells, and CD8 cells and altered NK cell function and interferon activity (Landay et al. 1991; Mawle et al. 1997).
- **Oxidative Stress and Nitric Oxide:** Research has identified elevations in nitric oxide, oxidative stress, mitochondrial dysfunction, NF-kappa B activity, inflammatory cytokines activity, vanilloid activity, and NMDA activity. Some scientists postulate a paradigm known as the NOO/ ONOO⁻ cycle as the underlying etiology of the aforementioned biochemical disorders and manifested symptoms (Pall 2007). At this time it is unclear whether the oxidative stresses are incidental or causal.

Diagnostic Approach

As CFS is diagnosed primarily based on history, and through exclusion of other causes for fatigue, limited laboratory testing is recommended: complete blood count with differential, erythrocyte sedimentation rate, chemistry panel, thyroid stimulating hormone and free T4, DHEA-sulfate, and cortisol. Other tests should be performed if indicated by physical exam and history.

Expensive immunologic tests and serologies are not recommended. Although infections may act as a trigger, an epidemiologic CDC study for over 40 organisms found no consistent association (Mawle et al. 1995). Therefore, checking serologies for EBV, CMV, or Lyme disease in the absence of a high index of suspicion does not influence treatment recommendations. (Straus et al, 1985). Although abnormalities have been noted in neuroimaging studies, they are of unclear significance and routine MRI and SPECT are not currently recommended (Schwartz et al. 1994). Finally, genetic panels are of great interest, but are not yet validated as diagnostic tests for CFS/FM.

Primary Care of Women with CFS/FM

Factors such as general disability and a focus on managing fatigue and pain may lead women with CFS/FM to skip recommended screening tests. It is incumbent upon the physician to incorporate age-appropriate screening for cervical, breast, and colon cancer. An additional challenge is treating common primary care issues such as hypertension, as patients with CFS/FM are often very sensitive to medication side-effects and may require starting at low doses with gradual titration.

Pregnancy and CFS/FM

There is very limited data of the impact of pregnancy on CFS/FM outcomes and vice-versa. The few studies available suggest an equal number of patients felt no change, improvement, or worsening of symptoms during and after pregnancy (Schacterle and Komaroff 2004). Many medications and supplements are not advised during pregnancy, necessitating a shift to safer therapies such as acupuncture, mind–body therapies, and homeopathy. High-quality prenatal vitamins and omega-3 fish oil should be recommended.

Overview of Pharmacologic Treatment of CFS/FM

Trials on medications for the indication of CFS/FM have increased over the past decade. The therapies are often neuromodulatory agents which target cells involved in sleep regulation and pain signaling. Many therapies are available for the conditions associated with CFS/FM such as IBS, interstitial cystitis, and dyspareunia, but these are addressed in other chapters and publications and will not be reviewed here.

ANTI-EPILEPTIC DRUGS ($\alpha_2\delta$ LIGANDS)

Pregabalin (Lyrica) was the first FDA-approved drug for FM. Both pregabalin and gabapentin (Neurontin) bind to the $\alpha_2\delta$ subunit of voltage-gated calcium channels of neurons, thereby inhibiting release of neurotransmitters such as glutamate and substance P. In 2007, two 14-week RCTs enrolled over 1100 patients that met ACR criteria for FM, had a pain visual analogue scale greater than 40 mm (0–100 mm), and mean numeric pain rating scale of at least 4 (0–10) (Crofford et al. 2005). Pregabalin was dosed at 150, 225, and 300 mg twice daily. Statistically significant improvements of more than 30% reduction in pain and sleep quality were seen beginning at week 1; higher doses also demonstrated improvement in global assessment and health status. The primary adverse effects leading to discontinuation were dizziness (6.4%) and somnolence (4%). Weight gain can be an issue at higher doses, often due to increased appetite and sugar cravings. A 6-month

DBPCT of pregabalin used an initial open-label treatment; only those patients who responded with more than or equal to 50% reduction in pain and scored as "much" or "very much" improved were eligible for randomization. In responders, beneficial effects in pain reduction persisted in about 2/3 of patients over the 6-month study. Improvements in sleep and mental functioning and fatigue were also noticed. Gabapentin has been studied in one trial with demonstrated efficacy but is not FDA approved for use (Arnold et al. 2007).

ANTIDEPRESSANTS

In June 2008, duloxetine HCL (Cymbalta) became the second FDA approved drug for FM. The approval was a result of two 3-month clinical trials totaling 874 patients (Arnold et al. 2004b). In both studies, compared with placebo, duloxetine was associated with more than a 30% reduction in pain as measured by the Brief Pain Inventory (BPI). Onset of pain relief began during the first week of treatment. Approximately 2/3 of patients in the treatment groups reported improved overall functioning on duloxetine 60 mg/day. Discontinuation from adverse effects (nausea, dry mouth, constipation, decreased appetite, sleepiness, increased sweating, and agitation) was 20% versus 12% in the placebo group.

OTHER MEDICATIONS

Other medications studied in FM/CFS with conflicting or negative results include galantine, intramuscular and intravascular immune globulin, acyclovir, fluoxetine, paroxetine, tricyclics, methylphenidate, hydrocortisone, fludrocortisone, antivirals, and NSAIDs. Cyclobenzaprine, tramadol, and acetaminophen seem to provide some relief in FM (Bennett et al. 2003; Tofferi 2004).

Integrative Therapies for Women Living with CFS/FM

Unlike many conditions where complementary therapies are chosen to supplement conventional therapy, in FM and CFS the paucity of treatments or desire to avoid dependence on addictive medications draws high number of patients to CAM therapies regardless of the level of evidence. For many of these women, the severity of symptoms fluctuates; moments of relative "wellness" give hope of return to former levels of functioning. Helping our patients maintain that hope, while keeping them from potentially harmful practices, is crucial to their continuing healing.

Integrative Medicine Perspective: Naturopathic Viewpoint

Naturopathic doctors strive to address the underlying individual cause, whether nutritional, environmental or biochemical. From my experience, in CFS/FM symptoms arise when specific cells are unable to perform normal cellular function. The first step in a naturopathic approach is to combine homeopathic drainage (to aid in detoxification of cellular metabolites) with the removal of identified underlying causes (to prevent further damage). Cells are then in an optimal position to absorb the nutrients found lacking in the body. By addressing imbalances, the body is able to restore a balanced physiology.

–Judy Fulop, ND

Botanicals and Supplements

A broad array of dietary supplements is employed in the management of CFS/FM. Very little research is available on supplements specifically for CFS/FM and small numbers, high dropout rates, and poor methodological quality limit most studies (Mannerkorpi et al. 2007). A few which show promise include the following.

D-RIBOSE

Based on the theory that mitochondrial energy is the core issue, D-ribose, a naturally occurring pentose carbohydrate, was given to 41 CFS/FM patients at a dose of 5 g three times daily for a total of 280 g. Sixty-six percent of patients showed a significant improvement in five visual analog scale (VAS) categories: energy, sleep, mental clarity, pain intensity, and well-being (Teitelbaum et al. 2006).

L-CARNITINE

This amino acid affects mitochondrial energy production by supporting free fatty acid transfer across mitochondrial membranes. Two studies on this compound and the related propionyl-L-carnitine, 2 g/day, are suggestive of benefit for general fatigue in CFS after 4–8 weeks of treatment (Plioplys and Plioplys 1997; Vermeulen and Scholte 2004).

MELATONIN

Patients with CFS/FM often have delayed circadian rhythmicity, contributing to sleep disturbances. A pilot study of melatonin, a chronobiotic drug, 5 mg orally for 3 months resulted in significant improvement in scores for fatigue, concentration, and activity in 8/29 patients (van Heukelom et al. 2006).

S-ADENOSYL METHIONINE (SAMe)

SAMe has analgesic, anti-inflammatory, and antidepressant effects. A PCT in patients with FM at doses of 800 mg/day for 6 weeks demonstrated statistically significant improvements in pain, fatigue, and morning stiffness but not in tender point score, isokinetic muscle strength, or mood evaluated by Beck Depression Inventory (Tavoni et al. 1987). A second crossover study of 17 patients with primary FM did show reduced number of trigger points and improved scores on both the Hamilton and SAD rating scales (Jacobsen et al. 1991).

5-HYDROXY-TRYPTOPHAN

5-Hydroxy-tryptophan (HTP) is the precursor compound in the synthesis of serotonin. There is some promising data that 5-HTP, typically given in doses of 50–150 mg in the evening, can reduce the number of tender points and improve anxiety, pain, sleep, and fatigue (Caruso et al. 1990; Nicolodi and Sicuteri 1996; Puttini and Caruso 1992). Episodes of eosinophilia-myalgia syndrome (EMS) in the 1980s from contaminated tryptophan, a very similar compound, have raised some safety concerns; though there have not been any instances of toxicity with 5-HTP. As with any supplement, patients should be guided toward high-quality products from reputable manufacturers.

DEHYDROEPIANDROSTERONE

The adrenal hormone dehydroepiandrosterone (DHEA) may work in the limbic system to regulate excitatory neurotransmission. In some people low DHEA levels create memory impairment and decreased concentration, which improve after supplementation. Typical doses in female patients are 5–15 mg/ day in the morning (Himmel and Seligman 1999; Kuratsune et al. 1998).

MAGNESIUM

Magnesium and malate, both needed for ATP formation, are sometimes recommended for FM/CFS, though limited data are available (Russell et al. 1995). When low red blood cell magnesium is documented, intramuscular magnesium sulfate 1 g weekly may improve energy levels and mood and reduce pain (Cox et al. 1991).

NADH

NADH (nicotinamide adenine dinucleotide hydrate) is a coenzyme essential to the production of ATP. In one study, some participants with CFS noted that 10 mg/day NADH taken for 4 weeks improved fatigue, other symptoms, and quality of life (Forsyth et al. 1999).

Nutrition

Nutrition plays a large role in the regulation of symptoms in FM/CFS patients (Werbach 2000). The most commonly recommended diets include the following.

ANTI-INFLAMMATORY DIET

Though FM is not related to inflammation, the principles of eating whole foods, high consumption of phytonutrient-rich fruits and vegetables and omega-3 rich protein sources is a healthy basic diet for all individuals.

VEGAN DIET

A 3-month study in Finland of a vegan diet consisting of fruits, legumes, seeds, nuts, and vegetables with elimination of coffee, tea, alcohol, sugar, and salt concluded with improvement of symptoms in pain, sleep, and overall wellness (Kaartinen et al. 2000). However, symptoms returned to baseline with resumption of a full diet.

ELIMINATION DIET

Food sensitivities can contribute to many CFS/FM symptoms such as fatigue, mental sluggishness, gastrointestinal, and genitourinary complaints. While many independent labs offer IgG testing for food sensitivities, the use of these tests is controversial. Alternatively, some providers recommend a trial of an elimination diet to identify the most frequent offending foods. An elimination diet may vary but often restricts sugar, alcohol, dairy products, wheat, eggs, citrus, soy, chocolate, coffee, and artificial sweeteners and additives. After a 3-week elimination, these foods are added back in, one at a time, every 4 days with monitoring for an exacerbation. For some people the elimination diet is an overwhelming challenge, and seeing the results from the IgG tests can be a motivating factor.

ADDITIVE ELIMINATION

Patients should avoid MSG (monosodium glutamate) and aspartame (NutraSweet). MSG (also found in labels as gelatin, hydrolyzed or textured protein, and yeast extract) is digested into the excitatory amino acid glutamate. Glutamate activates the NMDA receptors involved in the central nervous system's wind-up sensitization, known to be a problem in FM patients. Aspartame is converted into aspartate, another excitatory amino acid that can induce pain-amplifying receptors. Other common offenders include nitrates, nitrites, sulfites, preservatives, and coloring/flavoring additives.

CANDIDA DIET

Overgrowth of *Candida albicans*, or the "yeast syndrome," is a controversial diagnosis with scant scientific data. One study examined the impact of a low sugar, low yeast diet (LSLY) versus healthy eating diet in 52 individuals with CFS. Intention-to-treat analysis showed no statistically significant differences on levels of fatigue or quality of life (Hobday et al. 2008).

Physical Activity

The fatigue and pain of FM/CFS often make it challenging for patients to engage in an active lifestyle, and counseling needs to be done with empathy for those limitations. Some patients are able to exercise at full-intensity and duration from the outset, but others can do no more than 5 minutes at a stretch. Asking the patient her current maximal exertion and duration, and then working to increase that amount should be the starting goal. For deconditioned women or those with joint issues, an exercise physiologist or physical therapist with experience in FM/CFS can be invaluable.

AEROBIC EXERCISE

Graded exercise is an intervention reliably shown to have benefit in CFS/FM (Busch et al. 2002; Fulcher and White 1997; Powell et al. 2001). Research has shown reduced number of tender points, improved sleep and sense of well-being, increased serotonin, and reduced depression. A systematic review of randomized controlled trials (RCTs) concluded that aerobic exercise of low to moderate intensity, such as walking, biking, and pool exercise, can improve symptoms and distress in patients with FM/CFS (Jones et al. 2006). Aerobic exercise of moderate to high intensity has been shown to additionally improve aerobic capacity and tender point status.

MUSCLE STRENGTHENING

Strength training using free weights or elastic bands is associated with improvements in several measures including pain, number of tender points, and muscle strength, as well as a decrease in the mean score on the Beck Depression Inventory (Jones et al. 2002). A small number of patients experienced worsening symptoms during the study.

YOGA/TAI CHI

Benefits of yoga for FM patients have been examined in small pilot studies. Eight weekly sessions of relaxing yoga showed improvement in pain and functional assessments over time (da Silva et al. 2007). Tai Chi is a traditional Chinese discipline with both physical and mental components that appears to benefit varied chronic conditions such as rheumatoid arthritis; a pilot study in FM is currently underway (Wang et al. 2004).

Acupuncture and Traditional Chinese Medicine

Integrative Medicine Perspective: Traditional Chinese Medicine

Janet's progress provides an excellent example of how acupuncture must be individualized for the specific patient. Although acupuncture is very effective in treating the symptoms of CFS/FM especially pain, insomnia, fatigue, anxiety, and depression, the body's ability to take correction with acupuncture is individual.

Each acupuncture treatment gives the person a measured push to promote healing and decrease symptoms. The pace and intensity varies with each individual. With Janet, this was a challenge because with CFS there is a thin line between what promotes healing and what can be too much.

Virginia Burns, LAc and Ania Grimone, LAc

A 2007 systematic review on the use of acupuncture for FM found only five randomized clinical trials meeting criteria for inclusion (Mayhew and Ernst 2007). Two trials yielded negative results and three using electroacupuncture were positive. Well-conducted studies in peer-reviewed journals have conflicting results, with some claiming significant improvement in pain, fatigue, and energy and others showing no benefit (Assefi et al. 2005; Martin et al. 2006). Some of the differences may arise from difficulties inherent to acupuncture research, such as blinding techniques, and prescribed treatment protocols versus the more individual approach used in a clinical setting.

Mind–Body Medicine

Integrative Medicine Perspective: Health Psychology

In my experience of working with CFS/FM patients like Janet, it is important to maintain an overall biopsychosocial model of illness while looking at the unique factors that are impacting the individual within that model. Janet was experiencing a moderate reactive depression related to issues of competency and fears of lost capabilities. In addition, she had difficulty handling stresses when her needs competed with the demands of others. This conflict arose around her work, her personal creative endeavors, and in close interpersonal relationships. Our focus was on mind–body methods to reduce the resultant stress as well as cognitive approaches to managing the conflict and reaching a realistic balance around internal and external demands.

Howard Feldman, PhD

Patients with FM/CFS often fear being labeled as having a psychosomatic condition. It is important for the physician recommending psychotherapy and mind–body therapies to clarify their role in the overall treatment plan, validating the true physical nature of the illness. A systematic review of mind–body therapies for FM by the Cochrane Collaboration identified 13 eligible trials on autogenic training, relaxation exercises, mindfulness meditation, cognitive-behavioral training, hypnosis, guided imagery, biofeedback, or education (Hadhazy et al. 2000). The conclusion was that there is strong evidence that mind–body therapy is effective for self-efficacy, moderate evidence for improved quality of life, and inconclusive evidence for other outcomes such as pain. Similar positive results were noted for cognitive-based therapy and meditation-based stress reduction in CFS (Prins et al. 2001).

Manual and Manipulative Therapies

Integrative Medicine Perspective: Bodyworker and Energy Healer

Initially, most patients with CFS or FM including Janet are in too much pain for even superficial massage techniques. Treatments such as Cranial Sacral Therapy and Reiki have resulted in decreased pain and anxiety, improved energy, and greater relaxation. Both therapies are noninvasive and use very light touch.

Chris Wilson, CMT

Current research suggests gentle massage may lower anxiety and benefit sleep quality in CFS/FM (Field et al. 2002). In addition, after 5 weeks of biweekly therapy, substance P levels decreased and the patients' physicians assigned lower disease ratings and noted fewer tender points. A study using mechanical deep tissue massage (LPG technique) also showed reduction in tender points after 15 treatments by a physical therapist (Gordon et al. 2006). The deep tissue work of Rolfing showed benefit in one study, but for many patients the technique is too painful. In recommending manual therapies the physician should be aware that therapists vary considerably in technique, as well as knowledge about treating FM/CFS, making it imperative to refer to an experienced and well-qualified practitioner.

Energy Healing

QI GONG

The Traditional Chinese medicine energy therapy, qi gong, was examined in a pilot study of ten patients (Chen et al. 2006). Five to seven qi gong treatments over 3 weeks led to complete recovery in two patients and improvements in pain, depression, and function in the remaining subjects.

REIKI

Reiki, the Japanese-based energy field therapy is promoted as helpful for pain, sleep, immune function, and anxiety/depression. An NIH-funded study of Reiki and FM is ongoing.

DISTANCE HEALING

A European study of the effect of distance healing versus wait list on over 400 CFS patients did not demonstrate a statistically significant effect on mental and physical health (Walach and Bosch 2008).

Conclusion

Although FM is the second most common condition seen by rheumatologists, only 20% of cases are cared for in specialty clinics, leaving the bulk of the management to primary care providers. The first step in the patient's healing is for the clinician to enter into the relationship with acceptance and empathy. Next, simply educating her about the current scientific understanding and real nature of the disease can provide significant relief. Finally, recognize that the disease course will be a journey you and the patient will take together.

REFERENCES

Aaron LA, Burke MM, Buchwald D. Overlapping conditions among patients with chronic fatigue syndrome, fibromyalgia, and temporomandibular disorder. *Arch Intern Med.* 2000;160:221.

Afari N, Buchwald D. Chronic fatigue syndrome: a review. *Am J Psychiatry.* 2003;160:221–236.

Arnold LM, Goldenberg DL, Stanford SB, et al. Gabapentin in the treatment of fibromyalgia: a randomized, double-blind, placebo-controlled, multicenter trial. *Arthritis Rheum.* 2007;56:1336.

Arnold LM, Hudson JI, Hess EV, et al. Family study of fibromyalgia. *Arthritis Rheum.* 2004a;50(3):944.

Arnold LM, Lu Y, Crofford LJ, et al. A double-blind, multicenter trial comparing duloxetine to placebo in the treatment of fibromyalgia patients with or without major depressive disorder. *Arthritis Rheum.* 2004b;50:2974.

Assefi NP, Sherman KJ, Jacobsen C, Goldberg J, Smith WR, Buchwald D. A randomized clinical trial of acupuncture compared with sham acupuncture in fibromyalgia. *Ann Intern Med.* 2005;143(1):10.

Bates DW, Schmitt W, Buchwald D, et al. Prevalence of fatigue and chronic fatigue syndrome in a primary care practice. *Arch Intern Med.* 1993;153:2759.

Bennett RM, Kamin M, Karim R, Rosenthal N. Tramadol and acetaminophen combination tablets in the treatment of fibromyalgia pain: a double-blind, randomized, placebo-controlled study. *Am J Med.* 2003;114:537.

Bradley LA. Pathophysiologic mechanisms of FM and its related disorders. *J Clin Psychiatry.* 2008;69(Suppl 2):6.

Busch AJ, Barber KA.R., Overend TJ, Peloso PMJ, Schachter CL. Exercise for treating fibromyalgia syndrome. *Cochrane Database of Systematic Reviews.* 2007, Issue 3.

Caruso I, Sarzi Puttini P, Cazzola M, Azzolini V. Double-blind study of 5-hydroxytryptophan versus placebo in the treatment of primary fibromyalgia syndrome. *J Int Med Res.* 1990;18:201.

Chen KW, Hassett AL, Hou F, Staller J, Lichtbroun AS. A pilot study of external qigong therapy for patients with fibromyalgia. *J Altern Complement Med.* 2006;12(9):851.

Chew-Graham CA, Cahill G, Dowrick C, Wearden A, Peters S. Using multiple sources of knowledge to reach clinical understanding of chronic fatigue syndrome. *Ann Fam Med.* 2008;6(4):340.

Cohen H, Buskila D, Neumann L, Ebstein RP. Confirmation of an association between fibromyalgia and serotonin transporter promoter region (5-HTTLPR) polymorphism, and relationship to anxiety-related personality traits. *Arthritis Rheum.* 2002;46:845.

Cox IM, Campbell MJ, Dowson D. Red blood cell magnesium and chronic fatigue syndrome. *Lancet.* 1991;337:757.

Crofford LJ, Rowbotham MC, Mease PJ, et al. Pregabalin for the treatment of fibromyalgia syndrome: results of a randomized, double-blind, placebo-controlled trial. *Arthritis Rheum.* 2005;52:1264.

da Silva GD, Lorenzi-Filho G, Lage LV. Effects of yoga and the addition of Tui Na in patients with fibromyalgia. *J Altern Complement Med.* 2007;13(10):1107.

Demitrack MA. Neuroendocrine correlates of chronic fatigue syndrome: a brief review. *J Psychiatr Res.* 1997;31:69.

Field T, Diego M, Cullen C, Hernandez-Reif M, Sunshine W, Douglas S. Fibromyalgia pain and substance P decrease and sleep improves after massage therapy. *J Clin Rheumatol.* 2002;8(2):72.

Forsyth LM, Preuss HG, MacDowell AL, et al. Therapeutic effects of oral NADH on the symptoms of patients with chronic fatigue syndrome. *Ann Allergy Asthma Immunol.* 1999;82:185–191.

Fukuda K, Straus SE, Hickie I, et al. The chronic fatigue syndrome: A comprehensive approach to its definition and study. International Chronic Fatigue Syndrome Study Group. *Ann Intern Med.* 1994;121:953.

Fulcher KY, White PD. Randomized controlled trial of graded exercise in patients with the chronic fatigue syndrome. *BMJ.* 1997;314:1647.

Goldenberg DL, Simms RW, Geiger A, Komaroff AL. High frequency of fibromyalgia in patients with chronic fatigue seen in a primary care practice. *Arthritis Rheum.* 1990;33:381.

Gordon C, Emiliozzi C, Zartarian M. Use of a mechanical massage technique in the treatment of fibromyalgia: a preliminary study. *Arch Phys Med Rehabil.* 2006;87(1):145–147.

Hadhazy VA, Ezzo J, Creamer P, Berman BM. Mind-body therapies for the treatment of fibromyalgia. A systematic review. *J Rheumatol.* 2000;27:2911–2918.

Harth M, Nielson WR. The fibromyalgia tender points: use them or lose them? A brief review of the controversy. *J Rheumatol.* 2007;34:914.

Himmel PB, Seligman TM. A pilot study employing dehydroepiandrosterone (DHEA) in the treatment of chronic fatigue syndrome. [Abstract] *J Clin Rheumatol.* 1999;5:56.

Hobday RA, Thomas S, O'Donovan A, Murphy M, Pinching AJ. Dietary intervention in chronic fatigue syndrome. *J Hum Nutr Diet.* 2008;21(2):141.

Inanici F, Yunus MB. History of fibromyalgia: past to present. *Curr Pain Headache Rep.* 2004;8(5):369.

Jacobsen S, Danneskiold-Samsoe B, Andersen RB. Oral S-adenosylmethionine in primary fibromyalgia. double-blind clinical evaluation. *Scand J Rheumatol.* 1991;20:294.

Jones KD, Adams D, Winters-Stone K, Burckhardt CS. A comprehensive review of 46 exercise treatment studies in fibromyalgia (1988–2005). *Health Qual Life Outcomes.* 2006;4:67.

Jones KD, Burckhardt CS, Clark SR, et al. A randomized controlled trial of muscle strengthening versus flexibility training in fibromyalgia. *J Rheumatol.* 2002;29:1041.

Kaartinen K, Lammi K, Hypen M, Nenonen M, Hanninen O, Rauma AL. Vegan diet alleviates fibromyalgia symptoms. *Scand J Rheumatol.* 2000;29:308.

Kerr JR, Burke B, Petty R, et al. Seven genomic subtypes of chronic fatigue syndrome/myalgic encephalomyelitis: a detailed analysis of gene networks and clinical phenotypes. *J Clin Path.* 2008a;61(6):730.

Kerr JR, Petty R, Burke B, et al. Gene expression subtypes in patients with chronic fatigue syndrome/myalgic encephalomyelitis. *J Infect Dis.* 2008b;197(8):1171.

Kim E. A brief history of chronic fatigue syndrome. *JAMA.* 1994;272:1070.

Kuratsune H, Yamaguti K, Sawada M, et al. Dehydroepiandrosterone sulfate deficiency in chronic fatigue syndrome. *Int J Mol Med.* 1998;1:143.

Landay AL, Jessop C, Lennette ET, Levy JA. Chronic fatigue syndrome: clinical condition associated with immune activation. *Lancet.* 1991;338:707.

Mannerkorpi K, Henriksson C. Non-pharmacological treatment of chronic widespread musculoskeletal pain. *Best Pract Res Clin Rheumatol.* 2007;21(3):513.

Martin DP, Sletten CD, Williams BA, Berger IH. Improvement in fibromyalgia symptoms with acupuncture: results of a randomized controlled trial. *Mayo Clin Proc.* 2006;81:749.

Mawle AC, Nisenbaum R, Dobbins JG, et al. Seroepidemiology of chronic fatigue syndrome: a case-control study. *Clin Infect Dis.* 1995;21:1386.

Mawle AC, Nisenbaum R, Dobbins JG, et al. Immune responses associated with chronic fatigue syndrome: a case-control study. *J Infect Dis.* 1997;175:136.

Mayhew E, Ernst E. Acupuncture for fibromyalgia—a systematic review of randomized clinical trials. *Rheumatology (Oxford).* 2007;46:801.

Meeus M, Nijs J. Central sensitization: a biopsychosocial explanation for chronic widespread pain in patients with fibromyalgia and chronic fatigue syndrome. *Clin Rheumatol.* 2007;26(4):465.

Nicolodi M, Sicuteri F. Fibromyalgia and migraine, two faces of the same mechanism. Serotonin as the common clue for pathogenesis and therapy. *Adv Exp Med Biol.* 1996;398:373.

Offenbaecher M, Bondy B, de Jonge S, et al. Possible association of fibromyalgia with a polymorphism in the serotonin transporter gene regulatory region. *Arthritis Rheum.* 1999;42:2482.

Pall M. *Explaining "Unexplained Illnesses."* New York: Harrington Park Press; 2007.

Plioplys AV, Plioplys S. Amantadine and L-carnitine treatment of Chronic Fatigue Syndrome. *Neuropsychobiology.* 1997;35:16.

Powell P, Bentall RP, Nye FJ, Edwards RH. Randomized controlled trial of patient education to encourage graded exercise in chronic fatigue syndrome. *BMJ.* 2001;322:387.

Prins JB, Bleijenberg G, Bazelmans E, et al. Cognitive behaviour therapy for chronic fatigue syndrome: a multicentre randomised controlled trial. *Lancet.* 2001;357:841.

Puttini PS, Caruso I. Primary fibromyalgia syndrome and 5-hydroxy-L-tryptophan: a 90-day open study. *J Int Med Res.* 1992;20:182–189.

Russell IJ, Michalek JE, Flechas JD, et al. Treatment of fibromyalgia syndrome with Super Malic: a randomized, double blind, placebo controlled, crossover pilot study. *J Rheumatol.* 1995;22:953–958.

Schacterle RS, Komaroff AL. A comparison of pregnancies that occur before and after the onset of chronic fatigue syndrome. *Arch Intern Med.* 2004;164:401.

Schwartz RB, Garada BM, Komaroff AL. Detection of intracranial abnormalities in patients with chronic fatigue syndrome: comparison of MRI imaging and SPECT. *AJR Am J Roentgenol.* 1994;162:935.

Straus SE, Tosato G, Armstrong G, et al. Persisting illness and fatigue in adults and evidence of Epstein-Barr virus infection. *Ann Intern Med.* 1985;102:7.

Tavoni A, Vitali C, Bombardieri S, Pasero G. Evaluation of S-adenosylmethionine in primary fibromyalgia. *Am J Med.* 1987;83(Suppl 5A):107.

Teitelbaum JE, Johnson C, St Cyr J. The use of D-ribose in chronic fatigue syndrome and fibromyalgia: a pilot study. *J Altern Complement Med.* 2006;12(9):857.

Tofferi JK, Jackson JL, O'Malley PG. Treatment of fibromyalgia with cyclobenzaprine: a meta-analysis. *Arthritis Rheum.* 2004;51:9.

van Heukelom RO, Prins JB, Smits MG, Bleijenberg G. Influence of melatonin on fatigue severity in patients with chronic fatigue syndrome and late melatonin secretion. *Eur J Neurol.* 2006;13(1):55.

Vermeulen RC, Scholte HR. Exploratory open label, randomized study of acetyl- and propionylcarnitine in chronic fatigue syndrome. *Psychosom Med.* 2004;66:276.

Walach H, Bosch H. Effectiveness of distant healing for patients with chronic fatigue syndrome: a randomised controlled partially blinded trial. *Psychother Psychosom.* 2008;77(3):158.

Wang C, Collet JP, Lau J. The effect of Tai Chi on health outcomes in patients with chronic conditions: a systematic review. *Arch Intern Med.* 2004;164(5):493.

Werbach MR. Nutritional strategies for treating chronic fatigue syndrome. *Altern Med Rev.* 2000;5(2):93.

Wolfe F, Ross K, Anderson J, et al. The prevalence and characteristics of fibromyalgia in the general population. *Arthritis Rheum.* 1995;38(1):19.

Wolfe F, Smythe HA, Yunus MB, et al. The American College of Rheumatology 1990 criteria for the classification of fibromyalgia: Report of the Multicenter Criteria Committee. *Arthritis Rheum.* 1990;33:160.

29

Rheumatoid Arthritis

NISHA J. MANEK

CASE STUDY

Teresa was rehearsing for her first dance performance in a musical. Her ankles and feet became swollen, painful, and stiff. She could barely move in the mornings, and the first hour of rehearsals was particularly difficult. She thought she had overdone her training and sprained her joints. She also felt more tired. During the previous 2 weeks, she noticed swelling in her hands, and she could no longer remove her wedding ring. Her hands also felt numb and weak, so much so that she dropped a cup of coffee. Because her feet had been painful for 2 months and now her hands were bothering her, her mother insisted that Teresa see a physician.

Introduction

This chapter will familiarize the reader with the epidemiology, diagnosis, and conventional and integrative management of rheumatoid arthritis (RA). It also will address the sex bias of this disease, with a focus on reproductive and hormonal issues. The goal is to provide the clinician with a framework to approach disease management for women with RA, to plan a treatment program, and to discuss the evidence for the more common integrative modalities for treatment of RA.

Epidemiology

Rheumatoid arthritis is an autoimmune disorder of unknown etiology, characterized by chronic destructive synovitis. RA has an estimated prevalence in the United States of approximately 1% of the adult population (Helmick et al. 2008). The disorder is two to three times more prevalent in women than in men (Gabriel et al. 1999) and has a higher prevalence (>5%) in some Native American populations (Ferucci et al. 2005). Disease onset typically occurs during the fifth or sixth decade of life, although onset during the third or fourth decade is not uncommon (Gabriel et al. 1999).

Risk Factors

Rheumatoid arthritis is a multifactorial disease resulting from the interaction of genetic and environmental factors (Aho and Heliovaara 2004; Turesson et al. 2004). Family studies demonstrate a genetic predisposition to the development of RA; for first-degree relatives of patients with RA, RA develops at a rate about four times that in the general population. The genetic basis is associated with human leukocyte antigen class II alleles, especially with the subtype DRB1 (Turesson et al. 2004). As for environmental risk factors, only smoking has been epidemiologically determined to be a potential risk factor for RA (Aho and Heliovaara 2004; Costenbader et al. 2006; Criswell et al. 2006; Karlson et al. 1999; Turesson et al. 2004). Diet also appears to influence predisposition to RA, but a specific nutrient has not been identified (Aho and Heliovaara 2004; Karlson et al. 2003).

REPRODUCTIVE AND ENDOCRINE FACTORS

The greater prevalence of RA among women argues for an effect of sex hormones on the disease. Women with RA report decreased joint pain during the postovulatory phase of the menstrual cycle and during pregnancy when estradiol and progesterone levels are high (Ansar Ahmed et al. 1985; Firestein 2001). In contrast, during the postpartum period, when estrogen and progesterone levels fall, RA symptoms usually flare. The first few months of the postpartum period are a time of increased risk for development of RA (Mathur et al. 1979). Nulliparity has been associated with an increased risk of developing RA (Ansar Ahmed and Talal 1989; Cutolo and Lahita 2005; Persellin 1976–1977; Rudge et al. 1983), and in some studies oral contraceptives were protective against RA (Carette et al. 1989; Kay and Wingrave 1983; Linos et al. 1983; Vandenbroucke et al. 1982, 1986). Previous studies including the Nurses' Health Study, a prospective cohort study of 121,700 women, have yielded conflicting results regarding potential associations of postmenopausal hormones and risk of RA (Bijlsma et al. 1987; D'Elia et al. 2003; Hall et al. 1994; Hernandez-Avila et al. 1990; MacDonald et al. 1994; Merlino et al. 2003).

Sex hormone balance is crucial in the regulation of immune and inflammatory responses. Estrogens enhance humoral immunity, production of autoantibodies (rheumatoid factor and anticyclic citrullinated peptide), and proliferation of monocytes and macrophages, cells which in turn upregulate proinflammatory cytokines such as tumor necrosis factor α. Increased concentrations of estrogens (and low concentrations of androgens) occur in the synovial fluid of patients of both sexes with RA. Hydroxylated estrogen metabolites, in particular 16-α-hydroxyestrone, have mitogenic and cell-proliferative effects (Cutolo et al. 2006).

Making the Diagnosis

No single finding on physical examination or laboratory testing is pathognomonic of RA. Instead, the diagnosis of RA is a clinical one, requiring the collection of historical and physical features, as well as an alert and informed clinician. Early consultation with a rheumatologist is recommended to help solidify the diagnosis. Table 29.1 lists the classification criteria for RA (Arnett et al. 1988). It is critical to note that the first four criteria must be present for at least 6 weeks before a diagnosis of RA can be made.

Morning stiffness is a hallmark of inflammatory arthritis and is a prominent feature of RA. Quantifying the degree of stiffness is important for measuring changes in RA disease activity. Early in disease onset, patients may have significant functional impairment of the joints (Ramey et al. 1996). The distribution of involved joints is a critical clue to the underlying diagnosis and should be investigated with specific questions from the clinician (Table 29.2). Most patients report involvement of small joints, classically the proximal interphalangeal, metacarpophalangeal, and metatarsophalangeal joints, followed by the wrists, knees, elbows, ankles, hips, and shoulders, in roughly that order. Of particular importance, RA almost always spares the distal interphalangeal joint. The physical findings on joint examination can be subtle; however, with intermediate and late stages of RA, joint deformities become apparent.

Table 29.1. 1987 Revised Criteria for the Classification of RA

1. Stiffness in and around joints lasting ≥1 hour before maximal improvement

2. Arthritis of ≥3 joint areas simultaneously, observed by a physician

3. Arthritis of the proximal interphalangeal, metacarpophalangeal, or wrist joint

4. Symmetric arthritis

5. Presence of rheumatoid nodules

6. Positive test for serum rheumatoid factor

7. Radiographic changes characteristic of RA (erosions and/or periarticular osteopenia in hand and/or wrist joints

A person can be classified as having RA if ≥4 criteria are present at any time

Criteria 1–4 must be present for more than 6 weeks

Criteria 2–5 must be observed by a physician

Patients do not have to have a positive test for rheumatoid factor to receive a diagnosis of RA. However, seronegative patients must have other characteristic clinical features for RA to be diagnosed.

Abbreviation: RA, rheumatoid arthritis.
Source: Adapted from Arnett et al. (1988). Used with permission.

Table 29.2. Questions Clinicians Should Ask the Patient

What hurts as you get out of bed in the morning?

How long does it take to feel as limber as you are going to feel for the day? Can you estimate in minutes or hours?

When is your pain the worst (morning or evening)?

Do you smoke?

Do any members of your family have RA?

Can you:

    Turn faucet handles?

    Hold a hairbrush/toothbrush?

    Dress/bathe independently?

    Fix your own breakfast?

    Walk outdoors on flat ground?

What are the activities that you cannot do because of your symptoms?

Source: From Ramey et al. (1996).

It is crucial not to mistakenly label osteoarthritis as RA. The distal interphalangeal joints are spared in RA but are involved in osteoarthritis; both diseases are common and can coexist, particularly in elderly patients. A careful history and joint examination to ascertain the pattern of arthritis can help distinguish the two conditions.

CASE STORY

When Teresa sought medical care for her pain, she reported severe pain in the balls of her feet and that it felt like she was "walking on marbles." She had metatarsalgia due to subluxation of the metatarsophalangeal joints. Also, she was found to have clinical symptoms of carpal tunnel syndrome, which often occur with the onset of RA.

Diagnostic Tests

The presence of rheumatoid factor (RF) is a characteristic laboratory abnormality in RA. RF is positive in about 50% of cases at presentation, and about 20%–35% of cases will become positive within the first 6 months after diagnosis. RF is an antibody that recognizes IgG as its antigen. A positive RF test is associated with more severe joint disease and with extra-articular features.

Recently developed enzyme-linked immunosorbent assays for anticyclic citrullinated peptide antibodies have nearly the same sensitivity (45%–70%) as those for RF and are more specific for RA (>95%). Anticyclic citrullinated peptide antibodies are found earlier in the disease course and predict a more severe outcome.

Other laboratory tests useful in supporting the diagnosis of RA include synovial fluid analysis, measurement of acute-phase reactants (erythrocyte sedimentation rate [ESR], C-reactive protein [CRP]), and complete blood count. Elevation of ESR, CRP level, or both provides a surrogate measure of active inflammation and may be useful for estimating prognosis and gauging response to therapy. The most common abnormality in the complete blood count among patients with RA is normochromic, normocytic anemia (anemia of chronic disease). The degree of anemia is in proportion to the activity of the disease. Thrombocytosis also may be seen with uncontrolled inflammation. In RA, synovial fluid is inflammatory, with negative results on microbiologic culture and crystal analysis.

Imaging

Early in the disease, plain radiographs may show only soft tissue swelling or joint effusion. Periarticular osteopenia is characteristic of RA. Nearly 70% of patients have development of bony erosions within the first 2 years of disease (Kirwan 2001), which portends a progressive course. Erosions may be seen in virtually any joint but are most common in the metatarsophalangeal, meta-carpophalangeal, and wrist joints. Plain radiographs are useful for helping to establish prognosis and assessing joint damage longitudinally. Magnetic reso-nance imaging may demonstrate erosions much earlier than conventional radi-ography and offers superior detail in depicting articular structures. However, its cost precludes its widespread use in the routine assessment of patients.

Rheumatoid Arthritis as a Multisystem Disease

In addition to the joints, RA also can affect the skin, lungs, heart, kidneys, nerves, eyes, and muscles. The expected survival of patients with RA decreases by 3–10 years according to the severity of the disease and the age at RA onset. Most of the excess deaths are attributable to infection, cardiovascular disease, and respiratory diseases (Gonzalez-Gay et al. 2005; Mikuls 2003; Naz and Symmons 2007). Patients younger than 55 years who are seropositive for RF appear to be most at risk for cardiovascular disease; women in this group there-fore require particular attention in terms of disease management and risk factor modification (Naz et al. 2008). The increased mortality may stem from acceler-ated atherogenesis caused by RA-related chronic inflammation (Solomon et al. 2003). RA also increases the risk of lymphoma, which appears to correlate with the severity of articular disease (Baecklund et al. 2004; Wolfe and Michaud 2004). Patients with RA are at increased risk for osteoporosis, and this risk should be considered and managed early (Phillips et al. 2006).

Conventional Treatment

Early identification of RA and referral for treatment is essential. Aggressive dis-ease-modifying antirheumatic drug (DMARD) therapy should be initiated as soon as possible to decrease long-term functional disability (Tanaka et al. 2008). Nonsteroidal anti-inflammatory drugs (NSAIDs) and corticosteroids may be prescribed in the early stages. Corticosteroids have been shown, especially in the first 6 months after RA onset, to reduce radiographic disease progression. Low-dose corticosteroids (≤10 mg/day prednisone, or equivalent) may be used as a bridge therapy until longer-acting DMARDs become effective.

Methotrexate is the staple of DMARD treatment (Table 29.3), and a combination approach such as methotrexate and hydroxychloroquine is often prescribed (Saag et al. 2008). Close follow-up and repeat regular evaluations are necessary to assess response to treatment. For women who have an inadequate response to 3 months of aggressively dosed methotrexate, the addition of a tumor necrosis factor (TNF) inhibitor is highly effective and generally safe. No evidence suggests that one TNF inhibitor is superior to another, and the selection of TNF inhibitor is often based on patient preference.

I check the Health Assessment Questionnaire disability index of the patient (Stanford University School of Medicine 2003) at every visit. The Health Assessment Questionnaire is a strong clinical predictor of mortality; a change of 1 standard deviation results in an odds ratio for mortality of 2.3 (Wolfe et al. 2003).

For patients with RA, living with the disease requires that they manage symptoms, balance emotional states (Parker et al. 2003; VanDyke et al. 2004), adjust to changes in physical status and social activity (Katz and Yelin 2001), learn self-management strategies, and communicate with health professionals in various disciplines. An integrated, interdisciplinary care plan is shown in Table 29.4. Such a plan, in addition to conventional DMARD therapy, includes educational, social, vocational, and occupational support.

I regularly send my patients to the Arthritis Self-Management Program, which has been shown to increase exercise and to help decrease pain, disability, and physician and emergency room visits (Lorig et al. 1993).

CASE STUDY

Teresa gave up her career on stage as a dancer. Instead, she began to volunteer with youth groups, became active in her church, and learned as much as she could about her condition. She has become an empowering voice for self-care in RA and was recently invited to participate in the production of a video series on wellness solutions for arthritis. Her husband and mother also have become involved in learning about RA and are an important source of support for her.

Table 29.3. DMARDs Commonly Used to Treat RA

DMARD/Biologic Therapy	Primary Benefits	Disadvantages	Common Adverse Effects	Rare Adverse Effects	Laboratory Tests[a]
Methotrexate	Well-tolerated, once-weekly medication; *gold standard* for managing RA; administered with folic acid; slows radiographic damage	Contraindicated for potentially childbearing women; if used, need adequate contraception	Nausea, alopecia, fatigue, gingivitis, glossitis, oral ulcers, headaches, elevated LFTs; patients must not consume alcohol	Hepatotoxicity, pneumonitis, cytopenias	CBC, AST, albumin every 8 weeks
Hydroxychloroquine	Effective for mild disease and in combination with methotrexate	Takes 3–6 months to become effective; does not halt radiographic progression	Diarrhea, bloating, anorexia, rash	Retinopathy, neuromyopathy	Annual ophthalmologic exam
Sulfasalazine	Effective for mild to moderate disease; may be used in combination with other agents; slows radiographic progression	Contraindicated for patients who have sulfa allergies	GI effects, headache, rash	Cytopenias, hepatotoxicity	CBC every 2–4 weeks for 3 months, then every 3 months
Leflunomide	For moderate to severe disease; slows radiographic progression	Greater cost; long half-life; contraindicated for childbearing women	Diarrhea, nausea, anorexia, alopecia, fatigue, headache, elevated LFTs	Hepatotoxicity, pulmonary fibrosis	CBC, AST, albumin every 4–8 weeks

(continued)

Table 29.3. (Continued)

DMARD/Biologic Therapy	Primary Benefits	Disadvantages	Common Adverse Effects	Rare Adverse Effects	Laboratory Tests[a]
Infliximab	Highly effective for moderate to severe disease; slows radiographic damage	High cost; administered with methotrexate; infused every 6–8 weeks after loading doses	Injection-site reactions; increased risk of bacterial infection; safety in pregnancy unclear; avoid in nursing mothers	Opportunistic infection; reactivation of TB; lupus-like reactions; possible increase in lymphoma; demyelination	None unless patient also receiving other DMARDs
Etanercept	Highly effective for moderate to severe disease; slows radiographic damage	High cost; subcutaneous injections once or twice weekly	Injection-site reactions; increased risk of bacterial infection; safety in pregnancy unclear; avoid in nursing mothers	Opportunistic infection; reactivation of TB; lupus-like reactions; possible increase in lymphoma not yet determined; demyelination	None generally unless patient also receiving other DMARDs
Adalimumab	Highly effective for moderate to severe disease; slows radiographic damage	High cost; subcutaneous injections every other week or weekly	Injection-site reactions; increased risk of bacterial infections; safety in pregnancy unclear; avoid in nursing mothers	Opportunistic infection; reactivation of TB; lupuslike reactions; possible increase in lymphoma, demyelination	None unless receiving other DMARDs

Drug	Effectiveness	Administration/cost	Adverse effects	Serious adverse effects	Tests needed to monitor for adverse effects[a]
Anakinra	Effective in subsets of patients with RA; can be used in patients at risk for TB who cannot use a TNF antagonist; slows radiographic damage	High cost; daily subcutaneous injections; less effective than TNF antagonists at symptom relief	Injection-site reactions can be severe; increased risk of bacterial infections; safety in pregnancy unclear; avoid in nursing mothers	Cytopenias	CBC monthly for 3 months, then every 3 months
Abatacept	Effective in patients nonresponsive to methotrexate or TNF inhibitors; slows radiographic damage	High cost; administered as 30-minute infusion every 4 weeks	Mild to moderate infusion reactions; increased risk of bacterial infection (especially in patients with underlying lung disease)	Infections; possible increased risk of cancer	None unless patient also receiving other DMARDs
Rituximab	Effective in long-standing, active RA with inadequate response to TNF antagonist therapy; efficacy may persist many months after infusion	Administered as 2 separate 3–4-hour infusions 2 weeks apart; administration of IV methylprednisolone recommended minutes before infusion to prevent serious reactions; delay in clinical response	Mild to moderate infusion reactions; increased risk of bacterial infection	Severe infusion reactions; medications and supportive care measures should be available during infusion; repeat administration may be associated with lower immunoglobulin levels	CBC and platelet counts should be obtained at regular intervals and more frequently in patients with cytopenias

Abbreviations: AST, aspartase aminotransferase; CBC, compete blood count; DMARD, disease-modifying antirheumatic drug; GI, gastrointestinal tract; IV, intravenous; LFT, liver function test; RA, rheumatoid arthritis; TB, tuberculosis; TNF, tumor necrosis factor.

[a]Tests needed to monitor for adverse effects.

Table 29.4. A Comprehensive Care Plan for RA

	Approach		
Physical	*Educational*	*Psychological*	*Social*

Diagnostic procedures
Medication
Joint injections
Immunizations
   Influenza annually
   Pneumovax every 5
   years after 65 years
   Tetanus/diptheria
   every 10 years
Primary prevention of
coronary artery
disease (blood
pressure and lipid
control)
Osteoporosis
prophylaxis
Management of extra-
articular disease (e.g.,
sicca symptoms)
	Arthritis self-
	management
	Program
	Instruction regarding
	medication (dosages,
	adverse effects, and lab
	monitoring)
	Methods of compliance
	Smoking cessation
	Alcohol abstinence
	Use of orthotics/
	adaptive equipment
	Contraception in
	women of childbearing
	age
	Weight control
	  −Fasting in select
	  patients
	  −Juice fasting
	Diet and supplements
	  −Whole foods, limit
	  red meat intake
	  −ω-3 fatty acids
	  −γ-linolenic acid
		Aid in coping
		with:
		Depression
		  Anxiety
		  Anger
		  Low self-
		  esteem
		  Changes in
		  lifestyle
		Suggest:
		  Guided
		  imagery
		  Daily
		  meditation
		  Daily
		  journal
		  writing
			Finances for
			medical and daily
			living
			Avoidance of
			isolation
			  Therapeutic or
			  healing touch
			  Soft-tissue
			  massage
			Employment
			counseling
			Home care
			Sexual
			counseling

Splinting (e.g., wrist
splints for carpal
tunnel syndrome)
	Exercise
	  −Warm-water
	  exercise
	  −Tai Chi and Qigong
	  −Yoga with qualified
	  instructor		

Adaptive equipment Surgery			

Sexual Health, Fertility, and Pregnancy in RA

The burden imposed by RA on the patient and the family can be considerable, and intimate relationships can be strained because of chronic pain (Sterba et al. 2008). Both partners must understand the cyclic nature of RA (Kasle et al. 2008) and be responsive to each other's needs to decrease the risk of depressive symptoms. Contraception is necessary, especially if a woman is of childbearing age or is taking methotrexate or leflunomide, which are teratogenic.

Research is needed to establish the safety of biologic agents in pregnancy and lactation. Up to 75% of women with RA have remission of the disease during pregnancy, but this effect reverts in the postpartum period. Although TNF inhibitors are classified by the U.S. Food and Drug Administration as pregnancy category B, few would disagree that TNF inhibitors should be avoided just before or during pregnancy until more data are available (Golding et al. 2007). However, many patients risk permanent functional and structural disability if treatment is stopped for a prolonged period. A reasonable compromise for women with severe arthritis is to allow continuation of TNF inhibitors until the time of conception, with short-term use of low-dose prednisone permitted, as required, during the pregnancy. Given the known teratogenicity of methotrexate and leflunomide, TNF inhibitors might offer disease control while conception is attempted, which, for some, can be a lengthy interval. Appropriately timed withdrawal of methotrexate and leflunomide and continuation of TNF inhibitors until pregnancy allows some protection for the patient with what appears to be minimal risk to the fetus.

Integrative Therapies: A Look at the Evidence in RA

Patients with RA often use integrative treatment modalities, particularly herbal medicines, nutritional supplements (Resch et al. 1997), and modification of dietary habits. Evidence for the effectiveness of these treatments, however, is sparse. Therefore, recommendations for a particular integrative modality must be made in the context of each woman's needs and generally should be considered adjunctive to treatment with conventional DMARDs. Integrative modalities can, in many cases, offer the patient a sense of autonomy in the decision-making process for her treatment regimen. The different integrative treatments are summarized in Table 29.5.

Table 29.5. Evidence for Integrative Therapies for RA

Integrative Therapy	Recommendations	Comments
Botanicals and herbal medicine		
Boswellia serrata (Soeken et al. 2003)	Combination product (Articulin-F) used in studies of osteoarthritis	Use cautiously in patients with preexisting gastritis or GERD. Thus far, preliminary data in RA are negative; therefore, not recommended.
Cat's claw (*Uncaria tomentosa*) (Mur et al. 2002)	Optimal dose unknown	Preliminary data need confirmation in larger studies before cat's claw can be recommended as adjunctive treatment for RA.
γ-Linolenic acid (borage seed oil, evening primrose oil, black currant seed oil) (Soeken 2004)	Optimal dose and duration unknown	Pooled results show decreases in pain and morning stiffness compared with placebo. Mechanism of action of γ-linolenic acid appears to be suppressing the release of inflammatory mediators.
Ginger root (*Zingiber officinale*) (Srivastava and Mustafa 1992)	Dose unknown	No trial data in RA; ginger is used in Ayurvedic treatment for "rheumatism" and muscular aches. Generally, intake may be associated with dyspeptic symptoms.
Phytodolor (combination of *Populus tremula, Fraxinux excelsior, Solidago virgaurea*) (Gundermann and Muller 2007; Weiner and Ernst 2004)	Half strength to double strength for 4 weeks	Significant pain reduction achieved in trials using all strengths of Phytodolor, with no significant difference between them. Appears to have similar pain-relieving effects as traditional NSAIDs.
Resveratrol (grape extract) (Elmali et al. 2007)	No dose-ranging studies available	Preliminary data promising as an anti-inflammatory agent. Appears to exert effects via the NF-κ B pathway.
Turmeric (*Curcuma longa* rhizome) (Khanna et al. 2007)	No dose-ranging studies available	Studies in animal models of RA show promising results for curcumin as potential adjunctive treatment for human RA. Available in combination or single-herb preparation. Popular spice in Indian cuisine.

(continued)

Integrative Therapy	Recommendations	Comments
Thunder god vine (*Tripterygium wilfordii* Hook) (Cibere et al. 2003; Tao et al. 2002)	Trials used low dose (180 mg/d) or high dose (360 mg/d) for 20 weeks followed by open-label extension	Trials are small and require larger numbers for confirmation; most common adverse effect reported is diarrhea. Rare serious adverse effects include cytopenias; therefore, it must be taken under close physician supervision, and blood counts must be regularly checked.

Dietary methods, minerals, vitamins, and supplements

Fasting and vegetarianism (Pattison et al. 2004)	Whole-food diet with various fruits and vegetables; emphasis on oily fish such as wild salmon twice weekly	
		Long-term fasting is not recommended; risk of weight loss and malnourishment exists, especially because patients with RA may be catabolic.
Calcium (Khazai et al. 2008)	1200 mg/day	Can be taken in food (dairy) or as supplements. Especially recommended if receiving corticosteroid therapy.
Vitamin D (dietary and supplemental) (Kharzai et al. 2008)	800 IU of cholecalciferol daily	Vitamin D levels should be checked at least annually to ensure optimal 25(OH)D levels. Greater intake of vitamin D may be associated with a lower risk of RA in older women.
ὼ-3 Fish oil (Goldberg and Katz 2007)	3 g/day	Delay of therapeutic effect for up to 3 mo; use caution in patients taking anticoagulants, and more frequent coagulation checks advised.
Selenium (Peretz et al. 2001)	200 µg/day	Compared with placebo, no difference in RA activity observed.

(continued)

Table 29.5. (Continued)

Integrative Therapy	Recommendations	Comments
Exercise and physical activity		
Tai Chi/Qigong (Han et al. 2004)	Training required with an experienced tai chi teacher. Frequency, intensity, and duration of tai chi required to achieve improved joint function are not clear	Trials noted poor compliance with tai chi. Appears to be safe. A statistically significant and clinically important benefit of tai chi was demonstrated compared with controls. No detrimental effects on RA disease activity observed.
Yoga (Haslock et al. 1994)	Asanas, or postures, most beneficial for RA unknown	Must be done under supervision with a trained and certified yoga teacher. Probably useful in select patients if RA is controlled.
Alternative health systems		
Acupuncture and electroacupuncture (Casimiro et al. 2005)	Trials used weekly treatment for 5 weeks	Parameters of needling may vary from visit to visit and among different practitioners. Not recommended for RA based on current data.
Ayurveda (Park and Ernst 2005)	Mixtures vary in content, composition, and duration of use depending on the trial and practitioner	The weight of trial evidence has not been encouraging, and caution is required.
Homeopathy (Fisher and Scott 2001; Jonas et al. 2000)	Interventions reported in the literature varied widely (individualized or classic), and outcomes measured also varied	The small number of studies limits any definitive conclusion concerning any one type of homeopathic treatment in RA. In general, quality concerns exist for homeopathic clinical trials; therefore, homeopathy cannot be rigorously recommended for RA at this time.

(continued)

Integrative Therapy	Recommendations	Comments
Naturopathy (Dunn and Wilkinson 2005)	No trial data available	Combination of herbal and nutritional approach to treatment of inflammatory conditions. Unknown in which group of patients naturopathy is helpful.
Traditional Chinese medicine (He et al. 2008)	Practice varies with TCM practitioner	Research in China comparing conventional care with TCM for RA showed conventional care superior in achieving a therapeutic effect, as measured by American College of Rheumatology response; generally not recommended in combination with conventional care.
Mind–body practices		
Cognitive-behavioral therapy (Sharpe et al. 2008)	8 individual weekly therapist–client sessions	Program includes educational component plus self-management skills: relaxation training, attention diversion, goal setting, and management of flare-ups.
Mindfulness meditation	Daily practice for at least 30 minutes	RA patients with depressive symptoms benefited the most from meditation, including negative and positive affect and physicians' rating of joint tenderness. Daily diary may be used to assist with compliance with meditation.
Mindfulness-Based Stress Reduction Program (Pradhan et al. 2007)	8-week MBSR course and 4-month maintenance program	Significant improvements in psychological distress and well-being observed after MBSR plus a 4-month program of continued reinforcement. No effect on RA disease activity was observed.
Guided imagery and visualization	Daily practice recommended; programs vary in length but generally are a minimum of 20 minutes	Excellent audio recordings available; cost-effective; good adjunctive treatment for many patients; combines music with visualizations and affirmations.

(continued)

Table 29.5. (Continued)

Integrative Therapy	Recommendations	Comments
Massage and therapeutic touch	Effects vary and caution is required, especially with swollen joints. RA potentially can flare	Especially useful in elderly patients with chronic pain. Further studies needed for cost-effectiveness. May alleviate social isolation; may be expensive for many patients.
Spiritual and contemplative practices		
Prayer and worship (Bartlett et al. 2003; Keefe et al. 2001; McCauley et al. 2008)	Spiritual and religious practices vary widely	In some cases of negative coping mechanisms, referral to a counselor may be helpful. Also, a daily diary or journal can assist.
Structured writing (Smyth et al. 1999)	20 minutes of writing daily for 3 consecutive days of the week	Writing about stressful life experiences showed clinically relevant changes in health status of patients with RA at 4 month beyond those attributable to standard medical care; a simple psychological exercise can potentially reduce symptoms of a chronic disease.

Abbreviations: GERD, gastroesophageal reflux disease; MBSR, mindfulness-based stress reduction; NSAID, nonsteroidal anti-inflammatory drug; RA, rheumatoid arthritis; TCM, traditional Chinese medicine; 25(OH)D, vitamin D, 25-hydroxy.

ACUPUNCTURE

A Cochrane Review evaluated the use of acupuncture or electroacupuncture in patients with RA (Casimiro et al. 2005). Two randomized controlled trials (RCTs) ($n = 84$), 1 each for acupuncture and electroacupuncture, were reviewed. For acupuncture, no significant differences were observed in pain levels, number of swollen and tender joints, disease activity, CRP levels, or amount of pain medication needed compared with sham procedure. A short-term decrease in knee pain was reported for the trial of electroacupuncture, but the authors of the review believed that the trial was of low quality and may have overestimated how well acupuncture works. Another recent pilot study ($n = 36$) reported promising results that will lead to the design of a large-scale trial, which may help clarify the role for acupuncture in RA (Tam et al. 2007). At this time, poor trial data preclude recommendation of acupuncture for RA.

AYURVEDA AND TRADITIONAL CHINESE MEDICINE

A systematic review assessed the evidence from all RCTs on the effectiveness of Ayurvedic herbal medicine (Park and Ernst 2005). Three trials tested Ayurvedic medicines against placebo, and four trials compared different Ayurvedic preparations. Overall, the studies failed to show convincingly that such treatments are effective therapeutic options for RA (Park and Ernst 2005). Traditional Chinese medicine also has been compared with conventional Western care. Conventional care was more effective in the treatment of RA than traditional Chinese medicine with regard to efficacy, as measured by American College of Rheumatology response (He et al. 2008).

Thunder god vine (*Tripterygium wilfordii* Hook) is recommended in traditional Chinese medicine for many conditions. Three RCTs suggested that it has anti-inflammatory properties and efficacy in decreasing objective and subjective symptoms of RA (Cibere et al. 2003; Tao et al. 1989, 2002). However, toxicity is concerning, and the product used in the clinical trials is not readily available in the marketplace.

BOTANICAL MEDICINES

A Cochrane Review of herbal treatments for RA concluded that the use of γ-linolenic acid (GLA) appears to offer some potential benefit in RA, although further research is needed to establish optimum dosage and duration of treatment (Little and Parsons 2001). Another systematic review of the use of GLA included 14 RCTs; the findings suggested moderate support for GLA in reducing pain, number of tender joints, and stiffness (Soeken et al. 2003). Effect size by visual analog scale was 0.76 (95% confidence interval [CI], 0.37–1.15) for pain, 0.93 (95% CI, 0.47–1.38) for tender joint count, and 0.23 (95% CI, 0.02–0.90) for stiffness. Long-term safety data, efficacy, and potential drug interactions remain unknown for GLA.

Phytodolor (Steigerwald Arzneimittelwerk GMBH, Darmstadt, Germany), a proprietary medicine containing extracts of *Populus tremula*, *Fraxinus excelsior*, and *Solidago virgaurea*, has been evaluated in clinical trials. Phytodolor was as effective as standard NSAIDs in alleviating pain and improving joint function (Gundermann and Muller 2007; Weiner and Ernst 2004).

An extract of *Uncaria tomentosa* (cat's claw) was tested in 40 patients who were receiving treatment with sulfasalazine or hydroxychloroquine for their RA (Mur et al. 2003). After 24 weeks of treatment, a modest decrease in the number of painful joints with active extract was noted compared with placebo. This small preliminary study requires independent replication. Single RCTs reporting negative results exist for boswellia (*Boswellia serrata*) (Soeken et al. 2003), feverfew (*Tanacetum parthenium*) (Soeken et al. 2003), and willow (*Salix* spp) bark extract (Biegert et al. 2004). Ginger root (*Zingiber officinale*), used widely in Ayurveda and used by patients with various rheumatic conditions, has not been studied in RA (Srivastava and Mustafa 1992).

DIET

The question of the role of diet in prevention and treatment of RA is frequently asked by patients. Scientific data to illuminate this question are emerging. Pattison and colleagues (2004) reported the first prospective investigation of the association between meat intake and RA; their data suggest a link between meat intake and the risk of inflammatory polyarthritis or RA, but this has not been confirmed in other studies (Benito-Garcia et al. 2007). Many types of diets have been studied in association with RA. For example, long-term adherence to a Mediterranean-type diet may decrease the risk of RA and protect against a severe course of the disease (Skoldstam et al. 2003). Other dietary factors of interest include the lack of an association between coffee and tea consumption and risk of RA among women (Karlson et al. 2003; Mikuls et al. 2002), whereas available data suggest an inverse association between vitamin D intake (dietary and supplemental) and risk of RA (highest vs. lowest tertile: relative risk, 0.67 [95% CI, 0.44–1.00]; $P = .05$) (Merlino et al. 2004). RA is an independent risk factor for fracture development, and therefore adequate vitamin D and calcium intake are crucial for women with RA (Khazai et al. 2008). Other popular dietary recommendations include green tea, soy products, and avoidance of dairy, but no trial data exist. Extracts of pineapple (bromelain) (Walker et al. 2002), cherries (Marcason 2007), garlic, and ginger also have anecdotal evidence of efficacy against RA.

> The dietary advice I give each of my patients is to choose whole foods based on her own food preferences and habitual foods, which thereby facilitates her well-being (Gustafsson et al. 2005). Some clinicians advocate short-term fasting and juice fasting; in select women, especially if they are overweight, this can aid in disease control. I do not routinely advocate fasting because active RA is a catabolic disease, and malnourishment can be an issue. If the patient does fast, it must be done under close physician supervision.

ENERGY MEDICINE

Reiki and healing touch can be beneficial, especially for elderly women with RA. Few data exist on these modalities, however. In my experience, healing touch can offer a sense of well-being, relaxation, and acceptance in some patients.

EXERCISE AND PHYSICAL ACTIVITY

A Cochrane Review assessed the evidence for use of Tai Chi for treatment of RA (Han et al. 2004). Tai Chi appears to have beneficial effects on range of motion outcomes and functional status (Wang 2008). Qigong, a related technique of gentle exercise, also can be used to help maintain physical strength.

Few data exist on the use of yoga (Haslock et al. 1994), the Feldenkrais method, or pilates as exercise options for patients with RA. Personally, I have recommended these techniques to select women after their arthritis was in remission to help them maintain a good range of motion and flexibility. I also have recommended aquatherapy, and many fitness centers have an Arthritis Foundation program for water exercise in a warm pool under the supervision of a qualified instructor.

HOMEOPATHY

A review summarized three RCTs ($n = 266$) of homeopathic treatments for RA (Jonas et al. 2000). Two studies evaluated classic individualized homeopathy in patients with RA and did not show beneficial effects (odds ratio [95% CI], 2.04 [0.66–6.34]), whereas positive effects were reported in the third trial. No single homeopathic remedy emerged as more efficacious than the other. Another RCT found no evidence that homeopathy improves symptoms of RA over 3 months in patients taking NSAIDs or DMARDs (Fisher and Scott 2001). High-quality research is needed in this area to clarify which patients with RA may potentially benefit from homeopathy (Soeken 2004).

ITEMS WORN

Magnets are popular with many patients with RA. Studies of the wearing of static magnets found these not to be significantly different from wearing control devices (Segal et al. 2001). No data are available in support of the widely popular copper jewelry and crystals.

MIND–BODY

It is a well-observed phenomenon that stress can adversely affect RA. Mind–body practices are varied and include imagery, relaxation, meditation, and hypnotherapy. Most trials using hypnotherapy suggest that it can be useful in pain management; specifically, pain perception appears to be influenced positively (Torem 2007). No rigorous trials have been conducted of hypnotherapy for RA, but some anecdotal reports have recommended hypnotherapy as a treatment for juvenile RA (Cioppa and Thal 1974, 1975; Lovell and Walco 1989). Some of my own patients have taught themselves self-hypnosis; this requires patience and practice but can help in coping with symptoms of joint discomfort and pain (Yocum et al. 2000). Similarly, guided imagery and visualization can be used successfully (Walco et al. 1992). Some high-quality audio recordings are available, and for some women they can profoundly improve qualify of life.

Mindfulness meditation (Zautra et al. 2008) and the popular mindfulness-based stress reduction (MBSR) (Pradhan et al. 2007) have been studied in association with RA. Patients with RA who have chronic depression benefited most from mindfulness meditation across several measures, including negative and positive affect and physicians' ratings of joint tenderness (Zautra et al. 2008). Significant improvements in psychological distress (P = .04) and well-being (P = .03) were observed after an 8-week MBSR class plus a 4-month program of continued reinforcement, which indicates that MBSR may complement conventional disease management (Pradhan et al. 2007).

Cognitive-behavioral therapies (CBT) include the teaching of life and coping skills and the application of these skills in the patient's home and work environment (Ottonello 2007). Studies suggest that CBT is efficacious in RA for not only psychological adjustment but also physical functioning; it is also associated with fewer long-term doctor visits, resulting in decreased health care costs (Sharpe et al. 2008).

Other mind–body practices include muscle relaxation, music, spa therapy, and massage, which, although not rigorously tested in clinical trials, enjoy widespread popularity. Many patients have a standing appointment for massages or even receive a decreased cost for treatments because they go on a regular basis.

CASE STORY

Teresa regularly listens to a guided-imagery tape. She has avoided increases in medications such as corticosteroids in the short term because she is able to manage her level of joint pain with visualization. With practice, Teresa has developed this skill and goes to a "safe place" immediately whenever she perceives undue stress or pain.

SPIRITUAL PRACTICE AND PRAYER

Underwood and Teresi (2002) note that positive emotional experiences and expectations have been linked with favorable effects on immune functioning, independent of the negative effects of stress. Spirituality (defined as a psychological dimension around which individuals organize their lives, goals, values, and intentions) was an independent predictor of happiness and positive health perceptions, even after controlling for disease activity and physical functioning and for age and mood (Bartlett et al. 2003; McCauley et al. 2008). In contrast, negative religious coping (such as emotional venting) in persons with RA is significantly associated with depressive symptoms (VandeCreek et al. 2004) and can pose clinical challenges for the patient and her doctor. Religiously trained counselors may be helpful if the patient will accept a referral. Some patients may find it helpful to start a daily journal or diary to express their positive and negative emotions on paper (Keefe et al. 2001; Smyth et al. 1999).

Supplements

Fish oil is rich in the ω-3 polyunsaturated fatty acids (PUFAs) eicosapentaenoic acid and docosahexaenoic acid, which have been shown to have anti-inflammatory activity through interfering with prostaglandin metabolism (Goldberg and Katz 2007). Higher doses of ω-3 PUFAs (>2.7 g/day) were associated with improvements in morning stiffness and number of painful or tender joints; a minimum of 3 months of use is required for a therapeutic effect. Long-chain ω-3 PUFAs compete with other fatty acids for incorporation into phospholipids. Reducing the intake of ω-6 fatty acids (e.g., linoleic acid), which are metabolized to arachidonic acid and inflammatory eicosanoids, would be expected to increase the effectiveness of ώ-3 PUFA supplements (Adam et al. 2003). Of interest, α-linolenic acid (from flaxseed oil), which is a precursor of ώ-3 PUFAs, does not seem to have the same clinical effects (Nordstrom et al. 1995).

Green-lipped mussel (*Perna canaliculus*) has been shown to have anti-inflammatory effects (Halpern 2000), but a recent systematic review found little compelling evidence for the therapeutic use of freeze-dried green-lipped mussel powder for RA (Cobb and Ernst 2006).

Probiotics have been studied in RA, and oral administration of *Lactobacillus casei* has been shown to suppress arthritis in animal models by downregulating T-helper effector cell functions (So et al. 2008). A small RCT ($n = 21$) tested the effects of *Lactobacillus rhamnosus* but found no differences in results of clinical examination, the Health Assessment Questionnaire, ESR, or CRP compared with placebo (Hatakka et al. 2003).

Patients with RA may not be achieving the recommended daily intake of minerals such as calcium, zinc, and selenium (Stone et al. 1997); therefore, patients with RA should receive dietary education and/or supplementation. If the patient is taking methotrexate, folic acid is prescribed concurrently. Selenium has been tested in an RCT: no difference in pain, swollen joint count, or morning stiffness was noted compared with placebo, although both groups improved, demonstrating a placebo effect of the interventional trial (Peretz et al. 2001).

Other popular supplements include turmeric, a popular spice used in Asian cuisine. The active component, curcumin, has been studied in animal models of RA, with very promising results (Funk et al. 2006; Khanna et al. 2007). Resveratrol, the compound that gives red grapes the characteristic red color, has been shown to have anti-inflammatory properties (Elmali et al. 2007; Udenigwe et al. 2008). To date no trials have been conducted in human RA. I do, however, advise patients to try turmeric (or curcumin), provided they do not have a history of dyspepsia or are not taking warfarin, because of the potential for drug interactions.

Overall, the current evidence suggests that patients with RA should consume a diet rich in ώ-3 PUFAs, GLA, and vitamin D (Rennie et al. 2003).

Resources for Health Care Providers

The Arthritis Foundation's Guide to Alternative Treatments for Arthritis presents brief overviews of therapies, and the references cited in this chapter are from highly reputable journals (Foltz-Gray 2005). The Arthritis Foundation also maintains an informative Web site (2008) and a guide to alternative therapies online (http://www.arthritis.org/conditions/alttherapies). In addition, *Arthritis Today* magazine is published monthly by the Arthritis Foundation and prints annual supplement guides that present information on vitamins, herbs, and natural remedies.

The National Center for Complementary and Alternative Medicine maintains a helpful Web site with fact sheets and press alerts on complementary and alternative medicine therapies for arthritis (http://www.nccam.nih.gov).

Summary and Conclusions

Use of integrative therapies by women with RA can potentially improve the inflammation and associated symptoms. From the evidence presented here, it would be reasonable to consider Phytodolor, fish oil, and GLA supplements and gentle exercise such as Tai Chi. The effect sizes are moderate to small, and therefore integrative therapy should be considered adjuvant to conventional care. Importantly, mind–body techniques and CBT offer women with RA the skills to cope with and thrive with chronic illness. Effective health promotion requires a partnership between the patient, the family, and the community, as well as the health care provider. Integrative health care and open dialogue about integrative modalities are congruent with this goal.

REFERENCES

Adam O, Beringer C, Kless T, et al. Anti-inflammatory effects of a low arachidonic acid diet and fish oil in patients with rheumatoid arthritis. *Rheumatol Int.* 2003;23(1):27–36. Epub September 6, 2002.

Aho K, Heliovaara M. Risk factors for rheumatoid arthritis. *Ann Med.* 2004;36(4):242–251.

Ansar Ahmed S, Penhale WJ, Talal N. Sex hormones, immune responses, and autoimmune diseases: mechanisms of sex hormone action. *Am J Pathol.* 1985;121(3):531–551.

Ansar Ahmed S, Talal N. Sex hormones and autoimmune rheumatic disorders. *Scand J Rheumatol.* 1989;18(2):69–76.

Arnett FC, Edworthy SM, Bloch DA, et al. The American Rheumatism Association 1987 revised criteria for the classification of rheumatoid arthritis. *Arthritis Rheum.* 1988;31(3):315–324.

Arthritis Foundation. http://www.arthritis.org. Accessed August 2008.

Arthritis Foundation. "Alternative therapies." http://www.arthritis.org/alternatives.php. Accessed August 2008.

Baecklund E, Askling J, Rosenquist R, Ekbom A, Klareskog L. Rheumatoid arthritis and malignant lymphomas. *Curr Opin Rheumatol.* 2004;16(3):254–261.

Bartlett SJ, Piedmont R, Bilderback A, Matsumoto AK, Bathon JM. Spirituality, well-being, and quality of life in people with rheumatoid arthritis. *Arthritis Rheum.* 2003;49(6):778–783.

Benito-Garcia E, Feskanich D, Hu FB, Mandl LA, Karlson EW. Protein, iron, and meat consumption and risk for rheumatoid arthritis: a prospective cohort study. *Arthritis Res Ther*. 2007;9(1):R16.

Biegert C, Wagner I, Ludtke R, et al. Efficacy and safety of willow bark extract in the treatment of osteoarthritis and rheumatoid arthritis: results of 2 randomized double-blind controlled trials. *J Rheumatol*. 2004;31(11):2121–2130.

Bijlsma JW, Huber-Bruning O, Thijssen JH. Effect of oestrogen treatment on clinical and laboratory manifestations of rheumatoid arthritis. *Ann Rheum Dis*. 1987;46(10):777–779.

Carette S, Marcoux S, Gingras S. Postmenopausal hormones and the incidence of rheumatoid arthritis. *J Rheumatol*. 1989;16(7):911–913.

Casimiro L, Barnsley L, Brosseau L, et al. Acupuncture and electroacupuncture for the treatment of rheumatoid arthritis. *Cochrane Database Syst Rev*. 2005;(4):CD003788.

Cibere J, Deng Z, Lin Y, et al. A randomized double blind, placebo controlled trial of topical Tripterygium wilfordii in rheumatoid arthritis: reanalysis using logistic regression analysis. *J Rheumatol*. 2003;30(3):465–467.

Cioppa FJ, Thal AB. Rheumatoid arthritis, spontaneous remission, and hypnotherapy [letter]. *JAMA*. 1974;230(10):1388–1389.

Cioppa FJ, Thal AD. Hypnotherapy in a case of juvenile rheumatoid arthritis. *Am J Clin Hypn*. 1975;18(2):105–110.

Cobb CS, Ernst E. Systematic review of a marine nutriceutical supplement in clinical trials for arthritis: the effectiveness of the New Zealand green-lipped mussel Perna canaliculus. *Clin Rheumatol*. 2006;25(3):275–284. Epub October 12, 2005.

Costenbader KH, Feskanich D, Mandl LA, Karlson EW. Smoking intensity, duration, and cessation, and the risk of rheumatoid arthritis in women. *Am J Med*. 2006;119(6):503. e1–503.e9.

Criswell LA, Saag KG, Mikuls TR, et al. Smoking interacts with genetic risk factors in the development of rheumatoid arthritis among older Caucasian women. *Ann Rheum Dis*. 2006;65(9):1163–1167. Epub August 3, 2006.

Cutolo M, Capellino S, Sulli A, et al. Estrogens and autoimmune diseases. *Ann N Y Acad Sci*. 2006;1089:538–547.

Cutolo M, Lahita RG. Estrogens and arthritis. *Rheum Dis Clin North Am*. 2005;31(1):19–27.

D'Elia HF, Larsen A, Mattsson LA, et al. Influence of hormone replacement therapy on disease progression and bone mineral density in rheumatoid arthritis. *J Rheumatol*. 2003;30(7):1456–1463.

Dunn JM, Wilkinson JM. Naturopathic management of rheumatoid arthritis. *Mod Rheumatol*. 2005;15(2):87–90.

Elmali N, Baysal O, Harma A, Esenkaya I, Mizrak B. Effects of resveratrol in inflammatory arthritis. *Inflammation*. 2007;30(1–2):1–6.

Ferucci ED, Templin DW, Lanier AP. Rheumatoid arthritis in American Indians and Alaska Natives: a review of the literature. *Semin Arthritis Rheum*. 2005;34(4):662–667.

Firestein GS. Etiology and pathogenesis of rheumatoid arthritis. In: Ruddy S, Harris ED Jr, Sledge CB, eds. *Kelly's Textbook of Rheumatology*. 6th ed. Vol. 2. Philadelphia: W.B. Saunders Company; 2001:924.

Fisher P, Scott DL. A randomized controlled trial of homeopathy in rheumatoid arthritis. *Rheumatology (Oxford)*. 2001;40(9):1052–1055.

Foltz-Gray D. *Alternative Treatments for Arthritis*. Atlanta, GA: Arthritis Foundation; 2005.

Funk JL, Frye JB, Oyarzo JN, et al. Efficacy and mechanism of action of turmeric supplements in the treatment of experimental arthritis. *Arthritis Rheum*. 2006;54(11):3452–3464.

Gabriel SE, Crowson CS, O'Fallon WM. The epidemiology of rheumatoid arthritis in Rochester, Minnesota, 1955–1985. *Arthritis Rheum*. 1999;42(3):415–420.

Goldberg RJ, Katz J. A meta-analysis of the analgesic effects of omega-3 polyunsaturated fatty acid supplementation for inflammatory joint pain. *Pain*. 2007;129(1–2): 210–223. Epub March 1, 2007.

Golding A, Haque UJ, Giles JT. Rheumatoid arthritis and reproduction. *Rheum Dis Clin North Am*. 2007;33(2):319–343.

Gonzalez-Gay MA, Gonzalez-Juanatey C, Martin J. Rheumatoid arthritis: a disease associated with accelerated atherogenesis. *Semin Arthritis Rheum*. 2005;35(1):8–17.

Gundermann KJ, Muller J. Phytodolor: effects and efficacy of a herbal medicine. *Wien Med Wochenschr*. 2007;157(13–14):343–347.

Gustafsson K, Ekblad J, Sidenvall B. Older women and dietary advice: occurrence, comprehension and compliance. *J Hum Nutr Diet*. 2005;18(6):453–460.

Hall GM, Daniels M, Huskisson EC, Spector TD. A randomised controlled trial of the effect of hormone replacement therapy on disease activity in postmenopausal rheumatoid arthritis. *Ann Rheum Dis*. 1994;53(2):112–116.

Halpern GM. Anti-inflammatory effects of a stabilized lipid extract of Perna canaliculus (Lyprinol). *Allerg Immunol (Paris)*. 2000;32(7):272–278.

Han A, Robinson V, Judd M, Taixiang W, Wells G, Tugwell P. Tai chi for treating rheumatoid arthritis. *Cochrane Database Syst Rev*. 2004;3:CD004849.

Haslock I, Monro R, Nagarathna R, Nagendra HR, Raghuram NV. Measuring the effects of yoga in rheumatoid arthritis. *Br J Rheumatol*. 1994;33(8):787–788.

Hatakka K, Martio J, Korpela M, et al. Effects of probiotic therapy on the activity and activation of mild rheumatoid arthritis: a pilot study. *Scand J Rheumatol*. 2003;32(4):211–215.

He Y, Lu A, Zha Y, Tsang I. Differential effect on symptoms treated with traditional Chinese medicine and western combination therapy in RA patients. *Complement Ther Med*. 2008;16(4):206–211. Epub January 24, 2008.

Helmick CG, Felson DT, Lawrence RC, et al. Estimates of the prevalence of arthritis and other rheumatic conditions in the United States. Part I. *Arthritis Rheum*. 2008;58(1):15–25.

Hernandez-Avila M, Liang MH, Willett WC, et al. Exogenous sex hormones and the risk of rheumatoid arthritis. *Arthritis Rheum*. 1990;33(7):947–953.

Jonas WB, Linde K, Ramirez G. Homeopathy and rheumatic disease. *Rheum Dis Clin North Am*. 2000;26(1):117–123.

Karlson EW, Lee IM, Cook NR, Manson JE, Buring JE, Hennekens CH. A retrospective cohort study of cigarette smoking and risk of rheumatoid arthritis in female health professionals. *Arthritis Rheum.* 1999;42(5):910–917.

Karlson EW, Mandl LA, Aweh GN, Grodstein F. Coffee consumption and risk of rheumatoid arthritis. *Arthritis Rheum.* 2003;48(11):3055–3060.

Kasle S, Wilhelm MS, Zautra AJ. Rheumatoid arthritis patients' perceptions of mutuality in conversations with spouses/partners and their links with psychological and physical health. *Arthritis Rheum.* 2008;59(7):921–928.

Katz PP, Yelin EH. Activity loss and the onset of depressive symptoms: do some activities matter more than others? *Arthritis Rheum.* 2001;44(5):1194–1202.

Kay CR, Wingrave SJ. Oral contraceptives and rheumatoid arthritis. *Lancet.* 1983;1(8339):1437.

Keefe FJ, Affleck G, Lefebvre J, et al. Living with rheumatoid arthritis: the role of daily spirituality and daily religious and spiritual coping. *J Pain.* 2001;2(2):101–110.

Khanna D, Sethi G, Ahn KS, et al. Natural products as a gold mine for arthritis treatment. *Curr Opin Pharmacol.* 2007;7(3):344–351. Epub May 1, 2007.

Khazai N, Judd SE, Tangpricha V. Calcium and vitamin D: skeletal and extraskeletal health. *Curr Rheumatol Rep.* 2008;10(2):110–117.

Kirwan JR. Links between radiological change, disability, and pathology in rheumatoid arthritis. *J Rheumatol.* 2001;28(4):881–886.

Linos A, Worthington JW, O'Fallon WM, Kurland LT. Case-control study of rheumatoid arthritis and prior use of oral contraceptives. *Lancet.* 1983;1(8337):1299–1300.

Little C, Parsons T. Herbal therapy for treating rheumatoid arthritis. *Cochrane Database Syst Rev.* 2001;1:CD002948.

Lorig KR, Mazonson PD, Holman HR. Evidence suggesting that health education for self-management in patients with chronic arthritis has sustained health benefits while reducing health care costs. *Arthritis Rheum.* 1993;36(4):439–446.

Lovell DJ, Walco GA. Pain associated with juvenile rheumatoid arthritis. *Pediatr Clin North Am.* 1989;36(4):1015–1027.

MacDonald AG, Murphy EA, Capell HA, Bankowska UZ, Ralston SH. Effects of hormone replacement therapy in rheumatoid arthritis: a double blind placebo-controlled study. *Ann Rheum Dis.* 1994;53(1):54–57.

Marcason W. What is the latest research regarding cherries and the treatment of rheumatoid arthritis? *J Am Diet Assoc.* 2007;107(9):1686.

Mathur S, Mathur RS, Goust JM, Williamson HO, Fudenberg HH. Cyclic variations in white cell subpopulations in the human menstrual cycle: correlations with progesterone and estradiol. *Clin Immunol Immunopathol.* 1979;13(3):246–253.

McCauley J, Tarpley MJ, Haaz S, Bartlett SJ. Daily spiritual experiences of older adults with and without arthritis and the relationship to health outcomes. *Arthritis Rheum.* 2008;59(1):122–128.

Merlino LA, Cerhan JR, Criswell LA, Mikuls TR, Saag KG. Estrogen and other female reproductive risk factors are not strongly associated with the development of rheumatoid arthritis in elderly women. *Semin Arthritis Rheum.* 2003;33(2):72–82.

Merlino LA, Curtis J, Mikuls TR, Cerhan JR, Criswell LA, Saag KG. Iowa Women's Health Study. Vitamin D intake is inversely associated with rheumatoid arthritis: results from the Iowa Women's Health Study. *Arthritis Rheum.* 2004;50(1):72–77.

Mikuls TR. Co-morbidity in rheumatoid arthritis. *Best Pract Res Clin Rheumatol.* October 2003;17(5):729–752.

Mikuls TR, Cerhan JR, Criswell LA, et al. Coffee, tea, and caffeine consumption and risk of rheumatoid arthritis: results from the Iowa Women's Health Study. *Arthritis Rheum.* 2002;46(1):83–91.

Mur E, Hartig F, Eibl G, Schirmer M. Randomized double blind trial of an extract from the pentacyclic alkaloid-chemotype of Uncaria tomentosa for the treatment of rheumatoid arthritis. *J Rheumatol.* 2002;29(4):678–681.

National Center for Complementary and Alternative Medicine. http://nccam.nih.gov. Accessed August 2008.

Naz SM, Farragher TM, Bunn DK, Symmons DP, Bruce IN. The influence of age at symptom onset and length of followup on mortality in patients with recent-onset inflammatory polyarthritis. *Arthritis Rheum.* 2008;58(4):985–989.

Naz SM, Symmons DP. Mortality in established rheumatoid arthritis. *Best Pract Res Clin Rheumatol.* 2007;21(5):871–883.

Nordstrom DC, Honkanen VE, Nasu Y, Antila E, Friman C, Konttinen YT. Alpha-linolenic acid in the treatment of rheumatoid arthritis: a double-blind, placebo-controlled and randomized study: flaxseed vs. safflower seed. *Rheumatol Int.* 1995;14(6):231–234.

Ottonello M. Cognitive-behavioral interventions in rheumatic diseases. *G Ital Med Lav Ergon.* 2007;29(1 Suppl A):A19–A23.

Park J, Ernst E. Ayurvedic medicine for rheumatoid arthritis: a systematic review. *Semin Arthritis Rheum.* 2005;34(5):705–713.

Parker JC, Smarr KL, Slaughter JR, et al. Management of depression in rheumatoid arthritis: a combined pharmacologic and cognitive-behavioral approach. *Arthritis Rheum.* 2003;49(6):766–777.

Pattison DJ, Harrison RA, Symmons DP. The role of diet in susceptibility to rheumatoid arthritis: a systematic review. *J Rheumatol.* 2004;31(7):1310–1319.

Pattison DJ, Symmons DP, Lunt M, et al. Dietary risk factors for the development of inflammatory polyarthritis: evidence for a role of high level of red meat consumption. *Arthritis Rheum.* 2004;50(12):3804–3812.

Peretz A, Siderova V, Neve J. Selenium supplementation in rheumatoid arthritis investigated in a double blind, placebo-controlled trial. *Scand J Rheumatol.* 2001;30(4):208–212.

Persellin RH. The effect of pregnancy on rheumatoid arthritis. *Bull Rheum Dis.* 1976–1977;27(9):922–927.

Phillips K, Aliprantis A, Coblyn J. Strategies for the prevention and treatment of osteoporosis in patients with rheumatoid arthritis. *Drugs Aging.* 2006;23(10):773–779.

Pradhan EK, Baumgarten M, Langenberg P, et al. Effect of mindfulness-based stress reduction in rheumatoid arthritis patients. *Arthritis Rheum.* 2007;57(7):1134–1142.

Ramey DR, Fries JF, Singh G. The health assessment questionnaire 1995: status and review. In: Spilker B, ed. *Quality of Life and Pharmacoeconomics in Clinical Trials*. 2nd ed. Philadelphia: Lippincott-Raven; 1996:227–237.

Rennie KL, Hughes J, Lang R, Jebb SA. Nutritional management of rheumatoid arthritis: a review of the evidence. *J Hum Nutr Diet*. 2003;16(2):97–109.

Resch KL, Hill S, Ernst E. Use of complementary therapies by individuals with "arthritis." *Clin Rheumatol*. 1997;16(4):391–395.

Rudge SR, Kowanko IC, Drury PL. Menstrual cyclicity of finger joint size and grip strength in patients with rheumatoid arthritis. *Ann Rheum Dis*. 1983;42(4):425–430.

Saag KG, Teng GG, Patkar NM, et al. American College of Rheumatology 2008 recommendations for the use of nonbiologic and biologic disease-modifying antirheumatic drugs in rheumatoid arthritis. *Arthritis Rheum*. 2008;59(6):762–784.

Segal NA, Toda Y, Huston J, et al. Two configurations of static magnetic fields for treating rheumatoid arthritis of the knee: a double-blind clinical trial. *Arch Phys Med Rehabil*. 2001;82(10):1453–1460.

Sharpe L, Allard S, Sensky T. Five-year followup of a cognitive-behavioral intervention for patients with recently-diagnosed rheumatoid arthritis: effects on health care utilization. *Arthritis Rheum*. 2008;59(3):311–316.

Skoldstam L, Hagfors L, Johansson G. An experimental study of a Mediterranean diet intervention for patients with rheumatoid arthritis. *Ann Rheum Dis*. 2003;62(3):208–214.

Smyth JM, Stone AA, Hurewitz A, Kaell A. Effects of writing about stressful experiences on symptom reduction in patients with asthma or rheumatoid arthritis: a randomized trial. *JAMA*. 1999;281(14):1304–1309.

So JS, Kwon HK, Lee CG, et al. Lactobacillus casei suppresses experimental arthritis by down-regulating T helper 1 effector functions. *Mol Immunol*. 2008;45(9):2690–2699. Epub February 19, 2008.

Soeken KL. Selected CAM therapies for arthritis-related pain: the evidence from systematic reviews. *Clin J Pain*. 2004;20(1):13–18.

Soeken KL, Miller SA, Ernst E. Herbal medicines for the treatment of rheumatoid arthritis: a systematic review. *Rheumatology (Oxford)*. 2003;42(5):652–659.

Solomon DH, Karlson EW, Rimm EB, et al. Cardiovascular morbidity and mortality in women diagnosed with rheumatoid arthritis. *Circulation*. 2003;107(9):1303–1307.

Srivastava KC, Mustafa T. Ginger (*Zingiber officinale*) in rheumatism and musculoskeletal disorders. *Med Hypotheses*. 1992;39(4):342–348.

Stanford University. "ARAMIS: the Arthritis, Rheumatism, and Aging Medical Information System." July 2003. http://aramis.stanford.edu/downloads/HAQ37_pack.pdf. Accessed August 2008.

Sterba KR, DeVellis RF, Lewis MA, DeVellis BM, Jordan JM, Baucom DH. Effect of couple illness perception congruence on psychological adjustment in women with rheumatoid arthritis. *Health Psychol*. 2008;27(2):221–229.

Stone J, Doube A, Dudson D, Wallace J. Inadequate calcium, folic acid, vitamin E, zinc, and selenium intake in rheumatoid arthritis patients: results of a dietary survey. *Semin Arthritis Rheum*. 1997;27(3):180–185.

Tam LS, Leung PC, Li TK, Zhang L, Li EK. Acupuncture in the treatment of rheumatoid arthritis: a double-blind controlled pilot study. *BMC Complement Altern Med.* 2007;7:35.

Tanaka E, Mannalithara A, Inoue E, et al. Efficient management of rheumatoid arthritis significantly reduces long-term functional disability. *Ann Rheum Dis.* 2008;67(8):1153–1158. Epub October 30, 2007.

Tao XL, Sun Y, Dong Y, et al. A prospective, controlled, double-blind, cross-over study of Tripterygium wilfodii hook F in treatment of rheumatoid arthritis. *Chin Med J (Engl).* 1989;102(5):327–332.

Tao X, Younger J, Fan FZ, Wang B, Lipsky PE. Benefit of an extract of Tripterygium wilfordii Hook F in patients with rheumatoid arthritis: a double-blind, placebo-controlled study. *Arthritis Rheum.* 2002;46(7):1735–1743.

Torem MS. Mind-body hypnotic imagery in the treatment of auto-immune disorders. *Am J Clin Hypn.* 2007;50(2):157–170.

Turesson C, Weyand CM, Matteson EL. Genetics of rheumatoid arthritis: is there a pattern predicting extraarticular manifestations? *Arthritis Rheum.* 2004;51(5):853–863.

Udenigwe CC, Ramprasath VR, Aluko RE, Jones PJ. Potential of resveratrol in anticancer and anti-inflammatory therapy. *Nutr Rev.* 2008;66(8):445–454.

Underwood LG, Teresi JA. The daily spiritual experience scale: development, theoretical description, reliability, exploratory factor analysis, and preliminary construct validity using health-related data. *Ann Behav Med.* 2002;24(1):22–33.

VandeCreek L, Paget S, Horton R, Robbins L, Oettinger M, Tai K. 2004. Religious and nonreligious coping methods among persons with rheumatoid arthritis. *Arthritis Rheum.* 2004;51(1):49–55.

Vandenbroucke JP, Valkenburg HA, Boersma JW, et al. Oral contraceptives and rheumatoid arthritis: further evidence for a preventive effect. *Lancet.* 1982;2(8303):839–842.

Vandenbroucke JP, Witteman JC, Valkenburg HA, et al. Noncontraceptive hormones and rheumatoid arthritis in perimenopausal and postmenopausal women. *JAMA.* 1986;255(10):1299–1303.

VanDyke MM, Parker JC, Smarr KL, et al. Anxiety in rheumatoid arthritis. *Arthritis Rheum.* 2004;51(3):408–412.

Walco GA, Varni JW, Ilowite NT. Cognitive-behavioral pain management in children with juvenile rheumatoid arthritis. *Pediatrics.* 1992;89(6 Pt 1):1075–1079.

Walker AF, Bundy R, Hicks SM, Middleton RW. Bromelain reduces mild acute knee pain and improves well-being in a dose-dependent fashion in an open study of otherwise healthy adults. *Phytomedicine.* 2002;9(8):681–686.

Wang C. Tai Chi improves pain and functional status in adults with rheumatoid arthritis: results of a pilot single-blinded randomized controlled trial. *Med Sport Sci.* 2008;52:218–229.

Weiner DK, Ernst E. Complementary and alternative approaches to the treatment of persistent musculoskeletal pain. *Clin J Pain.* 2004;20(4):244–255.

Wolfe F, Michaud K. Lymphoma in rheumatoid arthritis: the effect of methotrexate and anti-tumor necrosis factor therapy in 18,572 patients. *Arthritis Rheum.* 2004;50(6):1740–1751.

Wolfe F, Michaud K, Gefeller O, Choi HK. Predicting mortality in patients with rheumatoid arthritis. *Arthritis Rheum.* 2003;48(6):1530–1542.

Yocum DE, Castro WL, Cornett M. Exercise, education, and behavioral modification as alternative therapy for pain and stress in rheumatic disease. *Rheum Dis Clin North Am.* 2000;26(1):145–159.

Zautra AJ, Davis MC, Reich JW, et al. Comparison of cognitive behavioral and mindfulness meditation interventions on adaptation to rheumatoid arthritis for patients with and without history of recurrent depression. *J Consult Clin Psychol.* 2008;76(3):408–421

30

Multiple Sclerosis

PATRICIA K. AMMON

CASE STUDY

Shannon was 36 when she was diagnosed with MS, although in hindsight she had been having symptoms for at least 5 years: intermittent numbness and tingling in various parts of her body, episodes of visual disturbances, episodes of extreme fatigue, and bouts of depression. She was 6 months postpartum, and developed extreme fatigue out of proportion to what may have been expected for a new mom. She also had feelings of numbness and tingling in her face, right arm, and left leg. She found herself being clumsy and dropping things. She went to see her gynecologist who diagnosed postpartum depression and placed her on fluoxetine. Fluoxetine did seem to help the fatigue slightly, but none of the other symptoms.

Growing frustrated with conventional medicine's approach to her symptoms, she came to see me, having heard of my reputation for dwelling deeply into causation of symptoms. After our visit, with careful history taking and in-depth neurologic examination, I discussed with her my concerns that this could be multiple sclerosis (MS). We discussed that MS is often diagnosed in the postpartum period (Salem 2004), and the rationale for treating MS from a hormonal standpoint. She started on Estriol at 4 mg BID, begun a supplement high in antioxidants, and had lab work for B12 and 25-hydroxyvitamin D. When her labs came back showing both B12 low and vitamin D level very low, we started B12 injections, 1 mg IM twice a week and 50,000 IU of vitamin D2 once a week (Alpert and Shaikh 2007). A magnetic resonance imaging (MRI) examination confirmed our diagnosis, showing demyelinating lesions in the periventricular areas, typical for MS. With her history and MRI, we elected not to do a lumbar puncture looking for oligoclonal bands. A neurologist reviewed her MRI, and agreed with the diagnosis. After discussion of the possible benefits of doing a purification regimen using Ayurvedic Panchakarma, Shannon elected to do this at a clinic in Boulder, Colorado, under the directorship of John Douillard, D.C., and had very positive results.

Now, after 10 years of diet modification, usually consistent supplement consumption, occasional purification Panchakarma (about once every 12–18 months), continuing B12 injections every 2 weeks, and vitamin D at 2000 IU/day (after labs showed a rising level of vitamin D to 75 nmol/L), she has been doing very well, with little to no symptoms of MS. She has stayed very physically active and has a wonderful attitude.

Women and Multiple Sclerosis: An Integrative Approach

INTRODUCTION

It is estimated that there are approximately 350,000 persons in the United States living with multiple sclerosis (MS), making it the most common neurologic disability in young adults. Approximately two-thirds of those diagnosed with MS are women (Beck et al. 2005). MS is a complex disorder with a wide range of individual symptoms. Theoretically, all individuals are endowed with the potential ability to evoke an autoimmune response to central nervous system (CNS) injuries (viral, bacterial, toxin, or direct injury). Axonal injury and inflammation may follow, leading to demyelination, which subsequently impairs the transmission of nerve impulses and results in fatigue, weakness, numbness, locomotor difficulty, pain, loss of vision, and other health problems. The inherent ability to control this response is correlated with the individual's ability to resist autoimmune disease induction (Haegert 2005).

ETIOLOGY

While the end result is the same—inflammation in the central nervous system leading to cell damage and cell death—the initiating trigger remains an area of intense study (Confavreux and Vukusic 2006). At present, there are four major theories of the cause of MS: immunologic, environmental, infectious agent, and genetic susceptibility.

Immunologic

The theory that MS is an organ-specific autoimmune disease, although unproven, is widely accepted. Antibodies against antigens located on the surface of the myelin sheath cause demyelination either directly or by complement-mediated processes. It has been suggested that priming of myelin-reactive T cells occurs as part of the disease process in MS. Primed T cells reactive to myelin antigens may develop a phenotype, making them more resistant to regulatory processes. That autoantigens can drive B-cell clonal expansion and contribute to autoimmunity has been demonstrated in other autoimmune conditions.

Environmental Factors

Our modern-day environment is overwhelmed with prooxidants from chemical pollution that can serve as endocrine disruptors to vaccines that stimulate the immune system. The possible connection between viral vaccines and MS is an area of controversy. Although immunity to tetanus appears to be protective against the development of MS (Verstraeten et al. 2005), there is even stronger evidence that hepatitis B vaccination can induce autoimmune attacks (Faure 2005). There is evidence that the timing of the exposure to an environmental agent plays a role, with exposure before puberty predisposing a person to develop MS later in life (Visscher et al. 1977). Several decades of research have documented that the incidence of MS increases with increasing distance from the equator. Possible explanations for this finding include genetic predisposition in population groups, dietary factors, and levels of the active form of vitamin D.

The relationship between mercury from dental fillings and MS is one of extreme controversy, with some studies concluding there is a clear relationship (Huggins and Levy 1998), and other studies showing a relationship between the

At present, there are too many similarities between mercury toxicity and MS symptoms to be ignored completely. That said, I rarely recommend that my patients have their mercury filling removed, unless there is another need, such as cracked filling. Removal can create more of a physiological stress by the mobilization of the mercury than the potential benefit a woman may derive.

extent of dental carries and MS, but no association between MS and the number of fillings (McGrother et al. 1999).

Infectious Agents

At least 16 different infectious agents have been implicated as causes of MS; however, none has been definitely proven to cause MS (Croxford et al. 2005). At present, the three agents receiving the most attention are human herpes 6 (HHV-6); *Chlamydia pneumoniae* (used to activate experimental allergic encephalitis—a mouse form of MS) (Du et al. 2002); and Epstein–Barr virus (EBV) (Krone et al. 2008).

Genetic Factors

Although most cases of MS are sporadic, susceptibility to develop MS is affected in part by genetic factors. The contribution of germ line genetic variants to disease expression may be modest as demonstrated by significant variations in the clinical expression of MS in monozygotic twins who both have the disease. It is likely that postgermline events influence the clinical expression of MS (Frohman et al. 2005a).

Integrative Therapy

Treatment modalities for MS aim to reduce oxidative damage and modulate the immune response. This is accomplished through dietary measures that reduce the potential for oxidative damage, introducing potent antioxidants that can cross the blood–brain barrier, utilizing supplements and hormones that modulate the immune response, and utilizing supplements that help restore normal brain function and repair.

Nutrition

As with many conditions, treatment begins with diet. The dietary influence on MS was first reported by Swank and associates in 1952. Swank noted that people living in colder climates tended to consume diets higher in fat than those living in tropical regions; this dietary difference was linked to higher incidence of MS in colder regions (Swank et al. 1952). As saturated fats and trans-fats are more susceptible to oxidation (Mayer 1999), they are more likely to provoke inflammation. Many of my recommendations come from David Perlmutter, MD, a board-certified neurologist, and leader in the field who practices in Naples, Florida (Perlmutter and Coleman 2004).

My prescription for nutrition includes the following:

- An anti-inflammatory diet (see Chapter 2 on nutrition).
- Consume less than 5% of energy from saturated fat.
- Consume less than 1% of energy from trans-fat. Trans-fat may be even more vulnerable to oxidation than saturated fat. By avoiding processed or packaged foods, it is possible to almost completely avoid trans-fats as they occur infrequently in nature.
- Increase intake of foods rich in omega-3 essential fatty acids: cold-water fish, nuts seeds, and dark green leafy vegetables. These foods reduce inflammation through their effect on prostaglandins and leukotrienes. If women find it more convenient to take supplements of these essential fatty acids, suggest a docosahexanoic acid (DHA) dose of 400–600 mg/day.
- Consider a reduced gluten/gluten-free diet. There are case reports of gluten sensitivity presenting as optic neuritis (Jacob et al. 2005). Other studies show an increase in some proteins from the gut in patients with MS and IgG against gliadin and gluten (Reichelt and Jensen 2004).
- Eliminate or significantly reduce alcohol intake. Alcohol is a potent trigger of the arachidonic acid cascade, leading to inflammation (Szabo 1999; Zahr et al. 2008).

Supplements

GLUTATHIONE

Endogenous glutathione provides the primary cellular defense against free radicals in people. Glutathione functions both as an antioxidant and as a detoxifying agent for a vast array of xenobiotics (Shaw and Bains 1997). The most effective way of raising intracellular levels of glutathione is by intravenous (IV) infusion.

I generally reserve using IV glutathione for patients who are having an exacerbation of symptoms. The dose is 600–800 mg diluted in 10–20 mL of sterile water, given IV two to three times a week. Precautions with using glutathione include respiratory distress, coughing, rhinorrhea, and vertigo. Because of its potential to irritate reactive airways, I always use caution when giving glutathione IV to patients with asthma, or others with allergic reactions.

Glutathione levels can also be raised by taking *N*-acetyl-cysteine, co-enzyme Q10, and alpha lipoic acid. *N*-acetyl-cysteine (NAC) taken orally raises glutathione levels. The dose is 2 g/day given in divided doses. Nausea and vomiting are common with doses higher than 2 g/day. Other side effects include diarrhea and an unpleasant odor.

Co-Q-10, like glutathione, is a potent antioxidant that easily crosses the blood–brain barrier. The optimal dose is around 300 mg/day; however, cost considerations may limit some women's ability to take this dose. Alpha-lipoic acid is rapidly absorbed from the gut, crosses the blood–brain barrier, and has powerful antioxidant activity. It not only augments the function of vitamins C, E, and glutathione (Packer et al. 1997) but also raises the body's level of glutathione. The dosage is 200–300 mg/day. Precautions include nausea, vomiting, skin rash, and urine with foul odor.

VITAMIN D

Long-term vitamin D deficiency can lead to paracrine effects such as type 1 diabetes, cancer, and MS (Alpert and Shaikh 2007). Researchers have speculated that large doses of vitamin D interact with T helper lymphocytes, which suppress the inflammatory response of the type 1 T helper lymphocytes to eliminate some of the autoimmune diseases that include MS (Cantorna 2006).

In my practice, I routinely measure 25-hydroxyvitamin D levels in any woman with MS. Several clinical studies have shown that a blood serum level of 75 nmol/L is necessary to support both the endocrine and autocrine functions of the body (Whiting and Calvo 2005). Supplementation of vitamin D is based on the patient's blood level, which ranges from 50,000 IU/week to 400 IU/day. Toxic levels of vitamin D (>350 nmol/L) result in hyperabsorption of intestinal calcium, and hypercalciuria, leading to renal calcinosis and renal injury (Robsahm et al. 2004). Clinical symptoms associated with vitamin D toxicity include polyuria, polydypsia, anorexia, nausea and vomiting, constipation, and hypertension.

CALCIUM

At 800 mg/day in humans, calcium has been shown to strongly affect the action of vitamin D for suppressing experimental autoimmune encephalomyelitis (EAE) in mice (Cantorna et al. 1999). EAE is an MS-like condition induced in laboratory mice to test treatment modalities (Zozulya and Wiendl 2008).

MAGNESIUM

Magnesium has a threefold role in MS. It is required for adequate levels of metabolized vitamin D products to be maintained in circulation. In addition, when dosed at 800 mg/day, magnesium has a mild effect on the muscle spasticity often associated with MS. Finally, an advantageous side effect of magnesium is its tendency to cause looser bowel movements, mitigating the constipation that commonly occurs among patients with MS. Should diarrhea develop, patients need to back off the dose of magnesium or balance it with calcium (which tends to constipate).

B COMPLEX VITAMINS

The B vitamins have been shown to aid in cognitive function, act as antioxidants, and decrease production of inflammatory cytokines (Bottiglieri 1996; Kumar et al. 2000). Deficiency of vitamin B12 and errors in vitamin B12 metabolism are known to cause demyelination of the CNS (Kira et al. 1994). Taking a multi-B vitamin assures sufficient thiamine, B12, and folic acid.

> While I will usually measure vitamin B12 levels in the newly diagnosed patient, serum levels do not always accurately reflect CNS levels. High doses of vitamin B12 given intramuscularly (IM) have been shown to improve brain stem nerve function in chronic, progressive MS (Reynolds 1992). The dose varies based on the patient's symptoms and response to the injections. I begin with 1 mg/week and average 1 mg two to three times a month. I recommend that my patients who are averse to injections use sublingual B12. A daily dose of 2500 µg SL will raise B12 levels.

INOSINE

Uric acid (UA) is a purine metabolite that selectively inhibits peroxynitrite-mediated reactions implicated in the pathogenesis of MS and other neurodegenerative diseases. The administration of UA is therapeutic in EAE. Raising UA levels in patients with MS, by oral administration of a UA precursor such as inosine may have therapeutic value (Scott et al. 2002). The usual starting dose is 500 mg twice a day. Dosages up to 3 g/day in divided doses have been used without adverse affects (Koprowski et al. 2001).

> Before using inosine, I routinely check UA levels as gout like symptoms can be induced when UA levels get too high.

BOTANICALS

Withania somnifera (Ashwagandha)

Ashwagandha is an Ayurvedic herb also known as winter cherry that is sometimes called Indian Ginseng in reference to its rejuvenative and tonic effects on the nervous system. Ashwagandha's antiinflammatory, antioxidant, anxiolytic, and antidepressant activities make this herb ideal for treating MS (Mishra et al. 2000; Panda and Kar 1997). The dosage for MS is 1–2 g of the whole herb in powdered form two or three times a day.

> Caution must be used in choosing a supplement supplier as some Ayurvedic herbs have been found to have high levels of contaminants such as lead (Saper et al. 2004). As a practitioner, you have the responsibility to be knowledgeable of the supplier's source to ensure your patient is not getting a contaminated product. I use Banyan Botanicals in my practice and I am satisfied with their quality control.

Hormones

Given that two-third of MS patients are women, it is logical to conclude that hormones play a role in disease initiation, progression, and potential disability (Shuster 2008). Studies on MS in pregnant women have shown that most women will have a significant decrease in symptoms during the pregnancy. A particular form of estrogen, estriol, is elevated during a pregnancy and at no other time in a woman's life. Research has shown that estriol causes an immune shift from T helper 1 to T helper 2 cells, leading to immune modulation and less inflammation (van den Broek et al. 2005). Studies have shown a decrease in symptoms and a decrease in gadolinium-enhancing lesions on MRI in women and men treated with estriol (Voskuhl 2002). Estriol is considered a weak estrogen, having little to no affect on bone health and minimal potential for endometrial hyperplasia (Head 1998). At present, estriol is only available through compounding pharmacies. The usual dose is 8 mg/day that can be given in divided doses.

Even though estriol is considered a weak estrogen, I am more comfortable using a small dose of progesterone when I prescribe estriol, usually 25–50 mg/day. At menopause, I usually continue the estriol at 8 mg/day and add estradiol at a dose of 0.5–1 mg BID as well as progesterone dosed at 25 mg/day in the woman without a uterus and 50–100 mg qd to BID in the women with intact uteri.

Menopause can be an extremely challenging time for any woman; for women with MS, where hormones play a significant role in the disease keeping hormones balanced is critical to a woman's well-being (Moore 2007).

As sexual dysfunction can be a particularly distressing symptom for a woman with MS, I always discuss this with my patients. With appropriate hormone replacement, many women find they can maintain sexual intimacy at a level they find desirable.

At menopause I check hormone blood levels for estradiol, progesterone testosterone and DHEA. These results and a woman's symptoms help guide the dosage.

TESTOSTERONE

Much like estriol's protective role in women, testosterone has been found to ameliorate MS symptoms in male *and* female patients (Voskuhl and Palaszynski 2001). The usual dosing for women is 2–5 mg/day of micronized bioidentical testosterone from a compounding pharmacy.

Dehydroepiandrosterone

Dehydroepiandrosterone (DHEA) serves as a metabolic intermediate in the pathway for synthesis of testosterone, estrone, and estradiol. It also affects lipogenesis, substrate cycling, peroxisome proliferation, mitochondrial respiration, protein synthesis, and thyroid hormone function (Suzuki et al. 1995). Researchers have found a clinical association between low DHEA levels and relapse in the MS patient (Du et al. 2001).

I use physiologic doses of DHEA when prescribing this hormone. For women, the dose is 10–30 mg/day. Whenever I use hormones of any kind, I carefully weigh the risks and benefits for each individual. All hormones can have potentially untoward effects and prescribing them requires careful monitoring with review of symptoms and blood tests for estradiol, progesterone, testosterone total and free, and DHEA-S.

Exercise

Exercise programs must be designed to activate working muscles but avoid overload that results in conduction block. Any exercise program must be individualized and adaptable to changing needs of the patient (Petajan and White 1999). Research shows that for people with MS, exercise capacity is reduced in response to a single bout of continuous exercise to maximal effort; however, minimally impaired people with MS often exhibit similar cardiorespiratory responses as healthy individuals during discontinuous exercise (Sutherland and Andersen 2001).

Aquatic activities are generally considered the most appropriate form of exercise for the MS population. Water can provide adequate support for those with gait and balance problems, allowing movement that may be difficult to achieve on land and keeping the body cool during exercise. Yoga techniques have been shown to improve circulation, balance, relaxation, flexibility, eyesight, and reduce muscle tension (www.americanyogaassociation.org).

Psychosocial Factors

Depression is common in MS, and death by suicide occurs seven times more frequently than in the general population. Combining counseling with bodywork therapies is a highly effective way to counter this depression. Antidepressant medications are often necessary.

Therapies to Consider

AYURVEDA

Considered by many scholars to be the oldest healing science, Ayurveda places great emphasis on prevention. It encourages the maintenance of health through close attention to balance in one's life, thinking, diet, lifestyle, and use of herbs. Just as everyone has unique fingerprints, each person has a particular pattern of energy that comprises her own constitution. Although any component of Ayurveda may be used in isolation (e.g., herbs), integrating all components of Ayurveda will have more of an optimal result. The purification and rejuvenation therapy called Panchakarma is an ideal therapy for patients with MS, because it includes treatment and education regarding diet and lifestyle.

TRADITIONAL CHINESE MEDICINE

MS is a complicated illness from the standpoint of traditional Chinese medicine (TCM). By addressing one component of MS (e.g., fatigue), it is possible to exacerbate another component (e.g., immune hyperreactivity). That said, TCM can be a helpful modality in the hands of an experienced practitioner familiar with MS. Beware of herbal combinations that may include an aspect of immune stimulation.

Pharmaceuticals

SYMPTOM MANAGEMENT

Depression can be so overwhelming in the MS patient that pharmaceuticals are required. With the multitude of agents available, it may take different trials to find the agent that works best for the individual. In my experience, fluoxetine at 20 mg/day has been the most beneficial, with the fewest side effects.

Bladder irritability with stress and urge incontinence is one of the most common concerns of many of my women patients. While oxybutynin and tolterodine tartrate are commonly prescribed, I have found that using very small doses of imipramine (10–25 mg/day) to be the most effective treatment with the fewest side effects. This dose can be divided during the day to achieve better bladder control.

Muscle spasticity is a fairly universal complaint with MS. Baclofen, at doses of 10 mg QID, is the most commonly used agent. In my practice, I more routinely use tizanidine at doses varying from 2 to 4 mg/day in divided doses. Clinical studies have shown tizanidine to be equal to baclofen or diazepam, with tolerability data favoring tizanidine (Kamen et al. 2008).

Fatigue is a universal complaint of the MS patient. I try to help patients manage fatigue with moderate, consistent exercise routines, B vitamins, and ensuring adequate rest. When these measures are not enough, I will rarely prescribe modafinil at 100 mg prn (Rammohan et al. 2002).

Pain, usually in the large muscles of the lower extremities, is incapacitating for some patients. The pain, which is difficult to characterize, can be experienced as a burning, deep discomfort throughout the body. Regular exercise, yoga, and relaxation techniques are my first management strategies. If insufficient, tizanidine can be helpful. Gabapentin can help neuropathic pain (Hays and Woodroffe 1999). Due to its high side effect profile, I will prescribe this at low doses (100–300 mg/day) on a prn basis.

Disease-Modifying Agents

There is evidence that intravenous and oral administration of corticosteroids shortens the duration of acute relapses (Barnes et al. 1997). There is no evidence that corticosteroids affect the overall degree of recovery or long-term course of the disease. The dosage for IV administration is 1 g/day for 3–5 days. Oral dosage regimens vary, with the most common regimen being prednisone 60 mg/day for 5 days, then 40 mg/day for 5 days, then 20 mg/day for 5 days, then 10 mg/day for 5 days. Side effects include congestive heart failure, hypertension, psychosis, osteoporosis, peptic ulcer, immune suppression with increased susceptibility to infection, and decreased carbohydrate tolerance.

Interferon beta-1b (Betaseron) and interferon beta-1a (Avonex and Rebif) were originally thought to increase the resistance of tissues, including those of the CNS, against viral infections. There are currently no data to suggest that viral inhibition underlies interferon beta effects on MS in any way (Frohman et al. 2005b). The precise mechanism for these drugs work is unknown, however, it is probable they have an immunomodulatory effect. Dosage is individualized and administration is either subcutaneously or intramuscularly. Side effects include injection site reaction, headache, fever, flu-like symptoms, pain, diarrhea, constipation, lymphocytopenia, elevation of liver enzymes, mayalgias, depression, and anxiety. There is also the high cost of these drugs to consider.

Glatiramer acetate (Copaxone) is a synthetic copolymer of the most prevalent amino acids in myelin basic protein. The drug is thought to work by mimicking myelin basic protein and thus redirecting inflammatory cells to the drug instead of the myelin. Dosage is generally 20 mg subcutaneously daily. Glatiramer is well tolerated by most patients, with local injection site reaction being the most prominent adverse reaction; the cost is also quite high.

Natalizumab (Tysabri) is a selective adhesion molecule inhibitor used for the treatment of relapsing forms of MS. Administered by IV infusion once a month, it was taken off the market shortly after FDA approval due to its side effects. Natalizumab is now being used only by neurologists in selective cases with careful monitoring.

Novantrone is an immunosuppressive drug used to treat cancer. It has received renewed attention in MS where it has been combined with glatiramer acetate in controlled studies. The dosage is individualized, with cardiotoxic effects being the major limitation associated with this drug (Arnold et al. 2008).

Low-dose naltrexone (LDN) is a pure opiate antagonist, licensed by the FDA for the treatment of alcohol and opioid addictions. It is currently available in the United States by off-label prescription, at a dose of 4.5 mg/day for the treatment of MS. This use has overwhelming anecdotal evidence that it prevents relapses in MS and reduces the progression of the disease. Although it is currently used worldwide, more clinical trials are needed to support its use (Agrawal, 2005). There are several other drugs in phase II and phase III clinical trials, including some that are given orally. Other studies are ongoing using combinations of approved drugs.

Summary

MS is a chronic inflammatory disease of the central nervous system that has multiple potential initiating causes. An event occurs in the CNS that increases production of free radicals causing oxidative damage to the myelin sheath and surrounding axons. An immune response is triggered, as it should be, but there is a defect in controlling that immune response resulting in an autoimmune situation. The key to prevention and treatment is to limit oxidative damage in the CNS and modulate the immune response to decrease inflammation. With the inflammation modulated, the nerve cells can then begin to heal with the help of nutrients. Recognizing the very real role of emotions and inflammation, maintaining a positive attitude is of the utmost importance.

REFERENCES

Agrawal YP. Low dose naltrexone therapy in multiple sclerosis. *Med Hypotheses.* 2005;64:721–724.

Alpert PT, Shaikh U. The effects of vitamin D deficiency and insufficiency on the endocrine and paracrine systems. *Biol Res Nurs.* 2007;9(2):117–129.

Arnold DL, Campangnolo D, Panitch H, et al. Glatiramer acetate after mitoxantrone induction improves MRI markers of lesion volume and permanent tissue injury in MS. *J Neurol.* 2008;255:1473–1478.

Barnes D, Hughes RAC, Morris R, et al. Randomized trial of oral and intravenous methylprednisolone in acute relapses of multiple sclerosis. *Lancet.* 1997;349:285–294.

Beck CA, Metz LM, Svenson LW, Patten SB. Regional variation of multiple sclerosis prevalence in Canada. *Mult Scler.* 2005;11:516–519.

Bottiglieri T. Folate, vitamin B12, and neuropsychiatric disorders. *Nutr Rev.* 1996;54:382–390.

Cantorna MT. Vitamin D and its role in immunology: multiple sclerosis, and inflammatory bowel disease. *Prog Biophys Mol Biol.* 2006;92:60–64.

Cantorna M, Humpai-Winter J, DeLuca H. Dietary calcium is a major factor in 1,25-dihydroxycholecalciferol suppression of experimental autoimmune encephalomyelitis in mice. *J Nutr.* 1999;129:1966–1971.

Confavreux C, Vukusic S. Natural history of multiple sclerosis: a unifying concept. *Brain.* 2006;129:606–616.

Croxford JL, Olson JK, Anger HA, Miller SD. Initiation and exacerbation of autoimmune demyelination of the central nervous system via virus-induced molecular mimicry: implications for the pathogenesis of multiple sclerosis. *J Virol.* 2005;79:8581–8590.

Du C, Khalil MW, Sriram S. Administration of dehydroepiandrosterone suppresses experimental allergic encephalomyelitis in SJL/J mice. *J Immunol.* 2001;167(12):7094–7101.

Du C, Yao S, Ljunggren-Rose A, Sriram S. *Chlamydia pneumoniae* Infection of the central nervous system worsens experimental allergic encephalitis. *JEM.* December 9, 2002.

Faure E. Multiple sclerosis and hepatitis B vaccination: could minute contamination of the vaccine by partial hepatitis B virus polymerase play a role through molecular mimicry? *Med Hypotheses.* 2005;65:509–520.

Frohman EM, Filippi M, Stuve O, et al. Characterizing the mechanisms of progression in multiple sclerosis. *Arch Neurol.* 2005a;62(9):1345–1356.

Frohman EM, Stuve O, Havrdova E, et al. Therapeutic considerations for disease progression in multiple sclerosis. *Arch Neur.* 2005b;62:1519–1530.

Haegert DG. Clinical multiple sclerosis occurs at one end of a spectrum of CNS pathology: a modified threshold liability model leads to new ways of thinking about the cause of clinical multiple sclerosis. *Med Hypotheses.* 2005;65:232–237.

Hays H, Woodroffe MA. Using gabapentin to treat neuropathic pain. *Can Fam Physician.* 1999;45:2109–2112.

Head KA. Estriol: safety and efficacy. *Alt Med Rev.* 1998;3(2):101–113.

Huggins HA, Levy TE. Cerebrospinal fluid protein changes in multiple sclerosis after dental amalgam removal. *Altem Med Rev.* 1998;3(4):295–300.

Jacob S, Zarei M, Kenton A, Allroggen H. Gluten sensitivity and neuromyelitis optica: two case reports. *J Neurol Neurosurg Psychiatry.* 2005;76:1028–1030.

Kamen L, Henney HR, III, Runyan JD. A practical overview of tizanidine use for spasticity secondary by multiple sclerosis, stroke, and spinal cord injury. *Curr Med Res Opin.* 2008;24(2):425–439.

Kira J, Tobimatsu S, Goto I. Vitamin B12 metabolism and massive dose methyl vitamin B12 therapy in Japanese patients with multiple sclerosis. *Int Med.* 1994;33:82–86.

Koprowski H, Spitsin SV, Hooper DC. Prospects for the treatment of multiple sclerosis by raising serum levels of uric acid, a scavenger of peroxynitrite. *Ann Neurol.* 2001;49:139.

Krone B, Pohl D, Rostasy K, et al. Common infectious agents in multiple sclerosis: a case control study in children. *Mult Scler.* 2008;14:4–5.

Kumar PD, Nrtsupha C, West BC. Unilateral internuclear ophthalmoplegia and recovery with thiamine in Wernicke syndrome. *Am J Med Sci.* 2000;320(4):278–280.

Mayer M. Essential fatty acids and related molecular and cellular mechanisms in multiple sclerosis: new looks at old concepts. *Folia Biolog (Praha).* 1999;45:133–141.

McGrother CW, Dugmore C, Phillips MJ, et al. Multiple sclerosis, dental carries and fillings: a case-control study. *Br Det J.* 1999;187:261–264.

Mishra LC, Singh BB, Dagenais S. Scientific basis for the therapeutic use of *Withania somnifera* (ashwagandha): a review. *Altern Med Rev.* 2000;5:334–346.

Packer L, Witt EH, Tritschler HJ. Alpha-lipoic acid as a biological antioxidant. *Free Radic Biol Med.* 1997;19:227–250.

Panda S, Kar A. Evidence for free radical scavenging activity of ashwagandha root powder in mice. *Indian J Physiol Pharmacol.* 1999;41:424–426.

Perlmutter D, Coleman C. *The Better Brain Book.* Penguin Books; 2004.

Petajan JH, White AT. Recommendations for physical activity in patients with MS. *Sports Med.* 1999;27.

Rammohan K, Rosenberg J, Lynn D, et al. Efficacy and safety of modafinil (Provigil ®) for the treatment of fatigue in multiple sclerosis: a two centre phase 2 study. *J Neurol Neurosurg Psychiatry.* 2002;72(2):179–183.

Reichelt KL, Jensen D. IgA antibodies against gliadin and gluten in multiple sclerosis. *Acta Neurol Scand.* 2004;110:239–241.

Reynolds EH. Multiple sclerosis and vitamin B12 metabolism. *J Neuroimmunol.* 1992;40:225–230.

Robsahm TE, Tretli S, Dahlback A, Moan J. Vitamin D3 from sunlight may improve the prognosis of breast-, colon- and prostate cancer (Norway). *Cancer Causes Control.* 2004;15:149–158.

Salem ML. Estrogen, a double-edged sword: modulation of TH1- and TH2-mediated inflammations by differential regulation of TH1/TH2 cytokine production. *Current Drug Targets Inflamm Allergy.* 2004;3(1):97–104.

Saper RB, Eisenberg DM, Phillips RS. Common dietary supplements for weight loss. *Am Fam Physician.* 2004;70(9):1731–1738.

Scott GS, Spitsin SV, Kean RB, Mikheeva T, Kiprowski H, Hooper DC. Therapeutic in experimental allergic encephalomyelitis by administration of uric acid precursors. *PNAS.* 2002;99(25):16303–16308.

Shaw CA, Bains JS. Neurodegenerative disorders in humans: the role of glutathione in oxidative stress-mediated neuronal death. *Brain Res Rev.* 1997;25:335–358.

Shuster EA. Hormonal influences in multiple sclerosis. *Curr Top Microbiol Immunol.* 2008;318:267–311.

Sutherland G, Andersen M. Exercise and multiple sclerosis: physiological, psychological, and quality of life issues. *J Sports Med Phys Fitness.* 2001;41:421–432.

Suzuki T, Suzuki N, Engleman EG, et al. Low serum levels of dehydroepiandrosterone may cause deficient IL-2 production by lymphocytes in patients with systemic lupus erythematosus (SLE). *Clin Exp Immunol.* 1995;99:251–255.

Swank RL, Lerstad O, Strom A. Multiple sclerosis in rural Norway: its geographical and occupational incidence in relation to nutrition. *N Engl J Med.* 1952;246:721–728.

Szabo G. Consequences of alcohol consumption on host defense. *Alcohol Alcohol.* 1999;34:830–841.

Using Yoga to help with multiple sclerosis. www.americanyogaassociation.org. Accessed June 28, 2009.

Van den Broek HH, Damoiseaux JG, De Baets MH, Hupperts RM. The influence of sex hormones on cytokines in multiple sclerosis and experimental autoimmune encephalomyelitis: a review. *Mult Scler.* 2005;11(3):349–359.

Verstraeten T, Davis R, DeStefano F. Immunity to tetanus is protective against the development of multiple sclerosis. *Med Hypotheses.* 2005;65:966–969.

Visscher BR, Detels R, Coulson AH, et al. Latitude, migration, and the prevalence of multiple sclerosis. *Am J Epidemiol.* 1977;106:470–475.

Voskuhl RR. Gender issues and multiple sclerosis. *Curr Neurol Neurosci Rep.* 2002;2:277–286.

Voskuhl RR, Palaszynski K. Sex hormones in experimental autoimmune encephalomyelitis: implications for multiple sclerosis. *Neuroscientist.* 2001;7:258–270.

Whiting SJ, Calvo MS. Dietary recommendations to meet both endocrine and autocrine needs of vitamin D. *J Steroid Biochem Mol Biol.* 2005;97:7–12.

Zahr NM, Mayer D, Vinco S, et al. In vivo evidence for alcohol-induced neurochemical changes in rat brain without protracted withdrawal, pronounced thiamine deficiency, or severe liver damage. Neuropsychopharmacology: Official publication of the American College of Neuropsychopharmacology. 2008 Aug 13.

Zozulya AL, Wiendl Heinz. The role of regulatory T cells in multiple sclerosis. Nature clinical practice. *Neurology.* 2008;4(7):384–398.

31

HIV

KAREN E. KONKEL

CASE STUDY

Suzanne was diagnosed with human immunodeficiency virus (HIV) in 2001, when she came to my office with oral thrush. She was not surprised, saying, "It was bound to catch up with me." Then aged 35, she had been using intravenous heroin since her late teens, initially as a way to cope with the death of her grandmother, who had raised her. Her first use "had me hooked," and she had been in and out of rehabilitation programs since then.

She now calls her diagnosis "the ultimate wake-up" and has successfully managed both her addiction and her HIV through the integration of complementary and conventional methods. She takes a standard three-drug antiretroviral medication regimen and has enhanced her general health over the intervening years through a regular practice of yoga, a whole food diet, and walking daily. She has finished school and will soon be certified as a drug and alcohol counselor.

While Suzanne's success in shifting her life's trajectory may be somewhat unusual, she is someone from whom we can learn and who offers an example of the benefits that can be reaped from taking an integrative approach to healing in the treatment of HIV/AIDS.

Introduction

A cquired immune deficiency syndrome (AIDS) was first recognized as an infectious disease in the early 1980s (KFF 2008; UCSF 2008). Within a few years, AZT, the first drug to treat the illness, became Food and Drug Administration (FDA)-approved. By 1995, the first protease inhibitor, saquinavir, was approved, and the era of multidrug "cocktails," also known as highly active antiretroviral therapy (HAART), began.

> I was in medical school in the early 1990s, when most of the patients on the hospital internal medicine service were young people dying of AIDS. Very little could be done beyond coordinating palliative care and offering emotional support. It was here that I learned the healing power of the physician–patient relationship.

Since then, much has changed. What was once a death sentence has become a chronic manageable disease, affecting many demographic groups, a significant one being heterosexual women. Offering an integrative approach to care may help women with HIV/AIDS live longer, healthier, and happier lives.

This chapter offers basic information about HIV, focusing on aspects unique to women, followed by an overview of conventional treatments, along with detailed evidence for additional therapies that can be integrated into conventional care to guide women to live well with HIV. Because of the tremendous complexity of HIV medicine, the reader is advised to consult an HIV specialist and to explore more comprehensive resources prior to providing treatment for HIV infection.

Epidemiology

Worldwide, 33.2 million people are living with HIV, of whom 15.5 million are women (UNAIDS 2007). In the United States in 2003, about 1 million people in the United States were living with HIV (CDC 2008). In 2005, 9708 women were diagnosed with HIV, representing about 26% of new cases (CDC 2008). Further, an estimated 95,959 women were living with AIDS, representing 23%

of the estimated total of 421,873. In comparison, in 1992, only 14% of those living with AIDS were women.

Although the prevalence of infection in women in general has increased, it has disproportionately affected certain ethnic groups. In 2005, black women were 23 times, and Hispanic women were four times, as likely as Caucasian women to be diagnosed with AIDS (CDC 2008). Of all women diagnosed with HIV/AIDS in 2005, 83% were non-Caucasian, and most were infected through heterosexual contact.

Circumstances Unique to Women

Many factors may influence the risk for women to become infected with HIV or create barriers to proper medical care once infected.

PHYSICAL TRANSMISSION OF THE VIRUS

When a couple is not using condoms, a woman is far more likely to be infected by a male partner than vice versa (Padian et al. 1991, 1997). Though sexual transmission from female to male is not highly efficient, HIV-infected women can easily transmit the virus through both pregnancy and breastfeeding.

PARTNER RELATIONSHIPS

There are several reasons why a woman may not expect or insist upon her partner using a condom, including perceived lack of self-efficacy, having an older sexual partner, or experiencing interpersonal violence within the relationship (DiClemente et al. 1996; Langille et al. 2007; Raiford et al. 2007; Teitelman et al. 2008). Further, a woman may believe her partner is monogamous, when in fact he may have other sexual partners, some of whom may be male. An outwardly heterosexual male who has covert sexual relationships with other men has been referred to as "being on the Down Low, or the DL" (Ford et al. 2007).

CAREGIVER ROLES

Women are often responsible for the care of children or others. Consequently, their own care may not be prioritized and therefore may be compromised.

SUBSTANCE USE

This is the second most common route of HIV infection in women (CDC 2008). Substance use is often deeply entangled with poverty, poor self-esteem, violence, and lack of resources, all of which will influence risks for HIV and receipt of inadequate health care.

LACK OF RESOURCES

Low socioeconomic status, inadequate access to transportation, un- or under-employment, and lack of health insurance are significant barriers to women receiving adequate preventive and proactive health care services (Anderson 2005).

PRIMARY MEDICAL CARE

Aside from considering the psychosocial and cultural issues particular to women with HIV, there are several areas of medical care that are unique. These include, but may not be limited to, cervical cancer screening, contraception, preconception counseling, and pregnancy and postpartum care. The breadth of these topics is beyond the scope of this chapter, and the reader is referred to other excellent resources in the field (Anderson 2005; AAHIVM 2007).

> The essence of integrative medicine is a healing patient–practitioner relationship. I find that such relationships are best forged by openly listening to a woman talk about her stressors, family and cultural roles, lifestyle and habits, self-perception, and other "nonmedical" concerns that she brings to the examination room.

Pathophysiology and Diagnosis

HIV is a retrovirus that selectively infects cells with CD4 receptors, primarily lymphocytes, monocytes, macrophages, and microglial cells in the brain. It can be transmitted through sexual contact, pregnancy and breastfeeding, transfusion of unscreened blood products, and sharps contaminated with HIV-infected blood or body fluids.

Once infection occurs, the virus rapidly destroys CD4-positive lymphocytes, primarily in the GI-associated lymphoid tissue, a change only gradually reflected in the peripheral blood where they are measured (Brenchley et al. 2004; Mehandru et al. 2004, 2006). This ultimately results in AIDS, which may manifest as opportunistic infections, cachexia, chronic diarrhea, prolonged fever, oropharyngeal candidiasis, generalized lymphadenopathy, lymphoma, dementia, and other illnesses (CDC 1992).

Infection may be suspected based upon AIDS symptoms, presence of risk factors, or the acute retroviral syndrome, which may include fever, sore throat, diarrhea, and myalgias. The 2006 CDC guidelines for HIV testing of adults, adolescents, and pregnant women in health care settings recommend routine HIV screening as long as people are notified and do not opt-out. State laws about HIV testing may vary; be familiar with local laws prior to testing.

Except for acute seroconversion, which requires testing for viral RNA, HIV infection is diagnosed by enzyme immunoassay, an antibody test, confirmed by Western Blot. Testing can be done on blood, saliva, and urine, and rapid 20-minute testing kits are available. Once the diagnosis is made, further evaluation is necessary to determine stage of infection and to initiate appropriate medical interventions.

Overview of Conventional Treatment of HIV Infection

Treatment of people with HIV/AIDS requires both primary care and HIV-specific care. Primary care addresses preventive needs, self-limited illness care, and management of chronic conditions other than HIV. HIV-specific care, especially treatment with HAART, is ideally provided by clinicians with expertise in the management of HIV (Landon et al. 2005). The risk for developing resistant infection is high if medications are not correctly chosen, and many of the medications have toxicities and drug interactions that require proficiency to monitor and manage.

Treatment with HAART involves an appropriately chosen combination of three or more antiretroviral medications with the goal of complete and ongoing suppression of viremia. Strict adherence to taking HAART is critical in avoiding the development of resistant infection. For this reason, medications are typically not started until a person's readiness for treatment has been assured.

Integrative Therapies for Women Living with HIV/AIDS

Early in the epidemic, when conventional medicine could offer little to treat HIV/AIDS, many people turned to complementary and alternative medicine

(CAM). However, despite the remarkable advances in treatment, the use of CAM by people with HIV remains prevalent. Since HAART was introduced, several studies have documented a prevalence of the use of CAM in HIV-positive populations ranging from 16% to 67% (Bica et al. 2003; Fairfield et al. 1998; Gore-Felton et al. 2003; Hsiao et al. 2003; Josephs et al. 2007). One study of HIV-positive women found that 60% were using CAM, most commonly vitamins (Mikhail et al. 2004). Clearly, women with HIV are seeking treatment options that either complement or replace conventional care.

The potential implications of CAM use integrated with conventional treatments, particularly HAART, are important to consider. For instance, drug–botanical interactions may negatively influence antiretroviral pharmacokinetics such that suppression of viral load is impaired, creating the potential for development of drug resistance (Lee et al. 2006; Mills et al. 2005; van den Bout-van den Beukel et al. 2006). Further, use of CAM may have an influence on adherence to conventional care. A study of HIV-infected women found that those using CAM in the form of "immunity boosters or vitamins" were 1.69 times more likely to miss a dose of HAART than those not reporting the use of CAM (Owen-Smith et al. 2007).

It is advisable for practitioners working with people with HIV to have a straightforward discussion about pros and cons of integrative therapies in managing HIV-related disease. The remainder of this chapter will therefore focus on a review of evidence about botanicals and supplements, nutrition, physical activity, acupuncture, mind–body medicine, and distant healing.

BOTANICALS AND SUPPLEMENTS

Some supplements have the capacity to influence the pharmacokinetics of HAART (Lee et al. 2006; Mills et al. 2005; van den Bout-van den Beukel et al. 2006). St. John's wort (*Hypericum perforatum*) lowers the levels of both protease inhibitors (e.g., indinavir) and non-nucleoside reverse transcriptase inhibitors (e.g., nevirapine), resulting in risk of viral resistance and drug failure (Zhou et al. 2004). Suspected similar interactions may occur with garlic and vitamin C, though evidence is limited. Milk thistle (*Silybum marianum*), goldenseal (*Hydrastis canadensis*), Echinacea (*Echinacea* spp.), ginkgo (*Ginkgo biloba*), and fish oil may also have interactions, but the clinical significance is uncertain (Lee et al. 2006; Mills et al. 2005; van den Bout-van den Beukel et al. 2006). Caution should be exercised with the use of supplements in those on HAART.

According to a Cochrane Review, there was insufficient evidence to support the use of herbal medicines for treatment of HIV (Liu et al. 2005). However, several herbal supplements included in that review had some evidence to support a positive effect. Further, other studies not considered in the Cochrane Review suggest that there are supplements that may have a beneficial effect in HIV. For instance, in a randomized controlled trial (RCT) of 450 HIV-infected subjects given 200 μg/day of high selenium yeast supplement, higher serum selenium levels were significantly associated with lower HIV viral loads and higher CD4 counts (Hurwitz et al. 2007).

The use of acetyl-L-carnitine (ALCAR) in HIV has been studied in at least two different contexts. First, a small pilot study ($n = 11$) suggested that intravenous ALCAR increased CD4 counts in patients who had declined HAART (Moretti 1998). More plentiful is research regarding the supplement's use for nucleoside antiretroviral-related peripheral neuropathy. One RCT found a significant reduction in neuropathic pain in those treated with intramuscular ALCAR 500 mg twice daily for 14 days (Youle et al. 2007). A small cohort study of 21 people with NRTI-related neuropathy treated with ALCAR found that after a mean of 4.3 years, 13 of the 16 people who remained in the study reported "very much or moderate" improvement in their symptoms (Herzmann et al. 2005). Another small open-label study ($n = 20$) of short-term use of 2000 mg/day of ALCAR reported a significant reduction in pain-intensity score over 4 weeks (Osio et al. 2006).

Polysaccharides extracted from various forms of algae are under study for potential benefit in HIV. Several in vitro studies have demonstrated suppression of HIV replication in the presence of such polysaccharides (Lee et al. 1999; Notka et al. 2003; Rechter et al. 2006). Clinical trials are lacking thus far.

> While the realm of natural products provides exciting possibilities for the development of novel antiretroviral therapies and adjunct treatments for HIV-related conditions, from a practical standpoint, until more is known about potential interactions, I generally steer patients who are on HAART away from such therapies.

NUTRITION

Consideration of nutrition is important in providing good HIV care. Not only can malnutrition and micronutrient deficiency impair immune function, HIV disease itself appears to cause lipid abnormalities, and some antiretroviral medications adversely affect metabolic parameters, most notably lipids and insulin sensitivity (Khalsa 2007; Wadhwa 2008). Psychosocial barriers, like poverty and homelessness, may impair adequate nutrition. Further, comorbidities such as thrush and poor dental health may affect one's ability to eat.

It is therefore important to take a proactive approach to nutrition counseling in patients with HIV. The use of a micronutrient supplement may increase CD4 counts and decrease disease progression and mortality (Fawzi et al. 2004; Jiamton et al. 2003; Kaiser et al. 2006). Many practitioners routinely recommend a daily multivitamin. Consider referral to a registered dietitian with expertise in HIV/AIDS nutrition. A straightforward approach to a healthier diet includes avoiding processed foods and additives, enhancing consumption of fruits and vegetables, whole grains, high-quality protein sources like beans, fish, legumes, and meats low in saturated fats, and choosing healthier fats like olive oil.

PHYSICAL ACTIVITY

Regular physical activity is important for maintaining good health. For women with HIV, it may be even more important. Aerobic exercise in HIV-positive people may produce a significant increase in CD4+ lymphocyte count (Perna et al. 1999). Two Cochrane Reviews concluded that progressive resistance and aerobic exercise appears to be medically safe and may be beneficial for people living with HIV, particularly in terms of weight, body composition, and cardio-pulmonary fitness (Nixon et al. 2001; O'Brien et al. 2004). The authors noted that future research should include more female participants.

In addition to aerobic and anaerobic exercise, there are plausible, though unproven, benefits of yoga and Tai Chi for those with HIV. Both practices can reduce stress and enhance one's sense of well-being. Given the stressors related to being a woman living with HIV, common sense suggests a likely benefit from these activities. The National Center for Complementary and Alternative Medicine at the National Institutes of Health has sponsored studies of yoga and Tai Chi in people with HIV, though results are not yet available (Clinicaltrials. gov 2008). Another study of Tai Chi in HIV concluded that participation in Tai Chi resulted in a significant improvement in quality of life (QOL) and reduction in HIV-related psychological distress (Robins et al. 2006).

ACUPUNCTURE

Studies of the use of acupuncture in HIV have included treatment of HIV-related neuropathy and HIV-related diarrhea, and enhancements in QOL. One RCT compared amitriptyline, acupuncture, and placebo for HIV neuropathy and found no benefit from either the drug or acupuncture in reducing pain (Shlay et al. 1998). Another study using acupuncture in a group setting to treat painful neuropathy found a significant reduction in pain and other subjective symptoms of neuropathy during a 5-week intervention (Phillips et al. 2004). A small pilot study of men ($n = 15$) experiencing HIV-related diarrhea found that over 4 weeks, the use of acupuncture and moxibustion (applying a heated herb to acupuncture points) decreased stool frequency and improved stool consistency (Anastasi and McMahon 2003).

Several studies have evaluated QOL in people with HIV following acupuncture. A pilot study ($n = 11$) found that an acupuncture intervention showed trends toward improvement in measures of HIV-related symptoms and QOL (Beal and Nield-Anderson 2000). Another pilot RCT ($n = 119$) incorporated the relaxation response (RR) with acupuncture. The acupuncture-only group had significant improvement in emotional QOL, while the acupuncture-RR group had significant improvements in emotional, spiritual, physical, and mental health measures of QOL (Chang et al. 2007).

MIND–BODY MEDICINE

This realm of CAM offers the greatest evidence for benefit to people with HIV, though most research has been done in men. A summary of some of the literature follows.

- A study of 36 HIV-infected African-American, Haitian, and Caribbean women noted that greater pessimism was related to lower natural killer (NK) cell cytotoxicity and cytotoxic/suppressor cells (Byrnes et al. 1998). Of 100 HIV-positive subjects followed longitudinally, those with attitudes of denial were more likely to become symptomatic, whereas those with a "fighting spirit" were less likely to progress (Solano et al. 1993).
- A meta-analysis of cognitive behavioral interventions for HIV suggested treatment-related improvements in depression, anxiety, anger, and stress, with limited evidence for an increase in CD4 count (Crepaz et al. 2008). An analysis of HIV-positive gay men who concealed their homosexuality reported that HIV progression advanced in direct proportion to the degree to which the men were "in the closet." The more "out" they were, the slower the disease progressed (Cole et al. 1996). A similar study demonstrated that men who consistently disclosed their HIV status and sexual orientation were more likely to have a rise in their CD4 count than those who did not (Strachan et al. 2007).
- A study of 25 HIV-infected gay or bisexual men randomly assigned to a control group or to a cognitive behavioral stress management (CBSM) group showed a small increase in naïve T cells in the CBSM

group, a 25% decline in naïve T cells in the control group, and the difference was not explained by baseline T cell count, viral load, or use of HAART (Antoni et al. 2002). Similarly, 49 gay HIV-infected men were randomized to a CBSM group or a control group. Those participating in CBSM maintained better psychosocial status and immunologic control of latent EBV infection up to 1 year later (Carrico et al. 2005). Another study of 10 HIV-positive gay men with CD4 < 400 were randomly assigned to a control group or to a relaxation treatment group. The treatment group showed significant improvement in anxiety, mood, self-esteem, and CD4 count, which was maintained at a 1-month follow-up (Taylor 1995).

Given the relatively ample evidence for mind–body medicine in the care of people living with HIV, including it in routine HIV care should be considered. A cost-effective way of doing so is through group visits, which can be used to teach stress management and relaxation strategies.

DISTANT HEALING

A fascinating double-blind randomized trial assessed the benefits of distant healing for people with advanced HIV (Sicher et al. 1998). Forty subjects with advanced HIV were pair-matched for age, CD4 count, and number of AIDS-defining illnesses and divided into treatment and control groups. Self-identified healers from various spiritual and secular traditions performed distant healing. After 6 months, a blinded chart review found that those in the treatment group acquired significantly fewer new AIDS-defining illnesses, had lower illness severity, had significantly improved mood, and required significantly fewer doctor visits, hospitalizations, and days of hospitalization. A later study failed to replicate the findings, though treatment group subjects were significantly more likely to correctly guess that they had been the recipients of distant healing (Astin et al. 2006).

REFERENCES

AAHIVM Fundamentals of HIV Medicine, 2007 Edition. Washington, DC: American Academy of HIV Medicine.

Anastasi JK, McMahon DJ. Testing strategies to reduce diarrhea in persons with HIV using traditional Chinese medicine: acupuncture and moxibustion. *J Assoc Nurses AIDS Care.* 2003;14(3):28–40.

Anderson J. *A Guide to the Clinical Care of Women with HIV/AIDS*. 2005 ed. Rockville, MD: U.S. Department of Health & Human Services, Health Resources & Services Administration, HIV/AIDS Bureau; 2005; Chapter 8.

Antoni MH, Cruess D, Klimas N, et al. Stress management and immune system reconstitution in symptomatic HIV-infected gay men over time: effects on transitional naive T-cells (CD4+CD45RA+CD29+). *Am J Psychiatry*. 2002;159:143–145.

Astin JA, Stone J, Abrams DI, et al. The efficacy of distant healing for human immunodeficiency virus—results of a randomized trial. *Altern Ther Health Med*. 2006;12(6):36–41.

Beal MW, Nield-Anderson L. Acupuncture for symptom relief in HIV-positive adults: lessons learned from a pilot study. *Altern Ther Health Med*. 2000;6(5):33–42.

Bica I, McGovern B, Dhar R, et al. Use of complementary and alternative therapies by patients with human immunodeficiency virus disease in the era of highly active antiretroviral therapy. *J Altern Complement Med*. 2003;9(1):65–76.

Brenchley JM, Schacker TW, Ruff LE, et al. CD4+ T cell depletion during all stages of HIV disease occurs predominantly in the gastrointestinal tract. *J Exp Med*. 2004;200(6):749–759.

Byrnes DM, Antoni MH, Goodkin K, et al. Stressful events, pessimism, natural killer cell cytotoxicity, and cytotoxic/suppressor T cells in HIV+ black women at risk for cervical cancer. *Psychosom Med*. 1998;60(6):714–722.

Carrico AW, Antoni MH, Pereira DB, et al. Cognitive behavioral stress management effects on mood, social support, and a marker of antiviral immunity are maintained up to 1 year in HIV-infected gay men. *Int J Behav Med*. 2005;12(4):218–226.

Centers for Disease Control and Prevention (CDC). http://www.cdc.gov/hiv/resources/factsheets/us.htm. Accessed April 4, 2008.

Centers for Disease Control and Prevention (CDC). http://www.cdc.gov/hiv/topics/women/resources/factsheets/women.htm. Accessed April 4, 2008.

Centers for Disease Control and Prevention (CDC). 1993 revised classification system for HIV infection and expanded surveillance case definition for AIDS among adolescents and adults. *MMWR Morb Mortal Wkly Rep*. 1992;41(RR-17):1–19.

Chang BH, Boehmer U, Zhao Y, Sommers E. The combined effect of relaxation response and acupuncture on quality of life in patients with HIV: a pilot study. *J Altern Complement Med*. October 2007;13(8):807–815.

Clinicaltrials.gov http://clinicaltrials.gov/ct2/show/NCT00029237?term=%28NCCAM%29+%5BSPONSOR%5D+%28tai+chi%29+%5BTREATMENT%5D&rank=10. Accessed April 27, 2008 and August 5, 2009.

Clinicaltrials.gov http://clinicaltrials.gov/search/term=(NCCAM)+%5BSPONSOR%5D+(yoga)+%5BTREATMENT%5D?recruiting=false. Accessed April 27, 2008 and August 5, 2009.

Cole SW, Kemeny ME, Taylor SE, et al. Accelerated course of human immunodeficiency virus infection in gay men who conceal their homosexual identity. *Psychosom Med*. 1996;58:219–231.

Crepaz N, Passin WF, Herbst JH, et al. Meta-analysis of cognitive-behavioral interventions on HIV-positive persons' mental health and immune functioning. *Health Psychol*. 2008;27(1):4–14.

DiClemente RJ, Lodico M, Grinstead OA, Harper G, Rickman RL, Evans PE. African-American adolescents residing in high-risk urban environments do use condoms: correlates and predictors of condom use among adolescents in public housing developments. *Pediatrics*. 1996;98(2 Pt 1):269–278.

Fairfield KM, Eisenberg DM, Davis RB, Libman H, Phillips RS. Patterns of use, expenditures, and perceived efficacy of complementary and alternative therapies in HIV-infected patients. *Arch Intern Med*. 1998;158(20):2257–2264.

Fawzi WW, Msamanga GI, Spiegelman D, et al. A randomized trial of multivitamin supplements and HIV disease progression and mortality. *N Engl J Med*. 2004;351:23–32.

Ford C, Whetten K, Hall S, Kaufman J, Thrasher A. Black sexuality, social construction, and research targeting "The Down Low" ("The DL"). *Ann Epidemiol*. 2007;17(3):209–216.

Gore-Felton C, Vosvick M, Power R, et al. Alternative therapies: a common practice among men and women living with HIV. *J Assoc Nurses AIDS Care*. 2003;14(3):17–27.

Herzmann C, Johnson MA, Youle M. Long-term effect of acetyl-L-carnitine for antiretroviral toxic neuropathy. *HIV Clin Trials*. 2005;6(6):344–350.

Hsiao AF, Wong MD, Kanouse DE, et al. Complementary and alternative medicine use and substitution for conventional therapy by HIV-infected patients. *J Acquir Immune Defic Syndr*. 2003;33(2):157–165.

Hurwitz BE, Klaus JR, Llabre MM, et al. Suppression of human immunodeficiency virus type 1 viral load with selenium supplementation: a randomized controlled trial. *Arch Intern Med*. 2007;167(2):148–154.

Jiamton S, Pepin J, Suttent R, et al. A randomized trial of the impact of multiple micronutrient supplementation on mortality among HIV-infected individuals living in Bangkok. *AIDS*. 2003;17(17):2461–2469.

Josephs JS, Fleishman JA, Gaist P, Gebo KA; HIV Research Network. Use of complementary and alternative medicines among a multistate, multisite cohort of people living with HIV/AIDS. *HIV Med*. 2007;8(5):300–305.

Kaiser Family Foundation (KFF). http://www.kff.org/hivaids/timeline/hivtimeline. cfm. Accessed March 28, 2008.

Kaiser JD, Campa AM, Ondercin JP, Leoung GS, Pless RF, Baum MK. Micronutrient supplementation increases CD4 count in HIV-infected individuals on highly active antiretroviral therapy: a prospective, double-blinded, placebo-controlled trial. *J Acquir Immune Defic Syndr*. 2006;42(5):523–528.

Khalsa A. Health Maintenance. In: *AAHIVM Fundamentals of HIV Medicine*, 2007 Edition. Washington, DC: American Academy of HIV Medicine. 2007:213–217.

Landon BE, Wilson IB, McInnes K, et al. Physician specialization and the quality of care for human immunodeficiency virus infection. *Arch Intern Med*. 2005;165:1133–1139.

Langille DB, Hughes JR, Delaney ME, Rigby JA. Older male sexual partner as a marker for sexual risk-taking in adolescent females in Nova Scotia. *Can J Public Health*. 2007;98(2):86–90.

Lee JB, Hayashi K, Hayashi T, Sankawa U, Maeda M. Antiviral activities against HSV-1, HCMV, and HIV-1 of rhamnan sulfate from *Monostroma latissimum*. *Planta Med*. 1999;65(5):439–441.

Lee LS, Andrade AS, Flexner C. Interactions between natural health products and anti-retroviral drugs: pharmacokinetic and pharmacodynamic effects. *Clin Infect Dis.* 2006;43(8):1052–1059. Epub September 8, 2006.

Liu JP, Manheimer E, Yang M. Herbal medicines for treating HIV infection and AIDS. *Cochrane Database Syst Rev.* 2005;3:CD003937.

Mehandru S, Poles MA, Tenner-Racz K, et al. Mechanisms of gastrointestinal CD4+ T-cell depletion during acute and early human immunodeficiency virus type 1 infection. *J Virol.* 2007;81(2):599–612. Epub October 25, 2006.

Mehandru S, Poles MA, Tenner-Racz K, et al. Primary HIV-1 infection is associated with preferential depletion of CD4+ T lymphocytes from effector sites in the gastro-intestinal tract. *J Exp Med.* 2004;200(6):761–770.

Mikhail IS, DiClemente R, Person S, et al. Association of complementary and alterna-tive medicines with HIV clinical disease among a cohort of women living with HIV/AIDS. *J Acquir Immune Defic Syndr.* 2004;37(3):1415–1422.

Mills E, Montori V, Perri D, Phillips E, Koren G. Natural health product-HIV drug interactions: a systematic review. *Int J STD AIDS.* 2005;16(3):181–186.

Moretti S. Effect of L-carnitine on human immunodeficiency virus-1 infection-associated apoptosis: a pilot study. *Blood.* 1998;91:3817–3824.

Nixon S, O'Brien K, Glazier RH, Tynan AM. Aerobic exercise interventions for adults living with HIV/AIDS. *Cochrane Database Syst Rev.* 2001;1:CD001796.

Notka F, Meier GR, Wagner R. Inhibition of wild-type human immunodeficiency virus and reverse transcriptase inhibitor-resistant variants by Phyllanthus. *Antiviral Res.* 2003;58(2):175–186.

O'Brien K, Nixon S, Glazier RH, Tynan AM. Progressive resistive exercise interventions for adults living with HIV/AIDS. *Cochrane Database Syst Rev.* 2004;4:CD004248.

Osio M, Muscia F, Zampini L, et al. Acetyl-l-carnitine in the treatment of painful anti-retroviral toxic neuropathy in human immunodeficiency virus patients: an open label study. *J Peripher Nerv Syst.* 2006;11(1):72–76.

Owen-Smith A, Diclemente R, Wingood G. Complementary and alternative medi-cine use decreases adherence to HAART in HIV-positive women. *AIDS Care.* 2007;19(5):589–593.

Padian NS, Shiboski SC, Glass SO, Vittinghoff E. Heterosexual transmission of Human Immunodeficiency Virus (HIV) in Northern California: results from a ten-year study. *Am J Epidemiol.* 1997;146:350–357.

Padian NS, Shiboski SC, Jewell NP. Female-to-male transmission of human immuno-deficiency virus. *JAMA.* 1991;266:1664–1667.

Perna FM, LaPerriere A, Klimas N, et al. Cardiopulmonary and CD4 cell changes in response to exercise training in early symptomatic HIV infection. *Med Sci Sports Exerc.* 1999;31(7):973–979.

Phillips KD, Skelton WD, Hand GA. Effect of acupuncture administered in a group setting on pain and subjective peripheral neuropathy in persons with human immu-nodeficiency virus disease. *J Altern Complement Med.* 2004;10(3):449–455.

Raiford JL, Wingwood GM, DiClemente RJ. Correlates of consistent condom use among HIV-positive African American women. *Women and Health.* 2007;46(2–3):41–58.

Rechter S, König T, Auerochs S, et al. Antiviral activity of Arthrospira-derived spirulan-like substances. *Antiviral Res.* 2006;72(3):197–206.

Robins JL, McCain NL, Gray DP, Elswick RK Jr, Walter JM, McDade E. Research on psychoneuroimmunology: tai chi as a stress management approach for individuals with HIV disease. *Appl Nurs Res.* 2006;19(1):2–9.

Shlay JC, Chaloner K, Max MB, et al. Acupuncture and amitriptyline for pain due to HIV-related peripheral neuropathy: a randomized controlled trial. Terry Beirn Community Programs for Clinical Research on AIDS. *JAMA.* 1998;280(18):1590–1595.

Sicher F, Targ E, Moore D II, Smith HS. A randomized double-blind study of the effect of distant healing in a population with advanced AIDS. Report of a small scale study. *West J Med.* 1998;169(6):356–363.

Solano L, Costa M, Salvati S, et al. Psychosocial factors and clinical evolution in HIV-1 infection: a longitudinal study. *J Psychosom Res.* 1993;37(1):39–51.

Strachan ED, Bennett WR, Russo J, Roy-Byrne PP. Disclosure of HIV status and sexual orientation independently predicts increased absolute CD4 cell counts over time for psychiatric patients. *Psychosom Med.* 2007;69(1):74–80. Epub December 13, 2006.

Taylor DN. Effects of a behavioral stress-management program on anxiety, mood, self-esteem, and T-cell count in HIV positive men. *Psychol Rep.* 1995;76(2):451–457.

Teitelman AM, Ratcliffe SJ, Morales-Aleman MM, Sullivan CM. Sexual relationship power, intimate partner violence, and condom use among minority urban girls. *J Interpers Violence.* 2008; 23: 1694–1712.

University of California at San Francisco (UCSF). http://www.library.ucsf.edu/collres/archives/ahp/chron.html. Accessed March 28, 2008.

UNAIDS. AIDS Epidemic Update: December 2007.

van den Bout-van den Beukel CJ, Koopmans PP, van der Ven AJ, De Smet PA, Burger DM. Possible drug-metabolism interactions of medicinal herbs with antiretroviral agents. *Drug Metab Rev.* 2006;38(3):477–514.

Wadhwa S. Epidemiology and pathogenesis of dyslipidemia and cardiovascular disease in HIV-infected patients. In: Rose BD, ed. *UpToDate.* Waltham, MA: UpToDate; 2008.

Youle M, Osio M; ALCAR Study Group. A double-blind, parallel-group, placebo-controlled, multicentre study of acetyl L-carnitine in the symptomatic treatment of antiretroviral toxic neuropathy in patients with HIV-1 infection. *HIV Med.* 2007;8(4):241–250.

Zhou S, Chan E, Pan SQ, Huang M, Lee EJ. Pharmacokinetic interactions of drugs with St John's wort. *J Psychopharmacol.* 2004;18(2):262–276.

32

Anxiety

ROBERTA LEE

CASE STUDY

April is a patient that I have worked with for 3 years. At 49 years, she had seen her share of difficult times. We had spent the last 3 months unraveling the significance of her difficulties on her health. A year ago, this mother of three robust children with a very supportive husband lost her youngest child to leukemia. The loss came suddenly. Her healthy son began experiencing illness after a viral illness, then chronic fatigue, and finally a devastating bone marrow cancer. The cancer was very aggressive and he failed chemotherapy, an unusual outcome. She felt very guilty about the loss. In her family, she was the major wage earner, spending an average of 30% of her time traveling as a business executive in sales. It was not a surprise to hear her express guilt concerning her absences in her son's life and this was compounded by profound grief—all very normal reactions for such a difficult situation. Early on, we decided that she and her family would benefit greatly in airing the feelings they were struggling with by having a family therapist. She continued these sessions but experienced many challenging symptoms despite her active involvement in making sense of this loss. The primary feeling she experienced was anxiety. She had reoccurring thoughts that she might lose one of her other children to cancer. When this dread surfaced, she noticed a particular order of sensations. The day before she would be irritable, that night she would have difficulty sleeping and wake-up from what seemed like hot flashes—and it all was much more dramatic on her travel away from home. When this happened, she also had a tougher time with her periods and her cycles seemed heavier. Often she would notice very dramatic bloating, cramping, and irritability several days before her period started. When I asked her what her diet was like— she sheepishly admitted that desserts and pasta were becoming a reward food on her travels—her weight was beginning to climb. She was "too tired" to keep up her walking routine and stopped her 45-minute walks, which she would do with a friend 4 days a week. I had her take the Hamilton Anxiety Rating test. The scoring was: mild anxiety: 18+, moderate anxiety: 25+: severe anxiety: 30+. April's score was 23. Her focus was "home and work, work and home"—gone were any lunches or even much conversation with any girlfriends. Much as she hated to admit it—she felt "imprisoned" by the routine. Lately, it was difficult to focus on work— she was simply too agitated.

Her treatment involved a full medical workup to exclude any medical diagnosis that would mimic these symptoms, for example, undiagnosed hypothyroidism or hypercortisolism. The next objective was to "rebalance her lifestyle routines." We put together a sleep ritual that included no emails, or other electronic communication 1 h prior to retiring, a hot bath and use of the essential oil of lavender (five drops in the tub). Her bedroom was cluttered and thus on one weekend, she made a commitment to remove all work-related things in the bedroom. Next when at home, we established a general time of retirement and wake-up. Her work life demanded frequent meals out and travel. We looked at her typical menus and selected potential food choices that were healthier. An exercise plan was formulated using a pedometer to assess distances achieved. She was able to initiate 10,000 steps 4 days a week. Several micronutrients were low on her physical: vitamin B12, magnesium, and vitamin 25-hydroxy cholecalciferol. She was advised to start the following supplements: magnesium glycinate 200 mg/day, vitamin D3 2000 IU/day, and vitamin B12 1000 µg/day sublingually. We reconstructed her diet and made a menu plan with the objective that she would stick to a Mediterranean diet increasing the use of olive oil, fish, whole grains, fruits, and vegetables. We blocked out her schedule so she had time to communicate regularly either in phone or in person with friends at least once a week. In 4 months, her HAM-A scale dropped to 10 (normal).

Introduction

Anxiety disorders affect approximately 40 million American adults or 18% of the population in a given year (Kessler et al. 2005). Anxiety disorders are categorized into subtypes: panic disorder, obsessive–compulsive disorder (OCD), posttraumatic stress disorder (PTSD), social phobia, specific phobia, and generalized anxiety disorder (GAD). Each anxiety disorder has different symptoms but all share a commonality of excessive dread and irrational fear. According to prevalence estimates, women are twice as likely as men to suffer from generalized anxiety, panic disorder, social phobias, and so on. This chapter will focus on GAD.

According to the DSM-IV criteria, the estimated lifetime prevalence of GAD is 4.1%. In a primary care setting, the prevalence of GAD is approximately 5%–8% (Kessler et al. 1994). Twice as many women as men suffer from GAD. Patients with GAD predominantly present with somatic symptoms (Hettema et al. 2005).

In the National Comorbidity survey, patients with GAD showed the following comorbid psychiatric diagnoses: social phobia 23.2% and 34.4%, specific phobia 24.5% and 35.1%, panic disorder 22.6% and 23.5%, and major depression 38.6% and 62.4% (Wittchen et al. 1994) (Table 32.1).

Approximately 40% of people with GAD have no comorbid conditions, but many develop another disorder as time evolves (Scheweitzer 1995). Psychiatric overlap is common. In fact, concurrent or coexistent organic or psychiatric disease is the rule rather than the exception in patients with GAD (Scheweitzer 1995). For example, panic disorder is common among patients with irritable bowel syndrome (Lydiard 1997). Anxiety disorders and depression frequently coincide—either can trigger the other. In the case of coexisting major depression, treatment of the depression is the primary objective. Subsequent visits will reveal whether the anxiety is relieved simply by addressing depression. Many persons coping with anxiety use alcohol or drugs to mask their distress. About 30% of people with panic disorder abuse alcohol, while roughly 17% use drugs (Pozuclo et al. 1999).

Pathophysiology

Generalized anxiety disorder is characterized by maladaptive responses to stressful stimuli and is multifactorial in etiology. Proposed theories include hypothalamic–pituitary–adrenal axis abnormalities with some link to the gut-brain neuropeptide cholecystokinin (Lydiard 1997). An imbalance of neurotransmitters—nor epinephrine, serotonin, γ-aminobutyric acid (GABA)—has also been postulated (Stewart et al. 2001). The amygdala is part of the limbic system and plays a primary role in the processing and memory of emotional reactions. The memories of danger and fear stored in the amygdala appear to be indelible, thus creating a pathophysiologic phenomenon that may progress to GAD (Stewart et al. 2001).

Genetic factors have a modest link in GAD. Some studies suggest a 30% heritability of GAD. Studies indicate genetic concordance with certain genetic loci that produce functional serotonin polymorphisms (Osher et al. 2000). The early environment also represents an important influence that affects genetic expression. One study reported that childhood adversity was associated with the emergence of GAD. Witnessing trauma in childhood was also linked with the development of GAD later in life (Kessler et al. 1997).

Medical causes may also be the primary reason for an anxiety state and should be excluded. These include hyperthyroidism and premenstrual syndrome (see the Table 32.1) among others. In addition, omitting unsuspected medications that cause over stimulation such as albuterol, caffeine, pseudophedrine, methylphenidate, phentermine, sibutramine, haloperidol, and acetazolamide, to name a few, is also suggested.

Table 32.1 provides medical conditions that may be contributing to a sensation of anxiety.

Diagnosis

The diagnostic criteria for GAD as defined by the DSM-IV require the following:

Excessive anxiety and worry about a number of events or activities, occurring more days that not for at least 6 months, that are out of proportion to the likelihood or impact of feared events.

The worry is pervasive and difficult to control.

The anxiety and worry are associated with three (or more) of the following six symptoms (with at least some symptoms present for more days than not for the past 6 months):

Restlessness or felling keyed up or on edge

Being easily fatigued

Difficulty concentrating or mind going blank

Irritability

Muscle tension

Table 32.1. Medical Conditions Often Associated with Symptoms of Anxiety

Cardiovascular	Hematologic
Acute myocardial infarction	Anemia
Angina pectoris	Chronic immune diseases
Arrhythmias	*Neurologic*
Congestive heart failure	Brain tumor
Hypertension	Delirium
Ischemic heart disease	Encephalopathy
Mitral valve prolapse	Epilepsy
Endocrine	Parkinson disease
Carcinoid syndrome	Seizure disorder
Cushing's disease	Vertigo
Hyperthyroidism	Transient ischemic attack
Hypothyroidism	*Respiratory*
Hypoglycemia	Asthma
Parathyroid disease	Chronic obstructive pulmonary disease
Pheochromocytoma	Pulmonary embolism
Porphyria	Dyspnea
Electrolyte imbalance	Pulmonary edema
Gastrointestinal	
Irritable bowel syndrome	
Gynecologic	
Menopause	
Premenstrual syndrome	

Source: Rakel D. *Integrative Medicine*. 2nd ed. In Lee R. "Chapter 4: Anxiety"

Sleep disturbance (difficulty falling or staying asleep, or restless unsatisfying Sleep)
Adapted from American Psychiatric Association *Diagnostic and Statistical Manual of Mental Disorders*. 4th ed. Washington, DC: American Psychiatric Association; 1994

Integrative Treatment

The following four steps are recommended for initial management of patients with GAD in conjunction with CBT, use of either conventional medications, or alternatively dietary supplements and botanicals. The approach focuses on addressing the mind–body–spirit continuum within the context of integrative care:

1. Remove exacerbating factors.
   Review of current medications and supplements that could contribute to anxiety (i.e., over-the-counter stimulants, botanical products designed for weight loss or "energy" enhancement). Caffeine and alcohol should be avoided.
2. Screen for diseases that mimic anxiety.
   Screening for underlying medical conditions that produce anxiety—for instance, hyperthyroidism or a withdrawal syndrome—should be done.
3. Institute physical activity.
   Physical activity (aerobic or anaerobic) at least 5 days out of 7 for 40 min that is enjoyable to the patient.
4. Improve nutrition.
   Nutritional support such as with omega-3 fatty acid supplementation (two to three servings of cold water fish per week, or flaxseed oil two tablespoons a day or 1000 mg of flaxseed oil in a capsule) is recommended.

Exercise

Numerous studies assessing the effects of exercise on anxiety have been published. The majority of these studies measured the effects of exercise on the presence of signs and symptoms of anxiety rather than with use of a diagnostic system like that of the DSM Paluska et al. 2000). Nonetheless, the results of most studies generally show a reduction in symptoms with increased physical activity.

Aerobic exercise programs produced a larger treatment effect than activities such as weight training and flexibility regimens, although both demonstrate effectiveness in the improvement of mood (Martinsen et al. 1989; Paluska et al. 2000). The duration of physical activity is relevant. In one study, programs exceeding 12 minutes for a minimum of 10 weeks were required to achieve significant anxiety reduction. The beneficial effect appeared to be maximal with 40 minutes per session (Paluska et al. 2000) and the benefits were lasting. In one study evaluating the long-term effects of aerobic exercise, participants at 1-year follow-up were found to have maintained the psychological benefits. Their exercise routines over the 12-month follow-up were either the same as those in the original study design or less intensive (DiLorenzo et al. 1999).

Why exercise improves mood is not completely understood. However, increased physical activity has been correlated with changes in brain levels of norepinephrine, dopamine, and serotonin, which may account for improved mood (Dunn et al. 1991). Many studies have shown significant endorphin secretion with increased exercise, with beneficial effects on state of mind. But blockade of endorphin elevation with antagonists such as naloxone during exercise does not correlate with decreased mental health benefits (Dunn et al. 1991). Some investigators have argued that the latter finding reflects flaws in methodologic design.

Nonetheless, the involvement of each patient in active recovery may confer a sense of independence, leading to increased self-confidence. In turn, the patient's ability to cope with challenging life events is increased. This is consistent with the integrative philosophy of healing. Furthermore, low incidence of side effects, low cost, and general availability make exercise a crucial component of integrative management.

The level of exertion and specific exercise prescription should be determined by the patient's level of fitness, interests in specific physical activities, and health concerns. Working with a health care practitioner is advised if a patient is initiating an exercise prescription and is sedentary.

Nutrition

In addition to recommending a wholesome diet, it is important to remove any foods or beverages that can exacerbate anxiety. The two primary offenders are caffeine and alcohol. Americans, on average, consume one or two cups of coffee a day, which represents approximately 150–300 mg of caffeine. People who are prone to feeling stress have reported that they experience increased anxiety from even small amounts of caffeine. With long-term use, caffeine has been linked with anxiety as well as depression. (Bruce et al. 1989) With long-term use, alcohol has been found to diminish levels of serotonin and catecholamines. Discontinuation of alcohol consumption is therefore suggested (Goodwin 1989).

Omega-3 Fatty Acids

Epidemiologic data suggest that omega-3 fatty acid deficiency correlates with increased anxiety. In animal studies, levels of polyunsaturated fats (PUFAs) and cholesterol metabolism have been shown to influence neuronal tissue synthesis, membrane fluidity, and serotonin metabolism (Maes et al. 1999). Studies in patients with major depressive disorder suggest that correction of the ratio of omega-6 to omega-3 consumption may improve mood. Given the evidence concerning neuronal tissue synthesis and serotonin metabolism, increased supplementation with omega-3 fatty acids seems reasonable as a dietary intervention (Bruinsma 2000). Recommending consumption of cold water fish (sardines, mackerel, tuna, salmon, herring) at least two or three times a week, taking a fish oil supplement (EPA 1 g/day), freshly ground flaxseed (two tablespoons daily), or flaxseed oil supplement (1000–2000 mg) would be appropriate.

Dietary Supplements

B VITAMINS

Deficiency of a number of vitamins, including the B vitamins, has been linked with mood disorders. Vitamin B6 (pyridoxine) and B12 (cobalamine) are important for the synthesis of S-adenosyl methionine (SAMe), the primary methyl donor in the production of brain neurotransmitters. B6 is important for the production of serotonin and has been linked with improvement in mood disorders, including anxiety, when supplemented (McCarty 2000). Although large-scale clinical studies are lacking, a trial of a B complex supplement seems advisable, especially in the elderly and persons taking medications that may deplete these vitamins (e.g., oral contraceptive or replacement estrogen) (Murray et al. 1999). Folic acid is a water-soluble B vitamin found in fruits, legumes, and green leafy vegetables. Folate is essential for normal brain function. Patients with low levels of folic acid do not respond well to selective serotonin reuptake inhibitors (SSRIs) (Alpert et al. 2000).

Dosage

The B complex vitamin should provide 100 mg of vitamin B6, 100 µg vitamin B12, and 400–600 µg folic acid.

Precautions

High doses of folic acid have been reported to cause altered sleep patterns, exacerbation of seizure frequency, gastrointestinal (GI) disturbances, and a bitter taste in the mouth. Serum vitamin B12 levels should be checked if folic acid supplementation is used, especially if megaloblastic anemia is noted in laboratory tests, as B12 deficiency can be masked by folic acid supplementation.

S-ADENOSYL METHIONINE

S-Adenosyl methionine (SAMe) is a biomolecule involved in the methylation of monoamines, neurotransmitters, and phospholipids such as phophatidyl-choline and phosphatidylserine. SAMe synthesis appears to be hampered in depressed patients. As depression is often a comorbid condition accompanying anxiety, SAMe may be considered an adjunctive addition in the treatment of anxiety.

Dosage

A total of 1200–1600 mg in divided doses was administered. Start with 200 mg twice daily for several days then increase to 400 mg twice daily for several days then 400 mg three times a day for several days and then, if necessary, increased to 400 mg four times a day (www.naturaldatabase.com 2008).

Precautions

Nausea is reported in some patients with initial use. SAMe is contraindicated in those with bipolar depression, as it can induce mania. Insomnia is a significant side-effect and some patients with predominantly anxiety and not depression, and may complain of increased agitation and irritability.

5-HYDROXYTRYPTOPHAN

5-Hydroxytryptophan (5-HTP) is an amino acid that serves as a precursor to serotonin. 5-HTP easily crosses the blood–brain barrier and effectively increases central nervous system (CNS) synthesis of serotonin, which may improve mood, anxiety, and sleep. Definitive, large-scale studies of efficacy and safety have not been conducted for 5-HTP, though small studies suggest that it superior to placebo in the treatment of depression.

Dosage

100–300 mg/day (www.naturaldatabase.com 2008).

Precautions

Years ago, L-tryptophan was linked to several cases of eosinophilic myalgia syndrome, a serious medical condition that involves the muscles, skin, blood, and other organs. Ultimately, the cause of this rare syndrome was due to a bacterial contaminant in the production process rather the amino acid itself.

Botanical Medicine

KAVA (PIPER METHYSTICUM)

In the realm of botanical medicine, kava is considered as a therapeutic option for the treatment of GAD in the United States and Europe. It is derived from the pulverized lateral roots of a subspecies of a pepper plant, *Piper methysticum*, and is indigenous to many Pacific islands. A review of seven small clinical trials found that kava was superior to placebo in the symptomatic treatment of GAD (Pittler et al. 2000).

The pharmacologically active constituents are the kava lactones, which have a chemical structure similar to that of myristicin, found in nutmeg (Shulgin 1973). These lipophilic lactone structures are present in the highest concentration in the lateral roots. Of the 15 isolated kava lactone structures, six are concentrated maximally in the root and vary depending on the variety of *P. methysticum* (Lebot et al. 1992). Kava's mechanism of action has not been completely elucidated, although the action seems similar to that of benzodiazepines.

Benzodiazepines exert their actions by binding to γ-aminobutyric acid (GABA) and benzodiazepine receptors in the brain; animal studies analyzing kava's anxiolytic action, however, show mixed and minor effects at both sites. Other studies indicate the kava constituents produce anxiolytic effects by altering the limbic system, especially at the amygdala and hippocampus (Pepping

1999). Other documented uses of kava have been as a muscle relaxant, anticonvulsant, anesthetic, and antiinflammatory agent.

Indication

Mild to moderate generalized anxiety.

Dosage

For anxiety, use a product that provides 50–70 mg kava lactones three times daily. For products with a standardized kava lactone concentration of 30%, this would be equivalent to 100–250 mg of dried root.

Precautions

Kava has been reported to cause acute hepatitis. Case reports occurred in those using predominantly ethanol and acetone kava extracts. Although underlying mechanisms are not well established or understood, commonsense dictates that kava should not be used in individuals who have liver problems or who drink alcohol on a daily basis (Blumenthal 2001). Liver tests should be routinely done in individuals who use kava on a daily basis, and patients should be counseled on the signs and symptoms of hepatotoxicity (jaundice, malaise, and nausea). Furthermore, kava should be discontinued from daily use after approximately 4 months. Kava interacts with many medications due to inhibition of CYP450 isozymes: CYP1A2 (56% inhibition), 2C9 (92%), 2C19 (86%), 2D6 (73%), 3A4 (78%), and 4A9/11. Inhibition of CYP450 isozymes is believed to be the most likely factor in causing kava-mediated adverse drug reactions via inhibition of drug metabolism (Mathews 2005).

Anecdotal reports have noted excessive sedation when kava is combined with other sedative medications (Almeida et al. 1996). Extrapyramidal side effects in four patients using two different preparations of kava were reported. Kava should be avoided in those with Parkinson syndrome (Schelosky et al. 1995). With heavy kava consumption, a yellow, ichthyosiform condition of the skin known as kava dermopathy has been observed. This condition is reversible with discontinuation of the kava (Norton 1994. The overdose potential appears low. In many cases, the rash, ataxia, redness of the eyes, visual accommodation difficulties, and yellowing of the skin reported in the literature from Australia and the Pacific region emerged after ingestion of up to 13 L/day, equivalent to

300–400 g of dried root per week. It should be noted that this amount represents a dose 100 times that of the recommended therapeutic dose (Schultz et al. 1998).

Pregnancy and Lactation

There are insufficient data to determine teratogenicity: for this reason, it is wise to avoid use of kava during pregnancy. Kava is present in the milk of lactating mothers; therefore, use is discouraged during breastfeeding (Brinker et al. 1998). Avoid use with other sedative medications.

VALERIAN (*VALERIANA OFFICINALIS*)

Valerian is another botanical that may be used for the treatment of GAD. The clinical efficacy of valerian has been evaluated mostly for treating sleep disturbances; fewer clinical studies assessing its use in anxiety are available. Nevertheless, it has been used in Europe for over a 1000 years as a tranquilizer and calmative. Valerian in combination with passionflower (*Passiflora incarnata*) or St. John's Wort (*Hypericum perforatum*) anxiety has been studied in small clinical trials for anxiety. One study compared valerian root and passionflower (100 mg of valerian root with 6.5 mg of passionflower extract) with chlorpromazine hydrochloride (Thorazine 40 mg/day) over a period of 16 weeks. In this study, 20 patients were randomly assigned to the two treatment groups after being identified as suffering from irritation, unrest, depression, and insomnia. Electroencephalographic changes in both groups consistent with relaxation were comparable; two psychological scales measuring these qualities demonstrated scores consistent with reduction in anxiety (Schellenberg et al. 1994). Another study evaluated anxiety in 100 patients receiving either a combination of 50 mg of valerian root plus 90–100 mg of standardized St. John's Wort for 14 days or 2 mg of diazepam twice daily in the first week and up to two capsules twice daily in the second week. The results showed reduction of anxiety in the phytomedicine treatment group to levels in healthy persons. Patients in the diazepam treatment group still had significant anxiety score (Panijel 1985).

Indication

Mild to moderate anxiety.

Dosage

For adults with anxiety, a dose of 150–400 mg valerian extract in the morning and another dose of 400–800 mg in the evening using a product standardized to 0.8% valerenic acid can be taken. Combinations with lemon balm (*Melissa officinalis*) and hops (*Humulus lupulus*) may also be considered. A combination of valerian and lemon balm was shown effective in treating restlessness and insomnia in children (Müller 2006) and alleviated anxiety in a double-blind randomized controlled trial of healthy volunteers subjected to laboratory-induced stress (Kennedy et al. 2006). Studies using the combination of valerian and hops suggest it is beneficial for improving sleep (Dimpfel and Suter 2008; Koetter et al. 2007; Morin et al. 2005; Reichert 1998).

Precautions

Valerian root is not suitable for the treatment of acute insomnia or nervousness, as it takes several weeks before a beneficial effect is obtained. An alternative that gives a more rapid response should be taken when valerian root initiated (DiLorenzo et al. 1999). There are occasional reports of headache and gastrointestinal complaints.

Mind–Body Medicine

RELAXATION TECHNIQUES

Relaxation training, stress reduction techniques, and breath work are of proven benefit. In fact, imaginal exposure is used as a tactic for repeated exposure to induce anxiety (in a gradual way). Patients learn through repeated exposure to cope with and manage their anxiety rather than eliminate it. A meta-analysis of relaxation techniques such as Jacobson's progressive relaxation, autogenic training, applied relaxation, and meditation were evaluated. Twenty-seven studies were included and the results showed consistent and significant efficacy of these modalities in reducing anxiety (Manzonie et al. 2008). Relaxation training paired with this interceptive therapy is useful. I often encounter patients who admit to their anxiety and are willing to confront and learn to cope with it but lack the ability to completely relax. Depending on their preferences, I help them choose a relaxation technique that reinforces a sense of calm. Therapies that can be used for this purpose are massage, sound therapy, aromatherapy, guided interactive imagery, and hypnosis. Because many patients have somatic sensations that accompany their anxiety, a complementary therapy that imparts a "remembrance" of a deeply relaxed state should also be reinforced on a more somatic-kinesthetic level.

Other Therapies to Consider

ACUPUNCTURE

Traditional medical systems (TMS) such as traditional Chinese medicine can be another option for the treatment of anxiety (Moyad et al. 1993). Several small trials showed a reduction of anxiety symptoms in patients using auricular acupuncture (Breier 1987). A study of 185 women with anxiety, depression, and substance abuse found that 21 days of auricular therapy provided significant reduction in anxiety and physical cravings for substances (Courbasson et al. 2007). Although the mechanisms are not well elucidated, these systems may somehow interface favorably to balance the autonomic nervous system (Arranz et al. 2007).

YOGA

Yoga, a physical and contemplative therapy, can be very calming for anxious individuals. A systematic review evaluated yoga for the treatment of anxiety. Eight studies were reviewed but the authors were unable to determine whether yoga was effective but the results were encouraging, suggesting a benefit of yoga on reducing anxiety symptoms (Kirkwood et al. 2005). A study of 130 subjects with moderate stress either underwent 10 weeks of 1-hour weekly yoga sessions or realxation therapy. Yoga was more effective in improving mental health but at the end of a 6-week follow-up both modalities were comparable in reducing stress (Smith et al. 2007).

MASSAGE

Touch is a universal stimulus that can bring great relaxation in anxiety. As children all of us have memories of touch that soothed us. Thirty-nine subjects with nausea, anxiety, and depressin undergoing chemotherapy for breast cancer received massage treatment for 20 minutes on five occasions. The findings indicated recution of nausea and anxiety (Billhult 2007).

DRUG THERAPY

Consideration of drug therapy depends on the degree of agitation and anxiety. A number of randomized trials have demonstrated the efficacy of antidepressants in the treatment of GAD, however, only a few have FDA approval for this condition. Venlafaxine (Effexor) is the only serotonin-norepinephrine reuptake inhibitor approved for GAD.

Agents approved for panic disorder, social phobia, and posttraumatic stress disorder are listed in Table 32.2 (Ciechanowski et al. 2007). Tricyclic antidepressants are an appropriate therapeutic option but are associated with significant anticholinergic, cardiovascular, and sedative effects. Most experts recommend a trial of at least 4 to 6 weeks to determine efficacy. AS less cardiotoxicity is associated with SSRIs, they may represent a better choice for patients with heart disease. Serotonin reuptake inhibitors have been reported to reduce libido, though the actual incidence of sexual dysfunction is not clear. Strategies for reducing sexual dysfunction include lowering the dose, switching to another SSRI or non-SSRI, or recommending a drug holiday.

Anxiolytics, particularly benzodiazepines, are commonly used for acute treatment of GAD. However, the risk of abuse and habituation must be carefully weighed when prescribing. The anxiolytic buspirone (BuSpar) lacks the problematic issue of drug dependence and excessive sedation (Ciechanowski et al. 2007) and may be a better option.

PSYCHOTHERAPY

The combination of psychotherapy alone, or in conjunction with supplements, botanicals, or prescription anxiolytic or antidepressant, is highly recommended, especially in GAD.

Two clinically proven forms are frequently used behavioral therapy and cognitive-behavioral therapy (CBT) (Hunot et al. 2007). Behavioral therapy focuses on changing the specific unwanted actions by using techniques to stop the undesired behavior. In addition, both behavioral therapy and CBT help patients understand their thinking patterns so that they can react differently to situations that make them anxious.

A meta-analysis found CBT more effective in reducing symptoms in patients with GAD than treatment as usual or waiting list. A controlled study evaluating patients newly diagnosed with GAD found that brief supportive psychotherapy had comparable outcomes to those who initially received benzodiazepines at

Table 32.2. Selected Drug Recommendations for Treatment of Anxiety

Drug	Initial Dose (in mg) (Range)	Frequency
Tricyclics		
Amitriptyline (Elavil)	25–50 (100–300)	qd
Desipramine (Norpramin)	25–50 (100–300)	qd
Imipramine (Tofranil)	25–50 (25–50)	qd
Nortriptaline (Pamelor)	25 (50–200)	
Selective serotonin reuptake inhibitors and mixed reuptake blockers		
Fluoxetine (Prozac)	10–20 (10–80)	qd
Fluvoxamine (Luvox)	50 (50–300)	qd
Paroxetine (Paxil)	10 (10–60)	qd
Sertraline (Zoloft)	50 (50–200)	qd
Others		
Venlafaxine (Effexor)	75 (75–375)	bid
Nefazodone (Serzone)	200 (200–600)	bid
Bupropion (Wellbutrin)	100 (200–450)	bid
Azapirones		
Buspirone (Buspar)	5 (15–60)	bid

Source: Adapted from *Depression Guideline Panel: Depression in Primary Care.* Vol. 2 AHCPR Publication No. 93–0551, Rockville, MD 1993.

3- and 6-month follow-up. Of note, visits to health care providers were not increased in the psychotherapy group. Outcomes were similar for CBT and supportive therapy (Ciechanowski et al. 2007).

Conclusion

In summary, GAD is a common complaint seen in primary care. The cause for GAD appears to be multifactorial and an integrated approach seems to be the most appropriate approach for most patients.

REFERENCES

Almeida JC, et al. Coma from the health food store: interaction between kava and alpra-zolam. *Ann Intern Med.* 1996;125:940–941.

Alpert JE, et al. Nutrition and depression: the role of folate, methylation and monoamine metabolism in depression. *J Neurol Neurosurg Psychiatry.* 2000;228–232.

Arranz L, Guayerbas N, Siboni L, Fuente M. Effect of acupuncture treatment on the immune function impairment found in anxious women. *Am J Chin Med.* 2007;35(1):35–51.

Billhult A, Berbom I, Stener-Vitorin E. Massage relieves nausea in women with breast cancer who are undergoing chemotherapy. *J Altern Complement Med.* 2007;13(1);53–57.

Blumenthal M. American Botanical Council announces new safety information on Kava. ABC Safety Release, December 20; 2001.

Blumenthal M, et al. *The Complete German Commission E Monographs: Therapeutic Guide to Herbal Medicines.* Austin, Tex, American Botanical Council; 1998.

Breier A, et al. Controllable and uncontrollable stress in humans: alterations in mood and neuroendocrine and psychophysiological function. *Am J Psychiatry.* 1987;244:11.

Brinker F, et al. *Herbal Contraindications and Drug Interactions.* 2nd ed. Sandy, Ore, Eclectic Medical Publications; 1998.

Bruce M, et al. Caffeine abstention in the management of anxiety disorders. *Psychol Med.* 1989;19:211–241.

Bruinsma K, et al. Dieting, essential fatty acid intake, and depression. *Nutr Rev.* 2000;4:98–108.

Ciechanowski P, Katon W, Schwenk T, Sokol H. Overview of generalized anxiety disorder. www.uptodayte.com, last updated October 23 2007. Accessed October 6, 2008.

Courbasson CMA, De Sorkin AA, Dullerd B, Van Wyk L. Acupuncture treatment for women with concurrent substance use and anxiety/depression: an effective alternative therapy? *Fam Community Health.* 2007;30(2):112–120.

DiLorenzo T, et al. Long-term effects of aerobic exercise on psychological outcomes. *Prev Med.* 1999;28:75–88.

Dimpfel W, Suter A. Sleep improving effects of a single dose administration of a valerian/hops fluid extract--a double blind, randomized, placebo-controlled sleep-EEG study in a parallel design using electrohypnograms. *Eur J Med Res.* 2008;13(5):200–204.

Dunn AL, et al. Exercise and the neurobiology of depression. *Exer Sport Sci Rev.* 1991;19:41–98.

Goodwin FK. Alcoholism research: delivering on the promise. *Public Health Rep.* 1989;103:569–574.

Hettema J, Prescott C, Myers J, Neale M, Kendler K. The structure of genetic and environmental risk factors for anxiety disorders in men and women. *Arch Gen Psych.* 2005;62;182–189.

Hunot V et al. Psychological therapies for generalized anxiety disorder. *Cochrane Database Syst Rev.* 2007:CD001848.

Kennedy DO, Little W, Haskell CF, Scholey AB. Anxiolytic effects of a combination of Melissa officinalis and Valeriana officinalis during laboratory induced stress. *Phytother Res.* 2006;20(2):96–102.

Kessler RC, Chiu WT, Demler O, Walters EE. Prevalence, severity, and comorbidity of twelve month DSM-IV disorders in the National Comorbidity Survey Replication (NCS-R). *Arch Gen Psychiatry.* 2005;626(6):617–627.

Kessler RC, Davis CG, Kendler KS. Childhood adversity and adult psychiatric disorder in the US National Comorbidity Survey. *Psycol Med.* 1997;27:1101.

Kessler RC, et al. Lifetime and 12-month prevalence of DSM-III –R psychiatric disorders in the United States. *Arch Gen Psychiatry.* 1994;51:8.

Kirkwood G, Rampes H, Tuffrey V, Richardson J, Pilkington K. Yoga for anxiety: a systematic review of the research evidence. *Br J Sports Med.* 2005;39(12):884–891.

Koetter U, Schrader E, Käufeler R, Brattström A. A randomized, double blind, placebo-controlled, prospective clinical study to demonstrate clinical efficacy of a fixed valerian hops extract combination (Ze 91019) in patients suffering from non-organic sleep disorder. *Phytother Res.* 2007;21(9):847–s851.

Lebot V, et al. *Kava—The Pacific Drug.* New Haven, CO: Yale University Press; 1992.

Lydiard RB. Anxiety and the irritable bowel syndrome: psychological, medical, or both? *J Clin Psychiatry.* 1997;58(suppl 13):51–58.

Maes M, et al. Lowered omega 3 polyunsaturated fatty acids in serum phospholipids and cholesteryl esters of depressed patients. *Psychiatry Res.* 1999;85:275–291.

Manzoni GM, Pagnigni F, CAstelnuovo G, Molinari E. Relaxation training for anxiety: a ten-years systematic review with meta-analysis. *BMC Psychiatry.* 2008;8:41.

Martinsen EW, et al. Aerobic and non-aerobic forms of exercise in the treatment of Anxiety disorders. *Stress Med.* 1989;115–120.

Mathews JM, et al. Pharmacokinetics and disposition of the kavalactone kawain: interaction with kava extract and kavalactones in vivo and in vitro. *Drug Metab Dispos.* 2005;33(10):1555–1563.

McCarty MF. High-dose pyridoxine in "anti-stress strategy. *Med Hypotheses.* 2000;54:803–807.

Morin CM, Koetter U, Bastien C, Ware JC, Wooten V. Valerian-hops combination and diphenhydramine for treating insomnia: a randomized placebo-controlled clinical trial. *Sleep.* 2005;28(11):1465–1471.

Moses J, et al. The effects of exercise training on mental well-being in the normal population: controlled trial. *J Psychosom Res.* 1989;33:47–61.

Moyad MA, et al. Ear acupuncture in psychosomatic medicine: the importance of Sanjiao (triple heater) area. *Acupunct Electrother Res.* 1993;18:185–194.

Müller SF, Klement S. A combination of valerian and lemon balm is effective in the treatment of restlessness and dyssomnia in children. *Phytomedicine.* 2006;13(6):383–387.

Murray M, et al. Affective Disorders. In: Pizzorno JE, Murray MT, eds. *Textbook of Natural Medicine.* 2nd ed. Churchill Livingstone; 1999.

Norton SA, et al. Kava dermopathy. *J Am Acad Dermatol.* 1994;31:89–97.

Osher Y, et al. Association and linkage of anxiety related traits with a functional polymorphism of the serotonin transporter gene regulatory region in an Israeli sibling pair. *Mol Psychiatry.* 2000;5:216–219.

Paluska S, et al. Physical activity and mental health: current conepts. *Sports Med.* 2000;29:167–180.

Panijel M. The treatment of moderate states of anxiety: randomized double-blind study comparing the clinical effectiveness of a phytomedicine with diazepam. *Therapiwoche.* 1985;41:4659–4668.

Pepping J. Alternative therapies: Kava: *Piper methysticum. Am J Health Syst Pharm.* 1999;56:957–960.

Pittler M, et al. Efficacy of kava extract for treating anxiety: systematic review and meta-analysis. *J Clin Psychopharmacol.* 2000;20:84–89.

Pozuclo L, et al. The anxiety spectrum: which disorder is it? *Patient Care.* 1999;33:13.

Rakel D. Anxiety. In Lee R. ed.*Integrative Medicine.* 2nd ed. Chapter 4. Philadelphia, PA: Saunders Elsevier; 2007.

Reichert R. Valerian [clinical monograph]. *Q Rev Nat Med Fall.* 1998;207–215.

Schellenberg R, et al. EEG—monitoring and psychometric evaluation of the therapeutic efficacy of Biral N in psychosomatic diseases. *Naturamed.* 1994;4:9.

Schelosky L, et al. Kava and dopamine antagonism. *J Neurol Neurosurg Psychiatry.* 1995;58:639–640.

Scheweitzer E. Generalized anxiety disorder: longitudinal course and pharmacologic treatment. *Psychiatric Clin North Am.* 1995;18:843–857.

Schultz V, et al. *Rational Therapy: A Physicians' Guide to Herbal Medicine.* Berlin: Springer-Verlag; 1998.

Shulgin AT. The narcotic pepper: the chemistry and pharmacology of *Piper methysticum* and related species. *Bull Narc.* 1973;25:59–74.

Shultz V, et al. Kava as an anxiolytic. In: *Rational Phytotherapy: A Physicians' Guide to Herbal Medicine.* Berlin: Springer-Verlag; 1998:65–73.

Smith C, Hancock H, Blake-Mortimer J, Eckert K. A randomised comparative trial of yoga nad relaxation to reduce stress and anxiety. *Complement Ther Med.* 2007;15(2);77–83.

Stewart SH, et al. Causal modeling of relations among learning history, anxiety sensitivity and panic attacks. *Behav Res Ther.* 2001;39:443–456.

Wittchen H, Zhao S, Kessler RC, Eaton WW. DSM-III-R generalized anxiety disorder in the National Comorbidity Sruvey. *Arch Gen Psychiatry.* 1994;51:1216.

www.naturaldatabase.com. Natural Medicines Comprehensive Database: Clinical Management Series: Natural Medicines in the Clinical Management of Anxiety. Accessed October 8, 2008.

33

Depression

NAOMI LAM AND SUDHA PRATHIKANTI

CASE STUDY

Gloria, a 43-year-old married female, presented for treatment of a long-standing depression that had worsened in the 6 months prior to her initial visit. She complained of occasional crying spells, anxiety, sadness, insomnia, and difficulty in concentrating. She stated that she had been "stress eating" and had gained about 15 pounds in the past 6 months. She noted that she sometimes felt "paralyzed, not able to make decisions" and felt she was "constantly second-guessing myself." She denied suicidal thoughts and stated that she was "somehow" able to function relatively well at work and at home despite her symptoms, which were "worse than I've ever had."

Gloria had a full-time job managing a large sales office, was raising two active teenage children, and had recently been diagnosed with hypertension and borderline diabetes. She described herself as the "emotional safety net" not only of her close-knit, large extended family but also of her office staff. In addition to her commitments at work and with family, she was also very active in her church. She was devoted to all of her responsibilities but often felt "a lot of guilt" because she felt "drained instead of nourished" by the many demands placed upon her.

Gloria felt strongly that she would like to avoid using pharmaceuticals. Although she had moderate symptoms of depression, she had never experienced a decrease in functioning, denied suicidal ideation, was very motivated, and had a healthy support network, I felt comfortable to move ahead without recommending medication in the initial treatment plan. I did advise her that should her symptoms worsen, we would need to discuss the possibility of medication. She agreed, and after reviewing her history and medication list, we developed a plan that eventually included traditional Chinese medicine, aerobic exercise, dietary supplementation, and mind–body medicine.

Gloria started a trial of S-adenosyl methionine (SAMe) and tried her best to limit herself to three healthy meals per day with adequate hydration. I advised her to limit her caffeine intake. Always "on the go" but not a big fan of exercise, Gloria was curious about yoga. She attended a few beginning hatha yoga classes at her local gym but soon dropped out due to feeling that "it just wasn't for me." She tried tai chi as well, but felt "it takes too much patience." We then agreed that a short daily walk in her neighborhood would be a healthy initial exercise regimen.

One month later, Gloria noted that she had stopped having crying spells. She attributed this to the SAMe, which had caused some gastrointestinal (GI) upset during the first week of treatment, but which she subsequently tolerated well. She noted that her short-lived contact with yoga had had surprising results: her insomnia had improved, with benefit from practicing savasana, or "corpse pose," at bedtime and when she awoke during the night. She was still having significant anxiety and some sadness during the day, and noted that her neck and shoulders were tight and painful. I recommended that she see an acupuncturist to address both the muscle pain and the mood symptoms. She began to lengthen her daily walks. I recommended that she try to increase her intake of fresh fruit and vegetables, and start taking omega-3 fatty acid supplements.

At her 8-week follow-up, Gloria felt that the SAMe was "definitely" helping with her mood. She also noted that with the changes she had made in diet and exercise, she had lost a couple of pounds, had more energy, and was sleeping better. Acupuncture had significantly decreased her muscle tension and pain, and she noted that the sessions were "incredibly healing and relaxing." We spoke in our sessions about the importance of self-care and about ways to reframe the guilt she felt about "spending so much time on me." She felt motivated to continue her treatment plan.

Four months into treatment, Gloria felt that her depression and anxiety had "mostly" resolved. She was eating and sleeping regularly, and took 1-hour walks approximately every other day. She had stopped seeing her acupuncturist but had incorporated a healthy diet and omega-3 fatty acid supplementation into her routine. We planned a gradual taper of SAMe. Her primary care doctor noted that her blood pressure and blood glucose had responded positively to these changes in her lifestyle. Gloria realized that she was gradually easing into a routine of self-care that helped her not only stay healthy, but also helped her to function more effectively as a caregiver.

Introduction

Over a lifetime, major depression affects women approximately twice as frequently as it does men (Kessler et al. 1993). The etiology of depression is unclear, but it appears to involve not only physiological and psychosocial but also genetic and environmental effects. Specific events in the reproductive life cycle of women—puberty, menses, childbirth, and menopause—appear to put women at higher risk of suffering from depression (Burt et al. 2002).

In addition to these hormonal risk factors, psychosocial stressors play an important role in this increased vulnerability to depression. Women are more likely than men to live in poverty, which is in itself a chronic stressor, and they are thus more likely to be exposed to stressors such as violence and crime (Nolen-Hoeksema 2000). Socialization into traditionally female roles, which tends to involve developing behaviors of nurturance, dependence, and passivity, is also postulated to have an impact on women's increased vulnerability to depression (Nolen-Hoeksema and Girgus 1994).

Given the rich and complicated intra- and interpersonal environment in which depression arises, it seems prudent to approach treatment with a holistic and flexible mindset. Integrative medicine lends itself very well to this approach. This chapter will present brief descriptions of the diagnosis and conventional treatment of depression, and will then focus on specific integrative treatments for depression, presenting evidence for women where available.

Diagnosis

Currently, patients suspected of suffering from depression are diagnosed in accordance with criteria set forth in the *Diagnostic and Statistical Manual*

Table 33.1. Diagnostic Criteria for Major Depressive Disorder

The patient experiences at least 5 symptoms from the following list during a 2-week period, nearly every day. One of the symptoms must be #1 or #2, as listed below:

1. Depressed mood most of the day
2. Markedly diminished interest in almost all activities most of the day
3. Significant weight loss when not dieting, OR weight gain; OR change in appetite
4. Changes in sleep patterns
5. Observable physical restlessness OR slowing down
6. Fatigue
7. Feelings of worthlessness, OR excessive guilt
8. Diminished ability to concentrate, OR noticeable indecisiveness
9. Recurrent thoughts of death (not just fear of dying), OR recurrent suicidal ideation without a specific plan, OR a specific plan for committing suicide, OR a suicide attempt

The symptoms are not due to bipolar affective disorder, a medical condition, or to the effect of drugs. They are not better explained by bereavement. They persist for longer than 2 months, OR they are characterized by marked functional impairment, extreme preoccupation with worthlessness, suicidal ideation, or psychotic symptoms (e.g., hallucinations, delusions).

of Mental Disorders (DSM-IV) (American Psychiatric Association 1994) (see Table 33.1).

However, in the day-to-day treatment of primary care patients, providers see women presenting with depressive symptoms in a large range of severity. For those women with mild-to-moderate symptoms, working with a caring primary physician who has access not only to antidepressant medications but also to information about integrative treatments can be an incredibly positive experience. It is important to note, however, that those women presenting with moderate to severe depression, who are at risk for further decompensation, should be referred to a psychiatrist for specialized management of their symptoms.

Conventional Treatment

A detailed description of the many and varied conventional treatments for depression is beyond the scope of this chapter. In brief, psychotropic medication (primarily antidepressants, anxiolytics, and sedative/hypnotics), physiologic modalities such as electroconvulsive therapy (ECT), and psychotherapy are the major types of psychiatric treatments aimed at lessening depressive symptoms.

As an integrative psychiatrist, I strive to optimize the balance between a woman's clinical need for medications, her attitudes and beliefs about medication, and her innate ability to cope with her feelings. I appreciate the value and benefits of pharmaceuticals and believe in their efficacy, especially in times of crisis. I also feel that if a woman does not believe that the medication will help, her depression may not respond optimally to this particular intervention. In the office, I take into consideration a woman's worries and concerns about taking medications, and incorporate education about their risks and benefits into treatment planning. Formulating a strategy that is clinically appropriate as well as sensitive to my patient's personal belief system is of utmost importance to me.

Commonly prescribed antidepressant medications include those belonging to the selective serotonin reuptake inhibitor (SSRI) class such as fluoxetine (Prozac), paroxetine (Paxil), sertraline (Zoloft), citalopram (Celexa), and escitalopram (Lexapro). Other frequently prescribed antidepressants include mirtazapine (Remeron), bupropion (Wellbutrin), and venlafaxine (Effexor), which have mixed receptor action.

Sexual side effects of antidepressant medications are of concern to many women and may affect approximately 30%–40% of patients taking them. These side effects include decreased libido, delayed orgasm, and anorgasmia. Strategies to address this situation include decreasing the dosage of medication, switching to another antidepressant medication, or adding an agent to decrease the sexual side effect If a patient is having an otherwise robust positive response to the medication, I might recommend lowering the dose or augmenting before I would encourage a switch. Common augmentation strategies include addition of buproprion, which affects noradrenergic and dopaminergic receptors, or yohimbine, which acts on α-2 adrenergic receptors. Of note, I find it vital to take a thorough history of the sexual side effect symptoms and course, as depression itself can cause decreased libido.

Pharmacologic and physiologic treatment approaches are purely biologically based, but an interesting intersection between conventional and integrative medicine occurs in the realm of psychotherapy. This intersection exists because most psychotherapeutic models require the practitioner to have an understanding not only of a patient's symptoms, but also her life history, relationships, personality, coping skills, beliefs, and values, in order to provide effective treatment. There is thus a long-standing tradition within conventional psychiatry of valuing a patient's entire life story. Sadly, in the setting of today's fast-paced medication management visits, and outside of psychotherapy treatment, that valuable part of the doctor–patient interaction is often absent.

In my integrative psychiatric practice, I feel fortunate to be able to approach patients with an eye for their uniqueness. Life circumstances, personality traits, genetic tendencies, and past experiences all shape a person's experience of depressed mood. I think that each woman presents with a singular depression that is a phenomenon distinct from any other patient's. This subjectivity, in my opinion, makes integrative approaches extremely well-suited to the treatment of depression. With integrative treatment in mind, I am able to formulate, together with my patients, individualized treatment plans that honor their particular strengths, interests, likes, and dislikes. This deeply personal way of supporting women through depression can provide a strong foundation upon which to build future treatment success.

Integrative Approaches

DIETARY SUPPLEMENTS AND BOTANICALS

St. John's Wort (Hypericum perforatum)

St. John's Wort is a flowering plant that is commonly used in Western Europe for treatment of mild to moderate depression and anxiety. In the United States, this herb is widely used and is easy to find in drugstores, health food stores, and grocery stores. Though many different preparations are available, not all are manufactured according to high-quality standards (see sidebar).

Hypericin and hyperforin are regarded as probable active compounds in St. John's Wort and are thus often used as marker compounds for standardization. However, to date no consensus regarding the identity of the active compound(s) has been reached. Authors of a recent review (Butterweck et al. 2007) concluded that multiple compounds are most likely responsible for pharmacologic activity.

St. John's Wort has been extensively studied as a possible treatment for depression, and the data have been inconsistent. According to the latest Cochrane Review (Linde 2005a), the effect size of St. John's Wort and placebo were nearly identical in pooled data from large trials. It was noted, however, that St. John's Wort extracts vary widely in pharmaceutical quality, and that the review data should not be generalized beyond those specific Hypericum products involved in the randomized controlled trials (RCTs) studied. A subanalysis in this Cochrane Review suggested that the herb is effective in treating mild depression, but not in addressing moderate or severe depression.

A few meta-analyses have compared St. John's Wort to tricyclic antidepressants, maprotiline, and SSRIs in depression (Linde et al. 1996; Linde, 2005b;

Roder et al. 2004; Whiskey et al. 2001). In these studies, the effect of St. John's Wort was equivalent to that of pharmacotherapy. Similarly, a recent RCT (Szegedi et al. 2005) indicated that St John's Wort 1800 mg/day was equivalent to paroxetine treatment in a group of patients with moderate to severe depression. Interestingly, in a large NIH-funded trial (Hypericum Depression Trial Study Group 2002), neither St. John's Wort nor sertraline was found to be more effective than placebo for moderate-to-severe depression. Taken together, the results of these studies seem to indicate that further research is needed to examine the efficacies of both herbal and pharmaceutical treatment of depression.

St. John's Wort may cause side effects similar to those of SSRIs including dry mouth, GI symptoms, anxiety, headache, fatigue, dizziness, or sexual dysfunction, though in clinical trials, it is better tolerated than SSRIs and the adverse effects are not significantly greater than placebo. St. John's Wort can also cause photosensitivity, and may increase the risk of serotonin syndrome when used in combination with serotonergic antidepressants. It is a cytochrome P450 (CYP450) inducer, and thus can alter blood levels of medications including oral contraceptives, cyclosporine, digoxin, warfarin, irinotecan, and antiretrovirals including indinavir and ritonavir.

The United States Pharmacopeia offers an online resource for those patients interested in finding dietary supplements manufactured to rigorous standards: www.uspverified.org

S-ADENOSYL METHIONINE

S-Adenosyl methionine (SAMe) is a ubiquitous biomolecule that is found in many metabolic pathways, including synthesis of monoamine neurotransmitters such as serotonin, dopamine, and norepinephrine. It has been used as an antidepressant in Western Europe for over 25 years.

SAMe has been extensively studied. Meta-analyses (Bressa 1994; Delle Chiaie et al. 2002) have shown that SAMe is better than placebo, and is equally effective as tricyclic antidepressants (TCAs), in the treatment of major depression. More recently, preliminary data (Mischoulon 2007) suggest that SAMe may have utility as an adjunct to SSRIs, and also that it may have a more rapid onset of action than conventional antidepressants.

SAMe has a side effect profile similar to that of SSRIs: anxiety, agitation, dry mouth, GI disturbances, headache, insomnia, palpitations, dizziness, and sweating. However, it does not cause the sexual side effects so commonly found with SSRI treatment. Bipolar patients taking SAMe are at risk of switching into hypomania, so concomitant treatment with a mood stabilizer is strongly recommended. As with SSRI treatment, the potential for serotonin syndrome exists in patients also taking tramadol, monoamine oxidase inhibitors (MAOIs), and meperidine.

SAMe is not covered by insurance and tends to be expensive. Thus, I have not found it useful to recommend to women on a limited income. However, I have seen positive results for those who can afford it, and who do not experience continued GI side effects. I generally ask women to start at 200 mg PO QAM and increase by 200 mg every 2–3 days in a BID dosing schedule, as tolerated, up to a maximum dosage of 1600 mg qd total. As SAMe can be activating, I advise taking the second dose in the mid-afternoon, no later than 4 PM. GI side effects can be mitigated by taking it with food.

FOLATE

Folate is a water-soluble B vitamin (vitamin B9) found in leafy green vegetables, fruit, and legumes. Epidemiological studies have found consistent associations between folate deficiency and depression. Theoretically, folate's action may be related to its role in the synthesis of SAMe (see above), which is a precursor to monoamine neurotransmitters. Active forms of folate, folinic acid, and methylfolate are preferred over folate in oral supplementation.

A review (Coppen and Bolander-Gouaille 2005) of two RCTs reported that folate augmentation improved response rates to conventional pharmacotherapy. One of these RCTs studied patients with folate deficiency and the other involved subjects with normal folate levels.

Side effects are rare. Folate supplementation should be paired with vitamin B12 supplementation (1 mg PO qd), as exogenous folate can mask the symptoms of B12 deficiency.

Study doses typically range from 0.4 to 1 mg PO qd along with a standard antidepressant medication. Folate is usually continued for the duration of antidepressant therapy.

OMEGA-3 FATTY ACIDS

Omega-3 fatty acids (eicosapentaenoic acid [EPA] and docosahexaenoic acid [DHA]) play many important roles in human metabolism, including that of supporting the growth and development of the nervous system. Epidemiological studies have linked low dietary consumption of omega-3s and increased prevalence of depression.

A recent large review (Parker et al. 2006) included RCTs examining potential effects of omega-3 fatty acid supplementation on mood. In this review, studies showing positive mood benefits involved use of EPA, or EPA/DHA combinations with EPA predominance, as augmentation to conventional pharmacotherapy. Negative studies looked at DHA, or EPA/DHA combinations with DHA predominance, as monotherapy or as adjunct therapy. The exact significance of this particular finding is unclear and deserves further research.

Omega-3 fatty acids are thought to exert their antidepressant effects by several possible mechanisms. They may contribute to neural cell stability and signal transduction by virtue of their integral role in neuronal membrane structure. They may promote secretion of brain-derived neurotrophic factor (BDNF), a peptide involved in promotion of neuronal longevity. Finally, they may help dampen the inflammatory cascades, which are seen in severe depression and which can adversely affect neurotransmitter metabolism.

Side effects include GI disturbance and fishy-tasting burps, both of which can be reduced by using high-quality preparations and keeping daily doses below 5 g qd. Omega-3 fatty acid supplementation, especially above 3 g qd, can cause excessive anticoagulation, so patients taking warfarin should be monitored. There is a small risk of inducing hypomania in bipolar patients, so in these cases concurrent treatment with a mood stabilizer is indicated.

I recommend that patients start with 500 mg PO qd of a high-quality supplement, taken with a meal containing fat, and increase as tolerated by 500 mg every 3–5 days in a BID dosing schedule up to 3 g PO qd.

5-HYDROXYTRYPTOPHAN

5-Hydroxytryptophan (5-HTP) is the immediate metabolic precursor to serotonin. The upregulation of serotonin biosynthesis is the potential mechanism of its antidepressant action. A recent review (Turner et al. 2006) reported mixed data regarding the possible mood benefits of 5-HTP in depression. Of the eleven RCTs studied, only five yielded statistically significant positive results. Of the five positive trials, three used 5-HTP as adjunct therapy to conventional pharmacotherapy, one used it as monotherapy, and one tested a combination of 5-HTP and dopamine versus placebo.

Further, larger studies are needed in order to clarify the potential utility of 5-HTP in the treatment of depression. It is important to recommend a high-quality product as there exists a theoretical risk of eosinophilic myalgia due to contamination. The recommended dosage of 5-HTP is 50–100 mg/day, though some studies have used up to 300 mg/day.

INOSITOL

Inositol, a naturally occurring isomer of glucose, is a key player in the second-messenger system modulating cell surface receptors for serotonin and other neurotransmitters. It is found in a variety of foods including citrus fruit, nuts, whole-grain cereals, and blackstrap molasses. The theoretical mechanism of its antidepressant action is via facilitating cellular responses to serotonin.

A recent review article (Taylor et al. 2004) identified four small RCTs studying inositol in depression. Three of the studies examined inositol versus placebo as adjunct to conventional pharmacotherapy, and showed no difference between the two groups. The fourth RCT yielded potential positive mood benefits for inositol monotherapy versus placebo.

Taking into consideration the paucity of data available, the role of inositol in the treatment of depression remains unclear, and further study is needed. Dosages typically used in studies are 10–12 g PO qd.

Mind–Body Approaches

MEDITATION

The general medical literature focuses upon two types of meditation, both of which are based in Eastern spiritual practices: concentration meditation and mindfulness meditation. There is little data addressing meditation as a primary treatment for major depression, rather existing studies investigated the benefits in medically ill patients with associated depressive symptoms and showed a potential positive effect (Goodale et al. 1990; Irvin et al. 1996; Jayadevappa et al. 2007; Speca et al. 2000). Two small studies of women with breast cancer (Targ and Levine 2002) and fibromyalgia (Sephton et al. 2007) with associated depression also showed mood benefits for meditation.

In one RCT (Sharma et al. 2005), depressed patients exhibited positive mood changes in response to concentration meditation as an adjunct to pharmacotherapy. Also, a recent review (Coelho et al. 2007) summarized data indicating that mindfulness-based cognitive therapy (MBCT), a psychotherapeutic model integrating meditation techniques with cognitive behavioral therapy (CBT) techniques, has potential benefit as an adjunct treatment to reduce risk of relapse in major depression.

Meditation is postulated to exert its effects by modulating the sympathetic and parasympathetic nervous systems. When undertaken with an experienced teacher, health risks are few. However, meditation is not indicated for individuals with a history of psychosis as meditative states can precipitate psychological crises in these patients.

> Where available, I have found it helpful to recommend beginning classes in mindfulness-based stress reduction (MBSR) or vipassana meditation. For those who feel more comfortable learning about meditation on their own, I recommend the book *Peace is Every Step*, a beautiful and accessible introduction to mindfulness meditation by the Vietnamese Buddhist monk Thich Nhat Hanh.

YOGA

Yoga, as practiced in the United States, involves breathing exercises (pranayama) and body postures (asanas). As yoga has entered mainstream American culture, many different types of yoga classes can now be found at local gyms and yoga centers. Some of these varieties include doing yoga in heated rooms, with or without vigorous pose changes. Most available studies in the literature have focused on pranayama in combination with gentle and rhythmic pose shifts.

One review examined the effect of yoga practice in patients with major depression (Pilkington et al. 2005). Though the studies were found to have significant design problems, the authors concluded that yoga has mood benefits in comparison to control groups. Data on depressed women's responses to yoga are scant. A small study (Michalsen 2005) indicated that Iyengar yoga improved depressive symptoms in a group of 24 female patients with "emotional distress," as quantified by the Center for Epidemiologic Studies Depression Scale.

Yoga is postulated to exert its effects by modulating the autonomic and the central nervous system. Performed under the guidance of an experienced teacher, it appears to be fairly safe.

> Beginning classes in hatha yoga or restorative yoga can be found at gyms, yoga centers, and sometimes temples or holistic health centers. In my experience, these forms of yoga are generally well-tolerated by patients. Even a short course of classes can provide benefits, as breathing exercises and poses can be used at home to provide anxiolysis and to ease the transition into sleep.

PROGRESSIVE MUSCLE RELAXATION

Progressive muscle relaxation (PMR) is a behavioral technique that was developed by Dr. Edmund Jacobson in the 1930s. It involves a protocol of step-by-step voluntary muscular contraction and then relaxation.

An elegant and interesting RCT (McLean and Hakstian 1979) showed an equivalent antidepressant effect for PMR and pharmacologic treatment; it also revealed that both of these interventions were inferior to behavior therapy. Two more recent small studies showed value for PMR as an adjunct to pharmacotherapy (Bowers 1990; Broota and Dhir 1990). There is also data suggesting that for patients with primary medical conditions and associated depression, PMR may provide mood benefits (Rodin et al. 2007; Stetter and Kupper 2002; Stiefel and Stagno 2004).

> More information on PMR, including step-by-step instructions for patients, can be found at http://www.guidetopsychology.com/pmr.htm

Traditional Chinese Medicine

ACUPUNCTURE

Acupuncture involves the use of fine needles and sometimes mild electrical current, or lasers, to stimulate specific points on the body, which are postulated to regulate and balance the flow of "qi."

Data from RCTs examining the effects of acupuncture compared to wait list control, sham acupuncture, and conventional treatment in patients with major depression have been analyzed in several review articles (Leo and Ligot 2007; Mukaino et al. 2005; Smith and Hay 2005). The authors of these articles concluded that the studies were methodologically poor, and meta-analysis did not reveal statistically significant differences between treatment groups. A more rigorously designed double-blind RCT examined laser acupuncture in the treatment of mild-to-moderate depression (Quah-Smith et al. 2005). This study showed positive mood benefits as a result of acupuncture treatment.

Data supporting the use of acupuncture in women with depressive symptoms consists mainly of small studies. A pilot study of acupuncture in the treatment of menopause-related symptoms, including depression, in tamoxifen-treated women yielded some preliminary positive results (Porzio et al. 2002). Another RCT examining a group of women with chronic neck and shoulder pain with associated depression revealed benefits for mood and quality of life (He et al. 2005).

As its benefits for analgesia and addiction are well known, and its healing effects for many other conditions are becoming acknowledged, acupuncture is becoming more easily accessible. Those curious about the intervention can find out more information by going online to http://nccam.nih.gov/health/acupuncture/. Information on each state's licensure requirements can be found at: http://acupuncture.com/statelaws/statelaw.htm. Local health care providers, schools of traditional Chinese medicine, or integrative medicine clinics, if available, can be a helpful referral resource for women seeking acupuncture treatment.

TAI CHI/QI GONG

Tai chi and qi gong are elements of traditional Chinese medicine that involve not only prescribed movements, but also regulated breathing and mental focus. Studies available in English are few, but one RCT found positive results for depressed geriatric patients participating in a program of tai chi (Chou et al. 2004). Another recent RCT showed mood benefits from qi gong in a group of depressed elderly patients (Tsang et al. 2006).

If available, local Chinese community centers or martial arts centers can be good resources for beginning tai chi and qi gong classes.

Other Integrative Approaches

AEROBIC EXERCISE

Most studies examining the effect of exercise on patients with depression have focused on walking, jogging, cycling, or swimming. A recent RCT looked at a large group of adults with major depression and found comparable improvements in mood among groups treated with sertraline alone, home exercise alone, or group exercise (Blumenthal 2007). All of the groups showed greater improvement than that found in the placebo-treated group. An RCT examining women with fibromyalgia found that a course of supervised exercise in warm water yielded mood benefits (Tomas-Carus et al. 2008).

Aerobic exercise is postulated to exert its antidepressant effects by increasing levels of monoamine neurotransmitters, upregulating endogenous endorphin production, increasing social contact if done in groups, and possibly by derailing negative thought patterns.

In my practice, I have found that enticing depressed women to exercise, if they are not already involved in regular activity, is quite difficult indeed. Often, the symptoms of decreased energy, psychomotor slowing, and decreased motivation are tenacious barriers. If my gentle suggestions are met with resistance, I will often wait until the depression is partially treated before returning to this particular intervention. I then advise women to build an exercise routine slowly. Taking its efficacy into consideration not only for mood but also for general health and weight loss, I have been happy to see that women often continue with regular exercise after their acute depression subsides.

MASSAGE THERAPY

Massage therapy involves the manipulation of soft tissue, using any of over 80 different techniques, with the goal of increasing well-being. In the United States, classical Swedish massage is the most common and involves the use of five distinct long and flowing strokes. Other common varieties include Shiatsu (a Japanese massage technique) and deep tissue massage.

There is little data available concerning massage therapy as treatment for major depression specifically, but authors of a meta-analysis of studies done on patients with primary medical conditions and associated depression concluded that a course of massage therapy may be as effective as a course of psychotherapy (Moyer et al. 2004).

Massage therapy is proposed to exert its antidepressant action through modulation of the parasympathetic nervous system, and/or by stimulating the release of endorphins or serotonin into the bloodstream via mechanical stimulation of tissue. In the hands of experienced practitioners, this intervention is quite safe.

PHOTOTHERAPY

In the darker winter months, the secretion of melatonin, a metabolic product of serotonin, is increased. Phototherapy suppresses melatonin secretion, which theoretically increases serotonin reserves, leading to an antidepressant effect. While phototherapy for seasonal affective disorder (SAD) is part of the conventional psychiatric armamentarium, this chapter examines the use of phototherapy in the treatment of nonseasonal depression.

A recent review article contained a meta-analysis of three RCTs, which indicated that for nonseasonal major depression, phototherapy alone provided significant reduction of depressive symptoms (Golden et al. 2005). As an adjunct to pharmacotherapy, no benefit was found in this study. An earlier review, however, did find positive effect from adjunctive phototherapy when meta-analysis was limited to RCTs of very high methodological quality (Tuunainen et al. 2004). Available data on phototherapy in depressed women was limited to a small RCT in which phototherapy showed benefit for patients with premenstrual dysphoric disorder (Lam et al. 1999).

Phototherapy appears to be most effective when patients are exposed to bright white light of 10,000 lux intensity, for 30 minutes in the early morning, every day for at least 1 week. Side effects include headache and eye irritation, and possible induction of hypomania in patients with bipolar disorder. Thus, close monitoring and concurrent treatment with a mood stabilizer is advised for bipolar patients.

Summary

Depression, while relatively common, is also a complex and infinitely variable disease entity. It is a true mind–body illness, marked by both physical and psychological manifestations, which are very well-suited to integrative medicine approaches. Of paramount importance in treatment is the heartfelt desire of the practitioner to be helpful and to respect the uniqueness of each patient. This treatment philosophy has a deeply positive impact upon depressed patients and upon their course of illness.

REFERENCES

Blumenthal JA. Exercise and pharmacotherapy in the treatment of major depressive disorder. *Psychosom Med.* 2007;69(7):587–596.

Bowers WA. Treatment of depressed in-patients: cognitive therapy plus medication, relaxation plus medication, and medication alone. *Br J Psychiatry.* 1990;156:73–78.

Bressa GM. S-adenosyl-l-methionine (SAMe) as antidepressant: meta-analysis of clinical studies. *Acta Neurol Scand Suppl.* 1994;154:7–14.

Broota A, Dhir R. Efficacy of two relaxation techniques in depression. *J Pers Clin Stud.* 1990;6:83–90.

Burt VK, Stein K. Epidemiology of depression throughout the female life cycle. *J Clin Psychiatry.* 2002;63(suppl)7:9–15.

Butterweck V, Schmidt M. St. John's wort: role of active compounds for its mechanism of action and efficacy. *Wien Med Wochenschr.* 2007;157(13–14):356–361.

Chou KL, Lee PW, Yu EC, et al. Effect of Tai Chi on depressive symptoms amongst Chinese older patients with depressive disorders: a randomized clinical trial. *Int J Geriatr Psychiatry.* 2004;19(11):1105–1107.

Coelho HF, Canter PH, Ernst E. Mindfulness-based cognitive therapy: evaluating current evidence and informing future research. *J Consult Clin Psychol.* 2007;75(6):1000–1005.

Coppen A, Bolander-Gouaille C. Treatment of depression: time to consider folic acid and vitamin B12. *J Psychopharmacol.* 2005;19(1):59–65.

Delle Chiaie R, Pancheri P, Scapicchio P, Delle Chiaie R, Pancheri P, Scapicchio P. Efficacy and tolerability of oral and intramuscular S-adenosyl-L-methionine 1,4-butanedisulfonate (SAMe) in the treatment of major depression: comparison with imipramine in 2 multicenter studies. *Am J Clin Nutr.* 2002;76(5):1172S–1176S.

American Psychiatric Association. *Diagnostic and Statistical Manual of Mental Disorders,* 4th ed. Washington, DC: American Psychiatric Association; 1994.

Golden RN, Gaynes BN, Ekstrom RD, et al. The efficacy of light therapy in the treatment of mood disorders: a review and meta-analysis of the evidence. *Am J Psychiatry.* 2005;162(4):656–662.

Goodale IL, Domar AD, Benson H. Alleviation of premenstrual syndrome symptoms with the relaxation response. *Obstet Gynecol.* 1990;75(4):649–655.

He D, Høstmark AT, Veiersted KB, Medbø JI. Effect of intensive acupuncture on pain-related social and psychological variables for women with chronic neck and shoulder pain—an RCT with six month and three year follow up. *Acupunct Med.* 2005;23(2):5.

Hypericum Depression Trial Study Group. Effect of Hypericum perforatum (St John's wort) in major depressive disorder: a randomized controlled trial. *JAMA.* 2002;287(14):1807–1814.

Irvin JH, Domar AD, Clark C, Zuttermeister PC, Friedman R. The effects of relaxation response training on menopausal symptoms. *J Psychosom Obstet Gynaecol.* 1996;17(4):202–207.

Jayadevappa R, Johnson JC, Bloom BS, et al. Effectiveness of transcendental meditation on functional capacity and quality of life of African Americans with congestive heart failure: a randomized control study. *Ethn Dis.* 2007;17(1):72–77.

Kessler RC, McGonagle KA, Swartz M, Blazer DG, Nelson CB. Sex and depression in the National Comorbidity Survey. I: lifetime prevalence, chronicity and recurrence. *J Affect Disord.* 1993;29:85–96.

Lam RW, Carter D, Misri S, Kuan AJ, Yatham LN, Zis AP. A controlled study of light therapy in women with late luteal phase dysphoric disorder. *Psychiatry Res.* 1999;86(3):185–192.

Leo RJ, Ligot JS Jr. A systematic review of randomized controlled trials of acupuncture in the treatment of depression. *J Affect Disord.* 2007;97(1–3):13–22.

Linde K, Berner M, Egger M, Mulrow C. St John's wort for depression: meta-analysis of randomised controlled trials. *Br J Psychiatry.* 2005b;186:99–107.

Linde K, Mulrow CD, Berner M, Egger M. St John's wort for depression. Cochrane *Database Syst Rev.* 2005a;(2):CD000448.

Linde K, Ramirez G, Mulrow CD, Pauls A, Weidenhammer W, Melchart D. St John's wort for depression—an overview and meta-analysis of randomised clinical trials. *Br Med J.* 1996;313(7052):253–258.

McLean PD, Hakstian AR. Clinical depression: comparative efficacy of outpatient treatments. *J Consult Clin Psychol.* 1979;47(5):818–836.

Michalsen A, Grossman P, Acil A, et al. Rapid stress reduction and anxiolysis among distressed women as a consequence of a three-month intensive yoga program. *Med Sci Monitor.* 2005;11(12):CR555–CR561.

Mischoulon D. Update and critique of natural remedies as antidepressant treatments. *Psychiatr Clin North Am.* 2007;30(1):51–68.

Moyer CA, Rounds J, Hannum JW. A meta-analysis of massage therapy research. *Psychol Bull.* 2004;130(1):3–18.

Mukaino Y, Park J, White A, Ernst E. The effectiveness of acupuncture for depression—a systematic review of randomised controlled trials. *Acupunct Med.* 2005;23(2):70–76.

Nolen-Hoeksema S. *The etiology of gender differences in depression: research trends and an integrative model.* Paper presented to the American Psychological Association Summit on Women and Depression, Wye River, MD, October 5–7, 2000.

Nolen-Hoeksema S, Girgus JS. The emergence of gender differences in depression during adolescence. *Psychol Bull.* 1994;115:424–443.

Parker G, Gibson NA, Brotchie H, Heruc G, Rees AM, Hadzi-Pavlovic D. Omega-3 fatty acids and mood disorders. *Am J Psychiatry.* 2006;163(6):969–978.

Pilkington K, Kirkwood G, Rampes H, Richardson J. Yoga for depression: the research evidence. *J Affect Disord.* 2005;89(1–3):13–24.

Porzio G, Trapasso T, Martelli S, et al. Acupuncture in the treatment of menopause-related symptoms in women taking tamoxifen. *Tumori.* 2002;88(2):128–130.

Quah-Smith JI, Tang WM, Russell J. Laser acupuncture for mild to moderate depression in a primary care setting—a randomised controlled trial. *Acupunct Med.* 2005;23(3):103–111.

Roder C, Schaefer M, Leucht S. Meta-analysis of effectiveness and tolerability of treatment of mild to moderate depression with St. John's Wort. *Fortschr Neurol Psychiatr.* 2004;72(6):330–343.

Rodin G, Lloyd N, Katz M, Green E, Mackay JA, Wong RK. Supportive Care Guidelines Group of Cancer Care Ontario Program in Evidence-Based Care. The treatment of depression in cancer patients: a systematic review. *Support Care Cancer.* 2007;15(2):123–136.

Sephton SE, Salmon P, Weissbecker I, et al. Mindfulness meditation alleviates depressive symptoms in women with fibromyalgia: results of a randomized clinical trial. *Arthritis Rheum.* 2007;57(1):77–85.

Sharma VK, Das S, Mondal S, Goswampi U, Gandhi A. Effect of Sahaj Yoga on depressive disorders. *Indian J Physiol Pharmacol.* 2005;49(4):462–468.

Smith CA, Hay PP. Acupuncture for depression. *Cochrane Database Syst Rev.* 2005;(2):CD004046.

Speca M, Carlson LE, Goodey E, Angen M. A randomized, wait-list controlled clinical trial: the effect of a mindfulness meditation-based stress reduction program on mood and symptoms of stress in cancer outpatients. *Psychosom Med.* 2000;62(5):613–622.

Stetter F, Kupper S. Autogenic training: a meta-analysis of clinical outcome studies. *Appl Psychophysiol Biofeedback*. 2002;27(1):45–98.

Stiefel F, Stagno D. Management of insomnia in patients with chronic pain conditions. *CNS Drugs*. 2004;18(5):285–296.

Szegedi A, Kohnen R, Dienel A, Kieser M. Acute treatment of moderate to severe depression with hypericum extract WS 5570 (St John's wort): randomised controlled double blind non-inferiority trial versus paroxetine. *BMJ*. 2005;330(7490):503.

Targ EF, Levine EG. The efficacy of a mind-body-spirit group for women with breast cancer: a randomized controlled trial. *Gen Hosp Psychiatry*. 2002;24(4):238–248.

Taylor MJ, Wilder H, Bhagwagar Z, Geddes J. Inositol for depressive disorders. *Cochrane Database Syst Rev*. 2004;(2):CD004049.

Tomas-Carus P, Gusi N, Häkkinen A, Häkkinen K, Leal A, Ortega-Alonso A. Eight months of physical training in warm water improves physical and mental health in women with fibromyalgia: a randomized controlled trial. *J Rehab Med*. 2008;40(4):248–252.

Tsang HW, Fung KM, Chan AS, Lee G, Chan F. Effect of a qigong exercise programme on elderly with depression. *Int J Geriatr Psychiatry*. 2006;21(9):890–897.

Turner EH, Loftis JM, Blackwell AD. Serotonin a la carte: supplementation with the serotonin precursor 5-hydroxytryptophan. *Pharmacol Ther*. 2006;109(3):325–338.

Tuunainen A, Kripke DF, Endo T. Light therapy for non-seasonal depression. *Cochrane Database Syst Rev*. 2004;(2):CD004050.

Whiskey E, Werneke U, Taylor D. A systematic review and meta-analysis of *Hypericum perforatum* in depression: a comprehensive clinical review. *Int Clin Psychopharmacol*. 2001;16(5):239–252.

34

Eating Disorders

CAROLYN COKER ROSS

CASE STUDY

Angela was admitted for treatment of bulimia nervosa and abuse of marijuana and cocaine. Her career as an actress had been affected recently by an increase in these behaviors after she began to have flashbacks or memories of childhood sexual abuse.

As a child, Angela was raised in a large Midwestern city by her mother. Her parents divorced when she was 5 years old, after which time her mother's alcohol use increased. Angela is the middle child and has two sisters. Angela is the only one of her siblings who attended college. As her mother's drinking increased, Angela found herself feeling more and more alone and "lost." While inebriated, her mother often raged at her children and was physically abusive to her older sister. Angela described her childhood years as "chaotic" and violent. Despite many career opportunities, Angela found herself having difficulty with people she worked with, which affected her access to roles she might have enjoyed playing. She reported that binging helped soothe her anxiety and made her forget her fears. After each binge, she felt like a failure, out of control, huge, fat, and ashamed. Purging helped her release some of these feelings—at least for a short while.

An integrative medicine treatment plan for this patient would include therapy to address issues associated with being an adult child of an alcoholic, which may include attendance at 12-step meetings (ACOA). The patient's therapy should include the use of dialectic behavior therapy to teach Angela skills of emotional regulation and distress tolerance. To address her bulimia, dietary supplements would be used to address nutritional deficiencies with the use of a multivitamin, magnesium and zinc; digestive issues with probiotics and digestive enzymes; and the need for mood stabilization with omega-3 fatty acids and a B complex vitamin. Massage and acupuncture can be used to decrease anxiety and depression. Starting the patient on a balanced diet with three meals a day and two protein snacks will help decrease binging. Medication may be warranted after the above for treatment of mood disorders.

Introduction

Eating disorders constitute a spectrum of disorders from anorexia to bulimia and binge eating disorder (BED) dating back to the fourth century AD with the first report of a high born Roman woman, a follower of St. Jerome who died from anorexia. Religious women were actually canonized for their fasting practices in the service of religion and were called "holy anorexics." Self-starvation reached epic levels during the Renaissance with approximately 181 deaths from anorexia between 1200 and 1600 AD. Many of these women were elevated to sainthood. In the late 1960s, the rate of eating disorders climbed with "fear of becoming fat" ranking as a rationale for self-starvation along with religious reasons or as a defense against sexuality (Bynum 1987).

Prior to that, however, Roman culture described a phenomenon similar to bulimia nervosa. "Eat, drink and be merry" included the use of "vomitoriums*" where a person could vomit and then return to the feast to continue eating and drinking. Ancient Egyptians used monthly purgatives to prevent sickness. Anorexia was identified as a medical diagnosis in 1870 and bulimia in 1903.

Currently, the American Psychiatric Association recognizes anorexia nervosa, bulimia nervosa, and eating disorder, not otherwise specified (which includes BED). Between 40% and 60% of those diagnosed with one eating disorder will crossover to another eating disorder diagnosis during their lifetime (Anderluh et al. 2008). Eating disorders, therefore, might best be considered a spectrum of illnesses rather than discrete and fixed diagnoses.

Over the past several decades, the incidence of eating disorders has increased. The lifetime prevalence as reported in a large-scale national study was 0.9% for

---

* There is conflicting evidence to support the use of the term vomitoriums by the Romans. The term "vomitorium" is actually in some accounts just the architectural term for stadiums and theatres that have passages for actors/participants to enter and leave. Aldous Huxley and others used the term vomitorium as I have above. It seems to be accepted that Romans did vomit after feasting and this is thought to be a standard part of the feasting experience. There are also pictures of ancient basins called "vomitoriums" which may have been used for this purpose.

anorexia nervosa (AN); 1.5% for bulimia nervosa (BN); 3.5% for BED in women. Women are three times more likely to develop anorexia or bulimia than men (Hudson et al. 2007). Sixty percent of those with BED, the most common of all eating disorders, are female and 40% male.

The average duration of bulimia and BED is approximately 8 years each (Hudson et al. 2007). Over time, approximately 50% of those with AN or BN will recover, 30% improve somewhat, and 20% will continue to be chronically ill.

There is no one known cause of eating disorders. Dieting may increase the risk of an adolescent female developing an eating disorder by seven fold (for moderate dieting) or eighteen fold (for severe dieting) (Patton et al. 1999). A study on the island of Fiji demonstrates the influence of Western culture on eating disorders. Three years after television was introduced, 80% of Fijian girls expressed a desire to lose weight with 11% using extreme measures such as self-induced vomiting to lose weight (Becker et al. 2002).

Genetics may also play a part. Relatives of an individual with anorexia are 11.3 times more likely to have anorexia and over four times more likely to develop bulimia than controls (Strober et al. 2000). BED also shows a familial predisposition (Bulik 2004). Twin studies show that if an identical twin has an eating disorder (anorexia or bulimia), the other twin's risk of developing an eating disorder is higher than it would be for fraternal twins or for a nontwin sibling (Costin 2007).

Anorexia Nervosa

Anorexia nervosa (AN) is associated with one of the highest mortality of any psychiatric diagnosis (Palmer 2003). There is an estimated 10% mortality in anorexics who have a 10-year disease history (American Psychiatric Association 1994). Co-occurring alcoholism or drug addiction can increase mortality in anorexics. Increasing numbers of mid-life women are developing AN for the first time or having a relapse of their eating disorder (Donaldson 1994).

The diagnosis of anorexia is made by a patient's inability to keep their body weight above 85% of normal, loss of three consecutive menstrual cycles, and severe body image distortion. Anorexics can either restrict food intake or they can combine restricting with binging and purging.

Bulimia Nervosa

Bulimia is different from anorexia in that it involves binging with compensatory behaviors to avoid weight gain. Binges are defined as eating large quantities of food in a small period of time. Compensatory behaviors can include compulsive exercise, self-induced vomiting, and the use of laxatives, diuretics or diet pills.

Bulimia nervosa (BN) usually begins after age 13 and its prevalence exceeds that of anorexia by the early adult years. There is a high comorbidity of substance use disorders (SUD) with a lifetime prevalence of 20%–40% (Lilenfeld 1997).

Binge Eating Disorder and Eating Disorder Not Otherwise Specified

Proposed DSM-IV criteria for BED include eating large quantities of food in a small period of time, loss of control over eating, and lack of a compensatory purge. Also common is remorse or shame after eating, eating very rapidly, and eating when not hungry and past the point of fullness. Up to 25% of overweight or obese individuals seeking weight loss treatment have BED (Pull 2004; Stunkard 2004).

Table 34.1. Eating Disorders — Medical Complications

	Anorexia	*Bulimia*	*Binge Eating Disorder*
Symptoms	Amenorrhea, constipation, headaches, fainting, cold intolerance	Bloating, fullness, lethargy, GERD, abdominal pain, sore throat, abnormal menses	Constipation, GERD, fatigue, abnormal menses, PCOS
Physical Findings	Cachexia, acrocyanosis, dry skin, hair loss, bradycardia, orthostatic hypotension, hypothermia, loss of muscle mass and subcutaneous fat, lanugo. Underweight	Knuckle calluses, dental enamel erosion, salivary gland enlargement, cardiomegaly (ipecac toxicity). Can be normal or overweight	Overweight or obese
Laboratory Findings	Hypoglycemia, leukopenia, elevated liver enzymes, euthyroid sick syndrome (low TSH, normal T3, T4), Osteopenia	Hypochloremic, hypokalemic or metabolic acidosis (from vomiting), hypokalemia (from laxatives/ diuretics,, elevated amylase(from vomiting)	Hyperlipidemia, hyperglycemia, Insulin resistance, Elevated androgens
ECG Findings	Low voltage, prolonged QT interval, bradycardia	Low voltage, prolonged QT interval, bradycardia	Variable

I am often asked: "What is the difference between binge eating disorder and compulsive overeating?" Those with BED tend to have more severe fluctuations in their weight, higher levels of body dissatisfaction, and tend to have started binging and dieting as a child (Sorbara 2002). Those with BED also have a higher incidence of depression and anxiety (Delgado 2002) and if you put them in a laboratory setting and give them permission to eat as much as they want, will tend to eat significantly more calories than those with CO (Walsh 2003).

Medical Complications

- The medical complications associated with eating disorders affect multiple systems of the body and many are related to nutritional deficiencies. Table 34.1 offers a summary of medical complications. For more detailed information; see Garner and Garfield (1997).

Treatment: Integrative Medicine Approach to Eating Disorders

The cornerstones of an integrative medicine approach can include:

- Medical treatment that focuses on reducing the risk of, detecting and treating complications of the disease, and on improving overall health status.
- Nutritional therapies to improve nutritional status, replace nutritional deficits, help women improve their relationship with food and improve digestion and absorption.
- The use of botanical therapies to treat insomnia and depression and reduce side effects of pharmacological therapies.
- Body movement to enable patients to reconnect with physical cues, learn healthy behaviors, and modify the hyperactivity of the HPA axis.
- Psychological testing to identify co-occurring diagnoses.
- Coping skills training including cognitive behavioral therapy and dialectical behavior therapy.
- Complementary and alternative therapies improve sleep and enable patients to experience deep states of relaxation, which modifies HPA axis hyperactivity, and also contribute to body awareness and acceptance.
- Prescription medications.

What keeps me from feeling hopeless about these life-threatening and difficult-to-treat diseases is the recognition that an eating disorder is a way of coping with something that the individual has difficulting tolerating—a history of trauma, abuse, neglect or their own emotional sensitivity. At all times, I keep in mind that there is a healthy self to work with and that this self is always striving to express its soul's purpose. I concentrate my efforts on connecting with and nurturing this soul self.

Medical Treatment

The most important initial therapy for all eating disorders is nutrition. For anorexics, weight restoration should include a weight gain goal of 1–2 pounds per week in an inpatient setting and 0.5–1 pound per week outpatient. Full weight restoration can reduce the risk of relapse significantly (Baran et al. 1995). Treatment by providers who are specialists in eating disorders has been shown to reduce mortality in eating disorder patients (Crisp et al. 1992).

Medication

The American Psychiatric Association advises that decisions about the use of medication should take a back seat to weight restoration, which may, by itself, improve symptoms of depression. Studies on antidepressants used in patients with anorexia have been hampered by high drop out rates and small numbers. To date there is no proven benefit in treating the acute phase of anorexia nervosa with medication. In contrast, antidepressants including tricyclics, selective serotonin reuptake inhibitors, and monoamine oxidase inhibitors have shown a statistically significant short-term benefit in reducing binge eating and purging in patients with bulimia and BED (Agras et al. 1987; Alger et al. 1991; American Psychiatric Association 2006; Leombruni et al. 2008; Walsh et al. 1988).

Nutritional Therapies

Ancel Keys in 1950 demonstrated the impact of starvation on behavior, and mood (Taylor and Keys 1950). Further research has confirmed his findings and demonstrated that nutrition affects all bodily functions including blood pressure, cholesterol, and resting heart rate (Kalm and Semba 2005).

Several studies have consistently demonstrated deficiencies in specific nutrients that affect energy, mood, and cognition. Those with eating disorders who restrict their intake may have deficiencies in calcium, iron, riboflavin, folic acid, vitamins A and C (Beaumont et al. 1981), vitamin B6, and the essential fatty acids (Langan and Farrell 1985; Rock and Vasantharajan 1995).

Nutritional approaches are focused on replacing missing nutrients and treating comorbid conditions.

ESSENTIAL FATTY ACIDS

In the obese patient, omega-3 fatty acid consumption has a beneficial effect on insulin sensitivity and glucose tolerance. Use of this supplement also lowers serum triglycerides (Ebbesson et al. 2005). Omega-3 fatty acids have been well studied in the treatment of major depression and bipolar disorder, which are comorbid in eating disorder patients (Adams et al. 1996; Cott and Hibbeln 2001; Hibbeln 1998, 2002; Noaghiul and Hibbeln 2003; Peet and Horrobin 2002). A small study demonstrated decreased aggressiveness and depressive symptoms in patients with borderline personality disorder, which is more prevalent in bulimic and BED patients (Zanarini and Frankenburg 2003).

Dosage and Side Effects

Over-the-counter preparations offer approximately 1 g of combined DHA and EPA, which can serve as a good starting dosage. Adverse effects include a theoretical increase in bleeding time. Side effects can include a fishy burp and stomach upset. It can be kept refrigerated or given at bedtime to avoid these side effects.

B VITAMINS

B vitamins are vital to human nutrition because they transport oxygen to the brain and offer protection from oxidative stress. B vitamins also convert glucose from our food into energy in the brain cells and assist in the manufacture of neurotransmitters. Deficiencies in vitamin B12 and folic acid have been found in patients with eating disorders and depression and have been implicated in poor responses to antidepressant medication (Coppen and Bolander-Gouaille 2005; Taylor et al. 2006) (Table 34.2).

Table 34.2. B Vitamins for Eating Disorders

	Recommended Daily Allowance for Women Over Age 19	Toxicity Related to High Doses
Folate	400–1000 μg/day	May cause seizures in those on antiseizure medications
B6	1.5 mg/day up to 100 mg/day	Neuropathy of arms and legs: reversible when supplementation is discontinued
Niacin	14 mg/day	Hyperuricemia, hyperglycemia, teratogenicity, maculopathy
B12	2.4 μg/day	None known

Dosage and Side Effects

Supplementation of all of the B vitamins is preferable to supplementing one or two. Folic acid supplementation should not exceed 1000 μg/day because large doses can mask B12 deficiency (Institute of Medicine 1998). Side effects include diarrhea and itching (B12), rash (folate) and flushing (niacin).

CALCIUM

Calcium is important in patients with eating disorders for prevention of bone loss and fractures. Bone loss can be the result of amenorrhea, use of laxatives, and alcohol abuse (Hirsch and Peng 1996; Marcus et al. 1985; U.S. Department of Agriculture 1994–1996). The mainstay of prevention and treatment of bone loss in anorexia is weight restoration, nutritional rehabilitation, and sponta-neous resumption of menstrual cycles (Golden 2003). Recommended dose of calcium is 1000–1200 mg/day from all sources. Excessive intake of calcium sup-plements can lead to hypercalcemia, decreased kidney function, and decreased absorption of other minerals.

VITAMIN D

Vitamin D has traditionally been recommended for bone health but recent studies show a role for vitamin D in enhancing immunity, maintaining muscle strength, and reducing the risk of diabetes. The obese patient (BMI >30) may have deficient circulating vitamin D because of sequestration in fatty tissue (Wortsman et al. 2000). For dose and potential side effects of vitamin D, see Chapter 36.

PROBIOTICS

Probiotics are products containing live microorganisms, which when administered in appropriate amounts confer a health benefit. Levels of probiotics can be decreased by the use of antibiotics, alcohol and drugs, stress, and chronic constipation. The two most common probiotics are Lactobacillus and Bifidobacterium. Research studies have shown that probiotics can reduce abdominal pain, distension, borborygmi, and flatulence in irritable bowel syndrome (Kajander et al. 2005) and can reduce the severity of constipation (Koebnick et al. 2003). In a study of eating disorder patients in an inpatient treatment program, the use of probiotics and digestive enzymes reduced digestive complaints from 15% to 5% (Ross et al. 2008).

Dosage and Side Effects

The usual dose of probiotics is 5–10 billion live bacteria. Adverse effects are rare and usually limited to patients with severe immune deficiency or pancreatitis.

Herbs

VALERIAN

Valeriana officinalis is effective in the treatment of anxiety due to social stress (Kohnen and Oswald 1988), generalized anxiety (Andreatini et al. 2002), and insomnia. When compared with placebo, taking valerian resulted in a decrease in slow-wave sleep onset but did not show any benefit over placebo in 14 other end points (Donath et al. 2000).

Dosage and Side Effects

The recommended starting dose of valerian for insomnia is 900 mg taken about 30 minutes before bedtime. Side effects include headache, gastrointestinal upset, dizziness, and low body temperature.

Mind–Body Therapies

Current research suggests that reversal or attenuation of the stress response plays a significant role in the treatment and prevention of disease. The hypothalamic-pituitary-adrenal axis is thought to be hyperactive in individuals with eating disorders perhaps as a result of childhood neglect or abuse (Birketvedt et al. 2006; Zonnevylle-Bender et al. 2005). Mind–body therapies such as biofeedback, meditation, progressive muscle relaxation, and guided imagery can help address this HPA axis hyperactivity.

Pop-Jordanova used biofeedback in treating anorexic and obese, binge eating preadolescent patients and found a reduction in nervous system activation (Pop-Jordanova 2000). Esplen used guided imagery to treat 50 bulimic women, which produced a 74% reduction in binging and a 75% reduction in self-induced vomiting (Esplen et al. 1998). A study of 55 women with bulimia showed decreases in vomiting, body dissatisfaction, and depression in those assigned to the stress management group as compared to nutritional management alone (Laessle et al. 1991).

Complementary and Alternative Therapies

There are few studies using complementary and alternative (CAM) therapies to treat eating disorders. A few studies on use of CAM in the co-occurring disorders are listed below and throughout this text. Other components of an integrative approach to eating disorders such as psychometric testing, exercise/body movement therapy, and skills training are more thoroughly covered in other books (Ross 2007; Ross, 2009).

MASSAGE THERAPY

A review of studies on massage therapy, including its use in eating disorders, shows that massage decreases levels of cortisol by an average of 31%, increases dopamine by 31%, and serotonin by 28% (Field et al. 2005). Massage therapy may decrease stress, lower anxiety, decrease body dissatisfaction, and increase dopamine and norepinephrine in women with anorexia (Anonymous 2001). In bulimics, massage may decrease depression and anxiety, lower cortisol, and raise dopamine levels (Field et al. 1998). Massage and other body-centered therapies have been useful in helping those with eating disorders shift their perception and reconnect to their bodies in a more positive way.

Given the paucity of research in the use of specific CAM therapies for treating eating disorders, I have quoted several of my ED patients' experiences of CAM therapies:

The meditation class helped me get back in touch with my spiritual connection, something I'd lost after my last relapse.

When I practiced the breathing exercises, I felt my breath moving into my belly and I experienced a difference between the 'flesh' of my belly which I'd worried about for so long (wanting to have a flat belly) and the gratitude I have for how my 'insides' all work together.

Massage was very spiritual for me and I found it vital to my recovery.

Outcomes

In a study of anorexic patients who were weight restored in an inpatient treatment center and were followed for a median of 15 months after discharge, 35% relapsed (defined as body mass index less than 17.5 for 3 months). The highest risk for relapse occurred from 6 to 17 months after discharge. The predictors of relapse included history of a suicide attempt; previous treatment for an eating disorder; severe obsessive-compulsive symptoms on admission; excessive exercise resumed immediately after discharge and ongoing weight and shape concerns at the time of discharge (Carter et al. 2004). Relapse for individuals with anorexia who were weight restored in treatment may also be related to how able they are to change their diets. Researchers found that continued avoidance of energy-dense foods and low diet variety were associated with poor outcomes (Schebendach et al. 2008).

Relapse from bulimia nervosa in a study of patients completing a day treatment program who achieved symptom control was 31% over the 2-year follow-up period. The majority of relapses occurred within the first 6 months. Predictors of relapse in this study included younger age, higher frequency of purging, and a higher score on the bulimia subscale of the Eating Attitudes Test before treatment and higher scores on the interpersonal distrust subscale of the Eating Disorder Inventory at the end of treatment. Frequency of binge eating, measures of self-esteem, depression, and social adjustment were not significantly correlated to relapse (Olmsted et al. 1994).

In a prospective study tracking the natural course of bulimia nervosa and eating disorder not otherwise specified (EDNOS), the probability of remission by 60 months was found to be 74% for bulimia and 83% for EDNOS. Among patients in remission, the probability of relapse was 47% for bulimia and 42% for

EDNOS (Grilo et al. 2007). The degree of body image distortion has also been shown to be a predictor for relapse in bulimics and anorexics (Keel 2005).

Studies on individuals with BED have shown some ability to predict risk of relapse on the basis of eating and shape concerns, depressive symptoms, and the overall severity of general psychopathology, including poor interpersonal skills pretreatment and at the mid-point of treatment (Dingemans et al. 2007; Hilbert et al. 2007).

Conclusion

Eating disorders comprise a spectrum of disorders that are difficult to treat and have a high risk for morbidity and mortality. The integrative medicine approach offers many options to explore. While research into these therapies is still in the early stages, the benefit to risk ratio is favorable. Recovery from an eating disorder is possible and the earlier individuals with these disorders are treated, the better the prognosis. The greatest value that physicians can offer to patients with eating disorders is the belief inherent in integrative medicine that the body, mind, and spirit all have the capacity for self-healing.

REFERENCES

Anonymous. Anorexia nervosa symptoms are reduced by massage therapy. *Eat Disord.* 2001;9:289–299.

Adams PB, Lawson S, Sanigorski A, Sinclair AJ. Arachidonic acid to eicosapentaenoic acid ratio in blood correlates positively with clinical symptoms of depression. *Lipids.* 1996;31:S157–S161.

Agras WS, Dorian B, Kirkley BG, Bruce A, John B. Imipramine in the treatment of bulimia: a double-blind controlled study. *Int J Eat Disord.* 1987;6:29–38.

Alger SA, Schwalberg MD, Bigaouette JM, Michalek AV, Howard LJ. Effect of a tricyclic antidepressant and opiate antagonist on binge-eating behavior in normoweight bulimic and obese, binge eating subjects. *Am J Clin Nutr.* 1991;53:865–871.

American Psychiatric Association. *Diagnostic and Statistical Manual of Mental Disorders.* 4th ed. Washington, DC: American Psychiatric Association; 1994.

American Psychiatric Association. *Practice Guideline for the Treatment of Patients with Eating Disorders.* 3rd ed. Washington, DC: American Psychiatric Association; 2006.

Anderluh M, Tchanturia K, RAbe-Hesketh S, Collier D, Treasure J. Lifetime course of eating disorders: design and validity testing of a new strategy to define the eating disorders phenotype. *Psychol Med.* 2008;1:1–10 [Epub ahead of print].

Andreatini R, Sartori VA, Seabra ML, Leite JR. Effect of valepotriates (valerian extract) in generalized anxiety disorder: a randomized placebo-controlled pilot study. *Phytother Res.* 2002;16:650–654.

Baran SA, Weltzin TE, Kaye WH. Low discharge weight and outcome in anorexia nervosa. *Am J Psychiatry.* 1995;152:1070–1072.

Beaumont PJ, Chambers TL, Rouse L, Abraham SF. The diet composition and nutritional knowledge of patients with anorexia nervosa. *J Hum Nutr.* 1981;35:265–272.

Becker A, Burwell S, Gilman D, et al. Eating behavior and attitudes following prolonged exposure to television among ethnic Fijian girls. *Br J Psychiatry.* 2002;180:509–514.

Bell RM. *Holy Anorexia.* Chicago, CA: University of Chicago Press; 1985.

Birketvedt GS, Drivenes E, Agledahl I, Sundsfjord J, Olstad R, Florholmen JR. Bulimia nervosa—a primary defect in the hypothalamic-pituitary-adrenal axis? *Appetite.* 2006;46:164–167.

Bulik CM. Role of genetics in anorexia nervosa, bulimia nervosa and binge eating disorder. In: Brewerton T, ed. *Clinical Handbook of Eating Disorders.* New York: Marcel Dekker; 2004.

Bynum CW. *Holy Feast and Holy Fast.* Berkeley: University of California Press; l987.

Carter JC, Blackmore E, Sutandar-Pinnock K, Woodside DB. Relapse in anorexia nervosa: a survival analysis. *Psychol Med.* 2004;34:671–679.

Coppen A, Bolander-Gouaille C. Treatment of depression: time to consider folic acid and B12. *J Psychopharmacol.* 2005;19:59–65.

Costin C. *The Eating Disorder Sourcebook.* 3rd ed. New York, NY: Mc Graw Hill; 2007.

Cott J, Hibbeln JR. Lack of seasonal mood change in Icelanders. *Am J Psychiatry.* 2001;158:328.

Crisp AH, Callender JS, Halek C, Hsu LK. Long-term mortality in anorexia nervosa. A 20-year follow-up of St. George's and Aberdeen cohorts. *Br J Psychiatry.* 1992;161:104–107.

Delgado CC, Morales Gorria MJ, Maruri Chimeno I, et al. Eating behavior, body attitudes and psychopathology in morbid obesity. *Actas Esp Psiquitr.* 2002;30:376–381.

Dingemans AE, Spinhoven P, van Furth EF. Predictors and mediators of treatment outcome in patients with binge eating disorder. *Behav Res Ther.* 2007;45:2551–2562.

Donaldson GA. Body image in women at midlife. Boston College Dissertation, 1994; 175 pp; AAT 9510315.

Donath F, Quispe S, Diefenbach K, Maurer A, Fietze I. Roots I. Critical evaluation of the effect of valerian extract on sleep structure and sleep quality. *Pharmacopsychiatry.* 2000;33:47–53.

Ebbesson SO, Risica PM, Ebbesson LO, Kennish JM, Tejero ME. Omega-3 fatty acids improve glucose tolerance and components of the metabolic syndrome in Alaskan Eskimos: the Alaska Siberia Project. *Int J Circumpolar Health.* 2005;64:396–408.

Esplen MJ, Garfinkel PE, Olmsted M, et al. A randomized controlled trial of guided imagery in bulimia nervosa. *Psychol Med.* 1998;28:1347–1357.

Field T, Hernandez-Reif M, Diego M, Schanberg S, Kuhn C. Cortisol decreases and serotonin and dopamine increase following massage therapy. *Int J Neurosci.* 2005;115:1397–1413.

Field T, Schanberg S, Kuhn C. Bulimic adolescents benefit from massage therapy. *Adolescence.* 1998;33:555–563.

Garner DM, Garfinkel PE (eds). *Handbook of treatment for eating disorders 2nd edition.* New York, NY. The Guilford Press; 1997.

Golden NH. Osteopenia and osteoporosis in anorexia nervosa. *Adolesc Med.* 2003;14:97–108.

Gordon CM, Nelson LM. Amenorrhea and bone health in adolescents and young women. *Curr Opin Obstet Gynecol.* 2003;15:377–384.

Grilo CM, Pagano ME, Skodol AE, et al. Natural course of bulimia nervosa and of eating disorder not otherwise specified: 5-year prospective study of remissions, relapses, and the effects of personality disorder psychopathology. *J Clin Psychiatr.* 2007;68:738–746.

Hibbeln JR. Fish consumption and major depression. *Lancet.* 1998;351:1213.

Hibbeln JR. Seafood consumption, the DHA content of mothers' milk and prevalence rates of postpartum depression: a cross-national, ecological analysis. *J Affect Disord.* 2002;69:15–29.

Hilbert A, Saelens BE, Stein RI, et al. Pretreatment and process predictors of outcome in interpersonal and cognitive behavioral psychotherapy for binge eating disorder. *J Clin Psychol.* 2007;75:645–651.

Hirsch PE, Peng TC. Effects of alcohol on calcium homeostasis and bone. In: Anderson J, Garner S, eds. *Calcium and Phosphorus in Health and Disease.* Boca Raton, FL: CRC Press; 1996:289–300.

Hudson JI, Hiripi E, Pope HG, Kessler RC. The prevalence and correlates of eating disorders in the national comorbidity survey replication. *Biol Psychiatry.* 2007;61:348–358.

Institute of Medicine. *Food and Nutrition Board. Dietary Reference Intakes: Thiamin, Riboflavin, niacin, Vitamin B6, Folate, Vitamin B12, Pantothenic Acid, Biotin, and Choline.* Washington, DC: National Academy Press; 1998.

Kajander K, Hatakka K, Poussa T. A probiotic mixture alleviates symptoms in irritable bowel syndrome patients: a controlled 6-month intervention. *Aliment Pharmacol Ther.* 2005;22:387–394.

Kalm LM, Semba RD. They starved so that others could be better fed: remembering Ancel Keys and the Minnesot Experiment. *Am Soc Nutr Sci J Nutr.* 2005;135:1347–1352.

Keel PK, Dorer DJ, Franko DL, Jackson SC, Herzog DB. Postremission predictors of relapse in women with eating disorders. *Am J Psychiatry.* 2005;162:2263–2268.

Kirsch I, Montgomery G, Sapirstein G. Hypnosis as an adjunct to cognitive-behavioral psychotherapy: a meta-analysis. *J Consult Clin Psychol.* 1995;63:214–220.

Koebnick C, Wagner I, Leitzmann P, Stern U, Zunft HJ. Probiotic beverage containing *Lactobacillus casei* improves gastrointestinal symptoms in patients with chronic constipation. *Can J Gastroenterol.* 2003;17:655–659.

Kohnen R, Oswald WD. The effects of valerian, propranolol and their combination on activation, performance and mood of healthy volunteers under social stress conditions. *Pharmacopsychiatry.* 1988;21:447–4488.

Laessle RG Beaumont PJ, Butow P, et al. A comparison of nutritional management with stress management in the treatment of bulimia nervosa. *Br J Psychiatry.* 1991;159:250–261.

Langan SM, Farrell PM. Vitamin E, vitamin A and essential fatty acid status of patients hospitalized with anorexia nervosa. *Am J Clin Nutr.* 1985;41:1054–1060.

Leombruni P, Piero A, Lavagnino L, Brustolin A, Campisi S, Fassino S. A randomized, double-blind trial comparing sertraline and fluoxetine 6-month treatment in obese patients with Binge Eating Disorder. *Prog Neuropsychopharmacol Biol Psychiatry.* 2008. [Epub ahead of print].

Lilenfeld LR, Kaye WH, Greeno CG, et al. Psychiatric disorders in women with bulimia nervosa and their first-degree relatives: effects of comorbid substance dependence. *Int J Eat Disord.* 1997;22:253–264.

Marcus R, Cann C, Madvig P, et al. Menstrual function and bone mass in elite women distance runners: endocrine and metabolic features. *Ann Intern Med.* 1985;102:158–63.

Noaghiul S, Hibbeln JR. Cross-national comparisons of seafood consumption and rates of bipolar disorders. *Am J Psychiatry.* 2003;160:2222–2227.

Olmsted MP, Kaplan AS, Rockert W. Rate and prediction of relapse in bulimia nervosa. *Am J Psychiatry.* 1994;151:738–743.

Palmer RL. Death in anorexia nervosa. *Lancet.* 2003;361:1490.

Patton GC, Selzer R, Coffey C, et al. Onset of adolescent eating disorders: population based cohort study over 3 years. *BMJ.* 1999;318:765–768.

Peet M, Horrobin DF. A dose-ranging study of the effects of ethyl-eicosapentaenoate in patients with ongoing depression despite apparently adequate treatment with standard drugs. *Arch Gen Psychiatry.* 2002;59:913–919.

Pop-Jordanova N. Psychological characteristics and biofeedback mitigation in preadolescents with eating disorders. *Pediatr Int.* 2000;42:76–81.

Pull CP. Binge eating disorder. *Curr Opin Psychiatr.* 2004;17:43–48.

Rock CL, Vasantharajan S. Vitamin status of eating disorder patients: relationship to clinical indices and effect of treatment. *Int J Eat Disord.* 1995;18:257–262.

Ross CC. *Healing Body, Mind and Spirit: An Integrative Medicine Approach to the Treatment of Eating Disorders.* Denver, CO: Outskirts Press; 2007.

Ross CC, *The Binge Eating and Compulsive Overeating Workbook.* Oakland, CA: New Harbinger Publications. 2009.

Ross CC, Herman P, Rojas J. Integrative medicine for eating disorders. *Explore J Sci Heal.* 2008;4(5):315–320.

Schebendach JE, Mayer LE, Devlin MJ, et al. Dietary energy density and diet variety as predictors of outcome in anorexia nervosa. *J Clin Nutr.* 2008;87:810–816.

Sorbara M, Geliebter A. Body image disturbance in obese outpatients before and after weight loss in relation to race, gender, binge eating, and age of onset of obesity. *Int J Eat Disord.* 2002;31:416–423.

Strober M, Freeman R, Lampert C, Diamond J, Kaye W. Controlled family study of anorexia nervosa and bulimia nervosa: evidence of shared liability and transmission of partial syndromes. *Am J Psychiatry.* 2000;157:393–401.

Stunkard AJ. Binge-eating disorder and the night-eating syndrome. In: Wadden TA, Stunkard AJ, eds. *Handbook of Obesity Treatment*. New York: The Guilford Press; 2004.

Taylor HL, Keys A. Adaptation to caloric restriction. *Science*. 1950;25(112):215–218.

Taylor MJ, Carney S, Geddes J, et al. *Folate for Depressive Disorders. Cochrane Review*. The Cochrane Library, Issue 2. Chichester, UK. John Wilen & Sons, Ltd; 2006.

U.S. Department of Agriculture. Results from the United States Department of Agriculture's 1994–1996 Continuing Survey of Food Intakes by Individuals/Diet and Health Knowledge Survey. 1994–1996. http://www.barc.usda.gov/bhnrc/foodsurvey/Products9496.html#foodandnutrientintakes

Walsh BT, Boudreau G. Laboratory studies of binge eating disorder. *Int J Eat Disord*. 2003;34 Suppl:S30–S38.

Walsh BT, Gladis M, Roose SP, Stewart JW, Stetner F, Glassman AH. Phenelzine versus placebo in 50 patients with bulimia. *Arch Gen Psychiatry*. 1998;45:471–475.

Wortsman J, Matsuoka LY, Chen TC, Lu Z, Holick MF. Decreased bioavailability of vitamin D in obesity. *Am J Clin Nutr*. 2000;72:690–693.

Zanarini MC, Frankenburg FR. Omega-3 Fatty acid treatment of women with borderline personality disorder: a double-blind, placebo-controlled pilot study. *Am J Psychiatry*. 2003;160:167–169.

Zonnevylle-Bender MJ, van Goozen SH, Cohen-Kettenis PT, Jansen Lucres MC, Annemarie VE, Herman VE. Adolescent anorexia nervosa patients have a discrepancy between neurophysiological responses and self-reported emotional arousal to psychosocial stress. *Psychiatr Res*. 2005;15;135:45–52.

35

Cardiovascular Health

VIVIAN A. KOMINOS

As I injected dye into the left main coronary artery, I immediately saw the critical lesion in the proximal left anterior descending. This was a typical "widow maker," the term that I had learned in medical school and training. But there was nothing typical about my patient. Beth was in her late forties and did not have the typical symptoms of chest tightness. Instead, she had noticed increasing fatigue for a year and, more recently, shortness of breath with exertion. She had seen two cardiologists before she came to me, and was told that it was all in her head. In fact, her regular exercise stress tests were normal and she was beginning to believe her doctors. Prior to her cardiac catheterization, I tried to reassure her that her nuclear stress test was probably not accurate due to breast tissue that sometimes obscures the anterior wall, but that we should just "take a look" to be certain there was no disease. In 1990, early in my practice, Beth taught me a lot and I vowed to learn all I could about women and heart disease.

Introduction

Cardiovascular disease (CVD) is the leading cause of death worldwide in both women and men (World Health Statistics 2007). In the United States, CVD accounts for one-third of all deaths in women but in some developing countries, it accounts for half of all the deaths in women over the age of 50 (Pilote et al. 2007). In the United States, more women than men die of CVD (American Heart Association 2008), a fact not known by many women and physicians. CVD kills almost 400,000 women each year in the United States, more than all cancers put together, yet many women still cite breast cancer as their chief medical concern (Christian et al. 2007).

Since CVD affects women differently than men, it is only fitting that CVD be examined separately for women. This chapter summarizes what is currently known about the most common forms of CVD, namely coronary heart disease (CHD) and hypertension, highlights gender-specific recommendations for CVD prevention, and discusses nutrition, supplements, pharmacotherapy, and the mind–body connection. All the recommendations that follow are obtained from data that has included women. Several studies that are repeatedly cited have been inclusive of women alone: the Nurses' Health Study (NHS), the Women's Health Study (WHS), and the Women's Health Initiative (WHI). These large prospective cohorts and trials have provided a wealth of information and have informed us that, fortunately, most CVD is preventable. The author hopes that this chapter will assist the reader in the prevention and treatment of CVD, the most common killer of women.

Risk Factors

Traditionally, risk stratification has been based on Framingham data which is limited in that it does not include family history and projects only a 10-year risk of myocardial infarction (MI) and CHD. The Framingham data is flawed in assessing risk especially among young nondiabetic women. According to Framingham, approximately 95% of women aged less than 70 years of age are at low risk (Wenger et al. 2008b). This does not reflect the reality that all women are at risk since more than a third of all women will ultimately die from CVD. The American Heart Association (AHA) has set forth evidence-based guidelines specifically designed for CVD prevention in women which more accurately risk stratifies women. Table 35.1 shows the classification of CVD risk in women.

Although diabetes is considered a CHD equivalent in men and women, it is a more powerful predictor in women than in men (Khaw et al. 2004). In premenopausal women, diabetes cancels out the protective role of endogenous estrogens. In young nondiabetic women, tobacco abuse is the strongest risk factor for CVD and yet many primary care physicians and gynecologists do not have the time to counsel their patients regarding smoking cessation. In women, 20% of CHD events occur in the absence of traditional risk factors (Khot et al. 2003). Hemoglobin A1c, high-sensitivity C-reactive protein (hsCRP), lipoprotein (a) [Lp(a)], apolipoproteins A-I and B-100, and parental history all added to the accuracy of predicting CHD events (Ridker et al. 2007). The metabolic syndrome is a cluster of risk factors associated with CVD (Table 35.2).

Table 35.1. Classification of CVD Risk in Women

Risk Status	Criteria
High risk	Established coronary heart disease Cerebrovascular disease Peripheral arterial disease Abdominal aortic aneurysm End-stage or chronic renal disease Diabetes mellitus 10-year Framingham global risk >20%*

At risk	≥1 major risk factors for CVD, including:
	    Cigarette smoking
	    Poor diet
	    Physical inactivity
	    Obesity, especially central adiposity
	    Family history of premature CVD (CVD at <55 years
	        of age in male relative and <65 years of age in female
	        relative)
	    Hypertension
	    Dyslipidemia
	    Evidence of subclinical vascular disease (e.g., coronary
	        calcification)
	    Metabolic syndrome
	    Poor exercise capacity on treadmill test and/or
	        abnormal heart rate recovery after stopping exercise.

Optimal risk	Framingham global risk <10% and a healthy lifestyle with no risk factors

*Or at high-risk on the basis of another population-adapted tool used to assess global risk.
Abbreviation: CVD, cardiovascular disease.
Source: Reprinted with permission from Mosca et al. (2007).

Table 35.2. Diagnosis of Metabolic Syndrome Requires at Least Three of the Following

Abdominal obesity: waist circumference >102 cm in men and >88 cm in women

Triglyceride level ≥150 mg/dL

HDL <40 mg/dL for men and <50 mg/dL for women

Systolic blood pressure ≥130 mm Hg or Diastolic blood pressure ≥85 mm Hg

Fasting glucose ≥110 mg/dL

It is becoming more prevalent in women than in men (Tonstad et al. 2007) and is rising in women of childbearing age (Ramos et al. 2008). There is increasing evidence that mind–body practices that reduce chronic stress, such as yoga, tai chi, and qigong, may improve insulin resistance and the metabolic syndrome (Innes et al. 2008).

Gender-Specific Issues Related to Heart Disease

Symptom presentation can be different in women than in men and women's awareness of CVD is still lacking (Christian et al. 2007). Although cardiovascular awareness among women has more than doubled since 1997 when surveys were first taken, there is still a large racial and ethnic gap and a majority of women surveyed, report confusion related to basic CVD prevention (Mosca et al. 2006). Recent data from the Women's Ischemia Syndrome Evaluation (WISE) has elucidated a pathophysiology of coronary artery disease (CAD) in women that differs from that of men. Diagnostic testing is often more difficult in women than in men due to hormone related ECG changes and breast attenuation artifact. Treatment in women does not always yield the same results as in men. All of these factors may explain why cardiac mortality for women is not decreasing as rapidly as for men (American Heart Association 2008).

SYMPTOMS IN CORONARY HEART DISEASE

Since over 60% of women who die suddenly from CHD do not have classic warning symptoms (American Heart Association 2008), and since 38% of women versus 25% of men will die within 1 year after a first heart attack, early recognition of symptoms and accurate diagnosis are paramount. Women, more often than men, initially present with angina instead of acute MI (Hemingway et al. 2008). Approximately 30% of all women with acute coronary syndrome do not present with chest pain versus approximately 20% of all men (Canto 2007). Women are more likely than men to present with other symptoms, such as upper back or neck pain, shortness of breath, palpitations, indigestion, or fatigue (Milner et al. 1999; Patel et al. 2004). Men are more likely to present with chest pain that radiates to the left arm and with diaphoresis (Arslanian-Engorgen et al. 2006). Women have reported prodromal symptoms of fatigue and shortness of breath that can occur up to 1 month prior to an acute MI (McSweeney et al. 2003). Despite the variance in symptoms, it is important to remember that the majority of women with CHD present with chest pain.

PATHOPHYSIOLOGY OF ATHEROSCLEROSIS

In the WISE study, women with chest pain and documented myocardial ischemia were found to have a lower incidence of obstructive CAD (Merz et al. 2006). When these women had persistent symptoms, they had a significant increased risk of MI or death even though there was minimal or no obstructive CAD. A vasculopathy is suggested as the source of ischemia. Instead of the traditional plaque that protrudes into the lumen, that is easy to visualize on coronary angiography, women may have intramural atherosclerosis as evidenced by intravascular ultrasound. In fatal acute coronary syndrome, women are more likely to have plaque erosion than plaque rupture (Merz et al. 2006). Women with coronary artery calcifications had greater mortality rates than men with the same coronary artery calcium score (Raggi et al. 2004).

NONINVASIVE DIAGNOSTIC TESTING

Since symptoms may be less reliable in women than in men, the threshold for diagnostic testing should be lower in women. However, there is lower utilization of stress testing in women than in men in all age groups (Mieres et al. 2005). The diagnostic accuracy of exercise electrocardiography is lower in women due to multiple factors including Bayesian factors (i.e., lower pretest probability), hormonal factors (estrogen has a "digoxin" like effect of ST segments), and anatomy (e.g., mitral valve prolapse). Exercise duration and the ability to exercise to maximal stress are the strongest prognostic indicators for both men and women (Mieres 2005). The inability to achieve five METS, the equivalent of the physical work that is required to perform activities of daily living signifies poor prognosis.

Clinical tip: In general, if a nondiabetic patient has a normal resting ECG, and is able to exercise, refer her for an exercise treadmill test. If she has diabetes, an abnormal rest ECG, or has poor exercise capacity, refer her for a stress test with cardiac imaging or a stress echocardiogram.

OUTCOME DIFFERENCES AND TREATMENT

Women less than 65 years old who present with an acute MI have 50%–100% higher mortality rates than age matched men (Alter et al. 2002; Vaccarino et al. 1999). The higher incidence of comorbid risk factors such as diabetes, renal failure, and heart failure explain only part of the mortality difference between women and men. No major mortality difference is seen in older women presenting with an acute MI when compared to age matched men (Vaccarino et al. 1999). When women present with unstable angina, they have better outcomes than men; when they present with non-ST segment elevation MI they fare about the same as men (Hochman 1999). Approximately one-third of all coronary artery bypass surgery (CABG) is performed on women. After CABG women fair worse than men even after adjusting for comorbid factors (Vaccarino et al. 2003). Women had twice the incidence of depression, almost twice the rate of hospital readmission, more physical symptoms and side effects, and lower physical function when compared to men. The majority of the studies reveal higher mortality rates in women than in men after CABG (Wenger et al. 2008b). Approximately one-third of all percutaneous coronary interventions (PCI) procedures are on women. For acute ST-segment elevation MI, PCI is superior to thrombolytics in both men and women (Lansky et al. 2005). In acute coronary syndrome, women had a reduction in death or MI with PCI if they were high-risk (elevated CPK-MB or troponin, higher TIMI risk score, high-sensitivity C-reactive protein (hsCRP) and brain natriuretic protein). For those women not at high-risk, the results are mixed. Although vascular complications are more common in women than in men, there has been overall improvement in outcomes in women undergoing PCI (Singh et al. 2008).

Aspirin Use in Women

PRIMARY PREVENTION

The WHS randomized 100 mg of aspirin every other day versus placebo in 39,876 women at low risk for CVD (Ridker et al. 2005). In a 10-year follow up there was a 17% reduction in ischemic strokes. In a subgroup analysis, women ≥65 years of age had a 26% reduction in CVD events, and 34% reduction in MI. In the NHS, a prospective observational study of 79,439 low risk women followed for 24 years, the group that self-selected to take aspirin had a significant relative risk reduction of 25% in all cause mortality and 38% in cardiovascular death (Chan et al. 2007). The benefit of aspirin in high-risk women has been well established in a meta-analysis of 287 studies (ATC 2002).

Clinical tip: Unless contraindicated, low-dose enteric coated aspirin should be given to all women >65 years old and all women at high-risk for CVD. Clopidogrel can be substituted if the woman is intolerant to aspirin.

SECONDARY PREVENTION

A reduction of mortality from the administration of low-dose aspirin was seen regardless of gender: 33 events were prevented for every 1000 women treated (ATC 1994). Based on evidence, low-dose aspirin should be recommended to women with no contraindications who have known CHD. Currently it is estimated that low-dose aspirin is used by only 50% of women who are aspirin eligible (Berger et al. 2006).

DUAL ANTIPLATELET THERAPY

In acute coronary syndrome, there is treatment benefit when adding clopidogrel to aspirin in both men and women (Yusef et al. 2001).

Nutritional Recommendations

Dietary patterns are diverse and affected by cultural background, socioeconomic status, and food availability. Epidemiologic data has shown that the Mediterranean, Anti-Inflammatory, and Indo-Mediterranean diets have a favorable effect on CVD. These diets are described elsewhere in the text. In general, a heart healthy diet incorporates whole grains, high fiber foods, and oily fish a few times a week, avoidance of trans fats, a limitation of saturated fats, the consumption of foods high in omega-3 fatty acids and sodium restriction. Specific nutritional recommendations follow.

OMEGA-3 FATTY ACIDS

In the NHS, there was a 38%–40% decreased risk of sudden myocardial death in the women that had the highest intake of omega-3 fatty acids, but there was no decrease in nonfatal CVD events after controlling for other risk factors (Albert et al. 2005; Hu et al. 2002). In Japan, where fish intake exceeds that of the United States, there was a strong inverse relationship seen between high dietary intake of fish (up to 8 servings a week) and risk of nonfatal MI and coronary events but no relationship was seen with fatal cardiac events (Iso et al. 2006). The inconsistent results have not been explained. Although the mechanisms by which omega-3 fatty acids may reduce sudden death are not understood, a recent cohort study found increased heart rate variability (HRV) in those adults who consumed the highest intake (Mozaffarian 2008). Omega-3 fatty acids are also indicated for treatment of hypertriglyceridemia and the prescription Lovaza has FDA approval for TG levels $\geq$ 500 mg/dL. In view of the proinflammatory state caused by our modern diets which have high ratios of omega-6 to omega-3 fatty acids intake, an increase in omega-3 rich foods from fish or flaxseed, canola, pumpkin seed, walnut, and soybeans is recommended both for primary and secondary prevention.

FIBER

Soluble fiber has been associated with lowering of total and LDL cholesterol, lowering of blood pressure, weight control, and improvement in insulin resistance and in clotting factors (Anderson and Hanna 1999). The NHS revealed that a 10 g/day increase in total fiber intake was associated with a significant decrease in risk of CHD events (Wolk et al. 1999). Another large prospective cohort study of women found that intake of dietary fiber was inversely associated with risk of MI and CVD but when adjusting for other CVD risk factors the association was not statistically significant (Liu et al. 2002). Nonetheless, due to the overwhelming evidence that high fiber diets prevent many of the risks associated with CVD, a diet with 5–10 g of soluble fiber is recommended by the Adult Treatment Panel III (Grundy et al. 2004). Good sources of soluble fiber include oat bran, psyllium, guar, and pectin.

SOY

Epidemiologic data has shown that postmenopausal women who consume diets rich in phytoestrogens, especially in the form of isoflavones, have a lower incidence of CVD (Kokubo et al. 2007). In addition, high intake of phytoestrogens has been associated with lower waist hip ratios and lower triglycerides (de Kleijn et al. 2002), and reduced fasting glucose levels, insulin levels, and inflammatory markers when compared to placebo (Atteritano et al. 2007). When soy nuts were added to a therapeutic lifestyle changes (TLC) diet in postmenopausal women, blood pressure and LDL cholesterol improved in hypertensive women and BP was reduced in normotensive women (Welty 2007). Although there is no conclusive evidence that soy has a beneficial or negative effect on CVD, based on epidemiologic data from Japan, it may be advisable to recommend that women obtain one serving of protein a day from natural soy foods such as tofu, tempeh, and soybeans.

TEA

The Rotterdam study revealed that fatal and nonfatal MI was lower in tea drinkers with a daily intake >375 ml (Geleijnse 2002). A prospective cohort revealed an inverse relationship between green tea consumption and cardiovascular mortality (Kuriyama 2006). This association was stronger in women than in men with the maximum benefit obtained with 3–4 cups of green tea a day. Concentrated catechins from green tea (500 mg or the equivalent of 6–7 cups of green tea) resulted in a significant decrease in plasma oxidized LDL (Inami et al. 2007). The consumption of at least 3 cups of tea per day was associated with less carotid plaque in women but not in men (Debette et al. 2008). The addition of milk counteracted the flow-mediated vasodilation that was seen plain black tea (Lorenz et al. 2007).

GARLIC

Garlic is the herbal supplement that has the most evidence for prevention or treatment of CVD mainly through its effects on lipids (Knox and Gaster 2007). The German Commission E has approved garlic for hyperlipidemia. A meta-analysis of 13 randomized, double-blind, placebo-controlled trials found garlic was superior to placebo in reducing cholesterol but that the decrease was small and of questionable clinical benefit (Stevinson et al. 2000). In a review of the more recent data, however, there is evidence that garlic has plasma lipid lowering abilities, anticoagulant, and antioxidant properties in vitro (Gorinstein et al. 2007). Herbalists have used garlic for hypertension and there is a meta-analysis that has shown its effectiveness (Silagy and Neil 1994).

NUTS

Three large prospective cohort studies have found an inverse relationship between nut consumption and CVD events (Albert et al. 2002; Fraser et al. 1992; Hu et al. 1998). In the NHS, women who consumed more than 5 oz of nuts a week had a significantly reduced risk of fatal and nonfatal CHD than women who consumed less than one ounce a month (Hu et al. 1998). Although nut consumption improves serum lipids, the 40%–50% CHD risk reduction that is found in the epidemiologic data cannot be explained by this factor alone. Other beneficial nutrients in nuts such as arginine, magnesium, folate, plant sterols, and soluble fiber along with omega-3 fatty acids and vitamin E also play a beneficial role (Vogel et al. 2005). It is important that patients understand that nuts are a high calorie food and that a serving size is only one ounce.

ALCOHOL

Moderate alcohol intake of 1–2 drinks a day has been shown to be related to decreased incidence of MI, of ischemic stroke, of peripheral vascular disease, and of death after an MI and CHF (Vogel et al. 2005). Although moderate alcohol does not result in increased morbidity, heavier intake poses significant hazards and can result in cardiomyopathy, hypertension, hemorrhagic stroke, arrhythmias, and sudden death. The risks and benefits must therefore be discussed with the patient.

Supplement Use in Cardiovascular Disease

Trials of supplement use have often yielded mixed or negative results. These are summarized in Table 35.3.

Table 35.3. Supplement Use in Cardiovascular Disease

Supplements with evidence for cardiovascular benefit and no deleterious effects	
Vitamin E: May be beneficial for older women and women with know CVD; recommended dose is 400 IU/day.	HOPE Study Investigators (2000): No detriment or benefit in a 4.5-year follow up. LEE et al. (2005): 7% (nonsignificant) risk reduction of CVD events; 26% (significant) reduction in subgroup aged >65. Cook et al. (2007): Mild reduction in subgroup of women with prior CVD.
Magnesium: Magnesium relaxes smooth muscle, stabilizes cardiac conductivity, and decreases neural excitability. Many in the Unites States have inadequate intakes especially the elderly and Caucasian and African American women (Ford and Mokdah 2003). Deficiency is also present in patients on diuretics. Dosage is usually 400 mg/day.	Appel et al. (1997): Prevention of hypertension in normotensives and lowering of BP in hypertensives with the DASH diet (see also: "Hypertension section.") Bashir et al. (1993): reduction in sustained ventricular tachycardia with supplement. Ma et al. (1995): Carotid artery thickness was inversely related to intake.

(continued)

Table 35.3. (Continued)

Supplements with evidence that is conflicting or lacking but for which there may be some benefit

Vitamin C	Kushi et al. (1996): Small, but nonsignificant increase in CHD mortality and stroke. Osganian et al. (2003): 28% reduction in fatal and nonfatal CHD event in those who took supplements versus diet alone. Knekt et al. (2004): 700 mg/day correlated to a 25% reduction in cardiovascular risk.
Vitamin D	Holick (2007): Deficiency is associated with higher risk for multiple diseases including CVD, CHF, some cancers, diabetes and autoimmune diseases; supplementation is encouraged for those who are deficient. Deficiency is more common in women than in men. Dosage is based on degree of deficiency; 1000 IU/day are recommended for the general population. Autier and Gangini (2007): Meta-analysis of 18 randomized trials: decrease in all cause mortality.
Coenzyme Q 10: Depletion is seen in patients on statins. Usual dosage is 200 mg/day.	Morisco et al. (1993): 38%–61% decrease in hospitalizations and pulmonary edema in patients with NYHA class II or IV CHF. Watson et al. (1999): No improvement in advanced CHF. Marcoff (2007): 200 mg of Coenzyme Q 10 are recommended for statin myopathy
L-Carnitine: Usual dosage is 3–6 g/day but it can potentiate the effect of warfarin.	Colonna and Iliceto (2000): Patients with an acute MI who received L-carnitine within 24 hours had improvements in LV volumes at 3, 6, and 12 months. There is no outcomes data regarding CVD events. Hiatt et al. (2001); Brevetti et al. (1999): In patients with peripheral vascular disease, there was improvement in maximum walking capacity and symptoms of claudication. Witte et al. (2001): Patients with CHF did not improve in terms of exercise capacity.

Supplements which may be harmful or have no proven benefit in cardiovascular disease

Beta-Carotene	ATBC Trial (1994): Increased lung cancer in male smokers. Rapola et al. (1996, 1998): Increased angina pectoris. Osganian et al. (2003): Increase in all-cause mortality and cardiovascular health.

(continued)

Supplements which may be harmful or have no proven benefit in cardiovascular disease	
Folic acid, vitamin B6, and vitamin B12: Prevention trials aimed at lowering homocysteine levels have not shown reduced CVD risk.	Bonaa et al. (2006): Increased cardiovascular events in folic acid plus B12 group. HOPE 2 Investigators (2006): Fewer patients had strokes; more were hospitalized with unstable angina; no CVD risk reduction in treatment groups. Lange et al. (2004): Increased in stent-restenosis.
L-Arginine	Blum et al. (2000): No increase in nitric oxide levels or decrease in inflammatory markers. Schulman et al. (2006): Study was stopped prematurely due to increased death rate in patient with acute MI with the treatment group.
Calcium	Bolland et al. (2008): Higher incidence of MI, TIA, stroke and sudden death in postmenopausal women treated with 1 g of elemental calcium. Hsia et al. (2007): No increase or decrease in cardiovascular risk.

Abbreviations: CHD, coronary heart disease; CHF, congestive heart failure; CVD, cardiovascular disease; LV, left ventricle; MI, myocardial infarction; NYHA, New York Heart Association; TIA, transient ischemic attack.

Herbal Preparations

Several drugs used for cardiovascular treatment have their origins in plants. These include aspirin, digoxin, atropine, reserpine, and amiodarone. Few herbal products available in the United States have undergone adequate testing for CVD. Table 35.4 summarizes the more common herbs. Red yeast rice is described under the "Hyperlipidemia" and garlic under the "Nutrition" sections of this chapter. Guggulipid and policosanol that are widely advertised as having lipid lowering abilities do not have good efficacy data.

Treatment of Hyperlipidemia

Lifestyle interventions should be the initial intervention and should always be part of drug and supplement therapy for the attainment of desirable lipid levels. A recent article states that women "should be aware of three numbers…100, 50, and 150; , LDL-C <100 mg/dL, HDL-C >50 mg/dL, and triglycerides ≤ 150 mg/dL" (Wenger et al. 2008a). For high risk women, those with known CHD or the CHD equivalent of diabetes, LDL-C goal should be <70.

Table 35.4. Herbal Preparations Used for the Treatment of Cardiovascular Disease

Herb	Disease	Method of Action	Dosing	Contraindication
Hawthorn (*Cratagus*)	CHF Reviewed in a meta-analysis of randomized trials	Increases stroke volume Reduces afterload Peripheral vasodilator	Minimum effective dose 300 mg of leaf extract (160–1800 mg of standardized extract used in trials)	Safer than digoxin; can be used with renal impairment, less arrhythmogenic potential Beware of combining it with digoxin, beta-blockers, and class III antiarrhythmics
Ginkgo biloba	Peripheral artery disease In a meta-analysis of 8 RPCDB trials pain-free walking increased by 34 m	Mechanism of action not known	120–160 mg/day	Can increase risk of bleeding; do not use with aspirin, warfarin, heparin, NSAIDS
Horse chestnut (*Aesculus hippocastanum*)	Chronic venous insufficiency: 14 RPC trials effective in decreasing lower leg volume and leg pain	Hydroxicoumarin derivative, glycosides escin, and aesculin	300 mg extract containing 50 mg aescin	Generally well tolerated

Abbreviations: CHF, congestive heart failure; NSAIDS, non-steroidal anti-inflammatory drug; RPC, randomized, placebo controlled; RPCDB, randomized, placebo-controlled double-blind

Source: Adapted from Vogel et al. 2005

HORMONAL INFLUENCES

Hormonal influences on lipoproteins are complex and help explain, at least partially, the increase of CVD after menopause. Prepubertal boys and girls are similar (Bittner 2005). During puberty, women's HDL-C rises and is maintained at roughly 10 mg/dL higher than men's HDL-C throughout their lifetime. However, many women with MI have HDL-C ≥60 mg/dL (Bittner et al. 2000), a level that is considered protective against CHD. During the premenopause years, lipoprotein levels vary and are affected by the menstrual cycle, pregnancy, and use of oral contraceptives. With oral contraceptives, triglycerides can increase by 13%–75% (Godsland et al. 1990), and LDL-C particle size can decrease (Foulon et al. 2001). In the postmenopausal years, total cholesterol increases, LDL-C particle size decreases and there is a greater increase in postprandial lipoproteins (Bittner 2005). Oral hormone replacement therapy decreases LDL-C and Lp(a) and increases HDL-C and triglycerides. Selective estrogen receptor modulators slightly affect lipoproteins, causing up to an 8% increase in triglycerides and up to 10% decrease in LDL-C (Barrett-Connor et al. 2002).

STATINS FOR SECONDARY PREVENTION

Statin therapy in women with established CHD significantly reduces CHD mortality, nonfatal MI, and revascularization. The effects of statins are similar in men and women and recent trials have provided evidence that women achieve the same clinical endpoints with statins as men (Bittner 2005). In the treating to new targets (TNT) study, in which 19% of the participants were women, there was a similar reduction in cardiovascular events with intensive lipid lowering in men and women (Wenger et al. 2008a).

Clinical tip: Supplementation with Coenzyme Q 10 (see Table 35.3) is recommended for statin and red yeast rice users.

STATINS FOR PRIMARY PREVENTION

The MEGA Study was the first trial to show a statistically significant reduction of CVD events in women (Mizuno et al. 2008). Women comprised over 68% of the 7832 participants in this prospective randomized, open label trial with a 10-year follow up. Among women randomized to receive pravastatin, there was a 26%–27% decrease in CVD events with the most benefit seen in women who were ≥60 years of age.

OTHER PHARMACOTHERAPY

Trials of clofibrate and colestipol have not included women. Trials on ezetimibe (Zetia) have shown similar success of lipid lowering in women and men but clinical outcome data is lacking.

The randomized, placebo-controlled JUPITER trial gave 20 mg of rosuvastatin to healthy women and men, without hyperlipidemia, with elevated hsCRP of ≥2 mg/L (Ridker et al. 2008). There was a 44% decrease in CVD events and death in the rosuvastatin group. This trial highlights the importance of screening for CVD risk with hsCRP and raises the question of whether the indications for statin use should be expanded. However, the trial has several limitations which should prevent an immediate rush to use statins in everyone with elevated hsCRP: it did not look at the effects of statins on normal levels of hsCRP; the long term safety of decreasing LDL cholesterol to 55 mg/dL, as was seen in this trial, in a healthy population is not known; levels of glycated hemoglobin and diabetes were higher in the rosuvastatin group; and CVD is affected by multiple factors in the participants other than hsCRP (Hlatky 2008).

> Statin use should be individualized to each patient's unique set of risk factors and preferences. I measure hsCRP in each of my patients and use it to help guide me for the prescription of statins along with aspirin use and lifestyle modification.

RED YEAST RICE

Red yeast rice (RYR) contains monacolin K (lovastatin) and eight other monacolins, along with sterols, isoflavones, and monounsaturated fatty acids. This family of substances probably explains why RYR is more effective at reducing cholesterol than what would be expected with the small amount of lovastatin that it contains. Based on a meta-analysis of randomized controlled trials of RYR, HDL-C can be raised by 15%–22%, LDL-C can be lowered by 27%–32%, and TG by 27%–38% (Liu et al. 2006). The recommended dosage is 1200 mg twice a day with meals. Side effects include headaches and GI discomfort. Lipid profiles and liver enzymes should be monitored 8 weeks after the initiation of RYR both to determine its effectiveness and to rule out any significant liver abnormalities. RYR is often well tolerated when statins are not. Outcome data with RYR is not available as it is for statins.

PHYTOSTEROLS

A dose of 1.8 to 2 g/day, divided over 2 meals, can result in a decrease of LDL-C by 9%–20% (Katan et al. 2003; Woodgate et al. 2006). HDL-C and Triglycerides are not affected. Plant stanols/sterols can be effectively combined with statins, niacin, or red yeast rice and are relatively safe with the exception of the rare person with familial sitosterolemia. There is no outcome data regarding phytosterol use and CVD.

NIACIN

Doses of up to 3000 mg/day, increased HDL-C by 30%, 21% decreased LDL-C by 21%, 44% decreased TG by 44%, and decreased Lp(a) by 26% (Goldberg et al. 2000). Niaspan is a prescription preparation which is long acting and can be used once a day. The "No Flush" over the counter preparations should not be used since they may not contain any free nicotinic acid that is responsible for the cholesterol-lowering effects. Besides flushing, side effects include GI disturbances, asthma exacerbation, acanthosis nigricans, and elevations in serum transaminases. Patients should be told of side effect of flushing, and of its usual improvement over the course of several weeks. Niacin should be taken in the evening, with dinner or a snack, up to 1 hour after taking an enteric coated low-dose aspirin in order to decrease flushing. Start dosing at 375–500 mg/day, increasing in increments of 250–500 mg every 2–3 weeks with careful monitoring of serum transaminases and lipid profiles. Niacin can be combined with statins or RYR and phytosterols.

FISH OIL

Omega-3 fatty acids are diverse in their effects on CVD risk reduction and are covered in greater detail in the "Nutrition" section of this chapter. They are effective in reduction of triglycerides and the prescription Lovaza has been approved for use in patients with triglyceride levels >/= 500 mg/dL. Omega-3 fatty acids reduce the syntheses and secretion of VLDL particles, and increase the removal of TG from VLDL and chylomicrons through upregulation of enzymes such as lipoprotein lipase (Bays et al. 2008). Omega-3 FA can be safely added to statin therapy. A randomized double-blind placebo-controlled trial shows a significant increase in HDL-C levels of 3.4%, and a decrease in non HDL-C (defined as total cholesterol minus HDL-C; or the sum of LDL-C and VLDL-C) levels by 9.0% when compared fish oil 4 g/day was combined with simvastatin versus simvastatin alone (Davidson et al. 2007). Dosages of 1–4 g/day are recommended.

Hypertension

One out of three adults in America has hypertension (Ong et al. 2007). Although hypertension affects men at younger ages than women, the rise in hypertension is steeper in women as they age. The overall prevalence of hypertension in men is slightly higher than in women (30.7 vs. 28.2); women are more aware then men when they are affected (67.6% vs. 66.7%); and more women are treated than men (58.0% vs. 52.1%). Yet fewer women than men have control of their hypertension (Ong et al. 2007). Women who have gestational hypertension have been shown to have higher risk for stroke and CVD later in life. Women who take oral contraceptives are two to three times more likely to have hypertension than women who are not on oral contraceptives, especially if they are older or obese (Chobanian et al. 2003).

Hypertension carries a significant decrease in life expectancy (Franco et al. 2005b) and contributes to the incidence of stroke, renal disease, CHD, and heart failure. Until the age of 50, diastolic and systolic blood pressures rise in tandem whereas after the age of 50 systolic blood pressure (SBP) continues to rise while diastolic blood pressure (DBP) falls or remains the same. Above the age of 60, elevated SBP has a higher relative risk for CHD than DBP whereas prior to the age of 50, DBP is a more potent risk predictor (Franklin et al. 2001). According to a meta-analysis, each 20 mm Hg increase in SBP over 115, and each 10 mm Hg in DBP over 75 doubles the risk of a fatal cardiovascular event with the absolute risk also rising with age (Lewington et al. 2002). The same meta-analysis found that decreases in BP bring about rapid decreases in CVD morbidity and mortality with a 50%–60% decrease in stroke death, and a 40%–50% decrease in CAD death for every 10 mm Hg decrease in SBP and 5 mm Hg decrease in DBP.

PREVENTION AND GUIDELINES FOR TREATMENT

In 2003, the Joint National Committee of Prevention, Detection, Evaluation and Treatment of High Blood Pressure (JNC 7) included the classification of prehypertension defined as a SBP between 120 and 139 mm Hg and/or DBP between 80 and 89 mm Hg (Chobanian et al. 2003). The risk of cardiovascular events increases 2.5 fold in women and 1.6 fold in men with prehypertension. As such, aggressive approaches for prevention and treatment must be employed. The initial approach to hypertension should include primary prevention with a goal blood pressure of 120/80 mm Hg. Guidelines for pharmacotherapy are discussed below.

DIET

Excess caloric intake and supraphysiologic intake of sodium contribute to hypertension. The fiber rich DASH diet which emphasizes whole grains, low-fat dairy, and nuts, and which is low in sodium and high in magnesium and potassium has been shown to be very effective in lowering BP to goal in 71% of patients with Stage 1 hypertension (Scetkey et al. 2004). When the DASH diet was used with lower sodium intake systolic BP was reduced by up to 7.1 mm Hg in nonhypertensive individuals and 11.5 mm Hg in hypertensive participants (Sacks et al. 2001). Twenty-four year follow data from over 80,000 women enrolled in the NHS revealed that there was a significant reduction in of CHD and stroke in those women who followed a DASH style diet (Fung et al. 2008).

MIND–BODY TECHNIQUES

Breathing exercises with device-guided breathing lower SBP by approximately 10 mm Hg and DBP by approximately 5 mm Hg (Meles et al 2004; Schein et al 2001). "Resperate" TM is such a device that has FDA approval. Biofeedback-assisted relaxation methods can be effective in select individuals who have high anxiety, rapid pulse, high urinary cortisol levels, and cool hand temperatures (McGrady et al. 1981, 1991). Transcendental meditation has been shown to reduce SBP by 4.7 mm Hg and DBP by 3.2 mm Hg (Anderson et al. 2008).

PHARMACOTHERAPY

Pharmacologic treatment, according to the JNC 7, is the same for women and men (Chobanian et al. 2003). Pharmacotherapy is indicated when the BP is ≥140/90 for all women or ≥130/80 for women who have chronic kidney disease or diabetes mellitus. A goal blood pressure of <130/80 mm Hg is recommended for those with a high risk of CHD (see Table 35.1), and <120/80 for those with left ventricular dysfunction (Rosendorff et al. 2007). Following are general guidelines for drug selection; however, the emphasis should be on obtaining goal BP.

1. General CAD prevention or high-risk for CAD: any effective drug or combination; evidence supports ACEI, ARB, CCB, or thiazide diuretic as first line therapy.
2. CAD: beta-blockers and ACEI or ARB.
3. Diabetes mellitus: ACE or ARB and additional therapy to achieve goal BP.
4. LV dysfunction: ACE or ARB, and beta-blockers, and aldosterone antagonist diuretics (for volume overload) and isosorbide dinitrates (African Americans); verapamil, diltiazem, clonidine, alpha-blockers are contraindicated.
5. Pregnancy/contemplation of pregnancy: ACE and ARB are contraindicated.

Exercise and the Heart

Both men and men achieve cardiovascular benefit from exercise. Data from the NHS and the WHI Obesity Study reveal that women in the highest quintiles of physical activity gain the most benefit when compared to sedentary women (Manson et al. 1999, 2002). Women who were sedentary had three times the risk of CVD or death when compared to women in the highest quintile of physical activity (Stevens et al. 2002). These studies revealed a strong dose-response gradient. Further, the benefit of exercise carried through every weight category (Stevens et al. 2002) and sedentary lifestyle remains an independent risk factor for CVD after multivariate analysis (Franco et al. 2005a).

Thirty minutes of moderate-intensity physical activity, defined as walking a brisk pace of 3 miles per hour on most days of the week, is the current recommendation by both the American College of Sports Medicine (Pate et al. 1995) and the Surgeon General's Report on Physical Activity (Department of Health and Human Services 1996). If patients cannot walk at a brisk pace, they should be encouraged to walk at a 2–2.9 mile/hr pace which reduces the risk of cardiovascular events by approximately 25% (Manson et al. 1999). Vigorous activity, examples of which include running, bicycling, swimming, tennis, and calisthenics, has added cardiovascular benefit. Since epidemiologic evidence has proven that the prescribed physical activity can prevent at least 30%–40% of the cardiovascular events that occur in women, it is of utmost importance that we give our patients a "prescription" for exercise.

Emotions and the Heart

Socioeconomic stress such as marital stress, caregiver strain, and financial hardship; and psychoaffective disorders such as depression, anxiety, anger, and hostility have been associated with and increased risk of CVD (Rozanski et al. 2005). The INTERHEART case-control study which included 12,461 men and women with acute MI in 52 countries and 14,637 matched controls, revealed that psychosocial stress was an independent risk factor for MI, regardless of geographic or ethnic background (Rosengren et al. 2004). Although there has been increasing data on the impact of stress on the heart, and although most physicians easily grasp this notion, they often fail to recognize depression in patients with CVD. In patients hospitalized with acute coronary syndrome who were depressed, only 24.5% of the patients were recognized by their physicians as being depressed (Amin et al. 2006). The current AHA guidelines recommend screening women with CVD for depression but no guidelines are given regarding treatment.

DEPRESSION

Epidemiologic studies support both major depression and depressive symptoms as a significant risk for CHD. Eleven cohort studies have shown that patients with depression have 2.5 times the risk of having an acute MI as nondepressed patients (Rugulies 2002). The presence of depression with a recent MI doubles the risk of death in both men and women, but the prevalence of depression in women is twice that of men (Naqvi et al. 2005). Diabetic women are more depressed than diabetic men, and depressed diabetic women have a more aggressive form of CVD than nondepressed diabetic women. Younger women with CHD have the highest prevalence of depression (Mallik et al. 2006) and have the highest risk of death after an acute MI.

Antidepressants

Tricyclic antidepressants (TCA) can slow intraventricular conduction thereby causing heart block or ventricular reentry arrhythmias (Glassman and Preud'homme 1993) and cause severe orthostatic hypotension (Glassman and Bigger 1981). Since TCA may cause a decrease in left ventricular function, they are contraindicated in patients with impaired LV function or CHD. In the SADHART trial, sertraline, a selective serotonin reuptake inhibitor (SSRI) has been shown to be safe in patients with CVD who have a major depressive disorder. In a double-blind, placebo-controlled trial that randomized 369 eligible patients to sertraline or placebo; sertaline did not reduce left ventricular ejection fraction, increase ventricular arrhythmias or heart block (Glassman et al. 2002). Sertraline was superior to placebo in the treatment of depression and there was a trend towards decreased cardiovascular events. However, the trial was a safety study and was not powered to determine if sertaline was effective for the reduction of cardiovascular events. It is the only prospective randomized control published to date. A recent review found that SSRI use was associated with decreased CVD morbidity and mortality in six studies, increased CHD events in two studies, and no significant effect in four studies (Von Ruden et al. 2008).

Psychological Intervention

There have been five large-scale behavioral intervention trials in cardiac patients that are summarized in Table 35.5. Although the results are mixed, the improvement in event-free survival was correlated to the successful reduction of psychological distress.

Exercise and Cardiac Rehabilitation

Lower depression scores have been seen in both ill and healthy people who are physically active (Lawlor and Hopker 2001). In a randomized, controlled study of 156 men and women with major depressive disorder followed for 16 weeks, exercise was as effective as sertraline in the treatment of depression (Blumenthal et al. 1999). In another randomized controlled trial in patients with CHD, exercise and stress management decreased depression, improved HRV, and improved flow mediated dilation (Blumenthal et al. 2005). Cardiac rehabilitation (CR) trials have shown a decrease in cardiovascular mortality when CR was successful in reducing psychosocial stress (Dusseldorp et al. 1999; Linden et al. 1996). Depressed patients who entered CR, had a 63% decrease in depression and a 73% decrease in cardiovascular morbidity and mortality over a 5-year period (Milani and Lavie 2007). Persistence of depression following CR, however, was associated with over a fourfold higher risk of cardiac mortality when compared to nondepressed patients. Only about half of all patients after acute MI participate in CR and women, especially minority and older women are 55% less likely to attend CR than men (Witt et al. 2004).

Table 35.5. Summary of Behavioral Intervention Trials in Cardiovascular Disease

Trial	Method	Result	References
Recurrent Coronary Prevention Project Study	862 post-MI patients randomized to group cognitive therapy or usual care	Therapy reduced Type A behavior and negative affect. 12.9% incidence of CV mortality and nonfatal MI in treatment group versus 21.2% in usual care.	Friedman et al. (1986)
Ischemic Heart Disease life Stress Monitoring Program	769 male patients after MI randomized to home-based stress-reduction program or usual care	Decrease in cardiac mortality of 47%, and decrease in depression scores in the treatment group when compared to control group. No decrease in hospitalizations for nonfatal cardiovascular events.	Frasure-Smith and Prince (1985)
Psychological Rehabilitation after Myocardial Infarction: Multicentre Randomised Controlled Trial	2328 post-MI patients, and their spouses, randomized to receive seven weekly outpatient group therapy sessions for stress reduction or usual care	At 12 months there were no differences in cardiac events; the program was not successful in reducing stress.	Jones and West (1996).
Randomized Trial follow-up to Ischemic Heart Disease Trial	1376 post-MI patients randomized to receive home-based therapy or usual care.	Higher cardiac (94% vs. 5.0%, $p = 0.064$) and all causes (10.3% vs. 5.4%, $p = 0.051$) mortality in women. No harm or benefit in men in the intervention group. The program did not have a statistically significant impact on depression and anxiety with reanalysis of the data showing that results could be attributed to inadequate psychological intervention	Cosette et al. (2001); Frasure-Smith et al. (1997)

(continued)

Table 35.5. (Continued)

Trial	Method	Result	References
Effects of Treating Depression and Low Perceived Social Support on Clinical Events after Myocardial Infarction: The Enhancing Recovery in Coronary Heart Disease Patients (ENRICHD) Randomized Trial	2481 post-MI patients who were depressed were randomized to receive cognitive behavioral therapy, plus group therapy if indicated, plus SSRIs for severe depression, or usual care.	No differences were seen in event-free survival however there were no significant differences among the treatment and control groups.	The ENRICHD Investigators (2003).

Abbreviations: CV, cardiovascular; MI, myocardial infarction; SSRD, selective serotonin reuptake inhibitors

ACUTE EMOTIONAL STRESS AND CARDIOMYOPATHY

The "Broken Heart" syndrome, or *Takotsubo* cardiomyopathy, occurs in the absence of obstructive coronary atherosclerosis and affects mostly postmenopausal women (Virani et al. 2007). There are no chronic symptoms, but an acute emotional or physical stressor initiates symptoms which clinically can be identical to an acute MI. Rapid and complete recovery of left ventricular dysfunction is a hallmark of this syndrome and if systolic function has not recovered in 4–6 weeks, a different diagnosis should be considered (Wittstein et al. 2007). Treatment includes usual care and medications but there is no consensus on how long to continue medications once LV function has recovered. The recurrence rate is approximately 3.5% (Gianni et al. 2006) but there is no data on prevention. Many questions remain regarding why it affects mostly women, and whether this syndrome represents an exaggeration of the normal stress response, or a pathologic defect?

PSYCHOLOGICAL STRESS AND VENTRICULAR ARRHYTHMIAS

The mechanism of ventricular arrhythmias (VA) can be understood: vagal efferents richly innervate atrial muscle and the SA and AV nodes and only sparsely innervate ventricular tissue. Sympathetic efferents are widespread throughout the heart. Therefore, the ventricles are vulnerable to sympathetic discharge. It is estimated that 20% of VA are precipitated by emotional stress. In patients with implantable cardiac defibrillators (ICD), anger was significantly more likely to be identified by patients prior to a shock and the VA was faster and more difficult to terminate (Lampert et al. 2002). There was a 37% increased incidence of sudden cardiac death (SCD) in patients with mild depression and a 77% increased risk of SCD in patients with severe depression when compared to controls (Empana et al. 2006).

PSYCHOLOGICAL STRESS AND ATRIAL ARRHYTHMIAS

Emotional stress is commonly cited by patients with atrial fibrillation and with palpitations from atrial ectopy. The Framingham Offspring Study revealed that anxiety predicted AF in men and correlated with increased overall mortality in men and women (Eaker et al. 2005). Examinations of HRV from holters revealed that there was higher sympathetic to parasympathetic activity until 10 minutes prior to the start of the AF (Ziegelstein 2007).

Acupuncture

Acupuncture has been used to treat stable angina (Richter et al. 1991), Raynaud's syndrome (Vogel et al. 2005), and hypertension (Chiu et al. 1997). The ability of acupuncture to inhibit sympathetic outflow may account for its effectiveness. The specific acupuncture points used for the treatment of CVD are the *Neiguan* or *Zusanli* acupoints which overlie the median and deep peroneal nerves (Guo et al. 1981). A placebo effect has been suggested. Since both acupuncture and the placebo effect involve the endogenous opioid system, there is a narrow window between what is placebo and a true response (Vogel et al. 2005). Further exploration is necessary regarding acupuncture's effectiveness in CVD.

Chelation

Evidence that chelation is beneficial is lacking in randomized trials. Yet chelation therapy with ethylenediamine tetraacetic acid (EDTA) has been used in the alternative treatment in patients with CHD since the 1950s. Initial studies with chelation were not controlled and even though there was initial symptom relief in 75% of patients with angina, by 18 months, one-third of the patients had died from their CVD and less than 40% of the remaining patients retained some benefit (Kitchell et al. 1963). Several other trials have shown no improvement in exercise time after treatment (Knudtson et al. 2002). No reputable cardiovascular society has endorsed chelation therapy. NCCAM in collaboration with NHLBI is in the process of studying the effect of chelation therapy and/or high-dose vitamin therapy in the treatment of CAD in a large, randomized, placebo-controlled trial known as TACT.

Summary

This chapter has outlined the unique nature of women's cardiovascular health and the author hopes that you will find the following brief summary for risk assessment and disease prevention helpful.

1. Listen to the woman. She is blessed with incredible intuitive powers after years of hormonal cycling and after being a caretaker for her family or friends. Be aware that typical symptoms of chest discomfort may or may not be present and that she may describe fatigue, or dyspnea as her anginal equivalent.

2. Determine her cardiovascular risk (Table 35.1).
3. Order appropriate diagnostic testing and/or refer to a cardiologist you trust. All diabetic women should see a cardiologist yearly.
4. Recommend appropriate preventive measures in ALL women:
   a. Nutritional counseling for weight reduction/maintenance, hypertension, or hyperlipidemia;
   b. exercise recommendations to improve physical conditioning, strength, flexibility, and balance;
   c. psychosocial intervention when appropriate;
   d. aspirin as outlined in this chapter;
   e. supplement use as outlined in this chapter, especially omega-3 fatty acids and magnesium;
   f. mind–body techniques for relaxation and stress management; and
   g. pharmacotherapy to achieve goal levels of blood pressure and lipids and to control diabetes.
5. Lastly, find joy in your practice so that you can be a better healer and improve your own cardiovascular health.

REFERENCES

Albert CM, Gaziano JM., Willett WC, Manson JE. Nut consumption and decreased risk of sudden cardiac death in the Physicians' Health Study. *Arch Intern Med.* 2002;162(12):1482–1387.

Albert CM, Oh K, Whang W, et al. Dietary alpha-linolenic acid intake and risk of sudden cardiac death and coronary heart disease. *Circulation.* 2005;112(21):3232–3238.

Alter DA, Naylor CD, Austin RC, Tu JV. Biology or bias: practice patterns and long-tern outcomes for man and women with acute myocardial infarction. *J Am Coll Cardiol.* 2002;39(12):1909–1916.

American Heart Association. 2008. *Heart Disease and Stroke Statistics—2008 Updates.* Dallas, TX: American Heart Association.

Amin AA, Jones AM, Nugent K, Rumsfeld JS, Spertus JA. The prevalence of unrecognized depression in patients with acute coronary syndrome. *Am Heart J.* 2006;152(5):928–934.

Anderson JW, Hanna TJ. Impact of nondigestible carbohydrates on serum lipoproteins and risk for cardiovascular disease. *J Nutr.* 1999;129:1457S–1466S.

Anderson JW, Liu C, Kryscio RJ. Blood pressure response to transcendental meditation: a meta-analysis. *Am J Hypertens.* 2008;21(3):310–316.

Antithrombotic Trialists' Collaboration (ATC). Collaborative meta-analysis of randomised trails of antiplatelet therapy for prevention of death, myocardial infarction, and stroke in high risk patients. *BMJ.* 2002;324(7329):71–86.

Antithrombotic Trialists' Collaboration (ATC). Collaborative overview of randomized trials of antiplatelet therapy: Prevention of death, myocardial infarction, and stroke by prolonged antiplatelet therapy in various categories of patients. *BMJ.* 1994;308:81–106.

Appel LJ, Moore TJ, Obarzanek E, et al. A clinical trial of the effects of dietary patterns on blood pressure. DASH Collaborative Research Group. *N Engl J Med.* 1997;336(16):1117–1124.

Arslanian-Engoren C, Patel A, Fang J, et al. Symptoms of men and women presenting with acute coronary syndromes. *Am J Cardiol.* 2006;98(9):1177–1181.

Atteritano M, Marini H, Minutoli L, et al. Effects of the phytoestrogen genistein on some predictors of cardiovascular risk in osteopenic, postmenopausal women: a 2-years randomized, double-blind, placebo-controlled study. *J Clin Endocrinol Metab.* 2007;92(8):3068–3075.

Autier P, Gandini S. Vitamin D supplementation and total mortality: a meta-analysis of randomized controlled trials. *Arch Intern Med.* 2007;167(16):1730–1737.

Barrett-Connor E, Grady D, Sashegyi A, et al. Raloxifene and cardiovascular events in osteoporotic postmenopausal women. *JAMA.* 2002;287(7):847–857.

Bashir Y, Sneddon JF, Staunton HA, et al. Effects of long-term oral magnesium chloride replacement in congestive heart failure secondary to coronary artery disease. *Am J Cardiol.* 1993;72(15):1156–1162.

Bays HE, Tighe AP, Sadovsky R, Davidson MH. Prescription omega-3 fatty acids and their lipid effects: physiologic mechanisms of action and clinical implications. *Expert Re Cardiovasc Ther.* 2008;6(3):391–409.

Berger JS, Roncaglioni MC, Avanzini F, Pangrazzi I, Tognoni G, Brown DL. Aspirin for the primary prevention of cardiovascular events in women and men: a sex-specific meta-analysis of randomized controlled trails. *JAMA.* 2006;295(3):306–313.

Bittner V. Perspectives on dyslipidemia and coronary heart disease in women. *J Am Coll Cardiol.* 2005;46:1628–1635.

Bittner V, Simon JA, Fong J, Blumenthal RS, Newby K, Stefanick ML. Correlates of high HDL cholesterol among women with coronary heart disease. *Am Heart J.* 2000;139:288–296.

Blum A, Hathaway L, Mincemoyer R, et al. Effects of oral L-arginine on endothelium-dependent vasodilation and markers of inflammation in healthy postmenopausal women. *J Am Coll Cardiol.* 2000;35:271–276.

Blumenthal JA, Babyak MA, Moore KA, et al. Effects of exercise training on older patients with major depression. *Arch Intern Med.* 1999;159(19):2349–2356.

Blumenthal JA, Sherwood A, Babyak MA, et al. Effects of exercise and stress management training on markers of cardiovascular risk in patients with ischemic heart disease. *JAMA.* 2005;293(13):1626–1634.

Bolland MJ, Barber PA, Doughty RN, et al. Vascular events in healthy older women receiving calcium supplementation: randomised controlled trial. *BMJ.* 2008;336(7638):262–266.

Bonaa KH, Njolstad I, Ueland PM, et al. Homocysteine lowering and cardiovascular events after acute myocardial infarction. *N Engl J Med.* 2006;354(15):1578–1588.

Brevetti G, Diehm C, Lambert D. European multicenter study on propionyl-L-carnitine in intermittent claudication. *J Am Coll Cardiol.* 1999;34:1618–1624.

Canto JG, Goldberg RJ, Hand MM, et al. Symptom presentation of women with acute coronary syndromes: myth vs. reality. *Arch Intern Med.* 2007;167(22):2405–2413.

Chan AT, Manson JE, Feskanich D, Stampfer MJ, Colditz GA, Fuchs CS. Long-term aspirin use and mortality in women. *Arch Intern Med.* 2007;167:562–572.

Chiu YJ, Chi A, Reid IA. Cardiovascular and endocrine effects of acupuncture in hypertensive patients. *Clin Exp Hypertens.* 1997;19(7):1047–1063.

Chobanian AV, Bakris GL, Clack HR, et al. The seventh report of the joint national committee on prevention, detection, evaluation, and treatment of high blood pressure: the JNC 7 report. *JAMA.* 2003;289(19):2560–2572.

Christian AH, Roasamond W, White AR, Mosca L. Nine-Year trends and racial and ethnic disparities in women's awareness of heart disease and stroke: An American Heart Association national study. *J Women Health.* 2007;16(1):68–81.

Colonna P, Iliceto S. Myocardial infarction and left ventricular remodeling: results of the CEDIM trial. L-carnitine Ecocardiografia Digitalizzata Infarcto Miocardico. *Am Heart J.* 2000;139(2 Pt 3):S124–S130.

Cook NR, Albert CM, Gaziano JM, et al. A randomized factorial trial of vitamins C and E and beta carotene in the secondary prevention of cardiovascular events in women: results from the Women's Antioxidant Cardiovascular Study. *Arch Intern Med.* 2007;167(15):1610–1618.

Cossette S, Frasure-Smith N, Lesperance F. Clinical implications of a reduction in psychological distress on cardiac prognosis in patients participating in a psychosocial intervention program. *Psychosom Med.* 2001;63(2):257–266.

Davidson MH, Stein EA, Bays HE, et al. Efficacy and tolerability of adding prescription omega-3 fatty acids 4 g/d to simvastatin 40 mg/d in hypertriglyceridemic patients: an 8-week, randomized, double-blind, placebo-controlled study. *Clin Ther.* 2007;29(7):1354–1367.

de Kleijn MJ, van der Schouw YT, Wilson PW, Grobbee DE, Jacques PR. Dietary intake of phytoestrogens is associated with a favorable metabolic cardiovascular risk profile in postmenopausal U.S. women: the Framingham study. *J Nutr.* 2002;132(2):276–282.

Debette S, Courbon D, Leone N, et al. Tea consumption is inversely associated with carotid plaques in women. *Arterioscler Thromb Vasc Biol.* 2008;28(2):353–359.

Department of Health and Human Services. 1996. *Physical activity and health: a report of the Surgeon General.* Atlanta: Department of Health and Human Services, Centers for Disease Control and Prevention, National Center for Chronic Disease Prevention and Health Promotion.

Dusseldorp E, van Elderen T, Maes S, Meulman J, Kraaij V. A meta-analysis of psychoeducational programs for coronary heart disease patients. *Health Psychol.* 1999;18(5):506–519.

Eaker ED, Sullican LM, Kelly-Hayes M, D'Agostino RB, Benjamin EJ. Tension and anxiety and the prediction of the 10-year incidence of coronary heart disease, atrial fibrillation, and total mortality: the Framingham offspring study. *Psychosom Med.* 2005;67:692–696.

Empana JP, Jouven X, Lemaitre RN, et al. Clinical depression and risk of out-of-hospital cardiac arrest. *Arch Intern Med.* 2006;166:195–200.

Ford ES, Mokdad AH. Dietary magnesium intake in a national sample of US adults. *J Nutr.* 2003;133(9):2879–2882.

Foulon T, Payen N, Laporte F, et al. Effects of two low-dose oral contraceptives containing ethinylestradiol and either desogestrel or levonorgestrel on serum lipids and lipoproteins with particular regard to LDL size. *Contraception.* 2001;64(1):11–16.

Franco OH, de Laet C, Peeters A, Jonker J, Mackenbach J, Nusselder W. Effects of physical activity on life expectancy with cardiovascular disease. *Arch Intern Med.* 2005a;165(20):2355–2360.

Franco OH, Peeters A, Conneux L, de Laet C. Blood pressure in adulthood and life expectancy with cardiovascular disease in men and women: life course analysis. *Hypertension.* 2005b;46(2):280–286.

Franklin SS, Larson MG, Khan SA, et al. Does the relation of blood pressure to coronary heart disease risk change with aging? *Circulation.* 2001;103(9):1245–1249.

Fraser GE, Sabate J, Beeson WL, Strahan TM. A possible protective effect of nut consumption on risk of coronary heart disease. *Arch Intern Med.* 1992;152(7):1416–1426.

Frasure-Smith N, Prince R. The ischemic heart disease life stress monitoring program: impact on mortality. *Psychosom Med.* 1985;47(5):431–445.

Frasure-Smith N, Lesperance F, Prince RH, et al. Randomised trial of home-based psychosocial nursing intervention for patients recovering from myocardial infarction. *Lancet.* 1997;350(9076):473–479.

Friedman M, Thorensen CE, Gill JJ, et al. Alteration of type A behavior and its effect on cardiac recurrences in post myocardial infarction patents: summary results of the recurrent coronary prevention project. *Am Heart J.* 1986;112(4):653–665.

Fung TT, Chiuve SE, McCullough ML, Rexrode KM, Logroscino G, Hu FB. Adherence to a DASH-Style diet and risk of coronary heart disease and stroke in women. *Arch Intern Med.* 2008;168(7):713–720.

Geleijnse JM, Launer LJ, Van de Kuip DA, Hofman A, Witteman JC. Inverse association of tea and flavenoid intakes with incident myocardial infarction: the Rotterdam Study. *Am J Clin Nutr.* 2002;75(5):880–886.

Gianni M, Dentali F, Grandi AM, Summer G, Hiralal R, Lonn E. Apical ballooning syndrome or takotsubo cardiomyopathy: a systematic review. *Eur Heart J.* 2006;27:1523–1529.

Glassman AH, Bigger JT. Cardiovascular effects of therapeutic doses of tricyclic antidepressants. *Arch Gen Psychiatry.* 1981;38(7):815–820.

Glassman AH, Preud'homme XA. Review of the cardiovascular effects of heterocyclic antidepressants. *J Clin Psychiatry.* 1993;54:16–22.

Glassman AH, O'Connor CM, Califf RM, et al. Sertraline treatment of major depression in patients with acute MI or unstable angina. *JAMA.* 2002;288(6):701–709.

Godsland IF, Crook D, Simpson R, et al. The effects of different formulations of oral contraceptive agents on lipid and carbohydrate metabolism. *N Engl J Med.* 1990;323(20):1375–1381.

Goldberg A, Alagona P Jr, Capuzzi DM, et al. Multiple-dose efficacy and safety of an extended-release form of niacin in the management of hyperlipidemia. *Am J Cardiol.* 2000;85(9):1100–1105.

Gorinstein S, Jastrzebski Z, Namiesnik J, Leontowicz H, Leontowicz M, Trakhtenberg S. The atherosclerotic heart disease and protecting properties of garlic: contemporary data. *Mol Nutr Food Res.* 2007;51(11):1365–1381.

Grundy SM, Cleeman JI, Merz NB, et al for the Coordinating Committee of the National Cholesterol Education Program. Implications of recent clinical trials for the National Cholesterol Education Program Adult Treatment Panel III Guidelines. *Circulation.* 2004;110:227–239.

Guo XQ, Jai RJ, Cao QY, Guo Zd, Li P. Inhibitory effect of somatic nerve afferent impulses on the extrasystole induced by hypothalamic stimulation. *Acta Physiolo Sin.* 1981;33:334–350.

Hemmingway H, Langenberg C, Damant J, Frost C, Pyörälä K, Carrett-Connor E. Prevalence of angina in women versus men. *Circulation.* 2008;117:1526–1536.

Hiatt WR, Regensteiner JG, Creager MA, et al. Propionyl-L-carnitine improves exercise performance and functional status in patients with claudication. *Am J Med.* 2001;110(8):616–622.

Hlatky MA. Expanding the Orbit of Primary Prevention—Moving Beyond JUPITER. *NEJM.* 2008;359(21): 2280–2282.

Hochman JS, Tamis JE, Thompson TD, et al. Sex, clinical presentation, and outcome in patients with acute coronary syndromes. *N Engl J Med.* 1999;341(4):226–232.

Holick MF. Vitamin D deficiency. *N Engl J Med.* 2007;357(3)266–281.

Hsia J, Heiss G, Ren H, et al. Calcium/vitamin D supplementation and cardiovascular events. *Circulation.* 2007;115(7):846–854.

Hu FB, Bronner L, Willett WC, et al. Fish and omega-3 fatty acid intake and risk of coronary heart disease in women. *JAMA.* 2002;287(14):1815–1821.

Hu FB, Stampfer MJ, Manson JE, et al. Frequent nut consumption and risk of coronary heart disease in women: prospective cohort study. *BMJ.* 1998;317(7169):1341–1345.

Inami S, Takano M, Yamamoto M, et al. Tea catechin consumption reduces circulation oxidized low-density lipoprotein. *Int Heart J.* 2007;48(6):725–732.

Innes KE, Selfe TK, Taylor AG. Menopause, the metabolic syndrome, and mind-body therapies. *Menopause.* 2008;15(5):1005–1013..

Iso H, Kobayashi M, Ishihara J, et al. Intake of fish and n3 fatty acids and risk of coronary heart disease among Japanese: the Japan Public Health Center-Based (JPHC) Study Cohort I. *Circulation.* 2006;113(2):195–202.

Jones DA, West RR. Psychological rehabilitation after myocardial infarction: multicentre randomized controlled trial. *BMJ.* 1996 313(7071) 1517–1521.

Katan MB, Grundy SM, Jones P, Law M, Miettinen T, Paoletti R, Stresa Workshop Participants. Efficacy and safety of plant stanols and sterols in the management of blood cholesterol levels. *Mayo Clin Proc.* 2003;78(8);965–978.

Khaw KT, Wareham N, Bingham S, Luben R, Welch A, Day N. Association of hemoglobin A1c with cardiovascular disease and mortality in adults: the European prospective investigation into cancer in Norfolk. *Ann Intern Med.* 2004;141(6): 413–420.

Khot UN, Khot MB, Bajzer CT, et al. Prevalence of conventional risk factors in patients with coronary heart disease. *JAMA.* 2003;290(7):898–904.

Kitchell JR, Palmon F, Aytan N, Meltzer LE. The treatment of coronary artery disease with disodium EDTA. *Am J Cardiol.* 1963;11:501–506.

Knekt P, Ritz J, Pereira MA, et al. Antioxidant vitamins and coronary heart disease risk: a pooled analysis of 9 cohorts. *Am J Clin Nutr.* 2004;80(6):1508–1520.

Knox J, Gaster B. Dietary supplements for the prevention and treatment of coronary artery disease. *J Altern Complement Med.* 2007;13(1):83–95.

Knudtson ML, Wyse DG, Galbraith PD, for the Program to Assess Alternative Treatment Strategies to Achieve Cardiac Health (PATCH) Investigators. Chelation therapy for ischemic heart disease: A randomized controlled trial. *JAMA.* 2002;287(4):481–486.

Kokubo Y, Iso H, Ishihara J, Okada K, Inoue M, Tsugane S. Association of dietary intake of soy, beans, and isoflavones with risk of cerebral and myocardial infarctions in Japanese populations: The Japan Public Health Center-Based (JPHC) Study Cohort I. *Circulation.* 2007;116:2553–2562.

Kuriyama S, Shimazu T, Ohmori K, et al. Green tea consumption and mortality due to cardiovascular disease, cancer, and all causes in Japan: the Ohsaki study. *JAMA.* 2006;296(10):1255–1265.

Kushi LH, Folsom AR, Prineas RJ, Mink PJ, Wu Y, Bostick RM. Dietary antioxidant vitamins and death from coronary heart disease in postmenopausal women. *N Engl J Med.* 1996;334(18):1156–1162.

Lampert R, Joska T, Burg MM, Batsford WP, McPherson CA, Jain D. Emotional and psychical precipitants of ventricular arrhythmia. *Circulation.* 2002;106:1800–1805.

Lange H, Suryapranato H, DeLuca G, et al. Folate therapy and in-stent restenosis after coronary stenting. *N Engl J Med.* 2004;350(26):2673–2681.

Lansky AJ, Hochman JS, Ward PA, et al. Percutaneous coronary intervention and adjunctive pharmacotherapy in women: a statement for healthcare professionals from the American Heart Association. *Circulation.* 2005;111:940–953.

Lawlor DA, Hopker SW. The effectiveness of exercise as an intervention in the management of depression: systematic review and meta-regression analysis of randomised controlled trials. *BMJ.* 2001;322(7289):763–767.

Lee IM, Cook NR, Gaziano JM, et al. Vitamin E in the primary prevention of cardiovascular disease and cancer: the Women's Health Study: a randomized controlled trial. *JAMA.* 2005;294(1):56–65.

Lewington S, Clarke R, Qizilbash N, Peto R, Collins R. Age-specific relevance of usual blood pressure to vascular mortality: a meta-analysis of individual data for one million adults in 61 prospective studies. *Lancet.* 2002;360(9349):1903–1913.

Linden W, Stossel C, Maurice J. Psychosocial interventions for patients with coronary artery disease: a meta-analysis. *Arch Intern Med.* 1996;156(7):745–752.

Liu J, Zhang J, Shi Y, Grimsgaard S, Alraek T, Fonnebo V. Chinese red yeast rice (*Monascus purpureus*) for primary hyperlipidemia: a meta-analysis of randomized controlled trials. *Chin Med.* 2006;23:1–4.

Liu S, Burin JE, Sesso HD, Rimm EB, Willett WC, Manson JE. A prospective study of dietary fiber intake and risk of cardiovascular disease among women. *J Am Coll Cardiol.* 2002;39(1):49–56.

Lorenz M, Jochmann N, von Krosigk A, et al. Addition of milk prevents vascular protective effects of tea. *Eu Heart J.* 2007;28(2):219–223.

Ma J, Folso AR, Melnick SL, et al. Associations of serum and dietary magnesium with cardiovascular disease, hypertension, diabetes, insulin, and carotid arterial wall thickness: the ARIC study. Atherosclerosis Risk in Communities Study. *J Clin Epidemiol.* 1995;48(7):927–940.

Mallik S, Spertus JA, Reid KJ, et al. Depressive symptoms after acute myocardial infarction: evidence for highest rates in younger women. *Arch Intern Med.* 2006;166(8):876–883.

Manson JE, Greenland P, LaCroix AZ, et al. Walking compared with vigorous exercise for the prevention of cardiovascular events in women. *N Engl J Med.* 2002;347(10):716–725.

Manson JW, Hu FB, Rich-Edwards JW, et al. A prospective study of walking as compared with vigorous exercise in the prevention of coronary heart disease in women. *N Engl J Med.* 1999;341(9):650–658.

Marcoff L, Thompson PD. The role of coenzyme Q10 in statin-associated myopathy. *J Am Coll Cardiol.* 2007;49:2231–2237.

McGrady A, Nadsady PA, Schumann-Brzezinski C. Sustained effects of biofeedback-assisted relaxation therapy in essential hypertension. *Biofeedback Self Regul.* 1991;16(4):399–411.

McGrady AV, Yonker R, Tan SY, Fine TH, Woerner M. The effect of biofeedback-assisted relaxation training on blood pressure and selected biochemical parameters in patients with essential hypertension. *Biofeedback Self Regul.* 1981;6(3):343–353.

McSweeney JC, Cody M, O'Sullivan P, Elberson K, Moser DK, Garvin BJ. Women's early warning symptoms of acute myocardial infarction. *Circulation.* 2003;108(21):2619–2623.

Meles E, Giannattasio C, Failla M, Gentile G, Capra A, Mancia G. Nonpharmacologic treatment of hypertension by respiratory exercise in the home setting. *Am J Hypertens.* 2004;17(4):370–374.

Merz CNB, Shaw LJ, Reis SE, et al. Insights from the NHLBI-sponsored women's ischemia syndrome evaluation (WISE) study. *J Am Coll Cardiol.* 2006;47(3):21S-29S.

Mieres JH, Shaw LJ, Arai A, et al. Role of noninvasive testing in the clinical evaluation of women with suspected coronary artery disease. *Circulation.* 2005;111:682–696.

Milani RV, Lavie CJ. Impact of cardiac rehabilitation on depression and its associated mortality. *Am J Med.* 2007;120(9):799–806.

Milner KA, Funk M, Richards S, Wilmes RM, Vaccarino V, Krumholz HM. Gender differences in symptom presentation associated with coronary heart disease. *Am J Cardiol.* 1999;84:396–399.

Mizuno K, Nakaya N, Ohashi Y, et al. Usefulness of Pravastatin in primary prevention of cardiovascular events in women: analysis of the management of elevated cholesterol in the primary prevention group of adult Japanese. *Circulation.* 2008;117:494–502.

Morisco C, Trim Arco B, Condor Elli M. Effect of coenzyme Q10 therapy in patients with congestive heart failure: a long-term multicenter randomized study. *Clin Investig.* 1993;71(Suppl):S134–S136.

Mosca L, Banka CL, Benjamin EJ, et al. Evidence-based guidelines for cardiovascular disease prevention in women: 2007 update. *Circulation.* 2007;115:1481–1501.

Mosca L, Mochari H, Christian A, et al. National study of women's awareness, preventative action, and barriers to cardiovascular health. *Circulation.* 2006;113:525–534.

Mozaffarian D, Stein PK, Prineas RJ, Siscovick DS. Dietary fish and omega-3 fatty acid consumption and heart rate variability in US adults. *Circulation.* 2008;117(9):1130–1137.

Naqvi TZ, Naqvi SS, Merz CN. Gender differences in the link between depression and cardiovascular disease. *Psychosom Med.* 2005;67:S15-S18.

Ong KL, Cheung BMY, Man YB, Lau CP, Lam KSL. Prevalence, awareness, treatment, and control of hypertension among United States adults 1999–2004. *Hypertension.* 2007;49:69.

Osganian SK, Stampfer MJ, Rimm E, et al. Vitamin C and risk of coronary heart disease in women. *J Am Coll Cardiol.* 2003;42(2):246–252.

Pate RR, Pratt M, Blair SN, et al. Physical activity and public health. A recommendation from the Centers for Disease Control and Prevention and the American College of Sports Medicine. *JAMA.* 1995;273(5):402–407.

Patel H, Rosengren A, Ekman I. Symptoms in acute coronary syndromes: does sex make a difference? *Am Heart J.* 2004;148(1):27–33.

Pilote L, Dasgupta K, Guru V, et al. A comprehensive view of sex-specific issues related to cardiovascular disease. *CMAJ.* 2007;176(6):S1–44.

Raggi P, Shaw LJ, Berman DS, Callister TQ. Gender-based differences in the prognostic value of coronary calcification. *J Women Health (Larchmt).* 2004;13(3):273–283.

Ramos RG, Olden K. The prevalence of metabolic syndrome among US women of childbearing age. *Am J Public Health.* 2008;98(6):1122–1127.

Rapola JM, Virtamo J, Haukka JK, et al. Effect of vitamin E and beta carotene on the incidence of angina pectoris. A randomized, double-blind, controlled study. *JAMA.* 1996;275(9):693–698.

Rapola JM, Virtamo J, Ripatti S, et al. Effects of alpha tocopherol and beta carotene supplements on symptoms, progression, and prognosis of angina pectoris. *Heart.* 1998;79(5):454–458.

Ridker PM, Buring JE, Rifai N, Cook NR. Development and validation of improved algorithms for the assessment of global cardiovascular risk in women. *JAMA.* 2007;297(6):611–619.

Ridker PM, Cook NR, Lee I, et al. A randomized trial of low-dose Aspirin in the primary prevention of cardiovascular disease in women. *N Engl J Med.* 2005;352:1293–1304.

Ridker PM, Danielson E, Fonseca F, et al for the JUPITER Study Group. 2008. Rosuvastatin to Prevent Vascular Events in Men and Women with Elevated C-Reactive Protein. *NEJM.* 2005;359(21):2195–2207.

Richter A, Herlitz J, Hjalmarson A. Effect of acupuncture in patients with angina pectoris. *Eur Heart J.* 1991;12(2):175–178.

Rosendorff C, Black HR, Cannon CP, et al. Treatment of hypertension in the prevention and management of ischemic heart disease. *Circulation.* 2007;115:2761–2788.

Rosengren A, Hawken S, Ounpuu S, et al. Association of psychosocial risk factors with risk of acute myocardial infarction in111 119 cases and 13 648 controls from 52 countries (the INTERHEART study): case-control study. *Lancet.* 2004;364:953–962.

Rozanski A, Blumenthal JA, Davidson KW, Saab PG, Kubzansky L. The epidemiology, pathophysiology, and management of psychosocial risk factors in cardiac practice. *J Am Coll Cardiol.* 2005;45(5):637–651.

Rugulies R. Depression as a predictor for coronary heart disease: a review and meta-analysis. *Am J Prev Med.* 2002;23(1):51–61.

Sacks FM, Svetsky LPO, Vollmer WM, et al. Effects on blood pressure of reduced dietary sodium and the dietar approaches to stop hypertension (DASH) diet. *N Engl J Med.* 2001;344(1):3–10.

Svetkey LP, Simons-Morton DG, Proschan MA, et al. Effect of the dietary approaches to stop hypertension diet and reduced sodium intake on blood pressure control. *J Clin Hypertension (Greenwich).* 2004;6(7):373–381.

Schein MH, Gavish B, Herz M, et al. Treating hypertension with a device that slows and regularses breathing: a randomised double-blind controlled study. *J Hum Hypertens.* 2001;15(4):271–278.

Schulman SP, Becker LC, Kass DA. L-Arginine therapy in acute myocardial infarction: the vascular interaction with age in myocardial infarction (VINTAGE MI) randomized clinical trial. *JAMA.* 2006;295:58–64.

Silagy CA, Neil HA. A meta-analysis of the effect of garlic on blood pressure. *J Hypertens.* 1994;12(4):463–468.

Singh M, Charanjit SR, Gersh BJ, et al. Mortality differences between men and women after percutaneous coronary Interventions. *JACC.* 2008;51(24): 2313–2322.

Stevens J, Cal J, Evenson KR, Thomas R. Fitness and fatness as predictors of mortality from all causes and from cardiovascular disease in men and women in the lipid research clinics study. *Am J Epidemiol.* 2002;156(9):832–841.

Stevinson C, Pittler MH, Ernst E. Garlic for treating hypercholesterolemia. *Ann Intern Med.* 2000;133(6):420–429.

The ATBC Cancer Prevention Study Group. The alpha-tocopherol, beta-carotene lung cancer prevention study: design, methods, participant characteristics, and compliance. *Ann Epidemiol.* 1994;4(1):1–10.

The ENRICHD Investigators. Effects of treating depression and low perceived social support on clinical events after myocardial infarction: the enhancing recovery in coronary heart disease patients (ENRICHD) randomized trial. *JAMA.* 2003;289(23):3106–3116.

The Heart Outcomes Prevention Evaluation (HOPE) 2 Investigators. Homocysteine Lowering with Folic Acid and B Vitamins in Vascular Disease. *N Engl J Med.* 2006;354(15):1567–1577.

The Heart Outcomes Prevention Evaluation (HOPE) Study Investigators. Vitamin E supplementation and cardiovascular events in high-risk patients. *N Engl J Med.* 2000;342(3):154–160.

Tonstad S, Sandvik E, Larsen PG, Thelle D. Gender differences in the prevalence and determinants of the metabolic syndrome in screened subjects at risk for coronary heart disease. *Metab Syndr Relat Disord.* 2007;5(2):174–182.

Vaccarino V, Lin ZQ, Kasl SV, et al. Gender differences in recovery after coronary artery bypass surgery. *J Am Coll Cardiol.* 2003;41:307–314.

Vaccarino V, Parsons L, Every NR, Barron HV, Krumholz HM. Sex-based differences in early mortality after myocardial infarction. *N Engl J Med.* 1999;341(4):217–225.

Virani SS, Khan AN, Mendoza CE, Ferreira AC, de Marchena E. Takotsubo cardiomyopathy, or broken-heart syndrome. *Tex Heart Inst J.* 2007;34:76–79.

Von Ruden AE, Adson DE, Kotlyar M. Effect of selective serotonin reuptake inhibitors on cardiovascular morbidity and mortality. *J Card Pharm Ther.* 2008;13(1): 32–40.

Vogel JHK, Bolling SF, Costello RB, et al. Integrating complementary medicine into cardiovascular medicine *J Am Coll Cardiol.* 2005;46:184–221.

Watson PS, Scalia GM, Galbraith A, Burstow DJ, Bett N, Aroney CN. Lack of effect of coenzyme Q on left ventricular function in patients with congestive heart failure. *J Am Coll Cardiol.* 1999;33:1549–52.

Welty RK, Lee KS, Lew NS, Zhou JR. Effect of soy nuts on blood pressure and lipid levels in hypertensive, prehypertensive, and normotensive postmenopausal women. *Arch Intern Med.* 2007;167(10):1060–1067.

Wenger NK. Drugs for cardiovascular disease prevention in women. *Drugs.* 2008;68 (3):339–358.

Wenger NK, Lewis SJ, Welty FK, Herrington DM, Bitner V. Beneficial effects of aggressive low-density lipoprotein cholesterol lowering in women with stable coronary heart disease in the Treating to New Targets (TNT) study. *Heart.* 2008a;94:434–439.

Wenger NK, Shaw LJ, Vaccarino V. Coronary heart disease in women: Update 2008. *Clin Pharmacol Ther.* 2008b;83(1):37–51.

Witt BJ, Jacobsen SJ, Weston SA, et al. Cardiac rehabilitation after myocardial infarction in the community. *J Am Coll Cardiol.* 2004;44:988–996.

Witte KKA, Clark AL, Cleland JGF. Chronic heart failure and micronutrients. *J Am Coll Cardiol.* 2001;37:1765–1774.

Wittstein IS. The broken heart syndrome. Cleveland *Clin J Med.* 2007;74(Suppl 1): S17–S22.

Wolk A, Manson JE, Stampfer MJ, et al. Long-term intake of dietary fiber and decreased risk of coronary heart disease among women. *JAMA.* 1999;281(21):1998–2004.

Woodgate D, Chan CH, Conquer JA. Cholesterol-lowering ability of a phytostanol softgel supplement in adults with mild to moderate hypercholesterolemia. *Lipids.* 2006;41(2): 127–132.

World Health Statistics. 2007. Geneva: World Health Organization; 2007. Available: www.who.int/whosis/whostat2007.pdf. Accessed April 25, 2008.

Yusef S, Zhao F, Mehta SR, Chrolavicius S, Tognoni G. Clopidogrel in unstable angina to prevent recurrent events trial investigators. Effects of Clopidogrel in addition to Aspirin in patients with acute coronary syndromes without ST-segment elevation. *N Engl J Med.* 2001;345:494–502.

Ziegelstein RC. Acute emotional stress and cardiac arrhythmias. *JAMA.* 2007;298:324–329.

36

Osteoporosis

LOUISE GAGNÉ

CASE STUDY

At age 52, Diana was diagnosed with osteopenia. Her T scores were –1.7 at the lumbar spine and –1.2 at the femoral neck. Diana had struggled with low-grade depression and anxiety for a number of years, but was otherwise in good health. She had experienced a sudden transition into menopause at age 48, following a hysterectomy and bilateral oophorectomy. She took a multivitamin irregularly and was on no prescription medications. Diana described her level of exercise as "close to zero." Routine blood work was unremarkable, other than her 25-hydroxy vitamin D (25(OH)D), which was in the deficient range at 13 ng/mL (32 nmol/L).

An integrative plan to support bone health was discussed with Diana. Over the following year, Diana began eating more fruits and vegetables, and more fish. She started taking supplements regularly and corrected her vitamin D deficiency. She began walking to work and purchased a self-hypnosis CD to help her unwind in the evening. A repeat dual X-ray absorptiometry (DEXA) scan showed no further bone loss and a small improvement in the lumbar spine T score.

Diana was relieved to hear her test results. She also expressed delight at how good she was feeling generally, stating she had "so much more energy." She had started to enjoy cooking and inviting friends over instead of "having popcorn for supper." Her mood had improved markedly. Diana felt motivated to further improve her bone density. It was suggested that she step up her exercise regime to include weight lifting 2–3 times/week. She was referred to a physiotherapist to review correct technique and to set up a structured exercise program.

> I love the "side benefits" that often happen for patients who embark on an integrative health program. In this case, Diana's bone health plan also enhanced her mood and increased her sense of overall well-being.

Introduction

Integrative medicine aims to support the health of the whole person and in doing so to promote healing in all body systems. Fragile bones do not exist in isolation. Thus, an integrative approach to osteoporosis includes an anti-inflammatory diet, appropriate supplements, exercise and mind–body practices, as well as pharmaceutical medicines when indicated.

Epidemiology

Osteoporosis is a significant cause of pain, disability, and death in aging populations throughout the world. More than 10 million Americans have osteoporosis and there are over 2 million osteoporosis-related fractures per year (Siris et al. 2001). Women are at higher risk and account for 75% of cases. Using the World Health Organization (WHO) criteria, 7% of postmenopausal women aged ≥50 years have osteoporosis and 40% have osteopenia. The costs to the U.S. health care system total over $16 billion annually (Riggs and Melton 1995).

Pathophysiology

Osteoporosis is a skeletal disorder characterized by low bone mass, increased bone fragility, and an increased risk of fracture. It is a multifactorial disease arising from genetic, hormonal, metabolic, mechanical, and immunological factors.

Bone mass reaches its peak around age 30 and begins to decline after age 40–50. However, repair and renewal of bone continues throughout adult life, with approximately 15% of bone mass turning over each year.

There are two major types of bone cells. Osteoblasts synthesize the organic bone matrix and its calcification. Osteoclasts reabsorb bone to provide for metabolic requirements and to allow for repair and remodeling to take place. Bone begins to deteriorate when bone resorption outpaces bone formation.

Screening and Diagnosis

ASSESSING BONE STRENGTH

Bone strength is determined by bone quality and bone density. Bone quality is influenced by its microarchitecture and the composition of the bone matrix and mineral (Compston 2006). Bone quality is not readily measured in a clinical practice setting. Bone mineral density (BMD) can be assessed using a DEXA scan.

Osteoporosis is defined as a BMD more than 2.5 standard deviations (SD) below the mean for young adults. Osteopenia is defined as a BMD 1–2.5 SD below the young adult mean. Established osteoporosis is diagnosed when the BMD falls more than 2.5 SD below the mean for young adults and there are one or more fragility fractures.

In some studies, BMD has been found to have poor fracture predictive value (Wainwright et al. 2005). However, in other studies, BMD has shown a strong correlation with fracture risk (Cummings et al. 1993; Guyatt et al. 2002). In reality, a wide overlap exists between the bone densities of women who will eventually suffer a fracture and those who will not (Marshall et al. 1996). Thus, other risk factors for osteoporotic fracture should be carefully assessed.

The North American Menopause Society (NAMS) recommends that BMD be measured in all women ≥65 years, in younger postmenopausal women with ≥1 risk factor, and in all women with medical conditions associated with an increased risk of osteoporosis (Borges and Bilezikian 2006).

Risk Factors for Osteoporotic Fracture

The focus of osteoporosis screening should be to reduce the risk of fracture. Thus, prevention programs should aim to ameliorate all modifiable factors related to fracture risk and not focus solely on BMD (see sidebar).

Factors that Increase Fracture Risk

Factors leading to poor bone strength and/or an increased risk of falls: nutritional deficiencies, smoking, high alcohol intake, excessive caffeine, premature menopause, malabsorption disorders, autoimmune disease, low body weight, small body frame, family history of osteoporosis, female gender, Caucasian or Asian descent, impaired vision, dizziness or balance problems, fainting or loss of consciousness, physical frailty, medication-related side effects, vitamin D deficiency. Medications: glucocorticoids, anticonvulsants, sedatives, anticholinergics, antihypertensives, heparin, cylcosporin, and medroxyprogesterone acetate.

The Role of Inflammation

There is growing evidence that osteoporosis is linked to chronic low-grade inflammation (Clowes et al. 2005; Ginaldi et al. 2005; Kim et al. 2007; Koh et al. 2005; Mundy 2007; Pfeilschifter 2003). Diets rich in anti-inflammatory compounds from fruits, vegetables, and omega-3 fatty acids have been found to decrease the risk of developing osteoporosis (Das 2000; Lanham-New 2006, 2008; New et al. 2000; Prynne et al. 2006; Tucker et al. 1999). Thus, an anti-inflammatory diet is a key element of an integrative bone health program.

Anti-inflammatory Diet

- 8–10 servings/day from a variety of deeply colored fruits and vegetables
- Healthy fats: extra virgin olive oil, avocados, nuts and fatty, cold water ocean fish
- Anti-inflammatory spices/herbs/teas such as: turmeric, ginger, rosemary, green tea
- Whole grain, low glycemic index carbohydrates
- Reduce consumption of partially hydrogenated oils, vegetables oils (safflower, sunflower, corn, soy), and saturated animal fats
- Avoid foods that provoke allergy or intolerance
- Cultivate healthy bowel flora

Nutrition for Bone Health

CALCIUM

Calcium is an essential nutrient for building and maintaining healthy bones. And yet, high calcium intakes do not ensure strong bones and low calcium intakes do not necessarily lead to weaker bones (Feskanich et al. 2003; Nordin 2000). Thus, calcium requirements must be assessed in light of calcium absorption versus calcium excretion.

Calcium is absorbed in the small intestine via a vitamin D–dependent transport mechanism. To improve calcium absorption and/or decrease calcium excretion: maintain 25(OH)D concentration $\geq$34 ng/mL (85 nmol/L) (Heaney et al. 2003), avoid excess animal protein (Barzel and Massey 1998), increase fruits and vegetables (Barzel and Massey 1998), keep dietary sodium <2400 mg/day (Harrington and Cashman 2003), avoid excess caffeine (Hallstrom et al. 2006), eat fewer highly refined carbohydrates (Thom et al. 1978), and ingest adequate essential fatty acids (Kruger and Horrobin 1997).

In the United States, calcium dietary reference intakes (DRIs) for women are 1300 mg/day from age 9–18, 1000 mg/day from age 19–50, and 1200 mg/day from age 50 onward.

Calcium citrate malate at a dose of 800 mg/day has been found to significantly reduce bone loss (Dawson-Hughes et al. 1990). However, milk consumption (Feskanich et al. 1997) and higher calcium intakes alone may not favorably impact fracture risk (Bischoff-Ferrari et al. 2007). Accordingly, calcium supplementation should be used along with vitamin D and other bone building foods. For most women, a total daily intake of at least 800 mg of elemental calcium is recommended.

VITAMIN D

Vitamin D is essential for calcium absorption and deficiency of this nutrient is common (Holick et al. 2005, 2006; Jacobs et al. 2008). Vitamin D supplementation of 700–800 IU/day has been shown to reduce fracture risk (Bischoff-Ferrari et al. 2005; Trivedi et al. 2003). Vitamin D also reduces the risk of falls (Bischoff-Ferrari et al. 2004a; Bischoff-Ferrari et al. 2006; Broe et al. 2007) and improves lower extremity function (Bischoff-Ferrari et al. 2004b) in older adults.

All women should be screened for vitamin D deficiency with a measurement of their serum 25(OH)D concentration. A value ≥34 ng/mL (85 nmol/L) is necessary for optimum calcium absorption (Heaney et al. 2003) and optimum fracture prevention is achieved at a level of 40 ng/mL (100 nmol/L) (Bischoff-Ferrari et al. 2005). Vitamin D supplements are an inexpensive and reliable way to ensure an optimum concentration. For most adults, at least 1000 IU/day is required(Bischoff-Ferrari 2007, 2008; Cannell et al. 2008; Vieth et al. 2007). Vitamin D_3 (cholecalciferol) is the preferred form to use (Armas et al. 2004) and should be taken with meals.

ESSENTIAL FATTY ACIDS

The dietary intake and ratio of essential fatty acids plays an important role in bone health. In animal studies, fish oils rich in omega-3 (n–3) fatty acids have been found to attenuate bone loss associated with estrogen withdrawal (Fernandes et al. 2003). Other studies have found that the n–3 fatty acid, eicosapentaenoic acid (EPA), enhances calcium absorption, reduces calcium excretion, and increases calcium deposition in bone (Kruger et al. 1998). Supplementation with calcium, EPA, and gamma linoleic acid (GLA) has resulted in increased lumbar and femoral bone density in women (Kruger et al. 1998). The optimum ratio of n–6 to n–3 fatty acids is ~1–2:1 (Simopoulos 2000).

PROTEIN

Protein is required for bone formation, and adequate intake is essential (Cooper et al. 1996). However, high levels of animal protein are associated with increased fracture rates and accelerated bone mineral loss (Abelow et al. 1992; Feskanich et al. 1996; Marsh et al. 1980). Lowering protein intakes to current RDA guidelines (0.8 g/kg) has been found to reduce urinary calcium excretion and lower markers of bone resorption (Ince et al. 2004). Several studies have also shown that an increased ratio of vegetable to animal protein is protective against fractures (Frassetto et al. 2000; Sellmeyer et al. 2001; Weikert et al. 2005). Thus, an adequate but not excessive intake of protein, including some vegetarian choices, is recommended.

VITAMIN K

Vitamin K plays a key role in carboxylating osteocalcin and other bone proteins (Pearson 2007). Epidemiological studies consistently show a strong link between higher vitamin K status and reduced fracture risk (Booth et al. 2000; Hodges et al. 1991).

Typical vitamin K intakes are below the levels associated with decreased fracture risk (Kaneki 2006). The current DRI for adult women is 90 µg, but amounts of 254 µg/day or higher may be needed for optimum bone health(Pearson 2007). The best sources of vitamin K are green leafy vegetables. Vitamin K is fat-soluble and foods rich in vitamin K should be eaten with some healthy fat, such as olive oil.

MAGNESIUM

Epidemiological studies have linked higher magnesium intakes with increased BMD (Ryder et al. 2005; Tucker et al. 1999). Some intervention trials of magnesium supplementation have also shown an increase in BMD as well as reduced fracture rates (Sojka and Weaver 1995; Stendig-Lindberg et al. 1993). The average magnesium intake is below the DRI of 320 mg/day. Magnesium deficiency may impair osteoblast function and induce bone resorption by osteclasts (Rude and Gruber 2004). Good sources of magnesium include nuts and seeds, soybeans, dark green leafy vegetables, and dairy products.

TRACE MINERALS

A number of trace minerals including zinc, copper, and manganese act as cofactors for specific enzymes related to bone metabolism (Gur et al. 2002). A varied, whole foods diet plus a good quality multivitamin/mineral supplement should ensure an adequate supply of these nutrients.

VITAMIN C

Vitamin C is a required nutrient for collagen formation and vitamin C deficiency is relatively common in the United States (Hampl et al. 2004). Vitamin C, along with calcium intakes ≥500 mg/day, appears to support an increase in BMD (Hall and Greendale 1998).

SOY

Studies of soy and its effects on bone have shown mixed results (Branca 2003). In one study, isoflavone-enriched foods showed no effect on BMD (Brink et al.

2008). Conversely, the Shanghai Women's Health Study found positive effects (Zhang et al. 2005). Notably, this study examined the intake of whole soy foods, rather than isolated isoflavones. The Shanghai study is also one of the few soy studies to examine fracture risk, as opposed to BMD or markers of bone turnover.

On the whole, evidence supports a beneficial effect of soy on bone health (Chiechi et al. 2002; Setchell and Lydeking-Olsen 2003). One to two servings per day of whole soy foods are recommended.

Substances that May Be Harmful to Bone Health

SODIUM

Average American diets exceed sodium intake guidelines and high salt diets are known to increase urinary calcium excretion (Harrington and Cashman 2003). Patients should be advised to keep their sodium intake <2400 mg/day.

CAFFEINE

Excessive caffeine intake is associated with a modest increase in the risk of osteoporotic fracture (Hallstrom et al. 2006). The increased risk occurs in women who consume >300 mg of caffeine/day (~4 cups of coffee), in conjunction with a low calcium intake. Excessive caffeine intake should be avoided.

VITAMIN A

Vitamin A (retinol) intakes of >3000 µg/day are associated with a significantly increased risk of hip fracture (Feskanich et al. 2002b). This increased risk exists for retinol intake from foods and from supplements (Melhus et al. 1998). Women should choose supplements that contain less than 3000 µg of retinol, or preferably, products that contain only beta-carotene and/or mixed carotenoids.

SMOKING

Cigarette smoking has been shown to increase the risk of fracture and the risk increases with the amount smoked (Cornuz et al. 1999; Kanis et al. 2005). Clearly, for many reasons, women should be encouraged not to begin smoking. Current smokers who quit will obtain benefits to their bone health after a period of 10 years (Cornuz et al. 1999).

ALCOHOL

Early, chronic, heavy alcohol consumption may be harmful to bone(Sampson 2002) yet low or moderate consumption of alcohol in adulthood appears to be protective (Berg et al. 2008). Moderate alcohol consumption has recognized benefits (Vogel 2002) and risks (Anonymous 2006; Mezzetti et al. 1998). All things considered, adult women should be advised to consume <7 alcoholic drinks per week.

Botanical Medicines

Numerous studies have examined the potential of herbal medicines to enhance bone health (Putnam et al. 2007). A study of Shen Gu mixture showed significant beneficial effects on bone (Mingyue et al. 2005). The Ayurvedic preparation, Reosto, has been found to significantly increase BMD (Shah and Kolhapure 2004). Black cohosh (*Actaea racemosa*) has been found to increase bone-specific alkaline phosphatase and stimulate osteoblast activity (Wuttke et al. 2006). *Dioscorea spongiosa* (Yin et al. 2004a, 2004b), *Astragalus membranaceus* (Kim et al. 2003), walnut extract (*Juglans regia* L.) (Papoutsi et al. 2008), and curcumin, a compound found in turmeric root (*Curcuma longa*) (Bharti et al. 2004) have also shown osteoprotective effects in laboratory and animal studies. Further research is needed to assess the role of botanical medicines in supporting bone health.

TEA (*CAMILLIA SINENSIS*)

Tea has anti-inflammatory effects, cardiovascular benefits, and cancer-protective properties (Gardner et al. 2007; De Bacquer et al. 2006). Tea drinking, unlike coffee, is not associated with deleterious effects on bone and, in fact, may be beneficial (Chen et al. 2003; De Bacquer et al. 2006).

The Mind–Body Connection

Chronic stress, through activation of the sympathetic nervous system (SNS), tends to exert catabolic effects on the body. In animal studies, chronic stress has been shown to stimulate bone resorption (Jia et al. 2006; Patterson-Buckendahl et al. 2007). Major depression (Cizza et al. 2001; Schweiger et al. 1994) and anorexia nervosa (Misra et al. 2008) are both associated with increased bone loss. Increased SNS input stimulates osteoclast activity and inhibits bone formation by osteoblasts (Togari et al. 2005).

Stress reduction, using mind–body practices such as meditation, self-hypnosis, guided imagery, breath work, or biofeedback games is highly recommended as part of an integrative plan to support bone health.

> Many of my patients enjoy listening to hypnosis or guided imagery CDs. There is nothing they need to do, other than to be in a safe, comfortable place. Busy women are delighted to hear that it is something they can do even while sleeping!

Exercise

Exercise is required to build and maintain strong bones. Exercise increases muscle mass and muscle mass is strongly correlated with bone density (Proctor et al. 2000). Muscle mass usually increases until age 30 and begins to decline after age 50. However, regular exercise at any age, even in the very elderly, can result in increased muscle strength, balance, and functional capacity (Evans 1997; Fiatarone et al. 1994).

Exercise training programs for women have been shown to consistently prevent or reverse bone loss in both the lumbar spine and the femoral neck (Wolff et al. 1999). The Bone Estrogen Strength Training (BEST) Study found that women who received 800 mg/day of calcium citrate, along with a structured exercise program, increased their BMD by ~2% (Cussler et al. 2005). Even women with established osteoporosis can improve their bone mass with a low impact exercise program (Todd and Robinson 2003). Hip fracture risk may be decreased by 41% by walking for ≥4 hours per week (Feskanich et al. 2002a). Back strengthening exercises can also lower vertebral fracture risk (Sinaki et al. 2002).

Recommended physical activities include walking, jumping, running, and weight training. Women should aim for 30–45 minutes of exercise, 5 or more times/week. Tai chi is highly recommended to reduce the number of falls in the elderly (Li et al. 2005; Voukelatos et al. 2007; Wolf et al. 1996).

Considerations in Younger Women

Peak bone mass is influenced by genetic factors and by diet and physical activity during youth. Regular physical activity and maintaining an ideal body weight are the most important modifiable factors in the development of optimum peak bone mass (Tom Lloyd et al. 2004).

Young women who use depot medroxyprogesterone acetate (DMPA) are at risk for bone loss (Walsh et al. 2008). However, BMD tends to recover after discontinuation of DMPA (Kaunitz et al. 2008). Smoking, heavy alcohol consumption, anorexia nervosa (Misra et al. 2008), late onset menarche, amenorrhea (Gordon and Nelson 2003), primary ovarian failure, and autoimmune diseases (Lloyd et al. 2002) are other risk factors that may interfere with bone growth.

Epidemiologic studies show that multiple pregnancies and periods of lactation are not associated with lower bone mass or increased fracture risk (Kalkwarf and Specker 2002; Melton et al. 1993).

Pharmaceuticals

In some circumstances, pharmacologic therapy for prevention or treatment of osteoporosis may be recommended. The NAMS guidelines recommend treatment in all postmenopausal women with prior vertebral or hip fracture or with hip or spine T scores <2.5 and in postmenopausal women with T scores between −2.0 to −2.5 and ≥1 additional risk factors(Borges and Bilezikian 2006). For fracture prevention, the number needed to treat (NNT) is generally much lower for women at high risk (Cranney et al. 2002). Low-risk women may wish to begin a comprehensive bone building program and continue to monitor their bone density prior to making a decision to begin medication.

The Role of Estrogen

Bone loss accelerates following menopause, as estrogen levels naturally fall. Postmenopausal hormone therapy (HT) has beneficial effects on bone, as well as other known benefits and risks (Fitzpatrick 2006; Nelson et al. 2002). In most cases, HT does not lead to overall health benefits and is not recommended to prevent or treat osteoporosis (Cauley et al. 2003; Force 2005). Use of HT should thus be individualized, based on an exploration of the risks and benefits for each woman.

Bisphosphonates

Bisphosphonates are the most commonly prescribed medications for the treatment of postmenopausal osteoporosis and are indicated for both prevention and treatment of this condition. Antiresorptive therapies reduce fracture risk by inhibiting the activity of osteoclasts and reducing bone turnover, thus increasing bone mass. High bone turnover is particularly relevant in the pathogenesis of vertebral fractures (Compston 2006).

Bisphosphonates may cause dyspepsia, nausea, esophagitis, and abdominal pain. There is also concern that they may impair microdamage repair and thus increase the brittleness of bone (Mashiba et al. 2000; Turner 2002). Alendronate and zoledronic acid are associated with an increased incidence of atrial fibrillation (Black et al. 2007; Heckbert et al. 2008). Osteonecrosis of the jaw is a serious, rare event associated with bisphosphonate use.

In observational studies, approximately 20% of women fail to respond to antiresorptive therapy, even with good compliance and supplementation with calcium and vitamin D. Without additional calcium and vitamin D, lack of clinical response may be as high as 28% (Adami et al. 2006).

Alendronate has been shown to increase BMD and to reduce the incidence of fractures of the spine and hip in women with osteoporosis (Bauer et al. 2004). Alendronate continues to be pharmacologically active in bone tissue for a number of years after treatment is stopped. Five years of therapy appears to be adequate for most women, although high risk women may benefit from a longer course of treatment (Black et al. 2006). The usual dose range is 35–70 mg once per week.

Risendronate also increases BMD and reduces vertebral and some nonvertebral fracture rates (Harris et al. 1999). After cessation of therapy, the beneficial effects of risendronate decline relatively rapidly (Watts et al. 2008). The usual dose is 35 mg once per week.

Ibandronate increases BMD and reduces vertebral fracture rates when compared with placebo (Chesnut Iii et al. 2004). Side effects are similar to bisphosphonates mentioned earlier (Harris et al. 2008). It may be given as monthly dose of 150 mg (McCarus 2006).

Zoledronic acid is particularly effective in reducing vertebral fractures and also reduces the risk of nonvertebral fractures. It is administered intravenously once a year at a dose of 5 mg (Black et al. 2007). Zoledronic acid may improve treatment compliance due to its convenient dosing schedule (Lewiecki 2008).

Selective Estrogen Receptor Modulators

Selective estrogen receptor modulators (SERMS) act as estrogen agonists on bone and lipid metabolism while also having estrogen antagonist actions on breast and endometrial tissue. Raloxifene has been shown to be effective at reducing postmenopausal bone loss and at reducing the risk of vertebral fractures (Ettinger et al. 1999). It also significantly reduces the risk of breast cancer and improves lipid profiles (Barrett-Connor et al. 2004). Raloxifene was found to have a favorable risk–benefit profile in the Multiple Outcomes of Raloxifene Evaluation (MORE) trial (Barrett-Connor et al. 2004). The usual dose is 60 mg/day. Side effects include deep vein thrombosis (DVT) and pulmonary embolism.

CALCITONIN

Calcitonin is produced by thyroid C cells and acts to inhibit bone resorption by inhibiting osteoclast activity. Calcitonin from salmon may be used to treat osteoporosis in women who are ≥5 years postmenopause. It is effective in reducing the pain associated with acute compression fractures of the vertebrae (Knopp et al. 2005) and may reduce the incidence of vertebral fractures. It is normally given as a daily intranasal spray of 200 IU. Side effects are usually minor and include flushing, nausea, and diarrhea.

TERIPARATIDE

Teriparatide (PTH 1–34) is a medication that includes a sequence of 34 amino acids contained in parathyroid hormone. Teriparatide has anabolic effects on bone, stimulating osteoblast cell proliferation. It is useful in reducing the incidence of new vertebral and nonvertebral fractures in postmenopausal women (Bilezikian et al. 2005; McCarus 2006; Reginster and Sarlet 2006). Teriparatide is given as a once daily subcutaneous injection (20 µg) for a period of ≤2 years. This therapy may be followed by an antiresorptive agent. Side effects include nausea and headaches.

STRONTIUM

Strontium ranelate is a promising medication that is currently being used in Europe for the treatment of postmenopausal osteoporosis. Several studies have found it to be an effective agent in reducing vertebral and nonvertebral fracture risk in both younger postmenopausal women and in the very elderly (O'Donnell et al. 2006; Seeman et al. 2006) Strontium ranelate acts both to stimulate bone formation and to reduce bone resorption. Adverse effects include nausea and diarrhea (Blake and Fogelman 2006).

Summary

Osteoporosis is best approached with a lifelong, comprehensive prevention program. Women of all ages should be aware of the diet and lifestyle choices that will support their bone health. The good news is that essentially the same strategies that help women to build healthy bones will also protect them against heart disease, diabetes, depression, and a host of other chronic conditions.

Recommendations to Build and Maintain Healthy Bones

1. An anti-inflammatory diet that includes an abundance of deeply colored fruits and vegetables, healthy fats, whole grains, and anti-inflammatory herbs, teas, and spices.
2. Elemental calcium intake from diet plus supplements totaling at least 800 mg/day.
3. A serum 25-OH vitamin D concentration in the range of 40 ng/mL (100 nmol/L).
4. A balanced ratio of *n*–6 to *n*–3 fatty acids.
5. Adequate but not excessive protein (0.8 g/kg) including some vegetarian protein sources.
6. One to two servings per day of whole soy foods.
7. A good quality multivitamin/mineral supplement.
8. Physical activity for 30–45 minutes most days of the week. Include weight bearing, aerobic and weight lifting exercise.
9. A daily mind–body practice.
10. Avoid smoking, excess alcohol, excess caffeine, and vitamin A (retinol) in amounts >3000 µg/day.
11. Reduce the risk of falls and, if possible, avoid medications that harm bone or increase the risk of falls.
12. Pharmaceutical therapies should be individualized and risks and benefits explored with each woman.

REFERENCES

Abelow BJ, Holford TR, Insogna KL. Cross-cultural association between dietary animal protein and hip fracture: a hypothesis. *Calcif Tissue Int.* 1992;50(1):14–18.

Adami S, Bone HG, Crepaldi G, et al. Fracture incidence and characterization in patients on osteoporosis treatment: the ICARO study. *J Bone Miner Res.* 2006;21(10):1565–1570.

Anonymous. Alcohol over time: still under control? For women, there's not much leeway between healthful and harmful drinking, especially as we get older. *Harv Women Health Watch.* 2006;13(11):1–3.

Armas LAG, Hollis BW, Heaney RP. Vitamin D2 is much less effective than vitamin D3 in humans. *J Clin Endocrinol Metab.* 2004;89(11):5387–5391.

Barrett-Connor E, Cauley JA, Kulkarni PM, Sashegyi A, Cox DA, Geiger MJ. Risk-benefit profile for raloxifene: 4-year data from the Multiple Outcomes of Raloxifene Evaluation (MORE) randomized trial. *J Bone Miner Res.* 2004;19(8):1270–1275.

Barzel US, Massey LK. Excess dietary protein can adversely affect bone. *J Nutr.* 1998;128(6):1051–1053.

Bauer DC, Black DM, Garnero P, et al. Change in bone turnover and hip, non-spine, and vertebral fracture in alendronate-treated women: the fracture intervention trial. *J Bone Miner Res.* 2004;19(8):1250–1258.

Berg KM, Kunins HV, Jackson JL, et al. Association between alcohol consumption and both osteoporotic fracture and bone density. *Am J Med.* 2008;121(5):406–418.

Bharti AC, Takada Y, Aggarwal BB. Curcumin (diferuloylmethane) inhibits receptor activator of NF-kappa B ligand-induced NF-kappa B activation in osteoclast precursors and suppresses osteoclastogenesis. *J Immunol.* 2004;172(10):5940–5947.

Bilezikian JP, Rubin MR, Finkelstein JS. Parathyroid hormone as an anabolic therapy for women and men. *J Endocrinolog Investig.* 2005;28(8 Suppl):41–49.

Bischoff-Ferrari HA. How to select the doses of vitamin D in the management of osteoporosis. *Osteoporos Int.* 2007;18(4):401–407.

Bischoff-Ferrari HA. Optimal serum 25-hydroxyvitamin D levels for multiple health outcomes. *Adv Exp Med Biol.* 2008;624:55–71.

Bischoff-Ferrari HA, Orav EJ, Dawson-Hughes B. Effect of cholecalciferol plus calcium on falling in ambulatory older men and women: a 3-year randomized controlled trial. *Arch Intern Med.* 2006;166(4):424–430.

Bischoff-Ferrari HA, Willett WC, Wong JB, et al. Fracture prevention with vitamin D supplementation: a meta-analysis of randomized controlled trials. *JAMA.* 2005;293(18):2257–2264.

Bischoff-Ferrari HA, Dawson-Hughes B, Willett WC, et al. Effect of Vitamin D on falls: a meta-analysis. *JAMA.* 2004;291(16):1999–2006.

Bischoff-Ferrari HA, Dietrich T, Orav EJ, et al. Higher 25-hydroxyvitamin D concentrations are associated with better lower-extremity function in both active and inactive persons aged > or =60 y. *Am J Clin Nutr.* 2004;80(3):752–758.

Bischoff-Ferrari HA, Dawson-Hughes B, Baron JA, et al. Calcium intake and hip fracture risk in men and women: a meta-analysis of prospective cohort studies and randomized controlled trials. *Am J Clin Nutr.* 2007;86(6);1780–1790.

Black DM, Schwartz AV, Ensrud KE, et al. Effects of continuing or stopping alendronate after 5 years of treatment: the Fracture Intervention Trial Long-term Extension (FLEX): a randomized trial. *JAMA.* 2006;296(24):2927–2938.

Black DM, Eastell R, Reid IR, et al. Once-yearly zoledronic acid for treatment of post-menopausal osteoporosis. *N Engl J Med.* 2007;356(18):1809–1822.

Blake GM, Fogelman I. Strontium ranelate: a novel treatment for postmenopausal osteoporosis: a review of safety and efficacy. *Clin Interven Aging.* 2006;1(4):367–375.

Booth SL, Tucker KL, Chen H, et al. Dietary vitamin K intakes are associated with hip fracture but not with bone mineral density in elderly men and women. *Am J Clin Nutr.* 2000;71(5):1201–1208.

Borges JLC, Bilezikian JP. Update on osteoporosis therapy. *Arq Bras Endocrinol Metabol.* 2006;50(4):755–763.

Branca F. Dietary phyto-oestrogens and bone health. *Proc Nutr Soc.* 2003;62(4):877–887.

Brink E, Coxam V, Robins S, et al. Long-term consumption of isoflavone-enriched foods does not affect bone mineral density, bone metabolism, or hormonal status in early postmenopausal women: a randomized, double-blind, placebo controlled study. *Am J Clin Nutr.* 2008;87(3):761–770.

Broe KE, Chen TC, Weinberg J, Bischoff-Ferrari HA, Holick MF, Kiel DP. A higher dose of vitamin d reduces the risk of falls in nursing home residents: a randomized, multiple-dose study. *J Am Geriatr Soc.* 2007;55(2):234–239.

Cannell JJ, Hollis BW, Zasloff M, Heaney RP. Diagnosis and treatment of vitamin D deficiency. *Expert Opin Pharmacother.* 2008;9(1):107–118.

Cauley JA, Robbins J, Chen Z, et al. Effects of estrogen plus progestin on risk of fracture and bone mineral density: the Women's Health Initiative randomized trial. *JAMA.* 2003;290(13):1729–1738.

Chen Z, Pettinger MB, Ritenbaugh C, et al. Habitual tea consumption and risk of osteoporosis: a prospective study in the women's health initiative observational cohort. *Am J Epidemiol.* 2003;158(8):772–781.

Chesnut CH III, Skag A, Christiansen C, et al. Effects of oral ibandronate administered daily or intermittently on fracture risk in postmenopausal osteoporosis. *J Bone Miner Res.* 2004;19(8):1241–1249.

Chiechi LM, Secreto G, D'Amore M, et al. Efficacy of a soy rich diet in preventing postmenopausal osteoporosis: the Menfis randomized trial. *Maturitas.* 2002;42(4):295–300.

Cizza G, Ravn P, Chrousos GP, Gold PW. Depression: a major, unrecognized risk factor for osteoporosis? *Trends Endocrinol Metab.* 2001;12(5):198–203.

Clowes JA, Riggs BL, Khosla S. The role of the immune system in the pathophysiology of osteoporosis. *Immunolog Rev.* 2005;208:207–227.

Compston J. Bone quality: what is it and how is it measured? *Arq Bras Endocrinol Metabol.* 2006;50(4):579–585.

Cooper C, Atkinson EJ, Hensrud DD, et al. Dietary protein intake and bone mass in women. *Calcif Tissue Int.* 1996;58(5):320–325.

Cornuz J, Feskanich D, Willett WC, Colditz GA. Smoking, smoking cessation, and risk of hip fracture in women. *Am J Med.* 1999;106(3):311–314.

Cranney A, Guyatt G, Griffith L, et al. Meta-analyses of therapies for postmenopausal osteoporosis. IX: Summary of meta-analyses of therapies for postmenopausal osteoporosis. *Endocr Rev.* 2002;23(4):570–578.

Cummings SR, Black DM, Nevitt MC, et al. Bone density at various sites for prediction of hip fractures. The Study of Osteoporotic Fractures Research Group. *Lancet.* 1993;341(8837):72–75.

Cussler EC, Going SB, Houtkooper LB, et al. Exercise frequency and calcium intake predict 4-year bone changes in postmenopausal women. *Osteoporos Int.* 2005;16(12):2129–2141.

Das UN. Essential fatty acids and osteoporosis. *Nutrition.* 2000;16(5):386–390.

Dawson-Hughes B, Dallal GE, Krall EA, et al. A controlled trial of the effect of calcium supplementation on bone density in postmenopausal women. *N Engl J Med.* 1990;323(13):878–883.

De Bacquer D, Clays E, Delanghe J, De Backer G. Epidemiological evidence for an association between habitual tea consumption and markers of chronic inflammation. *Atherosclerosis.* 2006;189(2):428–435.

Ettinger B, Black DM, Mitlak BH, et al. Reduction of vertebral fracture risk in postmenopausal women with osteoporosis treated with raloxifene: results from a 3-year randomized clinical trial. Multiple Outcomes of Raloxifene Evaluation (MORE) Investigators. [erratum appears in *JAMA.* 1999;282(22):2124]. *JAMA.* 1999;282(7):637–645.

Evans W. Functional and metabolic consequences of sarcopenia. *J Nutr.* 1997;127(5 Suppl):998S–1003S.

Fernandes G, Lawrence R, Sun D. Protective role of n-3 lipids and soy protein in osteoporosis. *Prostaglandins Leukot Essent Fatty Acids.* 2003;68(6):361–372.

Feskanich D, Willett WC, Stampfer MJ, Colditz GA. Protein consumption and bone fractures in women. *Am J Epidemiol.* 1996;143(5):472–479.

Feskanich D, Willett WC, Stampfer MJ, Colditz GA. Milk, dietary calcium, and bone fractures in women: a 12-year prospective study. *Am J Public Health.* 1997;87(6):992–997.

Feskanich D, Willett W, Colditz G. Walking and leisure-time activity and risk of hip fracture in postmenopausal women. *JAMA.*2002;288(18):2300–2306.

Feskanich D, Willett WC, Colditz GA. Calcium, vitamin D, milk consumption, and hip fractures: a prospective study among postmenopausal women. *Am J Clin Nutr.* 2003;77(2):504–511.

Feskanich D, Singh V, Willett WC, et al. Vitamin A intake and hip fractures among postmenopausal women. *JAMA.* 2002;287(1):47–54.

Fiatarone MA, O'Neill EF, Ryan ND, et al. Exercise training and nutritional supplementation for physical frailty in very elderly people. *N Engl J Med.* 1994;330(25):1769–1775.

Fitzpatrick LA. Estrogen therapy for postmenopausal osteoporosis. *Arq Bras Endocrinol Metabol.* 2006;50(4):705–719.

Force, U. S. Preventive Services Task Hormone therapy for the prevention of chronic conditions in postmenopausal women: recommendations from the U.S. Preventive Services Task Force.[summary for patients in *Ann Intern Med.* 2005;142(10):I59; PMID: 15897529]. *Ann Intern Med.* 2005;142(10):855–860.

Frassetto LA, Todd KM, Morris RC Jr, Sebastian A. Worldwide incidence of hip fracture in elderly women: relation to consumption of animal and vegetable foods. *J Gerontol A Biol Sci Med Sci.* 2000;55(10):M585–M592.

Gardner EJ, Ruxton CHS, Leeds AR. Black tea—helpful or harmful? A review of the evidence. *Eur J Clin Nutr.* 2007;61(1):3–18.

Ginaldi L, Di Benedetto M, De Martinis M. Osteoporosis, inflammation and ageing. *Immun Ageing.* 2005;2(1):14.

Gordon CM, Nelson LM. Amenorrhea and bone health in adolescents and young women. *Curr Opin Obstet Gynecol.* 2003;15(5):377–384.

Gur A, Colpan L, Nas K, et al. The role of trace minerals in the pathogenesis of postmenopausal osteoporosis and a new effect of calcitonin. *J Bone Miner Metab.* 2002;20(1):39–43.

Guyatt GH, Cranney A, Griffith L, et al. Summary of meta-analyses of therapies for postmenopausal osteoporosis and the relationship between bone density and fractures. *Endocrinol Metab Clin North Am.* 2002;31(3):659–679.

Hall SL, Greendale GA. The relation of dietary vitamin C intake to bone mineral density: results from the PEPI study. *Calcif Tissue Int.* 1998;63(3):183–189.

Hallstrom H, Wolk A, Glynn A, Michaëlsson K. Coffee, tea and caffeine consumption in relation to osteoporotic fracture risk in a cohort of Swedish women. *Osteoporos Int.* 2006;17(7):1055–1064.

Hampl JS, Taylor CA, Johnston CS. Vitamin C deficiency and depletion in the United States: the Third National Health and Nutrition Examination Survey, 1988 to 1994. *Am J Public Health.* 2004;94(5):870–875.

Harrington M, Cashman KD. High salt intake appears to increase bone resorption in postmenopausal women but high potassium intake ameliorates this adverse effect. *Nutr Rev.* 2003;61(5 Pt 1):179–183.

Harris ST, Watts NB, Genant HK, et al. Effects of risedronate treatment on vertebral and nonvertebral fractures in women with postmenopausal osteoporosis: a randomized controlled trial. Vertebral Efficacy with Risedronate Therapy (VERT) Study Group. *JAMA.* 1999;282(14):1344–1352.

Harris ST, Blumentals WA, Miller PD. Ibandronate and the risk of non-vertebral and clinical fractures in women with postmenopausal osteoporosis: results of a meta-analysis of phase III studies. *Curr Med Res Opin.* 2008;24(1):237–245.

Heaney RP, Dowell MS, Hale CA, Bendich A. Calcium absorption varies within the reference range for serum 25-hydroxyvitamin D. *J Am Coll Nutr.* 2003;22(2):142–146.

Heckbert SR, Li G, Cummings SR, Smith NL, Psaty BM. Use of alendronate and risk of incident atrial fibrillation in women. *Arch Intern Med.* 2008;168(8):826–831.

Hodges SJ, Pilkington MJ, Stamp TC, et al. Depressed levels of circulating menaquinones in patients with osteoporotic fractures of the spine and femoral neck. *Bone.* 1991;12(6):387–389.

Holick MF. High prevalence of vitamin D inadequacy and implications for health. *Mayo Clin Proc.* 2006;81(3):353–373.

Holick MF, Siris ES, Binkley N, et al. Prevalence of Vitamin D inadequacy among postmenopausal North American women receiving osteoporosis therapy. *J Clin Endocrinol Metab.* 2005;90(6):3215–3224.

Ince B, Avery, Anderson, Neer RM. Lowering dietary protein to U.S. Recommended dietary allowance levels reduces urinary calcium excretion and bone resorption in young women. *J Clin Endocrinol Metab.* 2004;89(8):3801–3807.

Jacobs ET, Alberts DS, Foote JA, et al. Vitamin D insufficiency in southern Arizona. *Am J Clin Nutr.* 2008;87(3):608–613.

Jia D, O'Brien CA, Stewart SA, Manolagas SC, Weinstein RS, et al. Glucocorticoids act directly on osteoclasts to increase their life span and reduce bone density. *Endocrinology.* 2006;147(12):5592–5599.

Kalkwarf HJ, Specker BL. Bone mineral changes during pregnancy and lactation. *Endocrine.* 2002;17(1):49.

Kaneki M. [Protective effects of vitamin K against osteoporosis and its pleiotropic actions]. *Clin Calcium.* 2006;16(9):1526–1534.

Kanis JA, Johnell O, Oden A, et al. Smoking and fracture risk: a meta-analysis. *Osteoporos Int.* 2005;16(2):155–162.

Kaunitz, Andrew M, Arias R, McClung M. Bone density recovery after depot medroxyprogesterone acetate injectable contraception use. *Contraception.* 2008;77(2):67–76.

Kim BJ, Yu YM, Kim EN, Chung YE, Koh JM, Kim GS. Relationship between serum hsCRP concentration and biochemical bone turnover markers in healthy pre- and postmenopausal women. *Clin Endocrinol.* 2007;67(1):152–158.

Kim C, Ha H, Lee JH, Kim JS, Song K, Park SW. Herbal extract prevents bone loss in ovariectomized rats. *Arch Pharmacol Res.* 2003;26(11):917–924.

Knopp JA, Diner BM, Blitz M, Lyritis GP, Rowe BH. Calcitonin for treating acute pain of osteoporotic vertebral compression fractures: a systematic review of randomized, controlled trials. *Osteoporos Int.* 2005;16(10):1281–1290.

Koh JM, Khang YH, Jung CH, et al. Higher circulating hsCRP levels are associated with lower bone mineral density in healthy pre- and postmenopausal women: evidence for a link between systemic inflammation and osteoporosis. *Osteoporos Int.* 2005;16(10):1263–1271.

Kruger MC, Horrobin DF. Calcium metabolism, osteoporosis and essential fatty acids: a review. *Progr Lipid Res.* 1997;36(2–3):131–151.

Kruger MC, Coetzer H, de Winter R, Gericke G, van Papendorp DH. Calcium, gamma-linolenic acid and eicosapentaenoic acid supplementation in senile osteoporosis. *Aging-Clin Exp Res.* 1998;10(5):385–394.

Lanham-New SA. Fruit and vegetables: the unexpected natural answer to the question of osteoporosis prevention? [comment]. *Am J Clin Nutr.* 2006;83(6):1254–1255.

Lanham-New SA. The balance of bone health: tipping the scales in favor of potassium-rich, bicarbonate-rich foods. *J Nutr.,* 2008;138(1):172S–177S.

Lewiecki EM. Intravenous zoledronic acid for the treatment of osteoporosis. *Curr Osteoporos Rep.* 2008;6(1):17–23.

Li F, Harmer P, Fisher KJ, et al. Tai Chi and fall reductions in older adults: a randomized controlled trial. *J Gerontol A Biolog Sci Med Sci.* 2005;60(2):187–194.

Lloyd T, Beck TJ, Lin HM, et al. Modifiable determinants of bone status in young women. *Bone.* 2002;30(2):416–421.

Lloyd T, Petit MA, Lin HM, Beck TJ. Lifestyle factors and the development of bone mass and bone strength in young women. *J Pediatr.* 2004;144(6):776–782.

Marsh AG, Sanchez TV, Midkelsen O, et al. Cortical bone density of adult lacto-ovo-vegetarian and omnivorous women. *J Am Diet Assoc.* 1980;76(2):148–151.

Marshall D, Johnell O, Wedel H. Meta-analysis of how well measures of bone mineral density predict occurrence of osteoporotic fractures. *BMJ.* 1996;312(7041):1254–1259.

Mashiba T, Turner CH, Hirano T, et al. Suppressed bone turnover by bisphosphonates increases microdamage accumulation and reduces some biomechanical properties in dog rib. *J Bone Miner Res.* 2000;15(4):613–620.

McCarus DC. Fracture prevention in postmenopausal osteoporosis: a review of treatment options. *Obstet Gynecolog Surv.* 2006;61(1):39–50.

Melhus H, Michaëlsson K, Kindmark A, et al. Excessive dietary intake of vitamin A is associated with reduced bone mineral density and increased risk for hip fracture. *Ann Intern Med.* 1998;129(10):770–778.

Melton LJ, Bryant SC, Wahner HW, et al. Influence of breastfeeding and other reproductive factors on bone mass later in life. *Osteoporos Int.* 1993;3(2):76–83.

Mezzetti M, La Vecchia C, Decarli A, et al. Population attributable risk for breast cancer: diet, nutrition, and physical exercise. [erratum appears in *J Natl Cancer Inst.* 2000;92(10):845]. *J Nat Cancer Inst.* 1998;90(5):389–394.

Mingyue W, Ling G, Bei X, Junqing C, Peiqing Z, Jie H. Clinical observation on 96 cases of primary osteoporosis treated with kidney-tonifying and bone-strengthening mixture. *J Tradition Chinese Med.* 2005;25(2):132–136.

Misra M, Prabhakaran R, Miller KK, et al. Weight gain and restoration of menses as predictors of bone mineral density change in adolescent girls with anorexia nervosa-1. *J Clin Endocrinol Metab.* 2008;93(4):1231–1237.

Mundy GR. Osteoporosis and inflammation. *Nutr Rev.* 2007;65(12 Pt 2):S147–S151.

Nelson HD, Humphrey LL, Nygren P, et al. Postmenopausal hormone replacement therapy: scientific review. *JAMA.* 2002;288(7):872–881.

New SA, Robins SP, Campbell MK, et al. Dietary influences on bone mass and bone metabolism: further evidence of a positive link between fruit and vegetable consumption and bone health? *Am J Clin Nutr.* 2000;71(1):142–151.

Nordin BC. Calcium requirement is a sliding scale. *Am J Clin Nutr.* 2000;71(6):1381–1383.

O'Donnell S, Cranney A, Wells GA, et al. Strontium ranelate for preventing and treating postmenopausal osteoporosis. [update of *Cochrane Database Syst Rev.* 2006;3:CD005326; PMID: 16856092]. *Cochrane Database Syst Rev.* 2006;(4):CD005326.

Papoutsi Z, Kassi E, Chinou I, Halabalaki M, Skaltsounis LA, Moutsatsou P. Walnut extract (*Juglans regia* L.) and its component ellagic acid exhibit anti-inflammatory activity in human aorta endothelial cells and osteoblastic activity in the cell line KS483. *Br J Nutr.* 2008;99(4):715–722.

Patterson-Buckendahl P, Pohorecky LA, Kvetnansky R. Differing effects of acute and chronic stressors on plasma osteocalcin and leptin in rats. *Stress.* 2007;10(2):163–172.

Pearson DA. Bone health and osteoporosis: the role of vitamin K and potential antagonism by anticoagulants. *Nutr Clin Pract.* 2007;22(5):517–544.

Pfeilschifter J. Role of cytokines in postmenopausal bone loss. *Curr Osteoporos Rep.* 2003;1(2):53–58.

Proctor DN, Shen PH, Dietz NM, et al. Relative influence of physical activity, muscle mass and strength on bone density. *Osteoporos Int.* 2000;11(11):944–952.

Prynne CJ, Mishra GD, O'Connell MA, et al. Fruit and vegetable intakes and bone mineral status: a cross sectional study in 5 age and sex cohorts. *Am J Clin Nutr.* 2006;83(6):1420–1428.

Putnam SE, Scutt AM, Bicknell K, Priestley CM, Williamson EM. Natural products as alternative treatments for metabolic bone disorders and for maintenance of bone health. *Phytother Res.* 2007;21(2):99–112.

Reginster JY, Sarlet, N. The treatment of severe postmenopausal osteoporosis: a review of current and emerging therapeutic options. *Treat Endocrinol.* 2006;5(1):15.

Riggs BL, Melton LJ III. The worldwide problem of osteoporosis: insights afforded by epidemiology. *Bone.* 1995;17(5 Suppl):505S–511S.

Rude RK, Gruber, HE. Magnesium deficiency and osteoporosis: animal and human observations. *J Nutr Biochem.* 2004;15(12):710–716.

Ryder KM, Shorr RI, Bush AJ, et al. Magnesium intake from food and supplements is associated with bone mineral density in healthy older white subjects. *J Am Geriatr Soc.* 2005;53(11):1875–1880.

Sampson HW. Alcohol and other factors affecting osteoporosis risk in women. *Alcoh Res Health J Natl Instit Alcohol Abuse Alcohol.* 2002;26(4):292–298.

Schweiger U, Deuschle M, Korner A, et al. Low lumbar bone mineral density in patients with major depression. *Am J Psychiatry.* 1994;151(11):1691–1693.

Seeman E, Seeman E, De Vernejoul MC, et al. Strontium ranelate reduces the risk of vertebral and nonvertebral fractures in women eighty years of age and older. *J Bone Miner Res.* 2006;21(7):1113–1120.

Sellmeyer DE, Stone KL, Sebastian A, et al. A high ratio of dietary animal to vegetable protein increases the rate of bone loss and the risk of fracture in postmenopausal women. Study of Osteoporotic Fractures Research Group. *Am J Clin Nutr.* 2001;73(1):118–122.

Setchell KD, Lydeking-Olsen E. Dietary phytoestrogens and their effect on bone: evidence from in vitro and in vivo, human observational, and dietary intervention studies. *Am J Clin Nutr.* 2003;78(3 Suppl):593S–609S.

Shah A, Kolhapure SA. Evaluation of efficacy and safety of Reosto in senile osteoporosis: a randomized, double-blind placebo-controlled clinical trial. *Ind J Clin Pract.* 2004;15(3):25–36.

Simopoulos AP. Human requirement for N-3 polyunsaturated fatty acids. *Poul Sci.* 2000;79(7):961–970.

Sinaki M, Itoi E, Wahner HW, et al. Stronger back muscles reduce the incidence of vertebral fractures: a prospective 10 year follow-up of postmenopausal women. *Bone.* 2002;30(6):836–841.

Siris ES, Miller PD, Barrett-Connor E, et al. Identification and fracture outcomes of undiagnosed low bone mineral density in postmenopausal women results from the National Osteoporosis Risk Assessment. *Am Med Assoc.* 2001;286:2815–2822.

Sojka JE, Weaver CM. Magnesium supplementation and osteoporosis. *Nutr Rev.* 1995;53(3):71–74.

Stendig-Lindberg G, Tepper R, Leichter I. Trabecular bone density in a two year controlled trial of peroral magnesium in osteoporosis. *Magnesium Res.* 1993;6(2):155–163.

Thom JA, Bishop A, Blacklock NJ. The influence of refined carbohydrate on urinary calcium excretion. *Br J Urol.* 1978;50(7):459–464.

Todd JA, Robinson RJ. Osteoporosis and exercise. *Postgr Med J.* 2003;79(932):320–323.

Togari A, Arai M, Kondo A. The role of the sympathetic nervous system in controlling bone metabolism. *Expert Opin Ther Targets.* 2005;9(5):931–940.

Trivedi DP, Doll R, Khaw KT. Effect of four monthly oral vitamin D3 (cholecalciferol) supplementation on fractures and mortality in men and women living in the community: randomised double blind controlled trial. *BMJ.* 2003;326(7387):469.

Tucker KL, Hannan MT, Chen H, et al. Potassium, magnesium, and fruit and vegetable intakes are associated with greater bone mineral density in elderly men and women. *Am J Clin Nutr.* 1999;69(4):727–736.

Turner CH. Biomechanics of bone: determinants of skeletal fragility and bone quality. *Osteoporos Int.* 2002;13(2):97–104.

Vieth R, Bischoff-Ferrari H, Boucher BJ, et al. The urgent need to recommend an intake of vitamin D that is effective. [comment]. *Am J Clin Nutr.* 2007;85(3):649–950.

Vogel RA. Alcohol, heart disease, and mortality: a review. *Rev Cardiovasc Med.* 2002;3(1):7–13.

Voukelatos A, Cumming RG, Lord SR, et al. A randomized, controlled trial of tai chi for the prevention of falls: the Central Sydney Tai Chi Trial. *J Am Geriatr Soc.* 2007;55(8):1185–1191.

Wainwright SA, Marshall LM, Ensrud KE, et al. Hip fracture in women without osteoporosis. *J Clin Endocrinol Metab.* 2005;90(5):2787–2793.

Walsh JS, Eastell R, Peel, NFA. Effects of Depot medroxyprogesterone acetate on bone density and bone metabolism before and after peak bone mass: a case-control study. *J Clin Endocrinol Metab.* 2008;93(4):1317–1323.

Watts NB, Chines A, Olszynski WP, et al. Fracture risk remains reduced one year after discontinuation of risedronate. *Osteoporos Int.* 2008;19(3):365–372.

Weikert C, Walter D, Hoffmann K, Kroke A, Bergmann MM, Boeing H. The relation between dietary protein, calcium and bone health in women: results from the EPIC-Potsdam cohort. *Ann Nutr Metab.* 2005;49(5):312–318.

Wolf SL, Barnhart HX, Kutner NG, McNeely E, Coogler C, Xu T. Reducing frailty and falls in older persons: an investigation of Tai Chi and computerized balance training. Atlanta FICSIT Group. Frailty and Injuries: cooperative Studies of Intervention Techniques. *J Am Geriatr Soc.* 1996;44(5):489–497.

Wolff I, van Croonenborg JJ, Kemper HC, Kostense PJ, Twisk JW. The effect of exercise training programs on bone mass: a meta-analysis of published controlled trials in pre- and postmenopausal women. *Osteoporos Int.* 1999;9(1):1–12.

Wuttke W, Gorkow C, Seidlova-Wuttke D. Effects of black cohosh (*Cimicifuga racemosa*) on bone turnover, vaginal mucosa, and various blood parameters in postmenopausal women: a double-blind, placebo-controlled, and conjugated estrogens-controlled study. *Menopause.* 2006;13(2):185–196.

Yin J, Kouda K, Tezuka Y, et al. New diarylheptanoids from the rhizomes of *Dioscorea spongiosa* and their antiosteoporotic activity. *Planta Med.* 2004a;70(1):54–58.

Yin J, Tezuka Y, Kouda K, et al. Antiosteoporotic activity of the water extract of *Dioscorea spongiosa. Biolog Pharm Bull.* 2004b;27(4):583–586.

Zhang X, Shu XO, Li H, et al. Prospective cohort study of soy food consumption and risk of bone fracture among postmenopausal women. *Arch Intern Med.* 2005;165(16):1890–1895.

37

Healthy Aging: The Whole Woman Approach

ELIZABETH R. MACKENZIE AND BIRGIT RAKEL

"Age has its own glory, beauty, and wisdom that belong to it. Peace, love, joy, beauty, happiness, wisdom, goodwill, and understanding are qualities that never grow old or die."

Joseph Murphy

Introduction

Aging is not a disease. Growing old is a natural process, the denouement in the narrative of a woman's life. The purpose of this chapter is to emphasize the potential for *healthy aging*. We know that our bodies change with age. Skin begins to lose its elasticity, wrinkles emerge, bones may become more brittle, muscle tone diminishes, and we gain weight more readily. Chronic conditions that have been forming for years may finally manifest as full-blown symptoms claiming our attention. Our energy levels may be lower, almost as though our vital force is leaking away. Still, there is potential for vibrant health if these challenges are approached with the proper perspective and if we are equipped with the best of integrative medicine. When thinking about how to support patients in their efforts to age healthfully, it is important for health professionals to move away from the perception of aging as a problem to be solved. As Andrew Weil, MD, has noted a crucial component of the healthy aging paradigm is to reconfigure the concept of aging.

I'm interested in the areas of our experience in which we value aging. I want to consider old trees, cheese, wine, whiskey, and steak. What are the qualities that we appreciate in aged things I think they include roundedness and smoothness as opposed to angularity and a kind of deep strength combined with mellowness (Weil 2001).

A key to healthy aging is the understanding that achieving good health does not necessarily mean having *perfect* health. It is possible to live fully while managing a chronic condition or coping with a disability. Wholeness does not require a perfect body, free from all flaws and disorders. However, the healthier we can get, the stronger we will feel in our bodies, and the more fully our lives can unfold. What we are after here is excellent energy, strong bodies, flexible forms, calm minds, and joyful spirits.

Women age differently, based on genetics, lifestyle, life events, social support, mental outlook, and other factors, both known and unknown. The life force is an important but often mysterious ally for health professionals. Most of us have met older women who are thriving despite a lifetime of smoking, drinking, and sedentary living, while others, conscientious about their health, are beset with illness. We can influence, but not control, health. The idea is to guide patients toward activities and interventions that will increase the probability of good health.

This is decidedly not an "antiaging" chapter, and we will not refer to "turning back the hands of time" or use similar metaphors. Actually, "antiaging" is a strange term, since we begin to age at birth. Being born sets the aging process in motion and only death can stop it. Our goals, as health professionals, should be to extend life while enhancing quality of life by preventing disease when possible and otherwise by managing it optimally.

The Conventional Approach to Aging

Conventional approaches to aging have strengths. Medicine is very good at screening, the treatment of acute illness, and dealing with advanced disease states. Cancer, for example, is no longer the "death sentence" it once was, and long-term survival rates for certain forms of cancer are quite high. However, it should be noted that *screening*, is not a good substitute for *prevention* and conventional medicine has not had a good track record on the health promotion side of the equation.

The biggest failing of conventional medicine with regard to aging, though, is its tendency to view aging as a pathology, rather than a natural stage in the lifecycle. The most obvious recent example is the conventional approach to menopause. For decades, hormone replacement therapy (HRT) was the standard response to changing hormonal levels in middle-aged women. At least two generations of American women were strongly encouraged to replace their hormones as they were tapering off during menopause. Then, the Women's Health Initiative (WHI) trial was stopped early when researchers realized that the risks of cardiovascular disease and breast cancer associated with hormone therapy were greater than its benefits (Heiss et al. 2008). This finding was confirmed when national breast cancer rates fell after a widespread cessation of HRT in response to media coverage (Heiss et al. 2008).

Nutrition and Aging

Eating fresh fruits and vegetables, whole grains and avoiding overly processed foods, is a central part of establishing a healthy diet. Specific considerations related to healthy aging include vegetarianism, calorie restricted diets, and the need for supplementation.

VEGETARIANISM

Some evidence suggests that vegetarianism promotes longevity. Singh et al. report that, "Current prospective cohort data from adults in North America and Europe raise the possibility that a lifestyle pattern that includes a very low meat intake is associated with greater longevity" (Singh et al. 2003). However, other large-scale European studies suggest that it may not be eschewing meat that is the critical factor, but adhering to a diet high in whole grains, vegetables, and fruit (Ginter 2008; Sabate 2003). Vegetarians do seem to have less incidence of ischemic heart disease, lower prevalence of obesity, and higher consumption of antioxidants (Ginter 2008). While these studies do not constitute a total indictment of meat consumption, they do point to the health benefits of reducing—but not necessarily eliminating—meat consumption, and focusing the diet on whole grains, vegetable, and fruits. Patients who choose to adhere to a strict vegetarian diet should make sure they are not deficient in essential nutrients. Lacto-ova vegetarians have an easier time getting enough protein and B vitamins than vegans. Most vegans will need to supplement their diet with sublingual B12 vitamins or use Brewer's yeast.

CALORIE RESTRICTED DIETS

Eating less as we age may promote longevity. Mice and fruit flies kept on a drastically calorie restricted diet lived significantly longer than their well-fed relatives. What this implies for human health is a bit speculative, but at least one study of elders in Okinawa seems to support the notion that consuming fewer calories in late life helps people live longer. Willcox et al. (2007) conducted a study of calorie restriction and longevity that found a strong correlation between the two. Calorie restriction (CR) refers to diets based on a 1400–2000 daily calorie intake (compared with the 2000–3000 calories considered normal). Although most CR studies have been performed using animal models, evidence is accumulating that "that CR provides a powerful protective effect against secondary aging in humans." For example "risk factors for atherosclerosis and diabetes are markedly reduced in humans on CR" (Holloszy and Fontana 2007).

Detoxification: Key to preventing disease or expensive hoax?

Although we may not like to reflect on this, we are surrounded by varying levels of potentially dangerous chemicals in the air, the water, the soil and our own bodies. "Different toxins accumulate in different tissues with many toxins being stored in lipid deposits where they can persist over the lifespan. It is possible that these toxins contribute to the development of cancers of the breast, prostate and leukaemias which all originate in fatty tissues" (Cohen 2007: 1009).

Many proponents of various detox programs believe that fasting, special diets, juices, colonics, saunas, sweat lodges, chelation therapy, and so on can be used to detoxify the body. There is little scientific evidence to support the effectiveness of detoxification programs (Cohen, "Detox or Sales Pitch" *Australian Family Physician* 2007). However, as women may be exploring these options on their own, physicians should be aware of these practices.

SUPPLEMENTS

Although it is optimal to receive all necessary vitamins and minerals through food, many older adults may need to supplement their diets. Here a few of the most popular supplements for older women.

Calcium

Calcium's main role as a supplement is in the treatment of osteoporosis. Dietary sources are calcium rich foods such as dairy, dark green leafy vegetable, and beans. Calcium supplementation in the elderly and postmenopausal women helps reduce bone loss (D evine et al. 1997; Napoli et al. 2007; Reid et al. 1993) Some studies have found that calcium may also lower blood pressure (Conlin et al. 2000; Wang et al. 2008). Calcium supplementation is safe when used orally, but some patients might experience GI symptoms such as nausea, constipation, and abdominal pain.

Vitamin D

Vitamin D has been in the news frequently in the recent past as it may play a critical role in providing protection from osteoporosis (Deane et al. 2007) and from cancer (Lappe et al. 2007; Schumann et al. 2007). Vitamin D supplementation may promote longevity in general (Autier and Gandini 2007). Populations who may be at a high risk for vitamin D deficiencies include the elderly, and those who have limited sun exposure.

Omega-3 Fatty Acids (Fish Oils)

Epidemiologic studies and randomized controlled trials have shown that taking recommended amounts of DHA and EPA in the form of dietary fish or fish oil supplements lowers triglycerides, reduces the risk of death, heart attack, dangerous abnormal heart rhythms, and strokes in people with known cardiovascular disease; slows atherosclerotic plaques; and lowers blood pressure (Kris-Etherton et al. 2003; Morris et al. 1993). The American Heart Association recommends that fish should be included in the diet for all individuals and fish oil supplements in those with a history of cardiovascular disease. Omega-3 fatty acids, particularly DHA, appear to reduce the risk of developing sight-threatening forms of age-related macular degeneration (SanGiovanni et al. 2008).

Glucosamine

Glucosamine is an amino-monosaccharide naturally produced in humans. It is believed to play a role in cartilage formation and repair, and thus useful in the treatment of arthritis (Reginster et al. 2001). Many studies, though not all, show glucosamine to be an effective intervention for relieving the symptoms of osteoarthritis (Vangsness et al. 2009). Typical dosage is 1500 mg/day, although obese patients may require larger dosages (derMarderosian and Briggs 2006).

Ginkgo (Ginkgo biloba)

Ginkgo biloba is widely used for its potential effects on memory and cognition. It has remained one of the top-selling dietary supplements in the United States for many years; however, when looking at the totality of the data, the evidence that ginkgo has predictable and clinically significant benefit for people with dementia or cognitive impairment is inconsistent and unreliable (Birks and Evans 2009). Since many of the ginkgo studies were small in size and short in duration, the National Institutes of Health funded the Ginkgo Evaluation of Memory (GEM) study that would follow more than 3000 participants for an average of 6 years. This study found that *G. biloba* at 120 mg twice a day of standardized extract was not effective in reducing either the overall incidence rate of dementia or Alzheimer's dementia in individuals 75 years and older with normal cognition or those with mild cognitive impairment (DeKosky et al. 2008). Though an increased risk of bleeding has been widely publicized, *G. biloba* appears to be safe in use with no excess side effects compared with placebo (Birks 2009).

Adaptogens

Perhaps the most useful herbs to support older women's overall health belong to the class entitled "adaptogens." These are generally considered to be those that have a modulating effect upon the neuroendocrine system, particularly during periods of stress. Primary botanicals in this class are ashwagandha (*Withania somnifera*), ginseng (*Panax ginseng*), rhodiola (*Rhodiola rosea*), schisandra (*Schizandra chinensis*), codonopsis (*Codonopsis pilosula*), as well as the reishi mushroom (*Ganoderma lucidum*). Since many of these plants/mushrooms are native to Asia and the Indian sub-continent, they have only recently come to the attention of Western researchers. A useful primer on this class of herbs is *Adaptogens: Herbs for Strength, Stamina, and Stress Relief* by David Winston and Steven Maimes (Rochester VT: Healing Arts Press, 2007).

Bodywork: The Importance of Alignment and Touch

Bodywork is an important part of the care of aging women. Massage, chiropractic, and more esoteric practices such as Alexander Technique, Feldenkrais Method, Bowen Work, and so on, may be useful allies in promoting healthy aging. For example, massage can alleviate insomnia, ease pain associated with misalignments, arthritis and tense muscles, speed recovery from surgery, improve blood and lymphatic circulation, and encourage deep relaxation (Kennedy and Chapman 2006). Because many older women are both touch deprived and coping with chronic pain, bodywork modalities should not be overlooked by physicians who care for them. Ideally, practitioners who are experienced with working with older clients are recommended.

Holistic Self-Care: Yoga, Tai Chi, Qigong, and Meditation

Many therapies are available to help women stay physically fit, emotionally balanced, and spiritually connected. A few practices address all three dimensions and receive special mention here: yoga, tai chi, qigong, and meditation. These are all activities that can be begun late in life, and have the added bonus of helping women learn to accept and love their bodies, while enhancing flexibility, balance, strength, cognitive function, and immunity. Health professionals and patients alike can benefit from the regular practice of these activities.

YOGA

"It might surprise you to learn that traditionally, the ideal age to begin the practice of yoga was said to be fifty-three, the age marking one's passage into a new stage of life, one of contemplation and self-discovery" (Alice Christensen, in Butera 2006 p. 199). The word *yoga* means "yoke" or "union" in Sanskrit, referring to the integration of mind, body, and spirit. Yoga can be practiced solely as a physical exercise, though this was not the traditional intent. There are eight "limbs" of yoga and only one of them refers to the physical poses or *asanas*. The other seven are restraint (*yama*), observances (*niyamas*), breath control (*pranayama*), sensory withdrawal (*pratyahara*), and finally concentration, meditation, and perfect concentration.

In the United States, most yoga classes focus on the *asanas* with some inclusion of *pranayama*. Many individuals prefer to work with instructors who understand the deeper dimensions of the practice, and can help them cultivate *prana* (the Sanskrit term for life force), while others are more comfortable approaching yoga as more of a physical exercise. The many different forms of yoga available today in the United States helps to ensure that older adults can find a style that works for them. Among the forms of yoga currently being taught are Iyengar, Ashtanga (or "Power Yoga"), Vinyasa (or "flow yoga"), Bikram (or "hot yoga"). Interviewing yoga instructors about their approach to teaching and the rigors of the class will help patients choose an appropriate style and level.

Yoga promotes health on many levels. Currently, the National Center for Complementary and Alterative Medicine (NCCAM) is funding studies on yoga and arthritis, insomnia, breast cancer, cancer and fatigue, cervical dysplasia, cardiovascular health, asthma, and smoking cessation. According to the NCCAM, scientific evidence suggests that yoga may

- improve mood and sense of well-being
- counteract stress
- reduce heart rate and blood pressure
- increase lung capacity
- improve muscle relaxation and body composition
- help with conditions such as anxiety, depression, and insomnia
- improve overall physical fitness, strength, and flexibility
- positively affect levels of certain brain or blood chemicals (http://nccam.nih.gov/health/yoga).

Yoga has become one of the most frequently studied of the mind–body practices, and a comprehensive review of all scientific findings on its health benefits is not possible here. Among the conditions associates with aging that yoga has been found to successfully ameliorate are coronary artery disease, musculoskeletal disorders, and hypertension (Butera 2006).

TAI CHI AND QIGONG

Like yoga, qigong is a practice that promotes a healthy body, mind, and spirit. Both qigong and tai chi are ancient practices rooted in the Chinese philosophy of balancing energies within the body itself and between the body and the environment.

Qi is the Chinese word for 'life energy'. According to Chinese medicine, qi is the animating power that flows through all living things. A living being is filled with it. A dead person has no more qi—the warmth, the life energy is gone.... However, health is more than an abundance of qi. Health implies that the qi in our bodies is clear, rather than polluted and turbid, and flowing smoothly, like a stream, not blocked or stagnant (Cohen, 1997: 3).

Both qigong and tai chi help the practitioner cultivate and circulate qi to support vibrant health. Qigong is the broader term; tai chi is actually a form of qigong. Both practices use slow, precise movements to encourage the flow of qi. Some forms of qigong emphasize breathing practices and movement, while others focus more on meditative activities.

The possible health benefits from the regular practice of qigong are numerous. Stress reduction, prevention of stroke, decreased hypertension, treatment of arthritis—these are among the many health-promoting effects found in the scientific study of qigong (Chen et al. 2006). Although many of these studies were conducted in China, some U.S. studies are beginning to explore the multiple health benefits of qigong, especially for aging populations. For example, a recent review of clinical trials found that qigong and tai chi "may help older adults improve physical function and reduce blood pressure, fall risk, and depression and anxiety" (Rogers et al. 2009).

MEDITATION

We do not usually associate meditation with physical fitness, but a regular practice can reduce the risk of developing cardiovascular disease (CVD) (Schneider et al. 2006), and may improve immunity (Davidson et al. 2003). From a mind–body perspective, this is not surprising. We would expect the quieting of the mind to help people better cope with stressors, and thus improve their physical health. Even more importantly, meditation assists people in accessing their core spiritual support, allowing them to draw upon inner reserves in times of stress and loss. Numerous studies have found that meditation improves physical, psychological, and spiritual well-being (Yuen and Baime 2006).

There are several forms of meditation practice common in the United States. One of the best known is transcendental meditation (TM). Introduced to Americans by the Maharishi Mahesh Yogi in the 1960s, TM is closely tied to the Indian Vedic tradition (Yuen and Baime 2006: 239). Practitioners are given a mantra (a syllable, word, or phrase) to chant as a tool to achieve a transcendent state of consciousness. Another increasingly popular form of meditation is Mindfulness Meditation (or Mindfulness Based Stress Reduction or MBSR). This form of meditation grew out of the Buddhist tradition, and was shaped by Jon Kabat-Zinn, PhD for use by health professionals and their patients. MBSR has been extensively studied and has been shown to promote health in a variety of ways, including reducing depression and anxiety, decreased perception of pain, less use of medication, better adherence to medical treatments, and increased motivation to make lifestyle changes (Ludwig and Kabat-Zinn 2008).

All three of these activities are holistic self-care practices that enhance the well-being of body, mind, and spirit. Aging women can integrate these practices into their lives to promote both mental and physical health, and because these are *self-care* practices, successfully initiating a regular practice has the added benefit of cultivating a subjective sense of empowerment.

Healthy Aging and Social Connection

It is hard to overestimate the importance of social connection for older adults. Giving and receiving social support may be one of the most important factors in maintaining health in old age (Giles et al. 2005; McReynolds and Rossen 2004).

In a groundbreaking study, Taylor et al. (2000) found that women responded to stress differently from men. Specifically, females' stress responses were characterized by "tend and befriend" activities, rather than "fight of flight" patterns (Taylor et al. 2000). The study found that during times of stress, women tended to engage in nurturing activities (called "tending" by the authors of the study) that "promote safety and reduce distress." They define "befriending" as the "creation and maintenance of social networks that may aid in this process" (Taylor et al. 2000). The researchers speculate that endorphins and oxytocin play roles in establishing the nurturing activity, while factors like learning and socialization reinforce the behavior. Both oxytocin and endorphins may also contribute to the formation and maintenance of social networks. Social connection may turn out to be a crucial part of our stress-buffering mechanism and healthy immune system functioning, and not just an important factor in psychological health.

These findings, coupled with decades of data on social support and health, suggest that social connection may be an important component of health promotion among older adults (Dupertuis et al. 2001; Fiori et al. 2006; Lyyra and Heikkinen 2006). Older adults are often isolated from their friends and families and must make a great effort to connect with others. Health professionals can support older patients by making recommendations that they seek out social connection, in the same way that they encourage exercise. This may be especially important for unmarried, widowed, and divorced women.

Spirituality and Health

Older adults experience loss on many levels: loss of physical functions, of energy and stamina, of career, status and identity, of independence, and loved ones. Many older women suffer as they lose their conventionally defined physical attractiveness, or their powerful social roles as mothers, homemakers, or professionals. A great number of older women outlive their husbands and must cope with the loss of their marriage, and some must witness the death of beloved adult children. As the popular saying has it, "Old age is not for sissies." Loss in the outer world offers us the opportunity to turn inward and start soul searching. A solid connection to one's spirituality is a proven psychological coping mechanism for dealing with loss (Pargament 1997).

Compared with younger populations, the aged often face negative stressors that are difficult to control.... The aged have a strong need to learn how to accept or to cope with pain, dependency, and their own mortality, while simultaneously enjoying what life still has to offer. For many persons, an acute awareness of the ephemeral nature of life can actually increase one's sense of joy (Ai and Mackenzie 2006).

From this perspective, the negative stressors associated with aging become catalysts for a journey of spiritual growth. Reframing their experience in this way can be enormously helpful to older adults coping with loss, and health professionals should not be reticent to discuss patients' spiritual lives. Although some women may not be open to discussing their spirituality with health professionals, studies indicate that the majority of patients welcome the opportunity (Ehman et al. 1999; McCord et al. 2004).

There is no standard algorithm for addressing the spiritual concerns of patients, and there are as many ways to encourage spiritual exploration as there are people. Patients with ties to traditional religions may just need some encouragement to participate more fully in their congregations. Others can be helped in their journey through meditation, yoga, tai chi or qigong all of which are in essence spiritual disciplines (see above). Gently inquiring into the kinds of activities that help your patient feel more at peace (e.g., walking in nature, gardening, caring for grandchildren) may provide important clues about where her spiritual home is located. The important thing is to acknowledge the connection between health and spirituality, and to let patients know that their moral, metaphysical, and spiritual concerns are an important dimension of their overall well-being. As Larry Dossey MD (2005) wrote, "We find ourselves in society that is spiritually malnourished and hungry for meaning." Health professionals seeking to care for whole persons have an obligation to respond to this hunger.

Conclusion

One of the most important things health professionals can do for their older patients is to introduce them to the idea that they can accept aging as a natural part of the life cycle, without resigning themselves to pain, dysfunction, or decrepitude. Coaching patients to adopt these lifestyle changes can set the stage for healthy aging while maximizing vitality, wholeness, and quality of life. It is appropriate to exhort older women to find ways to restore their vitality, while acknowledging the health challenges inherent in becoming old (Table 37.1).

Table 37.1. The Whole Woman Approach to Healthy Aging: A Clinician's Guide

1. One mind–body practice: meditation, yoga, tai chi, or qigong (daily)

2. Feasible and appropriate exercise routine (3+ days per week)

3. Establish or maintain social network (weekly)

4. Regular bodywork (monthly)

5. A nutrition/supplement plan tailored to the individual

6. Address spiritual concerns as appropriate

REFERENCES

Ai A, Mackenzie ER. Spiritual well-being the care of older adults. In: Mackenzie and Rakel, eds. *Complementary and Alternative Medicine for Older Adults.* New York, NY: Springer Publishing Company; 2006:276.

Autier P, Gandini S. Vitamin D supplementation and total mortality: a meta-analysis of randomized controlled trials. *Arch Intern Med.* 2007;167(16):1730–1737.

Birks J, Grimley Evans J. Ginkgo biloba for cognitive impairment and dementia. *Cochrane Database Syst Rev.* 2009;(1):CD003120.

Butera R. Yoga: an introduction. In ER Mackenzie and B Rakel, eds. *Complementary and Alternative Medicine for Older Adults.* New York, NY: Springer Publishing Company; 2006:199–213.

Chen K, Mackenzie ER, Hou F. The benefits of qigong. In: ER Mackenzie and B Rakel, eds. *Complementary and Alternative Medicine for Older Adults.* New York, NY: Springer Publishing Company; 2006:175–198.

Cohen K. *The Way of Qigong: the Art and Science of Chinese Energy Healing.* New York: Ballantine Books, 1997.

Cohen M. 'Detox': science or sales pitch? *Australian Family Physician.* 2007;36(12):1009–1010.

Conlin PR, Chow D, Miller ER 3rd, et al. The effect of dietary patterns on blood pressure control in hypertensive patients: results from the Dietary Approaches to Stop Hypertension (DASH) trial. *Am J Hypertens.* 2000;13(9):949–955.

Davidson RJ, Kabat-Zinn J, Schumacher J, et al. Alterations in brain and immune function produced by mindfulness meditation. *Psychosomatic Medicine.* 2003;65(4):564–570.

Deane A, Constancio L, Fogelman I, et al. The impact of vitamin D status on changes in bone mineral density during treatment with bisphosphonates and after discontinuation following long-term use in post-menopausal osteoporosis. *BMC Musculoskelet Disord.* 2007;8:3.

DeKosky ST, Williamson JD, Fitzpatrick AL, et al. Ginkgo biloba for prevention of dementia: a randomized controlled trial. *JAMA.* 2008;300(19):2253–2262.

derMarderosian A, Briggs M. Supplements and Herbs. In: ER Mackenzie and B Rakel, eds. *Complementary and Alternative Medicine for Older Adults.* New York, NY: Springer Publishing Company; 2006: 31–78.

Devine A, Dick IM, Heal SJ, et al. A 4-year follow-up study of the effects of calcium supplementation on bone density in elderly postmenopausal women. *Osteoporos Int.* 1997;7(1):23–28.

Dossey L. What does illness mean? In M Schlitz, T Amorok and M Micozzi, eds. *Consciousness and Healing: Integral Approaches to Mind-Body Medicine.* St. Louis MO: Elsevier/Churchill Livingstone, 2005:151.

Dupertuis LL, Aldwin CM, Bosse R. Does the source of support matter for different health outcomes? *J Aging Health.* 2001;13(4):494–510.

Ehman JW, Ott BB, Short TH, Ciampa RC, Hansen-Flaschen J. Do patients want physicians to inquire about their spiritual or religious beliefs if they become gravely ill? *Arch Intern Med.* 1999;159(15):1803–1806.

Fiori KL, Antonucci TC, Cortina KS. Social network typologies and mental health among older adults. *J Gerontol – Series B.* 2006;61:P25–P32.

Giles LC, Glonek GF, Luszcz MA, Andrews GR. Effect of social networks on 10 year survival in very old Australians. *J Epidemiol Community Health.* 2005;59(7):574–579.

Ginter E. Vegetarian diets, chronic diseases and longevity. *Bratislavske Lekarske Listy.* 2008;109(10):463–466.

Heiss G, Wallace R, Anderson GL, et al. Health risks and benefits 3 years after stopping randomized treatment with estrogen and progestin. *JAMA.* 2008;299(9):1036–1045.

Holloszy JO, Fontana L. Caloric restriction in humans. *Exp Gerontol.* 2007; 42(8):709–712.

Kennedy, Chapman. Massage therapy and older adults. In ER Mackenzie and B Rakel, eds. *Complementary and Alternative Medicine for Older Adults.* New York, NY: Springer Publishing Company; 2006:138–139.

Kris-Etherton PM, Harris WS, Appel LJ. Fish consumption, fish oil, omega-3 fatty acids, and cardiovascular disease. *Arterioscler Thromb Vasc Biol.* 2003;23(2):e20–e30.

Lappe JM, Travers-Gustafson D, Davies KM, et al. Vitamin D and calcium supplementation reduces cancer risk: results of a randomized trial. *Am J Clin Nutr.* 2007;85(6):1586–1591.

Ludwig DS and Kabat-Zinn J. Mindfulness in medicine. *JAMA.* 2008; 300(11):1350–1352.

Lyyra TM, Heikkinen RL. Perceived social support and mortality in older people. *J Gerontol – Series B.* 2006;61:S147–S152.

McCord G, Gilchrist VJ, Grossman SD, et al. Discussing spirituality with patients: a rational and ethical approach. *Ann Fam Med.* 2004;2(4):356–361.

McReynolds JL, Rossen EK. Importance of physical activity, nutrition and social support for optimal aging. *Clin Nurse Spec.* 2004;18(4):200–206.

Morris MC, Sacks F, Rosner B. Does fish oil lower blood pressure? A meta-analysis of controlled trials. *Circulation.* 1993;88(2):523–533.

Murphy J. *The Power of Your Subconscious Mind.* New York: Bantam Books; 2000(1963):259.

Napoli N, Thomson J, Civitelli R, Armamento Villareal RC. Effects of dietary calcium compared with calcium supplements on estrogen metabolism and bone mineral density. *Am J Clin Nutr.* 2007;85(5):1428–1433.

Pargament KI. *The Psychology of Religion and Coping.* New York: Guilford Press; 1997.

Reginster JY, Deroisy R, Rovati LC, et al. Long-term effects of glucosamine sulphate on osteoarthritis progression: a randomised, placebo-controlled clinical trial. *Lancet.* 2001;357(9252):251–256.

Reid I, Ames RW, Evans MC, et al. Effect of calcium supplementation on bone loss in postmenopausal women. *N Engl J Med.* 1993;328(7):460–464.

Rogers CE, Larkey LK, Keller C. A review of clinical trials of tai chi and qigong in older adults. *West J Nurs Res.* 2009;31(2):245–279.

Sabate J. The contribution of vegetarian diets to human health. *Forum Nutr.* 2003;56:218–220.

SanGiovanni JP, Chew EY, Agrón E, et al. The relationship of dietary omega-3 long-chain polyunsaturated fatty acid intake with incident age-related macular degeneration: AREDS report no. 23. *Arch Ophthalmol.* 2008;126(9):1274–1279.

Schneider RH, Walton KG, Salerno JW, Nidich SI. Cardiovascular disease prevention and health promotion with the TM program. *Ethn Dis.* 2006;16(3): S4, 15–26.

Schumann SA, Ewigman B. Double-dose vitamin D lowers cancer risk in women over 55. *J Fam Pract.* 2007;56(11):907–910.

Singh PN, Sabaté J, Fraser GE. Does low meat consumption increase life expectancy in humans? *Am J Clin Nutr.* 2003;78(3 Suppl):526S–532S.

Taylor SE et al. Biobehavioral responses to stress in females: tend-and-befriend not fight-or-flight *Psychol Rev.* 2000;107(3):411–429.

Vangness CT Jr, Spiker W, Erickson J. A review of evidence-based medicine for glucosamine and chondroitin sulfate use in knee osteoarthritis. *Arthroscopy.* 2009;25(10):86–94.

Wang L, Manson JE, Lee IM, Sesso HD. Dietary intake of dairy products ,and vitamin D and the risk of hypertension in middle-aged and older women. *Hypertension.* 2008;51(4)1073–1079.

Weil A. (interview with Bonnie Horrigan). On integrative medicine and the nature of reality. *Altern Ther Health Med.* 2001;7(4):103.

Willcox BJ, Willcox DC, Todoriki H, et al. Caloric restriction, the traditional Okinawan diet, and healthy aging: the diet of the world's longest-lived people and its potential impact on morbidity and life span. *Ann N Y Acad Sci.* 2007;1114:434–455.

Yuen E, Baime M. Meditation and healthy aging. In ER Mackenzie and B Rakel, eds. *Complementary and Alternative Medicine for Older Adults.* New York, NY: Springer Publishing Company; 2006:233–270.

38

Women's Health: An Epilogue

TIERAONA LOW DOG AND VICTORIA MAIZES

The course of women's lives has changed dramatically over the past 50 years, challenging the health care system to broaden its understanding of what constitutes "women's health." Women's health has typically been presented in a biologically defined manner, divided into functional, reproductive segments that revolve around menstruation. While this reproductive model has worked somewhat within the framework of conventional medicine, it falls short of recognizing the totality of women's experiences across the life span and has resulted in gaps in research, public policy, and delivery of comprehensive health care services to women. Women often see one provider during pregnancy, another for gynecological problems, a third for well-woman care, and an array of specialists who manage chronic diseases, with little coordination between services and caregivers. This fragmentation of services, if not unique to women, is more pronounced. And the emphasis that has been placed on reproduction has also, unfortunately, led to both a societal and medical attribution of all female emotions and behaviors to hormonal fluctuations rather than the economic, environmental, and social causes that so deeply affect women's lives. And it these areas that we would like to address in this final chapter.

Economics and Health

It is well known that the economic status of women is intimately intertwined with their health and well-being. While women have made tremendous gains toward economic equality over the last several decades, they remain disproportionately affected by poverty. In 2007, women's median annual paychecks reflected only 78 cents for every dollar earned by men; African American women

660

earned only 69 cents and Latinas 59 cents. If the rate of progress seen between 1995 and 2005 continues, women will not achieve wage parity for nearly 50 years (Institute for Women's Policy Research 2008).

The poverty rate for female single head of household families is 28.3%, more than double the rate for male single head of household families (DeNavas-Walt et al. 2007). Married women with dependent children are also disadvantaged, as they are more likely to work fewer hours for lower pay as they take time off for family responsibilities. Balancing work with personal and family health needs is a major stressor for many women. Studies show they remain the primary family caregivers, caring for sick children, parents, or partners, which often means working and earning less. These wage inequities follow women into their retirement years, reducing their Social Security benefits, pensions, savings, and other financial resources. Health insurance coverage is critical to women's economic stability as health problems can create major obstacles for the ability to work (Lee 2007). However, women often work in part-time and/ or low-wage positions that are least likely to offer health insurance and paid sick days. Taking time off to care for a sick child means loss of wages or even the loss of a job. It also means less time for personal health care. A 2004 survey found that 45% of nonelderly women on Medicaid reported fair or poor health, 13% had diabetes, 28% had asthma, and 40% suffered from anxiety or depression, all higher rates than women with private coverage (Salganicoff et al. 2005).

> "If the misery of the poor be caused not by the laws of nature, but by our institutions, great is our sin." Charles Darwin

Lack of access to preventive and early detection services increases the likelihood that women will suffer greater morbidity and mortality from a host of diseases. Uninsured women are more likely to receive a late-stage breast cancer diagnosis and are 30%–50% more likely to die from the disease. Uninsured women get Pap smears less often, putting them at up to a 60% greater risk for late-stage cervical cancers. Fortunately, public policies are being implemented to address these disparities. In 1990, the Center for Disease Control (CDC) created the National Breast and Cervical Cancer Early Detection Program to assist underserved and uninsured women obtain screening and diagnostic services. In October 2000, the Breast and Cervical Cancer Treatment Act, which gives states the option of providing full Medicaid benefits to uninsured women diagnosed with breast or cervical cancer by the CDC screening program, became law. However, this limited focus upon breast and cervical cancer falls far short of providing services and treatment for the vast number of diseases and chronic conditions that affect women.

Any discussion about the future of women's health must also address the societal structures within which women live. Social policies that promote a reasonably equitable distribution of wealth and provide basic health care and education are essential for improving the health of women in the United States and around the world.

Environmental Medicine

"In our every deliberation, we must consider the impact of our decisions on the next seven generations." Iroquois Confederacy

The current focus on risk management through health behaviors addresses many elements of disease prevention, but falls short in acknowledging the role that environmental factors may play in health. In the 1962 book *Silent Spring*, Rachel Carson, a marine biologist and environmentalist, increased public awareness to the harm that might occur due to the indiscriminate use of pesticides. She called attention to our growing reliance on chemicals for which safety is incompletely understood. Women know that their womb provides the first environment for their child and that the responsibility for the nourishment, safety, and well-being of their children falls primary to them. Women are increasingly concerned about the accumulating evidence that from the air we breathe, to the fish we eat and the water we drink, a broad range of compounds in the environment may be adversely affecting the health of our families and the health of our planet.

Clinicians know that excessive exposure to methylmercury can damage the nervous system, kidneys, and liver, as well as impair childhood development. Thus, we caution women and children to reduce their exposures (i.e., limit fish consumption). Long-term exposure to low levels of lead can result in serious neurological consequences, especially in children under the age of six. Lead was banned in U.S. residential paint in 1978 and leaded gasoline was gradually phased out. As a result, lead levels in children declined significantly from 1988 to 2004 (Jones 2009). But beyond these few examples, health care providers are relatively ignorant about the potential harm environmental toxins can have on human health. Of course, they are not alone. The Environmental Protection Agency (EPA) has required testing for less than 200 of the more than 62,000 chemicals that were in commerce prior to 1979, of which the majority have never been tested for safety. Another 20,000 chemicals have since been added to EPA's inventory (GAO 2005). It is an embarrassment that our regulatory standards regarding safety of industrial chemicals fall short of those in other countries, including all of the European Union countries (GAO 2007).

While there are zealots and skeptics on both sides of the issue, many scientists suspect that there may be a link between environmental toxins and some of our most prevalent medical conditions, such as asthma, autism, cancer, and infertility. Of particular concern are those compounds with the potential to disrupt normal endocrine, reproductive, central nervous, and immune function. Endocrine-disrupting compounds (EDCs), many which act like estrogens in the body, may be associated with decreasing sperm counts and increasing birth defects in males, as well as estrogen-driven cancers and gynecological disorders such as endometriosis, recurrent miscarriage, infertility, and polycystic ovary syndrome (Caserta 2008; McLachlan 2006; Wang and Baskin 2008).

Phthalates, a family of compounds used in making PVC (vinyl), cosmetics, fragrance, and medical devices, have been associated with early breast development and puberty in girls (Chou 2009; Jacobson-Dickman and Lee 2009). Urine samples taken from women in Taiwan, the United States, and the Netherlands clearly show that humans are chronically exposed to phthalates at levels higher than expected (Chou 2009; Hines 2009; Ye 2008). Bisphenol A (BPA), an ingredient of polycarbonate plastics and epoxy resins used to make food containers, shatter resistant baby bottles and coat metal in food cans, bottle tops, and water pipes, is a well-known EDC. BPA is equivalent to estradiol in its ability to activate responses via estrogen receptors associated with the cell membranes (Wozniak et al. 2005), stimulating rapid physiological responses at even very low picogram per ml (parts per trillion) concentrations.

BPA exposure in humans is widespread. Chronic, low level exposure occurs in virtually everyone living developed countries. A study in the United States detected BPA in 92.6% of people sampled ($n = 2517$), women had higher levels than men, and children had higher levels than adolescents (Calafat 2008). This is important, as acute toxicological studies in animals using only high doses of BPA do not adequately address this long-term low-level exposure in humans (Vom Saal et al. 2007).

"When an activity raises threats of harm to human health or the environment, precautionary measures should be taken even if some cause and effect relationships are not fully established scientifically. In this context the proponent of an activity, rather than the public, should bear the burden of proof. The process of applying the precautionary principle must be open, informed and democratic and must include potentially affected parties. It must also involve an examination of the full range of alternatives, including no action."

Wingspread Statement on the Precautionary Principle, January 1998.

Sensitivity to endocrine disruptors varies extensively across the life span, indicating that there are specific windows of increased susceptibility. Biomonitoring that assesses body burden, or the level of harmful chemicals in the body, should be expanded to track long-term low-level exposure to EDCs in women from infancy through old age to better determine at what point these crucial windows occur. As evidenced by studies that show reductions in exposure to secondhand smoke and serum lead levels, public policies can impact human exposure to environmental toxins. Tighter regulatory standards for evaluating the safety of new industrial compounds should be rapidly implemented to safeguard public health, as well as the health of other inhabitants of the earth.

For ideas on how to make simple and affordable changes to reduce exposure to environmental contaminants, visit www.womenshealthandenvironment. org.

Women and Research

Historically, scientists have paid little attention to the study of sex differences at the basic *cellular* and *molecular* levels, as well as in clinical trials. The research community assumed that beyond the reproductive system, such differences either did not exist or were not relevant. Clinicians have assumed that information obtained from clinical studies conducted on male subjects could simply be extrapolated to women. Yet, as researchers unravel the complex interplay between DNA, hormones, and environment, this assumption, even on a mechanistic level, seems almost childishly simplistic. For instance, the dominant model of human response to stress has been the "fight or flight" response. No one considered that there could be any significant difference in the way men and women physiologically respond to stress. However, research shows that stressors in women can also cause the release of oxytocin, a hormone that buffers the fight or flight response and encourages women to tend children and affiliate with others (Taylor 2000). This "tend and befriend" response to a threat reduces biological stress responses, including elevated heart rate, blood pressures, and hypothalamic pituitary adrenal axis stress responses, such as elevations in cortisol (Light et al. 2000). This may explain why women are more likely than men to seek out and use social support in all types of stressful situations, including health-related concerns, relationship problems, and work-related conflicts.

Understanding why the prevalence of disease can vary so dramatically between men and women is another area ripe for investigation. Women are two times more likely than men to suffer from depression, a statistic that holds true throughout the world (Weissman 1995). Differences in brain structure and function, and hormonal fluctuations across the reproductive cycle may differentially predispose women to depression. Research shows that estrogen modulates serotonin function and that women respond far better to serotonin reuptake inhibitors (SSRIs) than men (Young 2009) and premenopausal women respond far better than postmenopausal women (Kornstein 2000). However, gender differences in socialization, rates of violence against women, and women's disadvantaged social status are also very likely to contribute to the greater prevalence in women. Depression, like most conditions, is likely a combination of both biology and environment.

"While it is anatomically obvious why only males develop prostate cancer and only females get ovarian cancer, it is not at all obvious why, for example, females are more likely than males to recover language ability after suffering a left-hemisphere stroke or why females have a far greater risk than males of developing life-threatening ventricular arrhythmias in response to a variety of potassium channel-blocking drugs."

Institute of Medicine Report
    "Exploring the Biological Contributions to Human Health: Does Sex Matter?"

Sex and gender research is in its infancy. Prior to 1990, the National Institutes of Health devoted only 13% of its research funds toward studies of drug effects, diseases, and treatments that affect women as well as men, although women make up 52% of the world's population. Women of childbearing age were routinely excluded from research studies for fear that if a woman became pregnant during the trial, the treatment might pose a risk to the fetus and the researchers and/or drug manufacturer may be held liable. However, excluding such a vast number of women has led to considerable gaps in medical knowledge regarding the safety and effectiveness of treatments in fertile women. Women of reproductive age should be given the opportunity to share in both the benefit and burden of research (Wizemann and Pardue 2001).

Due to the glaring discrepancies in scientific research and the tireless work of women's health advocacy groups, the Office of Research on Women's Health (ORWH) was established in 1990 to ensure the inclusion of women and minorities in NIH-funded research. Its mission is to promote, stimulate, and support efforts to improve the health of women through biomedical and behavioral research on the roles of sex (biological characteristics of being female or male) and gender (social influences based on sex) in health and disease. A legislative mandate that women and minorities be included in all clinical research studies was incorporated into the NIH Revitalization Act of 1993.

There are tremendous opportunities and challenges that confront researchers who study the role of sex and gender in health and disease. New methodologies and models will need to be developed to enable scientists to investigate both male and female cell lines to determine whether stressors or medicines affect them differently. It is also critical that the editors of medical and scientific journals encourage authors to describe the sex ratios in their clinical trials and to what extent differences in outcomes were noted between the sexes. If no differences were identified, this should also be clearly stated. This type of research and reporting is crucial before generalized recommendations can be made for the public (IOM 2001).

Women's Voices

"Women have always been healers. They were the unlicensed doctors and anatomists of western history. They were abortionists, nurses and counselors. They were pharmacists, cultivating healing herbs and exchanging the secrets of their uses. They were midwives, travelling from home to home and village to village. For centuries women were doctors without degrees, barred from books and lectures, learning from each other, and passing on experience from neighbor to neighbor and mother to daughter. They were called 'wise women' by the people, witches or charlatans by the authorities. Medicine is part of our heritage as women, our history, our birthright."

Barbara Ehrenreich and Deirdre English
Witches, Midwives, and Nurses: A History of Women Healers

It seems fitting to close this chapter with an acknowledgment of all the women, named and unnamed, throughout history from ancient times to the present, across cultures and ethnicities, who have tended the sick and broken, helped bring countless children into the world, and gave comfort to those who were dying. The tradition of the female healer was largely oppressed for several centuries in Europe and the United States, when "formalized" medicine became the purview of men. Women were effectively shutout from medical schools; nursing became the profession many pursued. It has been a long, slow process but women are now making up a much greater proportion of physician numbers. In1970, only 7.1% of physicians in the United States were women (Kletke et al. 1990). By 2010, that number is projected to be 33% and almost half of those entering American medical schools today are women (Potterton et al. 2004). The number of men pursuing a nursing career is rising, yet it is women who dominate this "caring" profession. According to the National Sample Survey of Registered Nurses, 94.6% of registered nurses (RNs) in the United States are female, as are those practicing as nurse practitioners (HHS 2006). Women are well represented in some complementary medicine fields but not others. For instance, 85.9% of massage therapists are women (AMTA 2009), while 82% of chiropractic practitioners are male (ACA 2009). For the fields of naturopathy, herbal medicine and acupuncture the gender data are not readily available but it is clear that women, as they have done throughout history, continue to work to improve the health and ease the suffering of humankind.

> Confronting the multiplying challenges of health care, women physicians have joined the highest ranks of medical administration and research. As leaders, they make choices that benefit communities across America and around the world. As healers, they identify and respond to many of the most urgent crises in modern medicine, from the needs of underserved communities, to AIDS and natural and man-made disasters. Their influence reaches across the profession out into our lives, redefining women's roles and society's responsibilities. By changing the face of medicine, women physicians are changing our world.
>
> Changing the Face of Medicine: Celebrating America's Women
> Physicians National Library of Medicine 2005

While the numbers of women in medicine are increasing, many of the conditions that adversely affect the health of women can only be redressed by the creation and implementation of less discriminatory and more favorable social policies. In the 111th U.S. Congress, there are currently 75 women (17%) serving in the House of Representatives and 17 women (17%) in the Senate, the highest number of women to hold congressional office (WGR 2008). That the numbers are increasing is laudable but given that more than 50% of Americans are women, 17% representation is very low. It is critical that women's voices be heard at every level of government. The fact that a highly qualified woman, Hillary Clinton, ran for President of the United States in 2008 was an encouraging sign but there is still much work to be done.

A thoughtful examination of, and recommendations for, a more inclusive and expansive scientific agenda on women's health research is found in the ORWH Agenda for Research on Women's Health for the 21st Century. http://orwh.od.nih.gov/research/resagenda.html

Closing Remarks

If health is more than the absence of disease—if it is, rather, a harmonious interplay between the physical, emotional, social, and spiritual aspects of one's life—then a biopsychosocial, or integrative, approach to women's health is the only one that makes sense. Moving beyond a medical system that is primarily focused upon curing to one that also recognizes, embraces, and encourages healing is essential. Healing stretches beyond the boundaries of disease and cure into the realms of transcendence; purpose, hope, and meaning that form the very fabric of human experience and desire (Swinton 2001). A union that marries the social, political, cultural, geographical, and economic factors of women's lives with conventional biomedical care—placing each individual woman within the larger story of her own life and experience—allows us to more fully appreciate the dynamic and unique nature of health. It was from within this philosophical stance that this textbook on *Integrative Medicine and Women's Health* was written with the hope that it can serve as a model for helping improve the health and well-being of women across the life span and throughout the globe.

REFERENCES

American Chiropractic Association General Information about Chiropractic Care under Facts & Statistics about Chiropractic. Available at: http://www.acatoday.org/level1_css.cfm?T1ID=21. Accessed May 1, 2009.

American Massage Therapists Association: 2009 Massage Therapy Industry Fact Sheet. Available at: http://www.amtamassage.org/news/MTIndustryFactSheet.html. Accessed May 1, 2009.

American Medical Association. *Women in Medicine Data Source.* Chicago, IL: American Medical Association; 1997.

Calafat AM, Ye X, Wong LY, Reidy JA, Needham LL. Exposure of the U.S. population to bisphenol A and 4-tertiary-octylphenol: 2003–2004. *Environ Health Perspect.* 2008;116(1):39–44.

Caserta D, Maranghi L, Mantovani A, Marci R, Maranghi F, Moscarini M. Impact of endocrine disruptor chemicals in gynaecology. *Hum Reprod Update.* 2008;14(1):59–72.

Chou YY, Huang PC, Lee CC, Wu MH, Lin SJ. Phthalate exposure in girls during early puberty. *J Pediatr Endocrinol Metab.* 2009 Jan;22(1):69–77.

DeNavas-Walt, Carmen, Bernadette D. Proctor, Jessica Smith. U.S. Census Bureau, Current Population Reports, P60–233, *Income, Poverty, and Health Insurance Coverage in the United States: 2006.* Washington, DC: U.S. Government Printing Office; 2007.

General Accounting Office (GAO). Chemical Regulation: Approaches in the United States, Canada, and the European Union. GAO-06–217R, November 4, 2005.

General Accounting Office (GAO). Comparison of US and Recently Enacted European Union Approaches to Protect Against the Risks of Toxic Chemicals. GAO-07–825. August 2007.

Health and Human Services. 2004 National Sample Survey of Registered Nurses. Published 2006. Available at: http://bhpr.hrsa.gov/healthworkforce/rnsurvey04/. Accessed May 1, 2009.

Hines EP, Calafat AM, Silva MJ, Mendola P, Fenton SE. Concentrations of phthalate metabolites in milk, urine, saliva, and Serum of lactating North Carolina women. *Environ Health Perspect.* 2009 Jan;117(1):86–92.

Institute for Women's Policy Research: Still a Man's Labor Market: The Long-Term Earnings Gap. www.iwpr.org. Accessed August 10, 2009.

Jacobson-Dickman E, Lee MM. The influence of endocrine disruptors on pubertal timing. *Curr Opin Endocrinol Diabetes Obes.* 2009;16(1):25–30. Review.

Jones RL, Homa DM, Meyer PA, et al. Trends in blood levels and blood lead testing among US children aged 1 to 5 years, 1988–2004. *Pediatrics.* 2009;123(3):e376–e385.

Kletke PR, Marder WD, Silberger AB. The growing proportion of female physicians: implications for US physician supply. *Am J Public Health.* 2004;80(3):300–304.

Kornstein SG, Schatzberg AF, Thase ME, et al. Gender differences in treatment response to sertraline versus imipramine in chronic depression. *Am J Psychiatry.* 2000;157(9):1445–1452.

Lee S. *Keeping Moms on the Job: The Impacts of Health Insurance and Child Care on Job Retention and Mobility among Low-Income Mothers.* Washington, DC: Institute for Women's Policy Research; 2007.

McLachlan JA, Simpson E, Martin M. Endocrine disrupters and female reproductive health. *Best Pract Res Clin Endocrinol Metab.* 2006;20(1):63–75

The National Library of Medicine. Changing the Face of Medicine: Celebrating America's Women Physicians; 2005. Available at: http://www.nlm.nih.gov/exhibition/changingthefaceofmedicine/exhibition/changing.html Accessed May 1, 2009.

Potterton VK, Ruan S, Applegate K, Cypel Y, Forman HP. Why don't female medical students choose diagnostic radiology? A review of the current literature. *J Appl Commun Res.* 2004;1(8):583–590.

Salganicoff A, Ranji UR, Wyn, R. *Women and Health Care: A National Profile—Key Findings from the Kaiser Women's Health Survey.* Menlo Park, CA: Kaiser Family Foundation; 2005.

Taylor, S. E., Klein, L. C., Lewis, B. P., Gruenewald, T. L., Gurung, R. A. R, & Updegraff, J. A. (2000). Biobehavioral responses to stress in females: Tend-and-befriend, not fight-or-flight. *Psychological Review, 107,* 441–429.

Vom Saal FS, Akingbemi BT, Belcher SM, et al. Chapel Hill bisphenol a expert panel consensus statement: Integration of mechanisms, effects in animals and potential to impact human health at current levels of exposure. *Reprod Toxicol.* 2007;24:131–138.

Wang MH, Baskin LS. Endocrine disruptors, genital development, and hypospadias. *J Androl.* 2008;29(5):499–505.

Weissman MM, Olfson M. Depression in women: implications for health care research. *Science.* 1995;269:799–801.

Wizeman TM, Pardue ML, eds. *Exploring the Biological Contributions to Human Health: Does Sex Matter?* Committee on Understanding the Biology of Sex and Gender Differences, Board on Health Sciences Policy. Institute of Medicine. National Academy of Sciences, Washington, DC; 2001.

WGR Women in Government Relations: Record-Breaking Number of Women will Serve in the 111th Congress. Available at: http://www.wgr.org/news_events/index.cfm?fa=whatarticle&id=244. Accessed May 1, 2009.

Women in Government Relations. Record-Breaking Number of Women will Serve in the 111th Congress. Newsletter November 2008. http://www.wgr.org/news_events/index.cfm?fa=whatarticle&id=244. Accessed August 24, 2009.

Wozniak AL, Bulayeva NN, Watson CS. Xenoestrogens at picomolar to nanomolar concentrations trigger membrane estrogen receptor-a mediated Ca++ fluxes and prolactin release in GH3/B6 pituitary tumor cells. *Environ Health Perspect.* 2005;113:431–439.

Ye X, Pierik FH, Hauswer R, et al. Urinary metabolite concentrations of organophosphorous pesticides, bisphenol A, and phthalates among pregnant women in Rotterdam, the Netherlands: the Generation R study. *Environ Res.* 2008 Oct;108(2):260–267.

Young EA, Kornstein SG, Marcus SM, et al. Sex differences in response to citalopram: a STAR*D report. *J Psychiatr Res.* 2009;43(5):503–511.

INDEX

Note: Page references in *italics* refer figures and tables, respectively.

Bisphenol A (BPA), 663
Bisphosphonate
for bone health, 633–634
Black cohosh (*Actaea racemosa, Cimicifuga racemosa*)
for breast cancer, 359–360
for menopause, 371
for premenstrual syndrome, 177
Bone health, 22, 23. *See also* Osteoporosis
anti-inflammatory diet for, 626
botanicals for, 631
estrogen, role of, 633
harmful substances for, 630–631
mind–body medicine for, 631–632
nutrition for, 627–630
pharmacologic therapy for, 633
and physical activity, 55
recommendations, 636
selective estrogen receptor modulators for, 634–635
younger women, considerations, 632–633
Bone strength
assessing, 625
Boric acid
for vulvovaginal candidiasis, 192
Botanical therapy
for breast cancer, 359–360
for cardiovascular disease, 599, 600
for CFS/FM, 462–463
for depression, 559–663
for endometriosis, 292, 292–293, 294
for generalized anxiety disorder, 544–546
for HIV, 526–527
for irritable bowel syndrome, 419–420
during labor and delivery, 220–221
for menopause, 370–375
during mid/late pregnancy, 213
for migraine, 437–438
for multiple sclerosis, 512
for nausea and vomiting of pregnancy, 209–210
for premenstrual syndrome, 175–177, 178
for rheumatoid arthritis, 491–492
for urinary tract infections, 406–408
for uterine fibrosis, 327–329
for vaginitis, 195, 196

Botulinum toxin
for migraine, 442
BPA. *See* Bisphenol A
Breast and Cervical Cancer Treatment Act, 661
Breast cancer, 348–362
acupressure for, 361
acupuncture for, 361
botanical therapy for, 359–360
diagnosis and treatment of, 352–356, 353, 355–356
massage for, 361–362
mind–body therapies for, 74, 361
nutrition for, 356–359
physical activity and, 356
population screening for, 351–352
prevention strategies for, 351
relative risk for, 349–350, 350
Breast milk expression, methods of, 224
Breastfeeding, 223
Breathwork
definition of, 67
Buchu (*Agathosma betulina*)
for urinary tract infections, 408
Bulimia nervosa (BN), 573–575
BV. *See* Bacterial vaginosis

Caffeine
bone health, harmful to, 630
and generalized anxiety disorder, 541
for premenstrual syndrome, 171
Calcitonin
for bone health, 635
Calcium
for bone health, 627
for eating disorders, 579
for healthy aging, 649
intake during pregnancy, 205–206
for multiple sclerosis, 510
for premenstrual syndrome, 174
Calorie restricted diet
for healthy aging, 648–649
Cancer
breast, 348–362
cervical, 335–345
dietary supplements for, 36

Expressive writing
definition of, 67

Fatty acids
for bone health, 628
for eating disorders, 578
Fertility. *See also* Infertility in women
mind–body therapies for, 73
Fetal alcohol syndrome, 204
Feverfew (*Tanacetum parthenium*)
for migraine, 438
Fiber
for cardiovascular disease, 595
insoluble, 9
soluble, 8–9
Fibromyalgia
and chronic fatigue syndrome (FM/
CFS), 454–469
botanical therapy for, 462–463
definition and symptomatology of, 456
diagnostic approach for, 459
dietary supplements for, 462–463
energy healing for, 469
epidemiology of, 456
manual therapies for, 468–469
mind–body medicine for, 467–468
nutrition for, 464–465
pathophysiology for, 456–459
pharmacologic treatment for, 460–461
physical activity for, 466–467
pregnancy and, 460
primary care for, 459–460
homeopathic treatment for, 145–146
and physical activity, 56
spinal manipulative therapy for, 157–158
Fish oil. *See also* Omega-3 fatty acids
for breast cancer, 362
for cardiovascular disease, 603–604
for healthy aging, 650
for migraine, 435–436
for rheumatoid arthritis, 495–496
Five-element acupuncture, 106. *See also*
Acupuncture
Flaxseeds
for menopause, 369
Flexibility training, *51*

Flexion distraction technique, 156, 157
FM. *See* Fibromyalgia
Folic acid (folate), 202
for cervical cancer, 338, 339, 341
for depression, 561
for perinatal depression, 239
during pregnancy, 205
Forgiveness, 85
Functional hypothalamic amenorrhea
(FHA), 254–256
cognitive behavioral therapy for, 264
depression and, 261
HPT axis suppression and, 258–259
hypnotherapy for, 264
metabolic stress and, 260
ovulation induction
with clomiphene citrate for, 263
with gonadotropin for, 263
personality factors and, 262–263
psychosocial stress and, 260–261

Gabapentin (Neurontin), 460, 461
GAD. *See* Generalized anxiety disorder
Gamma-linolenic acid (GLA), 491
Gamma-oryzanol
for menopause, 370
Gardasil
for cervical cancer, 340
Garlic (*Allium sativum*)
for cardiovascular disease, 596
Generalized anxiety disorder (GAD),
535–550
botanical therapy for, 544–546
categorization of, 537
diagnosis of, 538, 539
dietary supplements for, 542–544
exercise, 540–541
medical conditions associated with, *539*
mind–body medicine for, 547–548
nutrition for, 541
pathophysiology for, 537–538
psychotherapy for, 549–550
during pregnancy and lactation,
546–547
Genistein
for uterine fibrosis, 326